# THE COMPLETE GUIDE TO NUTRITIONAL HEALTH

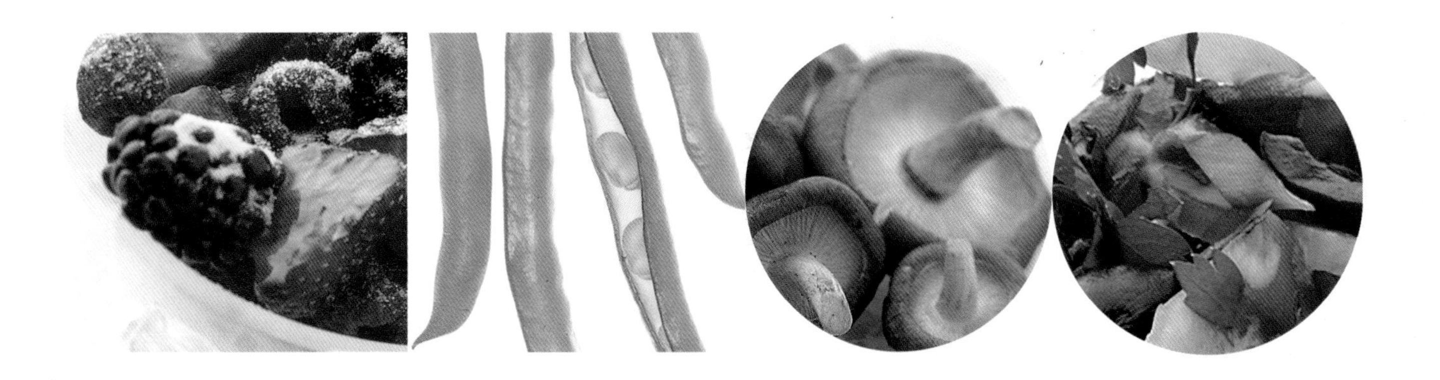

**The Complete Guide to Nutritional Health**
Pierre Jean Cousin and Kirsten Hartvig

Conceived, created and designed by Duncan Baird Publishers Ltd
Sixth Floor
Castle House
75–76 Wells Street
London W1T 3QH

Material from this book was first published in the UK and Ireland in 2001 and 2002 by Duncan Baird Publishers Ltd in two separate volumes: *Food is Medicine* and *Eat for Immunity*



Managing Editor: Judy Barratt
Editor: Richard Emerson
Editorial Assistant: Jessica Hughes
Managing Designer: Manisha Patel
Designers: Steve Painter, Suzanne Tuhrim, Joy Wheeler
Commissioned Photography: William Lingwood
Stylists: David Morgan, Helen Trent, Sunil Vijayakar

British Library Cataloguing-in-Publication Data:
A CIP record for this book is available from the British Library

ISBN: 1-84483-010-1

10 9 8 7 6 5 4 3

Typeset in Helvetica Neue
Colour reproduction by Scanhouse, Malaysia, and Colourscan, Singapore
Printed and bound in Singapore by Imago

PUBLISHER'S NOTE: *The Complete Guide to Nutritional Health* is not intended as a replacement for professional medical treatment and advice. The publishers and authors cannot accept responsibility for any damage incurred as a result of any of the therapeutic methods contained in this work. If you are suffering from a medical condition and are unsure of the suitability of any of the therapeutic methods in this book, or if you are pregnant, it is advisable to consult a medical practitioner. Essential oils must be diluted in a base oil before use. They should not be taken internally and are for adult use only. The detox programme should be avoided by children, elderly people, and women who are pregnant or breast-feeding.

The abbreviation BCE is used in this book:
BCE Before the Common Era (the equivalent of BC)

PIERRE JEAN COUSIN and KIRSTEN HARTVIG

# THE COMPLETE GUIDE TO NUTRITIONAL HEALTH

MORE THAN 600 FOODS AND RECIPES FOR OVERCOMING ILLNESS AND BOOSTING YOUR IMMUNITY

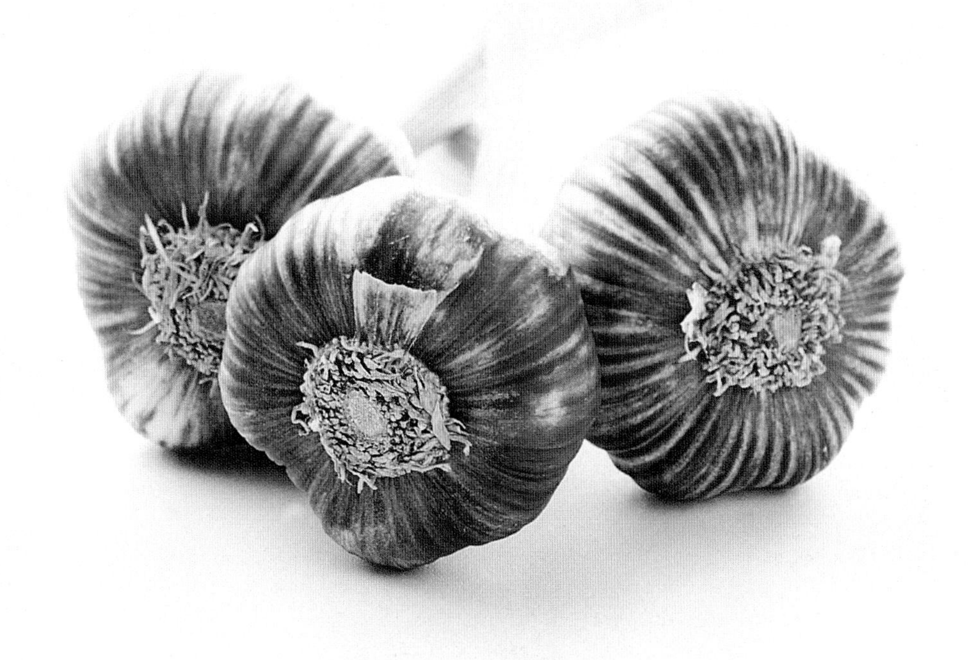

DUNCAN BAIRD PUBLISHERS

LONDON

# contents

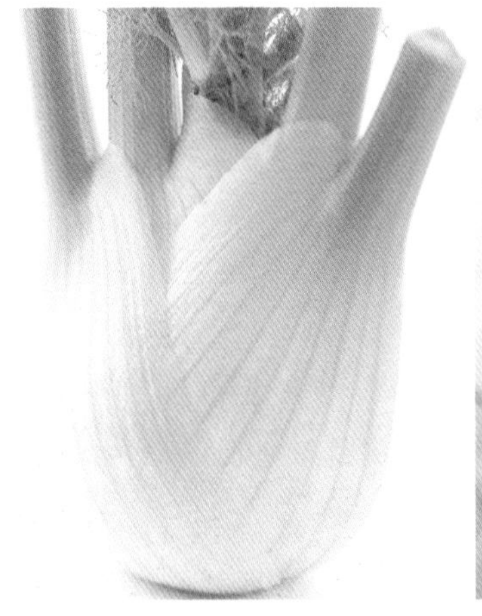
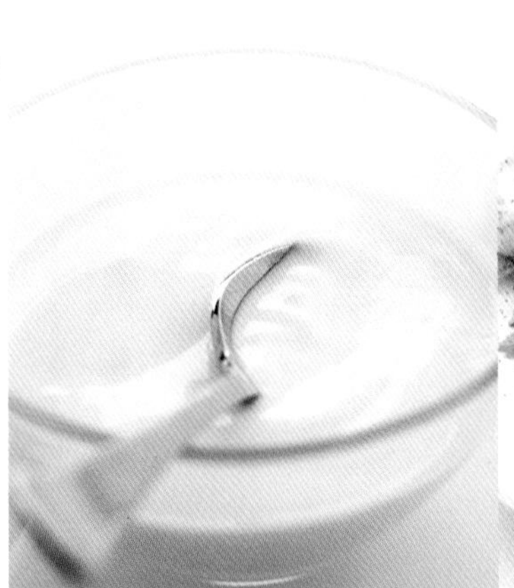
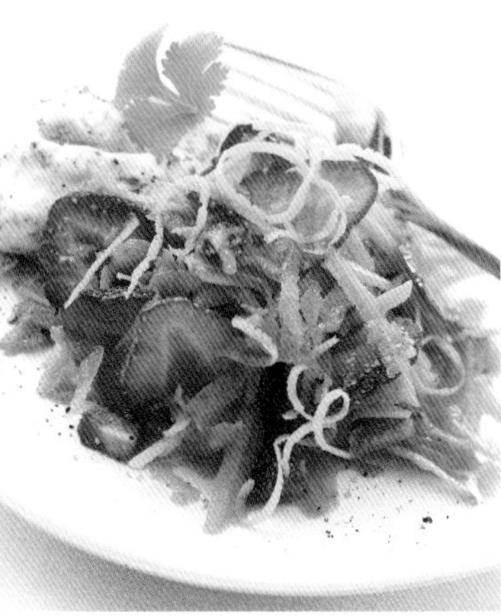
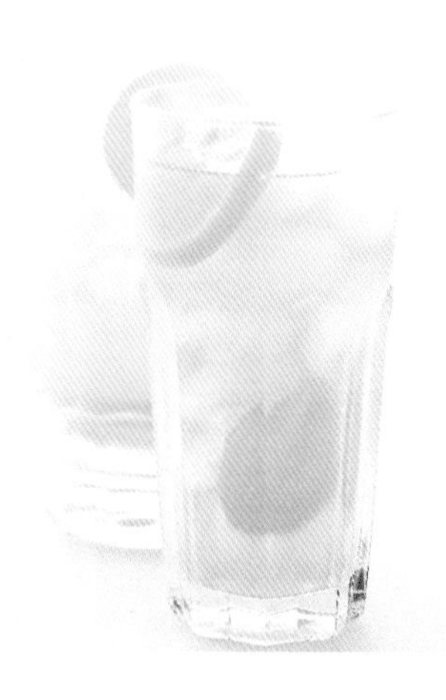

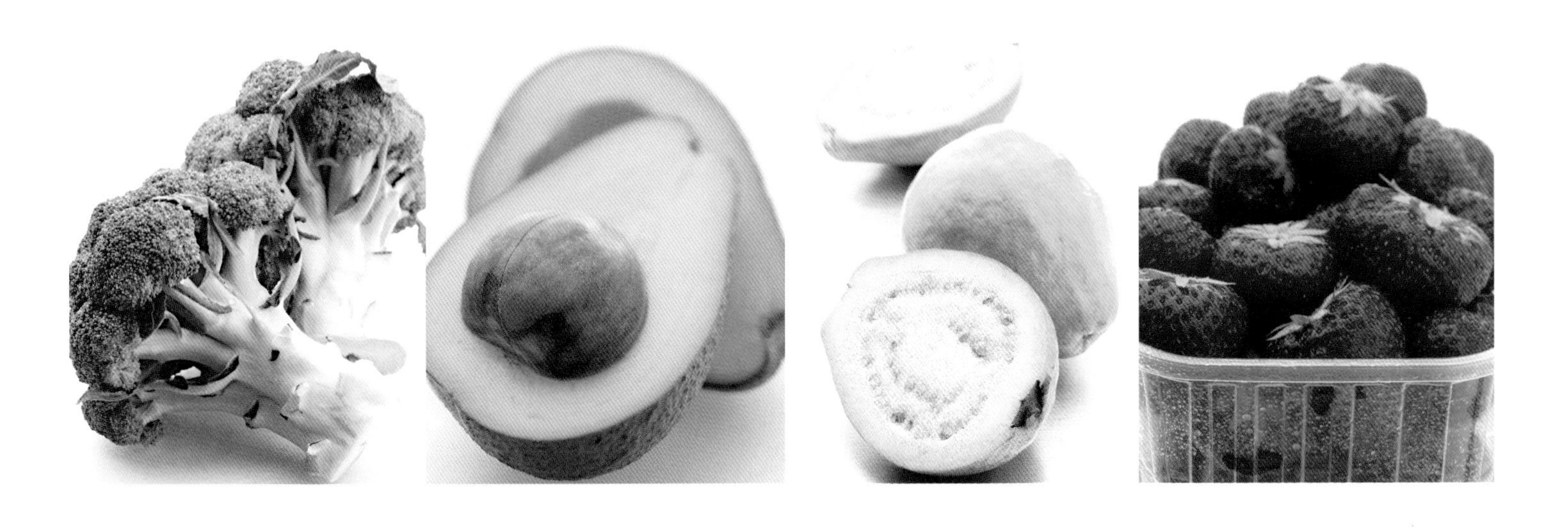

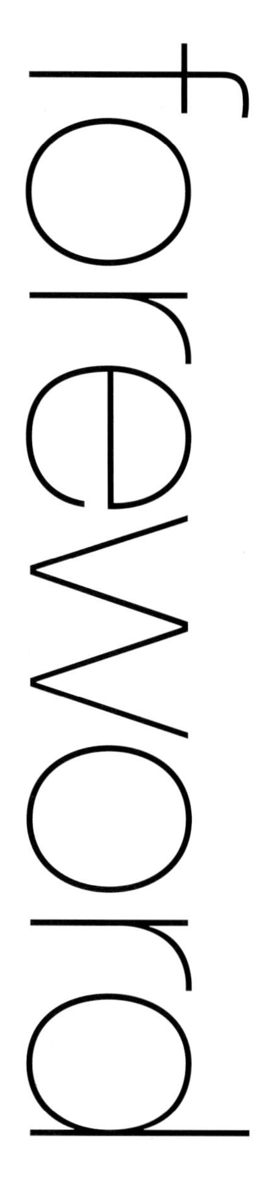


Readers who digest and act on the advice in this book are likely to improve their enjoyment of life into middle and old age. I hope that, as you read this foreword, you think of yourself not just as an individual, but as a member of a family and community, whose choices and actions affect others.

In general, people live longer, and also suffer from disease for more of their lives, than ever before in history. In rich countries, such as those in North America and Western Europe, people on average suffer some serious disability for around a quarter of their lives, and often die from diseases likely to cause intense suffering in the last years of their lives.

It is true that older people are more vulnerable to all sorts of diseases. But disease is not an inevitable function of ageing. I am writing this foreword during a visit to the headquarters of the World Health Organization (WHO) in Geneva. Colleagues here envision a world in which it is normal to live a long, healthy and active life and to die of old age in good health.

## feed the mind, body and spirit

If you want to change the world, begin with yourself, within your community. *The Complete Guide to Nutritional Health* is full of useful information and good advice. Its most important message can be expressed in a few words: food and nutrition is crucial to health. And as health is not only physical but also mental, emotional and spiritual, it might be better to say that the nature and quality of what we eat and drink are the most important determinants of our state of being.

This is an old truth to which writers such as Pierre Jean Cousin and my colleague and friend Kirsten Hartvig are bearing new witness. Everybody now knows that the incidence of tooth decay, constipation, gut diseases, obesity, high blood pressure, diabetes, osteoporosis, stroke, heart disease and most cancers, in all populations and communities, is mostly determined by food and nutrition, together with tobacco habits and level of physical activity. In 2002, the WHO launched a new initiative designed to prevent chronic diseases throughout the world, with that message.

Everybody also knows that secure, adequate and varied food supplies are essential to prevent deficiency diseases; and nutritional deficiency not only remains a massive public health issue in Africa and Asia, but is also quite common among impoverished people who live in rich countries like the United States.

Furthermore, a vital message for families, and most of all for parents, is that exclusive breast-feeding until 6 months old, followed by weaning on to nutrient-dense plant-based diets, gives babies and young children the best protection against infectious diseases at the time, and also throughout life.

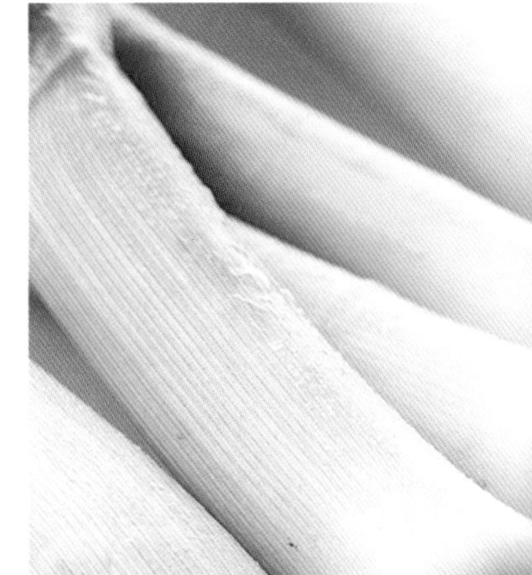

## natural and fresh is best

But that is not all! As the authors of *The Complete Guide to Nutritional Health* show, diets based on fresh or minimally processed foods (above all wholegrain, starchy foods combined with pulses, such as beans, and a variety of vegetables and fruits, which are rich in vitamins, minerals, phytochemicals and essential fats and fibre), and which are correspondingly low in highly processed foods, total fat, saturated fat, sugar, salt and also alcohol, protect the health of all systems of the body. And yes, this includes the nervous system – of which the brain is one part, the source of our thoughts, feelings and beliefs.

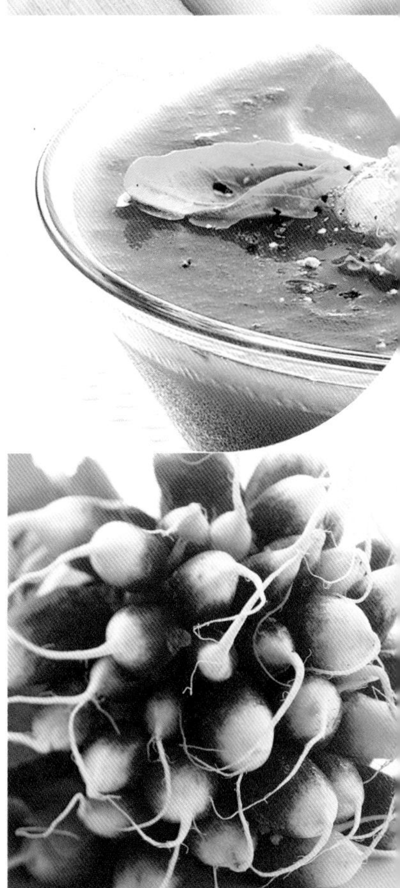

Before automation, peoples' livelihoods depended on manual labour, and so height and weight and therefore physical strength were desirable. Some people still suppose that the best diets for humans, and especially children, are those that promote growth. In fact, *homo sapiens* evolved to grow and mature slowly, and in more affluent countries diets high in protein, fat and often sugar, have created increasingly unhealthy and obese populations.

Those of us who are lucky enough to be economically and socially secure, with homes and work, and who enjoy international travel, electronic technology, and shops full of fresh foods, do not want to revert to any kind of primeval existence. What we can achieve now is the best of all worlds. Pierre Jean and Kirsten have assembled, summarized and displayed a vast amount of knowledge, designed to convince you that excellent food and nutrition is the rational way to avoid disease,

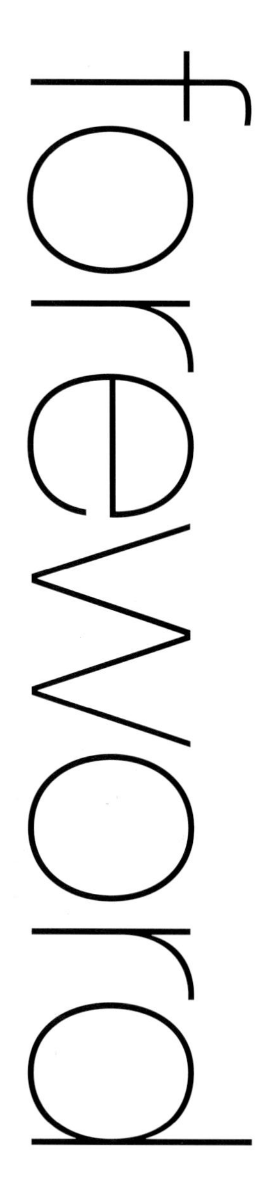

and also that natural foods and drinks contain prudent remedies for most illnesses. Don't be daunted by the detail. The fundamental message is simple – the basic nourishment for your body, mind and spirit, and that of your family and community, is in your local supermarket now.

**Geoffrey Cannon**

Author, *The Politics of Food*
Chief editor, *Food, Nutrition and the Prevention of Cancer: a Global Perspective*
Advisor on food and nutrition policy, Ministry of Health, Brazil

## how to use this book

*The Complete Guide to Nutritional Health* brings together the knowledge and experience of two renowned experts on the links between good food and good health. Pierre Jean Cousin is a practising herbalist and acupuncturist with a thriving complementary medicine practice based in Kensington, London. Kirsten Hartvig is a registered naturopath. She lives in the French Pyrenees with her husband Nic Rowley. Since 1994, they have been running retreats and courses in Denmark and France on the subjects of healthy eating, natural health and healing.

In this book, the two authors give their own unique insights into the subject of nutrition. Pierre Jean looks at how various foods, including fruits, vegetables, dairy products and fish, can help prevent and treat a wide range of common ailments. Kirsten takes a wholly vegetarian approach to nutritional health, focusing on the way that the right choice of foods can strengthen the immune system, thereby enabling the body's innate defensive mechanisms to combat disease.

In both Part One, Food is Medicine, and Part Two, Eat for Immunity, the two authors have listed their personal choices of "superfoods" they regard as having exceptional health-promoting qualities. Shown right are the symbols used to highlight some important facts about these foods. For the most part, the products selected by the two nutritionists are not rare or exotic fruits and vegetables that are difficult to obtain, but everyday items available from most food shops or supermarkets. On the following pages you can read all about their medicinal properties, and then use the handy cross-references to discover a whole host of delicious and nutritious recipes that present these medicinal foods at their mouth-watering best. The recipes are for four people, unless otherwise stated, with the exception of the juices, syrups and herbal drinks.

In other sections, Pierre Jean and Kirsten describe a wide range of common ailments and offer their personal suggestions for the best combination of foods to prevent or treat these disorders.

But this book is about health, not illness. By using *The Complete Guide to Nutritional Health* to develop your understanding of the therapeutic value of fresh, natural, nutrient-packed foods, you will go a long way to ensuring life-long good health and vitality – not to mention enjoyable mealtimes – for you and your family.

**Bon appetit!**

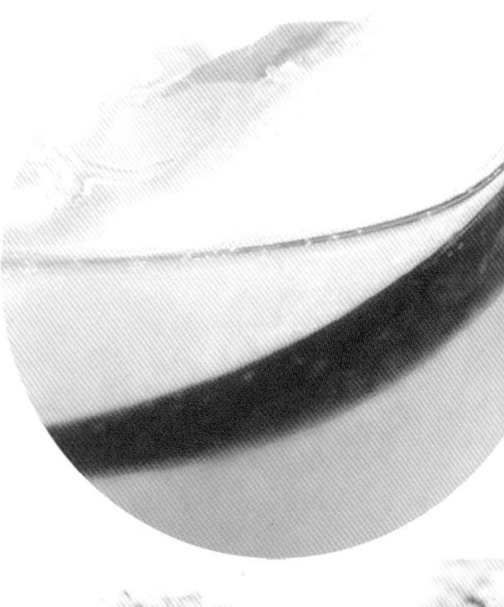

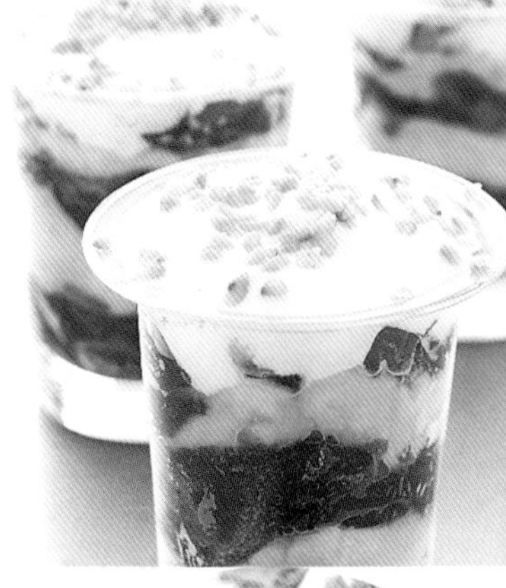

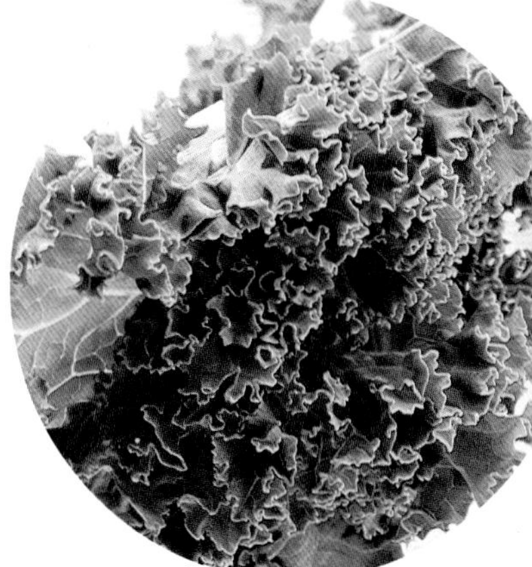

KEY TO SYMBOLS USED IN FOOD IS MEDICINE

★ IMPORTANT NUTRIENTS AND OTHER ACTIVE INGREDIENTS

● BODY SYSTEM AND AILMENT

! WARNING

✓ BENEFICIAL FOODS AND OTHER RECOMMENDATIONS

✗ FOODS, DRINKS AND PRACTICES TO AVOID

KEY TO SYMBOLS USED IN EAT FOR IMMUNITY

★ IMPORTANT NUTRIENTS AND OTHER ACTIVE INGREDIENTS

✓ IMMUNE-BOOSTING ACTION AND OTHER BENEFICIAL PROPERTIES

! WARNING

💡 INTERESTING FACTS AND HANDY HINTS

USEFUL CONVERSIONS FROM METRIC TO IMPERIAL

| Metric | | Imperial |
|---|---|---|
| 25 g | = | 1 oz |
| 100 g | = | 3.5 oz |
| 500 g | = | 18 oz |
| 1 kg | = | 2.25 lb |
| 25 ml | = | 1 fl oz |
| 100 ml | = | 4 fl oz |
| 600 ml | = | 20 fl oz / 1 pint |
| 1 litre | = | 36 fl oz |
| 1 tsp | = | 5 ml |
| 1 tbsp | = | 15 ml |

# part one: food is medicine

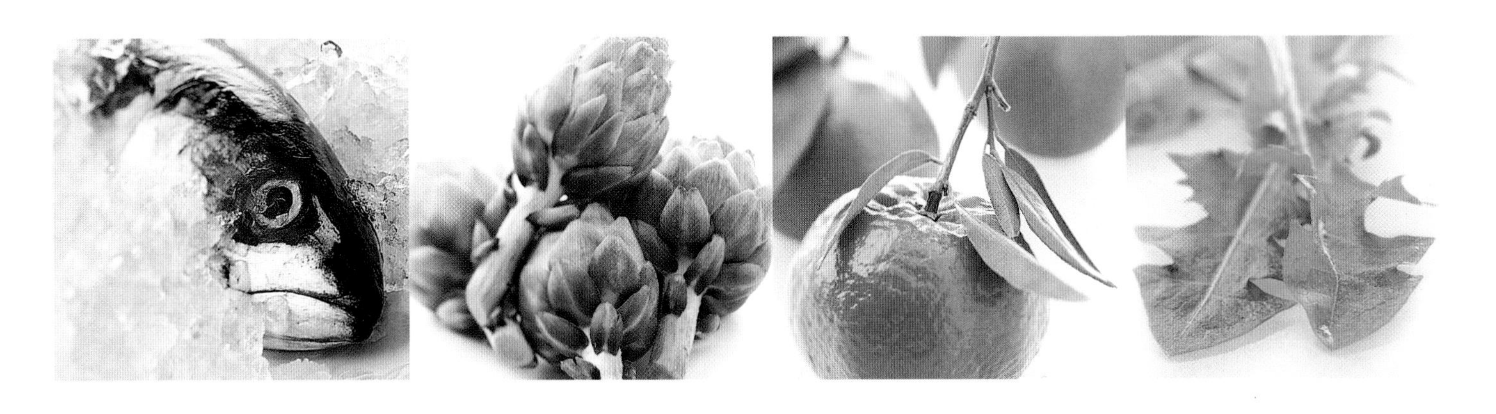

pierre jean cousin

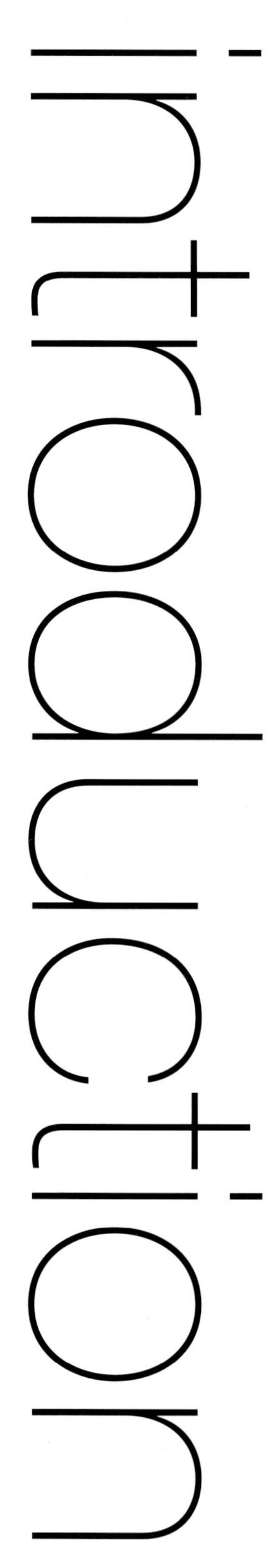


One of the most important ways in which we can influence our health is by monitoring what we eat. Eating unhealthily – too much animal fat, salt, sugar and artificial additives – can cause irreparable damage to our bodies, especially to the cardiovascular system and the kidneys. Eating healthily can increase vitality, immunity and life expectancy. We can also influence the health of future generations by teaching our children healthy eating habits.

Food can be used not only to prevent illness but also to treat it. Throughout the ages, and in all cultures, food has played an important role in healing the sick. Yet in contemporary Western societies the emphasis in healthcare has moved from traditional methods, such as diet, to modern medical techniques and a reliance on pharmaceuticals. As a result, self-help dietary remedies are rarely considered. As an experienced practitioner of a range of complementary therapies, I firmly believe in bringing the healing power of foods back to where it belongs – in our homes.

## the principles of healthy eating

The mainstay of a healthy diet is plenty of unrefined complex carbohydrates and fiber. Foods such as beans, lentils, potatoes, wholewheat pasta, wholegrain bread and cereals should make up – quite literally – the bulk of our diet. Protein-rich foods, such as meat or fish, can be added to this carbohydrate base in small amounts. Contrary to popular belief, we don't need very much protein for good health and it is not necessary to eat meat, fish and dairy products as a daily source of protein. The other essential ingredients in a healthy diet are vitamins, minerals and phytochemicals (biologically-active substances in plants), which are found in abundance in fruit and vegetables, and essential fatty acids from nuts, seeds, oily fish and oils such as olive oil.

This basic template for healthy eating closely matches the traditional diet that is – or was – eaten in many cultures. Civilizations throughout history have relied upon a combination of cereals and pulses for their staple diet. In Asia this combination is rice and soy; in America corn and beans; in Europe wheat, rye, barley, oats or buckwheat and beans, lentils or other pulses; and in Africa it is wheat, millet or sorghum and beans or chickpeas. Traditionally, a variety of fruit and vegetables (often eaten raw) has complemented this diet, together with small amounts of meat and fish when available. Fermented foods, such as cheese, yoghurt, curd, fish sauce, pickled vegetables, cider, beer and wine – all of which have a beneficial effect on the intestine – also feature in the traditional diet. This diet is ideally suited to the human body – it is rich in friendly bacteria, fiber and nutrients and helps to maintain a healthy biological balance in the intestine.

It is very easy to adopt the healthy eating habits that are characteristic of such diets by following these simple common-sense measures:

- Buy more fresh fruit and vegetables (they are rich in antioxidants – substances that help to prevent degenerative disease such as cancer and heart disease), cereals, pulses and fish.
- Cut down on meat, dairy products and convenience food.
- Replace meat with oily fish.
- Tailor food intake to match your actual calorie needs (for most people this means eating less).
- Buy a cook book that focuses on the Mediterranean diet.
- Reduce your intake of sugar, coffee, tea, fizzy drinks and alcohol.
- Eat at regular intervals (up to five times a day if this suits your needs).

- Eat food that is in season and, ideally, locally produced according to organic principles.
- Make sure that your diet is as varied as possible.
- Use fresh ingredients as often as possible; avoid canned or dried food that contains additives.
- Be flexible in your eating – aim for balance and enjoyment. Avoid rigid dietary programmes.

# how the modern diet fails

These principles of healthy eating contrast starkly with the diet that is increasingly common in the West. Whereas the diet of our pre-industrial ancestors was rich in fresh produce, the modern diet, which has evolved over the last 50–60 years, is characterized by food that contains preservatives, colourants, taste enhancers, sugar, caffeine and even traces of fertilizers, pesticides, antibiotics, hormones and metals. This leads to a proliferation of unhealthy bacteria in the gut, an accumulation of toxins in the body, poor digestion and an increased likelihood of allergies, cardiovascular disease and a range of cancers, including breast and bowel cancer.

In the West, food is abundant (the amount produced far exceeds our needs) and relatively cheap owing to modern production and processing techniques. These techniques have created what has been termed "food industrialization" – the production of large amounts of food quickly and cheaply at the expense of quality and nutritional content. Paradoxically, although we now have more choice in what we can eat, less time is devoted to the selection, preparation and consumption of food. Our diets often consist of a limited number of ingredients that we continue eating out of routine and convenience.

Much of the food that we buy is impoverished. For example, when fresh produce is out of season in one country, it is often imported from another, and much of its vitamin content is lost during transit or storage in refrigerators or on supermarket shelves.

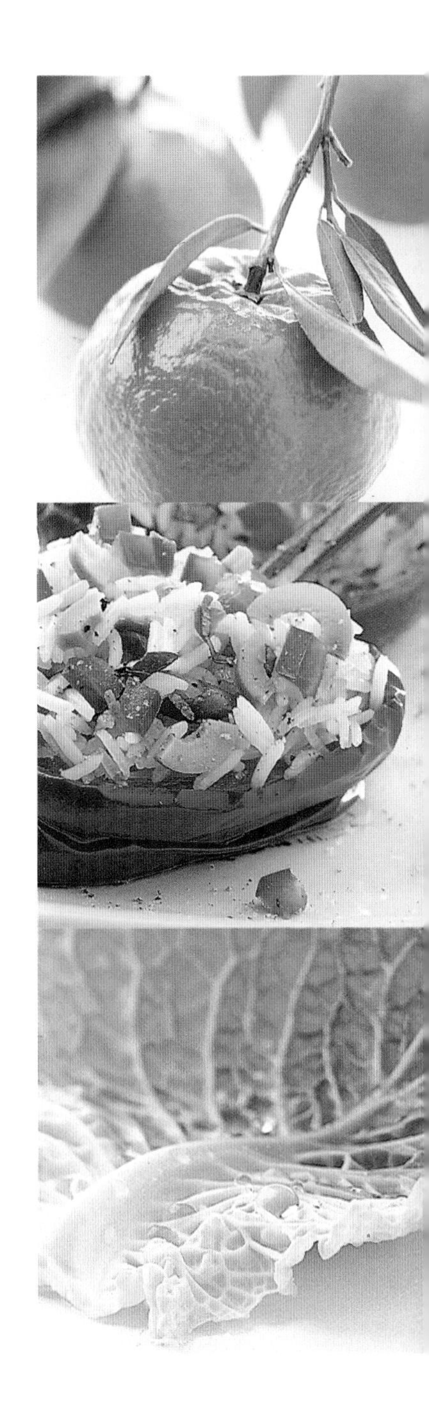

Goodness is also depleted in the process of sterilization: in order to make fresh food "safe" and prolong shelf-life by eliminating micro-organisms, it is often sterilized or irradiated – yet this procedure renders it, quite literally, lifeless. Although all unhealthy, disease-causing bacteria are killed in the process, all the "good" bacteria and ferments are also destroyed. These are important for digestion and in maintaining a healthy and balanced environment in the intestine. Most milk, for example, is pasteurized, with the result that it does not contain natural ferments and is difficult for many people to break down and digest. Milk products that have not been pasteurized, such as live yoghurt (which is full of lactobacilli bacteria), are well tolerated by most people. Another consequence of sterilization is that, if food is left out of the refrigerator for too long or is reheated too many times, micro-organisms, such as listeria, will re-establish themselves. Without competition from good bacteria, unhealthy ones can proliferate unchecked and cause disease.

Industrialized food production is partly responsible for a range of contemporary health problems, such as male hormone imbalance (linked to the misuse of hormones in animals), the advent of antibiotic-resistant strains of bacteria (linked to the routine addition of antibiotics to animal feed), salmonella in poultry and eggs (linked to poor living conditions among animals), and Creutzfeldt-Jacob disease (linked to bovine spongiform encephalopathy or BSE, a disease affecting cows that is caused by contaminated cattle feed). Genetic modification of food is the

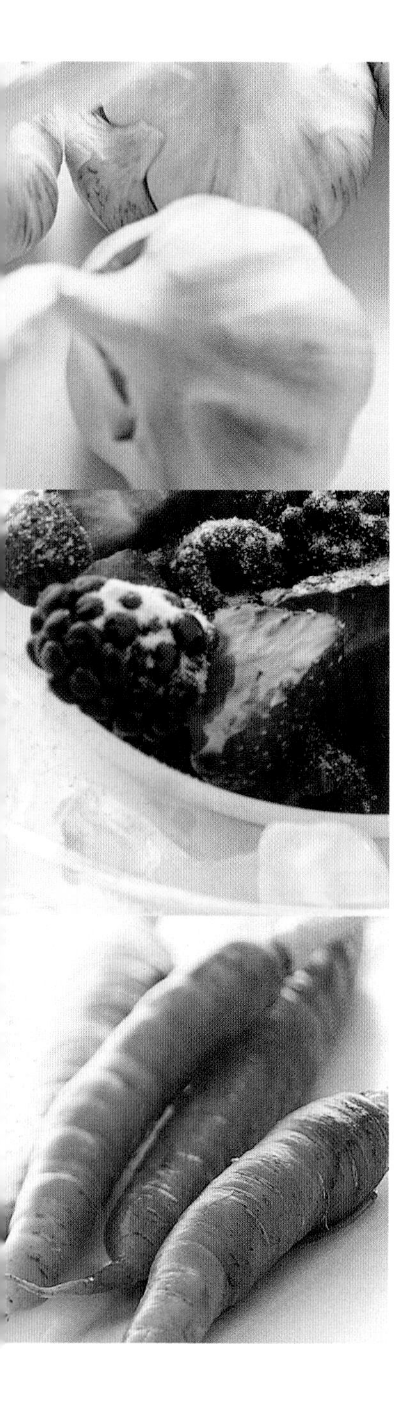

latest in a catalogue of food-production experiments that I believe may have harmful, long-term effects on human health and the environment. The defensive attitude of scientists who argue that "no evidence exists that genetically-modified (GM) food is unsafe" needs to be challenged – this kind of negative statement does not constitute proof that GM food is safe.

Owing to the wide-ranging effects of food industrialization it is important that, as consumers, we make informed choices about what we buy – not just favouring foods that are unprocessed and grown according to organic principles, but also excluding products that are nutritionally empty and preserved and enhanced in artificial ways.

# the medicinal value of food

Our knowledge of the healing power of food is based upon thousands of years of tradition and empirical observation. Modern scientific research now confirms the curative abilities of foods that have been used therapeutically through the ages. A huge variety of foods is known to contain compounds that have medicinal properties. For example, the potent antibacterial action of allicin, a substance found in garlic, is well documented. So too are the protective and healing properties of antioxidants and essential oils found in fruit, vegetables, herbs and spices. Some pharmacologically-active ingredients are extracted from food and sold in tablet form. Cynarin, for example, is an active ingredient that is extracted from artichoke. An extensive body of research has shown that this substance can play an important role in treating liver disease and help damaged liver tissue to regenerate. The great advantage of using food as medicine is that food is readily available to all of us and can be self-administered with relative safety. Food cures work in a purely holistic way by enhancing the body's natural functions and encouraging it to heal itself.

# using Part One – Food is Medicine

The aim of Food is Medicine is to provide inspiration and practical advice that will help you to adopt healthy eating habits and to use food in medicinal ways. Food is Medicine is divided into four chapters. The first chapter, Guide to Healing Foods, lists more than 140 common foods, their nutrients and their most important medicinal properties. It also identifies seven "star" foods that are renowned for their beneficial properties. Chapter two, Foods for Common Ailments, specifies the foods that can play a part in treating over 80 common medical conditions. The third chapter, Healing Recipes, is a collection of recipes that use medicinal foods in interesting and delicious combinations. The final chapter, Diet in Practice, offers a practical guide to vitamins and minerals and the foods in which they are found. It also explains how to detoxify your body with a simple diet based on fruit, vegetables, juices and herbal infusions.

Most of the recipes and techniques that I have selected are straightforward to make or carry out, and use easily available ingredients. The recipes can be used in three different ways:

- As everyday dishes for people who are healthy, but interested in preserving their long-term well-being by incorporating health-giving foods in their diet.
- As remedies for acute and chronic illnesses. The recipes for juices (pages 117–119) and medicinal drinks (pages 123–131) will be the most useful as they are the most medicinally potent.

Food remedies can be used in conjunction with conventional medical treatment to manage or heal a variety of severe or chronic complaints. The time that it takes to witness improvements depends on your ailment and state of health – try to be patient and persevere with food remedies. Illnesses that are stress-related are also amenable to dietary treatment.

- As first-aid treatments and for symptom relief. Some of the foods used in the recipes can alleviate problems such as indigestion and period pain. Others can be applied to the skin as remedies for bites, burns, stings and skin problems, such as eczema, or as beauty treatments.

Some of the medicinal-drink recipes contain alcohol in the form of wine or vodka. Although in large quantities alcohol is bad for health, it is an excellent solvent that concentrates the active ingredients of plants. Macerating a herb such as basil in vodka, for example, preserves its medicinal compounds in a form that is easy and convenient to take (basil is good for indigestion, nausea and to ease feelings of bloatedness). Most medicinal drinks that contain alcohol need be taken in only small doses or for a short period of time – just long enough to help a particular symptom or condition. The medicinal infusions and decoctions often fall into the category of traditional herbal medicine rather than dietary remedies. Since all of the medicinal drinks are potent, they should be used with caution and should not be given to children unless the recipe states that this is acceptable. If you are in doubt about whether it is appropriate to treat yourself with herbal or food remedies, or you are worried about a health problem, consult your doctor.

In a few recipes, a little cream may be added to the finished dish – this is entirely optional. If you have a health problem such as lactose intolerance, use soya milk and soya yoghurt instead of milk products. If you suffer from hypertension, high cholesterol, heart disease or diabetes, you should avoid adding sugar, salt and fat to any of the recipes.

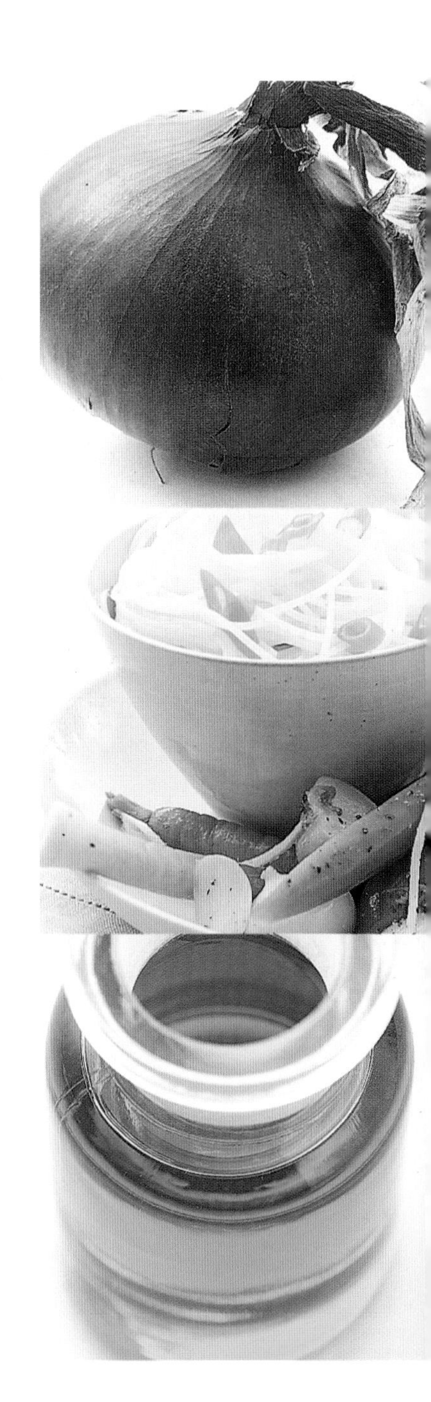

## selecting and harvesting ingredients

Whenever possible, use organically-grown fruit and vegetables, make sure they are fresh and avoid keeping them in a refrigerator for too long. When buying meat, buy organically-produced, free-range or farm-raised meat; buy small quantities of quality cuts rather than larger amounts of cheaper meat. Try to buy fish on the same day that it is delivered to your fishmonger.

If possible, try to harvest wild ingredients from your garden or local countryside. When picking ingredients, such as borage leaves, nettles and dandelion leaves, choose young plants that are growing away from main roads, rail tracks, and paths that are regularly used by animals. Make sure that you can confidently identify the plants that you need and that what you pick is in good condition and fit for consumption. You can cultivate many herbs, such as camomile, lemon balm, savory, mint, basil, thyme and rosemary, in your garden or in pots on a patio or balcony. When harvesting wild fruit, such as berries, choose bushes and trees that are not exposed to pollution from roads. Collect only undamaged, ripe fruit and don't be tempted to eat it on the spot – it must be washed thoroughly, and preferably cooked.

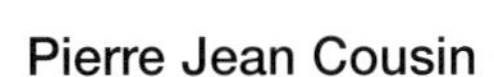

**Pierre Jean Cousin**

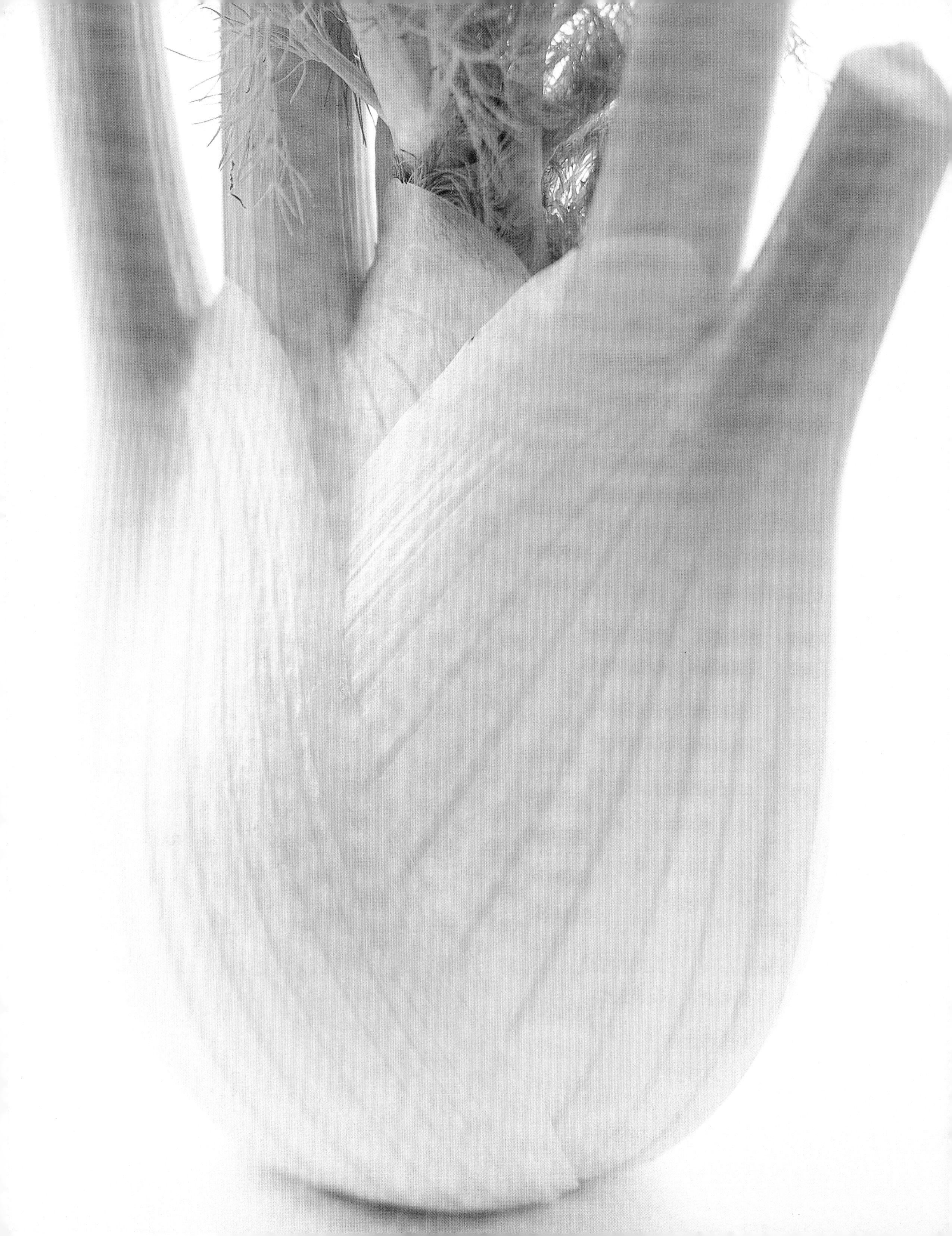

chapter one

# guide to healing foods

Many people consider food as fuel – they need it simply to keep them going through the day. But food can also prevent and treat illness, offering an astounding medicine-chest of natural remedies that come with little or no risk. The foods in this section are arranged by type to help you to make informed choices about which specific foods may be beneficial to you. Included are seven star foods – true wonders of nature that we should all include in our diet to boost and protect good health.

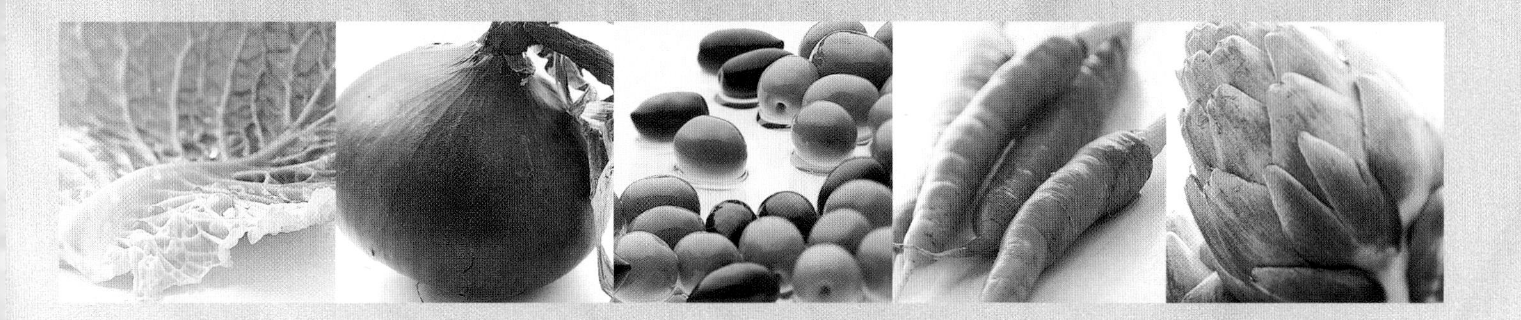

# vegetables, cereals and pulses

## ROOT VEGETABLES

### POTATO

★ VITAMINS B, C, FOLIC ACID, COPPER, PHOSPHORUS, POTASSIUM, SULPHUR, CARBOHYDRATE

● DIGESTIVE SYSTEM Diabetes, gastritis, peptic ulcers.

Potatoes are good for mild digestive problems. Potato juice, mixed with equal amounts of carrot and cabbage juice and a little lemon juice to taste, can ease the symptoms of gastritis and peptic ulcers. The juice or pulp of raw potatoes can be applied directly to burns, insect bites, eczema and boils. Germinated or green potatoes should not be eaten as they may cause stomach upset. RECIPES *chicken breasts with celeriac mash (page 106), dandelion, bacon and potato cakes (page 106), potato and watercress mash (page 109), potatoes with herb sauce (page 111).*

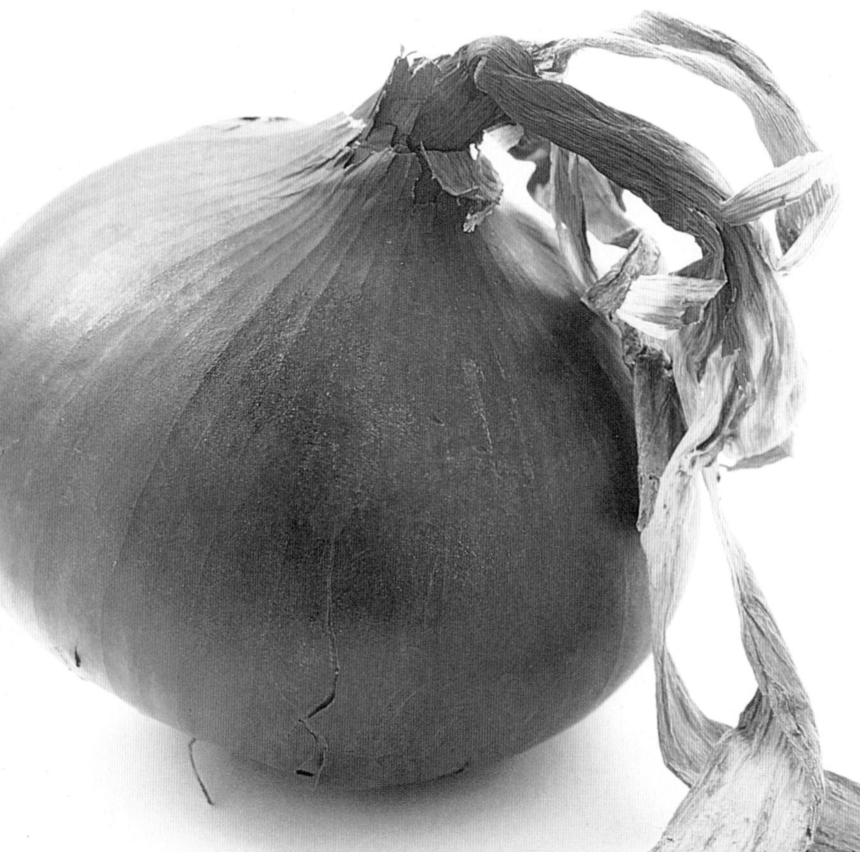

### PARSNIP

★ VITAMINS C, FOLIC ACID, E, PHOSPHORUS, POTASSIUM, CARBOHYDRATE, FIBRE

Parsnips belong to the same family as carrots and parsley. They contain small quantities of essential oils (mostly terpenes) that are thought to have anti-cancer properties.

### TURNIP

★ VITAMINS A, B, C, FOLIC ACID, CALCIUM, IRON, MAGNESIUM, PHOSPHORUS, POTASSIUM, SULPHUR, NATURAL SUGAR

Turnips, together with several other vegetables, such as broccoli, cabbage, brussels sprouts, cauliflower and swede, are cruciferous (see Broccoli, page 22). Both the root and the young leaves of the turnip can be eaten (the root can be eaten raw, grated in salads). RECIPES *young turnip salad (page 98), pickled turnips (page 120).*

### ONION AND SHALLOT

★ VITAMINS A, B, C, MAGNESIUM, PHOSPHORUS, POTASSIUM, SULPHUR COMPOUNDS, BIOFLAVONOIDS, ESSENTIAL OIL, NATURAL SUGAR

● BONES AND JOINTS Arthritis (rheumatoid), gout, rheumatism.

● BLOOD AND CIRCULATION Arteriosclerosis.

● DIGESTIVE SYSTEM Diabetes, diarrhoea.

● IMMUNE SYSTEM Colds, influenza.

● WOMEN'S HEALTH Period pain.

Onions have antibiotic and anti-fungal properties, can block tumour formation, reduce levels of blood cholesterol and prevent blood clots forming. They ease fluid retention and promote the elimination of urea. Onions are beneficial to both the digestive and circulatory systems. They can be juiced or used in a decoction for the treatment of digestive problems, diarrhoea, coughs, colds and flu. Onions can be eaten raw (macerating in olive oil makes them more palatable). Onion juice can be drunk mixed with water or carrot juice; it can also be applied neat to insect stings, warts and boils. RECIPES *onions in cider (page 109).*

### BEETROOT

★ VITAMINS A, B, C, IRON, MAGNESIUM, MANGANESE, POTASSIUM, ZINC, ASPARAGIN, BETAINE, BIOFLAVONOIDS, NATURAL SUGAR

● BLOOD AND CIRCULATION Anaemia.

Beetroot is nutritious, easy to digest and a rich source of minerals. It contains betaine, a substance that regulates gastric pH and facilitates digestion. Beetroot can be eaten raw, chopped or grated in salads, or drunk as a juice (one glass per day for a month is the recommended dosage for improving digestive function). The leafy tops of the beetroot plant can be cooked in soups; they are rich in vitamins and minerals and good for the liver.

RECIPES *borscht (page 92), beetroot and celery juice (page 119), pickled beetroot (page 120).*

### CELERIAC

★ VITAMINS A, B, C, IODINE, IRON, MAGNESIUM, MANGANESE, POTASSIUM, ANTIOXIDANTS

● BLOOD AND CIRCULATION Hyperlipidaemia.

Celeriac is the root of a variety of celery plant; it helps to lower levels of blood cholesterol and reduce the risk of bowel cancer.

RECIPES *chicken breasts with celeriac mash (page 106).*

### RADISH (RED AND BLACK)

★ FOLIC ACID, SULPHUR, RAPHANOL, WATER

● BONES AND JOINTS Arthritis (rheumatoid).

● DIGESTIVE SYSTEM Dyspepsia.

● RESPIRATORY SYSTEM Cough, whooping cough.

Although radishes are of poor overall nutritional value, they contain an active ingredient called raphanol that promotes bile flow and the emptying of the gallbladder. There are different types of radish. Black radishes are much larger than the common red variety and contain a greater concentration of raphanol. A combination of carrot and black radish juice is recommended for people with poor liver function and gallbladder problems such as gallstones – mix equal amounts of juice in a 150 ml glass. Both black and red radishes are best eaten raw in salads. A syrup of black radish can be used as an expectorant cough mixture that is appropriate for whooping cough. The young leaves of red radishes contain valuable minerals and are an excellent addition to soups.

RECIPES *radish and kumquat salad (page 96), escarole salad (page 99), black radish salad (page 99), black radish syrup (page 130).*

### LEEK

★ VITAMINS B, C, CALCIUM, IRON, MAGNESIUM, MANGANESE, PHOSPHORUS, POTASSIUM, SILICA, SULPHUR

● BONES AND JOINTS Arthritis (rheumatoid), gout.

● KIDNEYS AND BLADDER Bladder stones.

Leeks belong to the same family as garlic and onion, and contain smaller amounts of the same active ingredients. Leeks are diuretic, laxative, antiseptic and are excellent for a healthy digestive tract. Leek juice can be used externally on abscesses, skin inflammation, stings and bites. A leek macerated in vinegar for 24 hours is an effective remedy for corns and calluses – apply to the affected area overnight and repeat if necessary.

RECIPES *buckwheat with leek sauce (page 103), leek and chive mimosa with polenta (page 105), leek syrup (page 130).*

*continues on page 22*

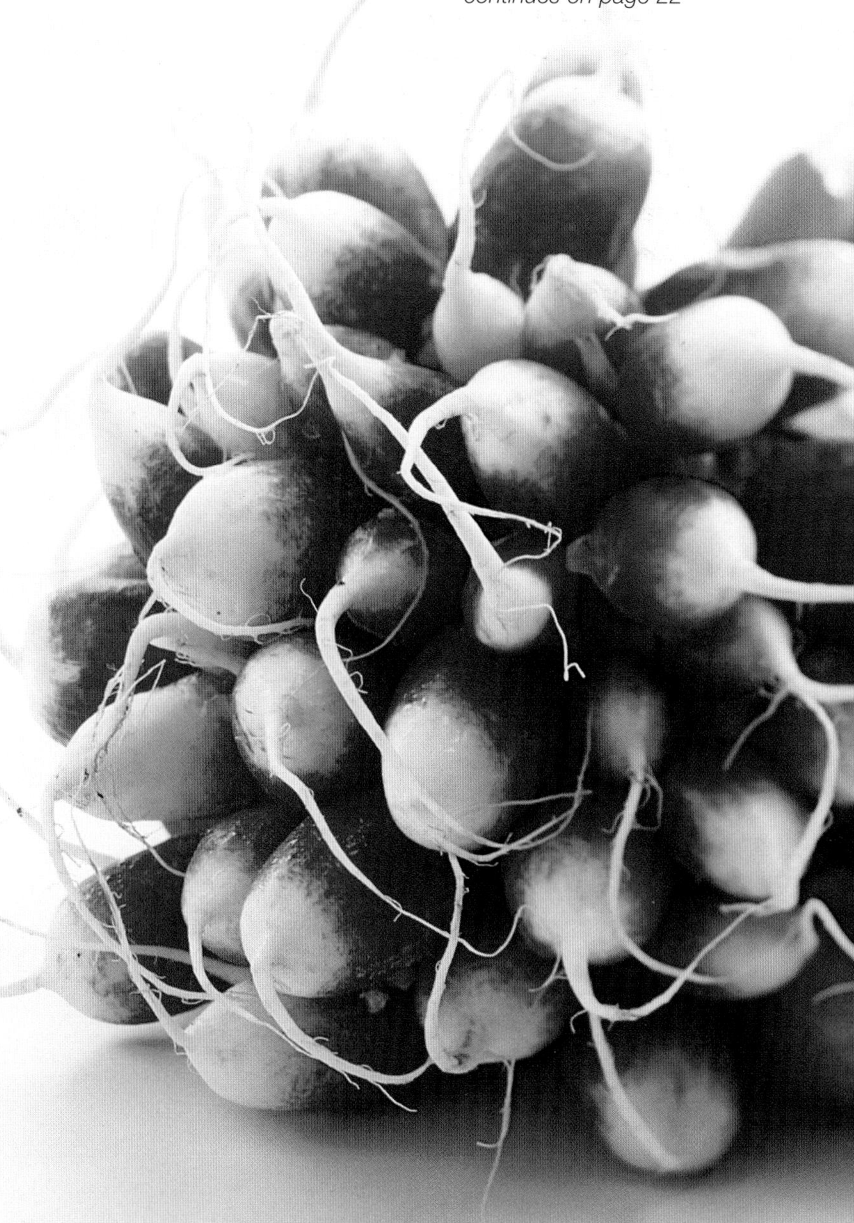

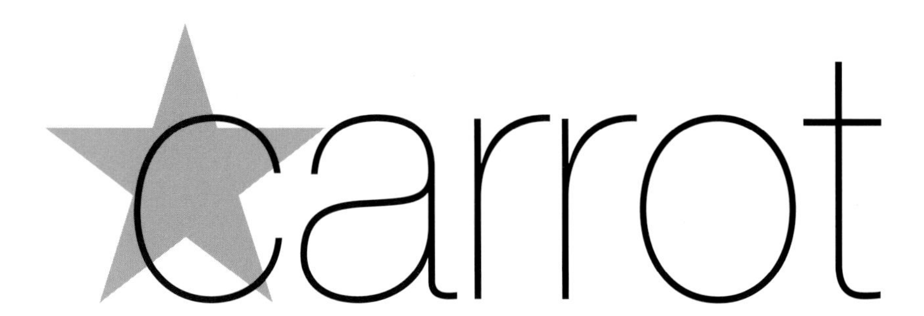

# carrot

**CARROTS ARE RICH IN ANTIOXIDANTS AND PROTECT THE BODY FROM CERTAIN TYPES OF CANCER. THEY BOOST THE IMMUNE SYSTEM AND ARE USEFUL IN TREATING A RANGE OF AILMENTS, FROM POOR NIGHT VISION TO STOMACH ULCERS.**

## The properties of carrot

The medicinal properties of carrots were known to the Greeks and Romans. Carrots then were long, thin yellow roots with a strong scent. Modern carrots, which originated in Holland in the 17th century, tend to be orange-coloured, plump and short.

Carrots are one of the most precious vegetables in a medicinal kitchen – they contain vitamin A, folic acid, iron, potassium, magnesium, manganese, sulphur, copper, carotenes and pectin. Their high fibre and fluid content makes them gently laxative and good for constipation, but they also have astringent properties that makes them good for diarrhoea – they can be used as a remedy for either problem in children. A treatment for diarrhoea in adults consists of eating boiled carrots and boiled rice and drinking black tea. The young leaves of carrots are rich in minerals and can be added to soups or cooked with cereals as a tonic for children or people recovering from illness.

Raw carrots inhibit the activity of listeria and salmonella, and thus help to prevent or reduce the risk of food poisoning. Carrots are recommended for chronic fatigue, anaemia, poor immune defences, poor night vision, stomach ulcers and intestinal problems. They can also promote lactation in nursing mothers. Carrot juice contains more medicinally-active ingredients than cooked carrots and the juice is recommended for young children. Raw carrots were traditionally given to horses suffering from bronchitis.

Carrots should be peeled to remove organophosphates (and other artificial residues from pesticides and fertilizers) that may accumulate in the outer part of the vegetable. If possible, buy organically-grown carrots that are free from organophosphates and fertilizers.

## Long-term health benefits

Carrots are an excellent source of antioxidants and are known to have a protective action against lung and other types of cancer. A diet that includes plenty of carrots also lowers unhealthy levels of cholesterol in the blood – preventing the build up of fatty deposits in artery walls – and boosts the body's immune system.

Carrots are a cheap and easily available source of antioxidants and, ideally, they should be consumed two or three times a week either raw in salads (or as snacks) or in juice form.

## Medicinal preparations

Carrot seeds can be made into a medicinal infusion (page 124) that stimulates appetite and digestion, and is both diuretic and carminative (relieves flatulence). Externally, carrot juice can be mixed with other ingredients, including cucumber, strawberries and chervil, to make a beauty treatment that rejuvenates the face and neck. An external application of carrot juice can also help to alleviate eczema and acne.

## STAR FOOD PROFILE

- **BLOOD AND CIRCULATION** Anaemia.
- **DIGESTIVE SYSTEM** Diarrhoea, flatulence, peptic ulcers.
- **NERVOUS SYSTEM, MIND AND EMOTIONS** Mental fatigue.
- **SKIN, HAIR AND NAILS** Acne, dermatitis and eczema.

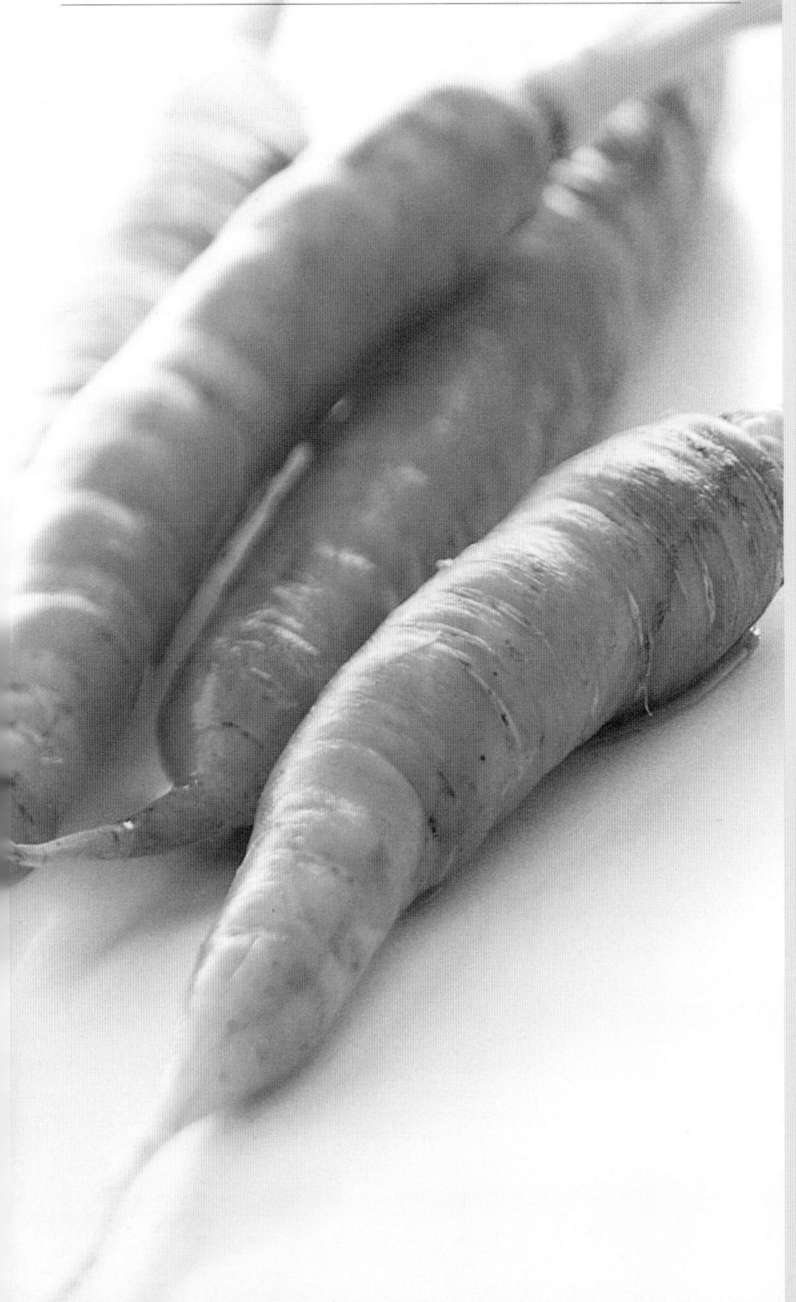

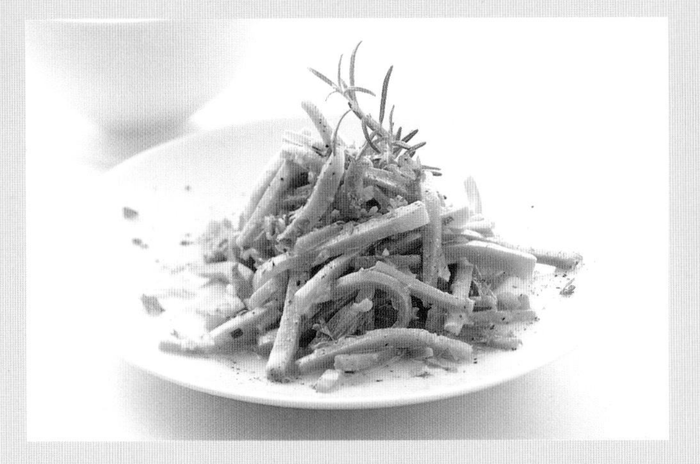

# carrots with rosemary

30 g butter
1 red onion, sliced
1 kg carrots, peeled and sliced
1 heaped tbsp finely chopped rosemary
5 tbsp fresh cream or yoghurt
Salt and pepper
To garnish: 1 tbsp chopped parsley

In a saucepan, melt the butter and add the onion, carrots and rosemary. Cover and let the ingredients cook slowly in their own juices for 30 minutes or until the carrots are tender. Add a little water if the saucepan becomes dry. When the carrots are cooked, add the cream or yoghurt and season to taste. Garnish with parsley and serve.

# carrot salad

500 g carrots, grated
Juice of 1 lemon
Juice of 1 orange
Pinch of salt

Mix the ingredients in a large bowl. Cover and chill before serving.

# carrot, cabbage and sweet pepper juice

4 medium carrots, roughly chopped
½ cabbage, core removed and quartered
1 red or green pepper, de-seeded
2 small shallots

In a juicer, process the ingredients, adding water if necessary. Chill and serve soon after making.

# GREEN AND LEAFY VEGETABLES

## BROCCOLI

★ **VITAMINS A, C, FOLIC ACID, E, CALCIUM, IRON, ZINC**

● **BLOOD AND CIRCULATION** High blood pressure.

Broccoli, together with several other vegetables, such as turnips, cabbage, brussels sprouts, cauliflower and swedes, belong to the cruciferous family. They are rich in antioxidants and are believed to reduce the risk of certain types of cancer, including lung and colon cancer. Avoid overcooking broccoli as approximately half of its beneficial substances may be destroyed in the process.

RECIPES *broccoli and green bean juice (page 119).*

## BRUSSELS SPROUT

★ **VITAMIN A, C, FOLIC ACID, E, IRON, POTASSIUM**

See Broccoli, above.

RECIPES *brussels sprouts with chestnuts (page 110).*

## CAULIFLOWER

★ **VITAMINS C, FOLIC ACID, E, POTASSIUM, ZINC, CAROTENES**

● **BONES AND JOINTS** Arthritis (rheumatoid).

See Broccoli, above.

RECIPES *pickled cauliflower (page 120).*

## GREEN BEAN

★ **VITAMIN A, FOLIC ACID, COPPER, PHOSPHORUS, SILICA, CARBOHYDRATE, CHLOROPHYLL**

● **BONES AND JOINTS** Arthritis (rheumatoid), gout, rheumatism.

● **KIDNEYS AND BLADDER** Kidney stones.

Green beans have diuretic properties which help kidney function and prevent water retention. They stimulate the production of white blood cells (needed to defend the body against infection) and are gently cardio-tonic. For rheumatism, water retention or as a general cardio-tonic, green beans should be eaten every day for a month (the cooking water can be also be drunk or used as a stock for soup). Alternatively, half a glass of green bean juice every morning for four to five weeks has the same medicinal benefits.

RECIPES *green bean salad (page 97), green beans with dijon mustard (page 111), green bean and garlic juice (page 119), broccoli and green bean juice (page 119).*

## CHARD

★ **VITAMINS A, B, FOLIC ACID, IRON**

Chard is a form of beet that is grown for its green leaves. It has diuretic and laxative properties and is useful for treating kidney and bladder inflammation. The cooked leaves can be used in a poultice for burns, abscesses and boils.

## DANDELION

★ **VITAMINS A, B, C, FOLIC ACID, CALCIUM, IRON, MANGANESE, POTASSIUM, SILICA, BIOFLAVONOIDS, BITTER PRINCIPLE, CHLOROPHYLL, INULIN**

● **BLOOD AND CIRCULATION** Anaemia, hyperlipidaemia.

● **DIGESTIVE SYSTEM** Colitis, constipation, gallstones.

● **KIDNEYS AND BLADDER** Kidney stones.

● **SKIN, HAIR AND NAILS** Eczema.

Dandelion leaves are recommended for people with poor liver function, gallbladder or kidney stones. The young leaves can be used in salads or cooked in the same way as other green leafy vegetables. When choosing young dandelion plants for salads or soups, include the young flower buds. The fresh sap from the dandelion is said to be an effective topical treatment for verrucae. Dandelion root is widely used in herbal medicine for its diuretic and detoxifying properties.

RECIPES *dandelion, bacon and potato cakes (page 106), dandelion infusion (page 123).*

## NETTLE

★ **VITAMINS A, C, CAROTENE, CALCIUM, IRON, MAGNESIUM, POTASSIUM, SILICA, SULPHUR**

● **BONES AND JOINTS** Arthritis (rheumatoid), gout, rheumatism.

● **BLOOD AND CIRCULATION** Anaemia.

● **DIGESTIVE SYSTEM** Diarrhoea.

Nettles are a novel addition to many recipes. They are diuretic, astringent and depurative; they promote the elimination of uric acid, stimulate liver function, appetite and bile flow; and they help combat infection. Nettles can be used as a fortifying ingredient in recipes for children and people recovering from illness. They are also good for diminishing menstrual and other types of bleeding. RECIPES *nettle soup (page 94), nettle risotto (page 103), halibut steak with nettle butter (page 107).*

### SPINACH

★ VITAMIN C, FOLIC ACID, IRON, ZINC, CAROTENE

Spinach is rich in antioxidants and stimulates pancreas function. The juice is a powerful tonic; an infusion of the seeds is good for mild constipation (cover 10 g of seeds in 250 ml boiling water, infuse for 10 minutes then strain); and the leaves can be used as a topical treatment for burns or eczema. Avoid over-consumption of spinach as it may reduce calcium absorption. People who suffer from gout, arthritis or inflammation of the digestive tract should not eat excessive amounts of spinach.

RECIPES *lamb with spinach and lentils (page 105), spicy spinach, prunes and beans (page 107), red mullet with raw spinach salad (page 109).*

### WATERCRESS

★ VITAMINS A, B, C, E, IODINE, IRON, MANGANESE, PHOSPHORUS, ZINC

● BONES AND JOINTS Arthritis (rheumatoid), rheumatism.

● BLOOD AND CIRCULATION Anaemia.

● DIGESTIVE SYSTEM Intestinal parasites.

● RESPIRATORY SYSTEM Bronchitis.

Watercress stimulates the appetite and has tonic, depurative, diuretic, expectorant and anti-cancer properties. It is good for lack of energy. Watercress leaves or juice can be applied to the skin to ease inflammation, ulcers and boils, eliminate freckles and heal scars. The juice or the cooking water is a good hair tonic.

RECIPES *cottage cheese with watercress (page 101), potato and watercress mash (page 109).*

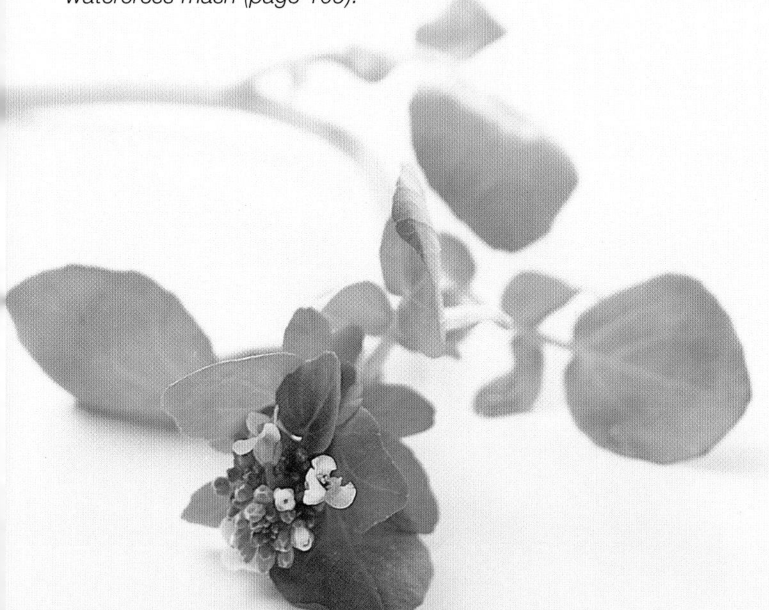

# SALAD VEGETABLES

### LETTUCE

★ VITAMINS A, C, D, FOLIC ACID, E, IRON, MANGANESE, POTASSIUM, ZINC, LACTUCARIUM

● NERVOUS SYSTEM, MIND AND EMOTIONS Insomnia.

During the Middle Ages lettuce was served at the start of a meal in order to stimulate the appetite. Because it is rich in fibre it helps food to pass quickly through the intestines, and aids digestion. Lettuce contains lactucarium, a substance that has sedative and analgesic properties, and is thought to be useful in the treatment of mild insomnia. Lettuce seeds are the most valuable part of the plant from a medicinal perspective. A decoction of the seeds is helpful for asthma, bronchitis, spasmodic cough and insomnia. A decoction of lettuce leaves can be used externally as an anti-inflammatory treatment for conjunctivitis and acne.

RECIPES *lettuce and basil juice (page 119), lettuce-seed decoction (page 126).*

### LAMB'S LETTUCE

★ VITAMINS A, B, C, FOLIC ACID, IRON, CHLOROPHYLL, FIBRE

● BONES AND JOINTS Arthritis (rheumatoid).

● BLOOD AND CIRCULATION Anaemia, arteriosclerosis.

● DIGESTIVE SYSTEM Constipation, gastroenteritis.

● KIDNEYS AND BLADDER Bladder stones.

Lamb's lettuce is recommended for digestive problems. It has detoxifying and slight diuretic properties, it facilitates the elimination of urea (which prevents the formation of uric acid crystals) and is said to be good for respiratory disorders, probably by helping the elimination of mucus. Lamb's lettuce is best eaten raw in salads but can also be cooked or taken in juice form.

### ROCKET

★ VITAMINS A, B, C, FOLIC ACID, IRON, CHLOROPHYLL, FIBRE

● DIGESTIVE SYSTEM Dyspepsia.

Rocket was once considered to be an aphrodisiac and its cultivation in monasteries was forbidden. It is widely used in Italian cuisine and can be used in salads or lightly cooked with pasta and ravioli. It has tonic properties and stimulates appetite and digestion.

*continues on page 26*

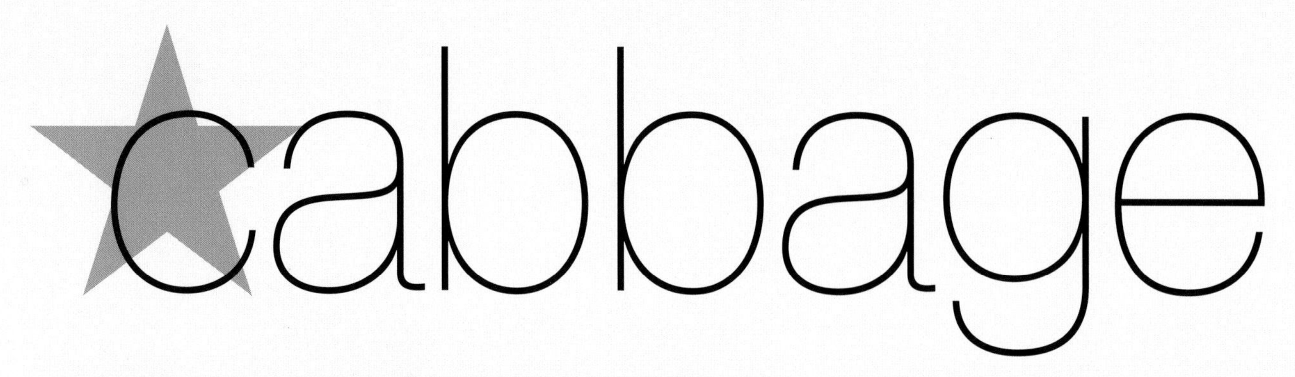

# cabbage

**CABBAGE IS A LONG-ESTABLISHED REMEDY FOR A VARIETY OF DIGESTIVE AILMENTS. IT IS ALSO RICH IN ANTIOXIDANTS AND CAN STRENGTHEN THE IMMUNE SYSTEM AND HELP THE BODY TO OVERCOME INFECTION.**

### The history of cabbage

The therapeutic benefits of the common cabbage have been known and appreciated across Europe for thousands of years: the Slavs, Celts, Basques and Germans all used cabbage for both food and medicine and the Romans considered it to be a panacea for almost any disease. It is thought that cultivation of the cabbage plant may go back as far as the Neolithic period. Cabbage belongs to the cruciferous family of vegetables, which also includes broccoli and turnip. There are many different colours, sizes and varieties of cabbage.

### The properties of cabbage

Cabbage is rich in vitamins A, B, C, K and E, potassium, sulphur and copper. It also contains a variety of antioxidants that help to reduce the risk of bowel cancer and cardiovascular disease. Cabbage is anti-inflammatory, diuretic and helps to lower blood sugar. Medicinal uses of cabbage focus on digestive ailments such as gastritis, stomach ulcers, colitis and diverticulitis. Research shows that cabbage juice is an effective treatment for stomach ulcers. A recommended remedy for inflammation of the digestive tract is a small glass of cabbage juice every morning for a few weeks. Cabbage juice is also a natural cleansing and purifying agent.

An immune system stimulant, cabbage is good for treating common colds and catarrh, laryngitis and other upper respiratory tract infections. The abundance of sulphur compounds in cabbage also makes it an effective remedy for rheumatism and arthritis. Cabbage contains a small amount of a substance called glucobrassinin which reduces the activity of the thyroid gland. Excessive consumption of cabbage among people who receive insufficient iodine may lead to a mild and rare form of hypothyroidism.

### Cabbage in the diet

Many of the active ingredients contained in cabbage are lost in prolonged cooking; raw cabbage and cabbage juice are of greater medicinal value. A good way of eating raw cabbage is chopped and pickled in the form of sauerkraut. This contains a high concentration of lactobacilli – bacteria that are beneficial to the intestines.

### Using cabbage externally

Cabbage leaves made into a poultice can be applied externally to heal wounds, fractures, sprains, burns, and joint inflammation caused by rheumatism, arthritis and gout. The juice can be applied to the skin in the treatment of eczema and acne. Cabbage leaves placed on the eyes can relieve local inflammation.

## STAR FOOD PROFILE

- **BONES AND JOINTS** Arthritis (rheumatoid), rheumatism.
- **BLOOD AND CIRCULATION** Raynaud's disease.
- **DIGESTIVE SYSTEM** Colitis, diverticulitis, gastritis, peptic ulcers.
- **RESPIRATORY SYSTEM** Asthma, cough.

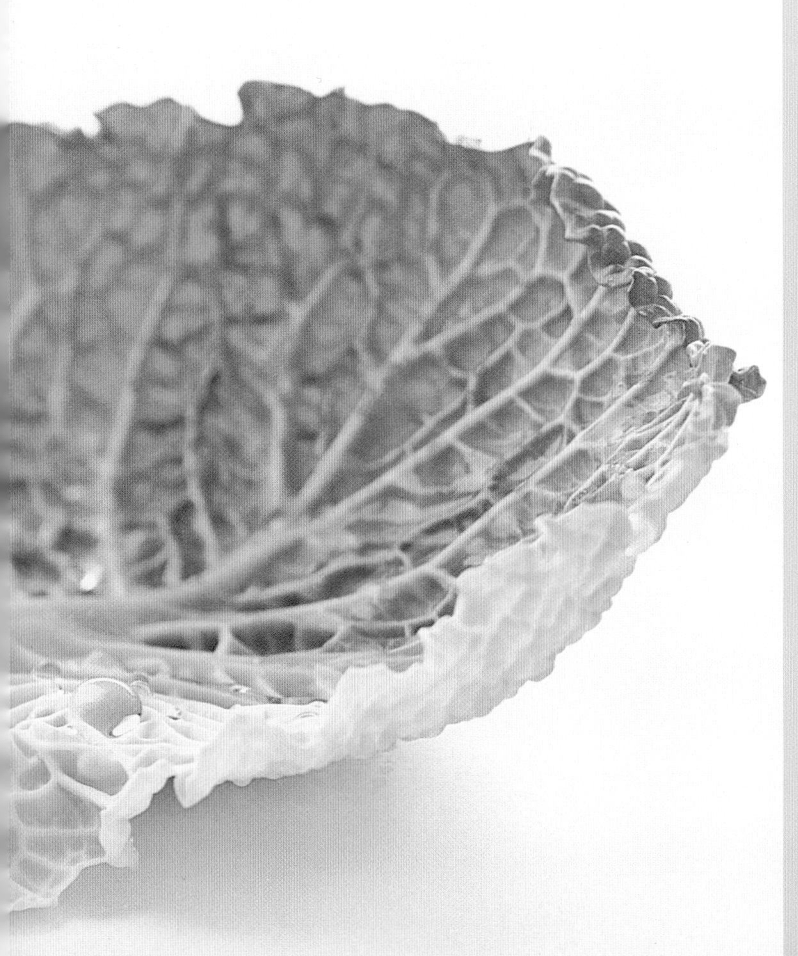

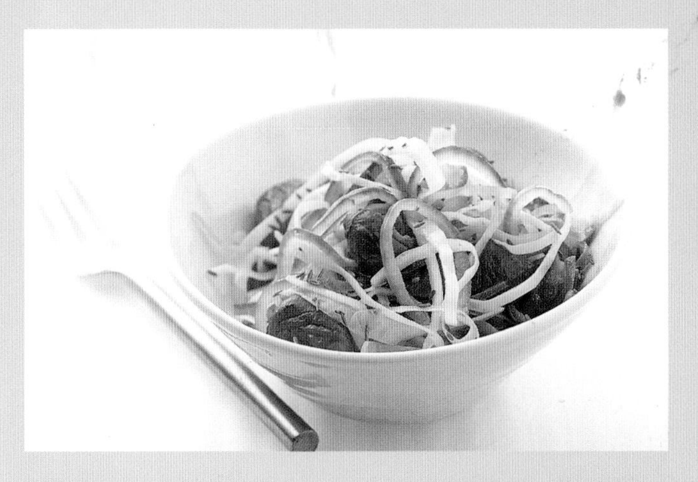

# cabbage with chestnuts

This dish goes well with roast pork.

1 medium-sized white cabbage (or red cabbage or Brussels sprouts)
2 tbsp olive oil
4 medium-sized red onions, sliced
300 g chestnuts, peeled and cooked
To garnish: cumin seeds

Chop the cabbage into thin strips, then blanch in salted, boiling water for a few minutes. In another large pan, soften the onions in the olive oil over a low heat, then add the cabbage and chestnuts, and cook for a further 5 minutes. Sprinkle over some cumin seeds before serving hot.

# cabbage, carrot and blueberry juice

2 parts fresh cabbage juice
2 parts fresh carrot juice
1 part blueberry juice

Combine the juices thoroughly. Chill and serve.

## CELERY

★ **VITAMINS A, B, C, CALCIUM, MAGNESIUM, MANGANESE, POTASSIUM, ESSENTIAL OIL**

● **BONES AND JOINTS** Gout, rheumatism.

● **KIDNEYS AND BLADDER** Kidney or bladder stones.

● **IMMUNE SYSTEM** Sore throat.

Celery is beneficial for digestive problems and poor appetite. It is best eaten raw in salads or juiced with carrots or green vegetables and is particularly easy to digest in soup form. Fresh celery juice is antiseptic so it can help to ease mouth ulcers and sore throats. The juice can also be mixed with an equal amount of carrot juice and applied to the skin to promote healing. Celery is very low in calories so it is a useful part of a weight-loss diet.

RECIPES *celery with wine and herbs (page 110), cabbage, carrot and celery juice (page 119), beetroot and celery juice (page 119).*

## CUCUMBER

★ **VITAMINS A, B, C, IODINE, MANGANESE, SULPHUR**

● **BONES AND JOINTS** Gout, rheumatism.

● **DIGESTIVE SYSTEM** Ulcerative colitis.

Cucumbers have a very high water content; they are diuretic, anti-inflammatory, help to dissolve uric acid and are good for intestinal health. They should be eaten with the skin on (whenever possible buy organically produced, unwaxed cucumbers). Cucumber flesh or juice can be used externally to reduce inflammation and to hydrate and protect the skin. A face mask can be made from blending 1 tablespoon of fresh cream with equal amounts of cucumber, melon and pumpkin seeds in a food processor. The cream should be applied to the face, left for 30 minutes and then rinsed off.

RECIPES *pineapple and cucumber salad (page 99), cucumber salad (page 99), rice with cucumber balls (page 109), cucumber and lettuce heart juice (page 119).*

## PEPPER

★ **VITAMINS A, C, ANTIOXIDANTS**

● **BONES AND JOINTS** Rheumatism.

● **DIGESTIVE SYSTEM** Diarrhoea, dyspepsia, wind.

The colour of a pepper – green, yellow or red – indicates its stage of maturity. Sweet peppers can be eaten raw in salads and grilled or roasted in a variety of Mediterranean dishes. Hot peppers are used in spicy dishes such as curry; they contain up to 1 per cent capsaicin, a pungent-smelling and -tasting substance that is beneficial for the heart and circulation.

RECIPES *stuffed peppers (page 104).*

## TOMATO

★ **VITAMINS A, B, C, FOLIC ACID, TRACE ELEMENTS, ANTIOXIDANTS**

● **BONES AND JOINTS** Arthritis (rheumatoid), rheumatism.

● **DIGESTIVE SYSTEM** Cholecystitis, constipation, gallstones.

● **KIDNEYS AND BLADDER** Bladder stones.

Tomatoes help to dissolve urea, preventing the formation of uric acid crystals. They reduce inflammation of the digestive tract and bacterial activity in the bowel. Many commercially available tomatoes are grown too quickly in hot-houses or are genetically modified. Organically-produced varieties of tomato offer greater medicinal benefits.

RECIPES *tomato coulis (page 103), polenta with basil tomato sauce (page 105), celery and tomato juice (page 118).*

## COURGETTE

★ **VITAMINS A, B, C, MAGNESIUM, PHOSPHORUS, POTASSIUM, ZINC, CAROTENES**

● **DIGESTIVE SYSTEM** Dyspepsia, gastroenteritis.

● **NERVOUS SYSTEM, MIND AND EMOTIONS** Insomnia.

Courgettes are gentle on the intestines, mildly laxative, diuretic and can alleviate bladder and kidney inflammation. They are recommended for diabetic people who manage their illness through diet. Courgettes can be eaten raw in salads or lightly cooked. Courgette juice can be mixed with other vegetable juices and drunk daily. The juice (or the mashed flesh) can be applied to the skin as a remedy for inflammation and abscesses – add clay to make a beauty mask.

RECIPES *courgette cake (page 103).*

## SALAD LEAVES

★ **VITAMINS B, C, FOLIC ACID, K, IRON, MAGNESIUM, BIOFLAVONOIDS**

Salad leaves, such as chicory, escarole, frisée and endive, have mild diuretic properties and contain a bitter compound that is good for the liver and gallbladder. They are an important source of nutrients. Chicory root may be dried and roasted and used as a caffeine-free alternative to coffee. Endive is grown without light and has little nutritional value.

RECIPES *escarole salad (page 99).*

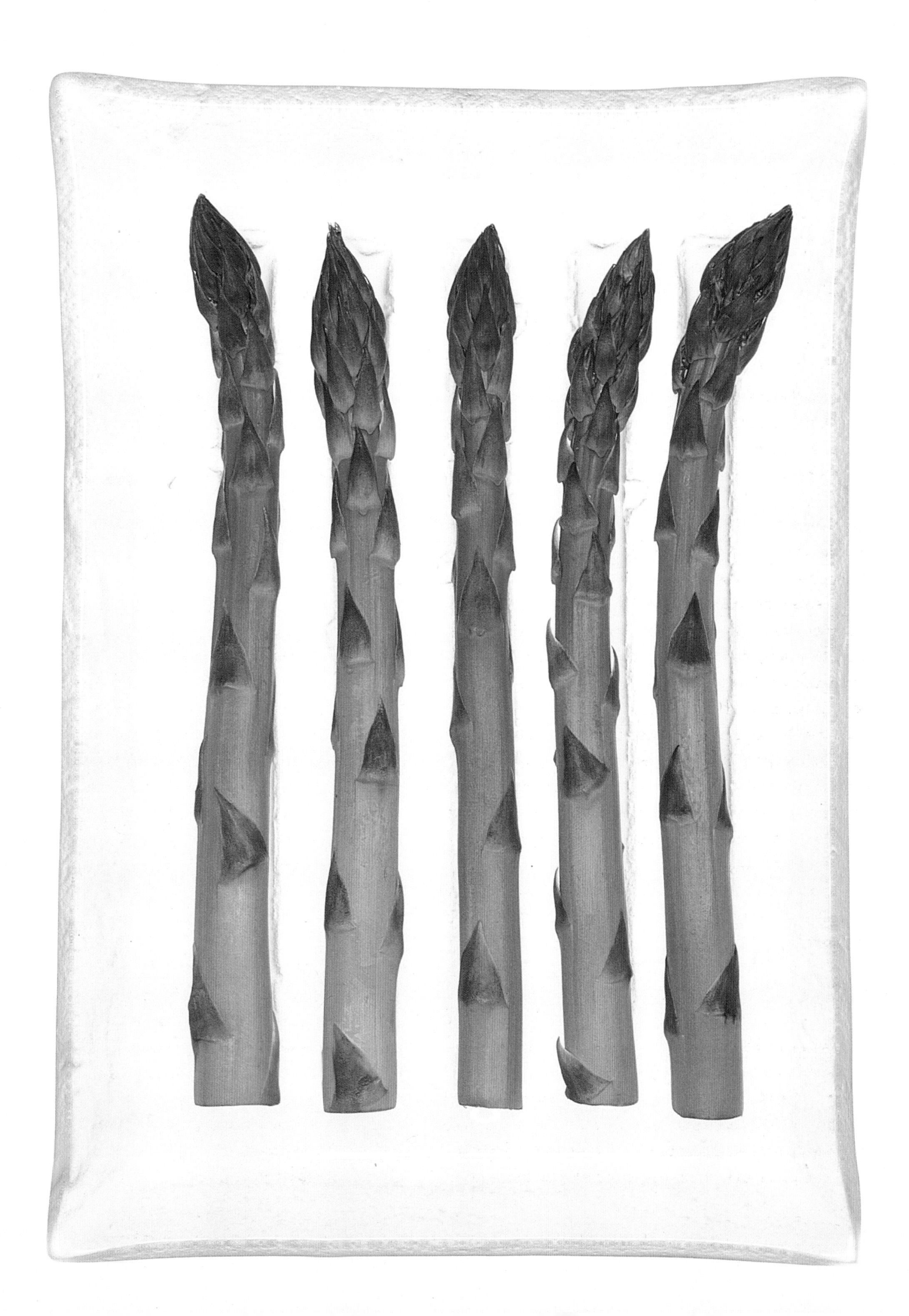

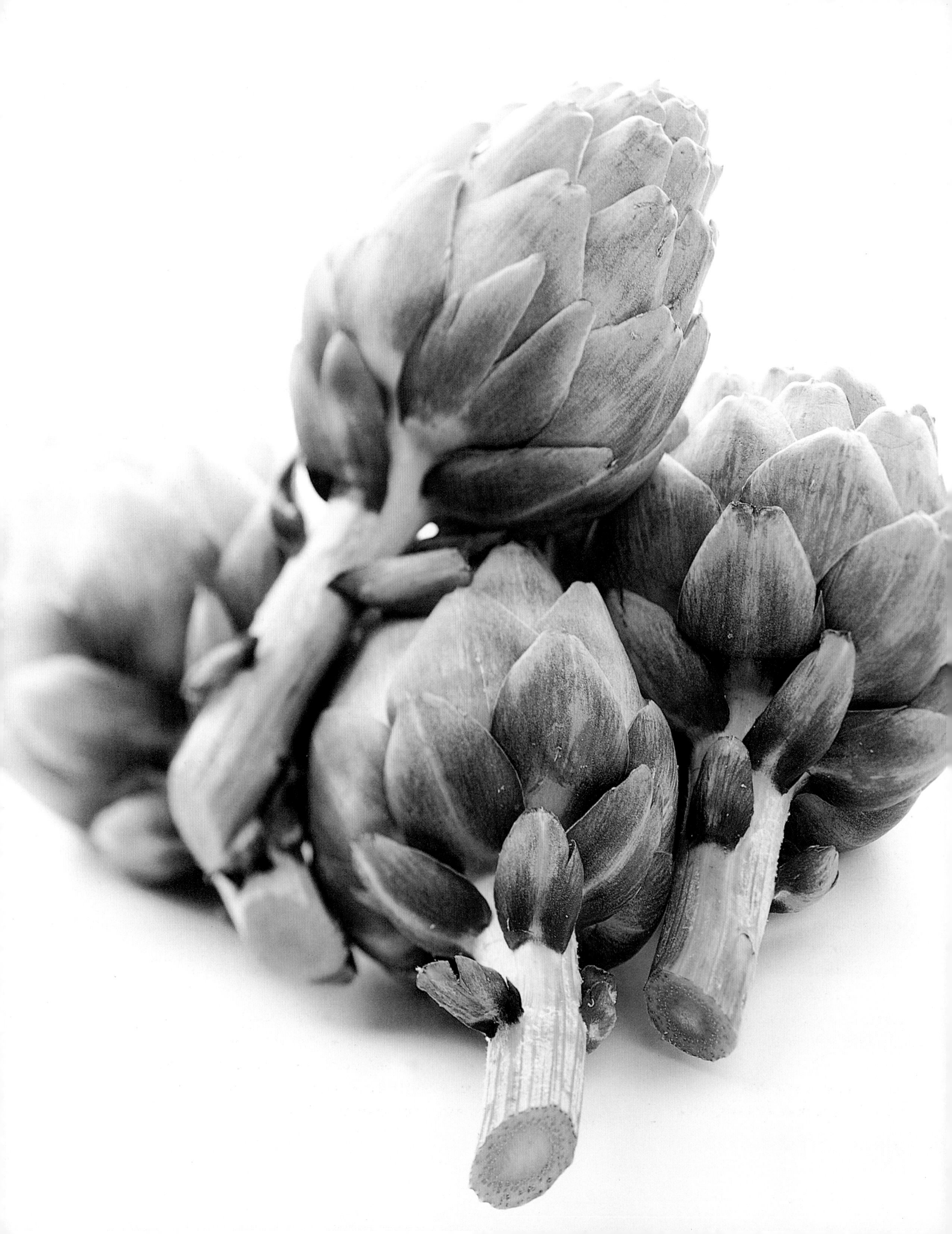

# GOURMET VEGETABLES

## ASPARAGUS

★ VITAMINS A, B, C, FOLIC ACID, COPPER, FLUORIDE, MANGANESE, POTASSIUM, ASPARAGINE

● **BLOOD AND CIRCULATION** Arteriosclerosis, high blood pressure, hyperlipidaemia.

● **DIGESTIVE SYSTEM** Constipation.

Asparagus is diuretic, low in calories, and, owing to its high fibre content, is good for intestinal health. It inhibits bacterial activity in the intestines, promotes lactation and has anti-cancer properties. Asparagine is an active ingredient in asparagus that has an irritant effect – for this reason, asparagus should be avoided by people suffering from ailments that involve inflammation, such as gout, rheumatism and cystitis. Asparagus may be grated and eaten raw in salads, although it is more commonly boiled or steamed until tender.

RECIPES *warm asparagus salad (page 99), asparagus syrup (page 131).*

## ARTICHOKE

★ VITAMINS A, B, C, IRON, MANGANESE, PHOSPHORUS, CYNARIN

Artichoke contains substances that are proven to be beneficial to the kidneys (by promoting diuresis) and to the liver (by promoting detoxification). Artichoke improves the secretion of bile and its emulsification and therefore aids the digestion of fat. It also helps to lower levels of blood cholesterol. Some types of young artichokes can be eaten raw in salad; other varieties should be steamed or boiled (the cooking water contains most of the bitter active ingredient and should be drunk for maximum benefit).
An infusion made with artichoke leaves can alleviate liver and kidney problems. Artichoke buds are detoxifying and can help to alleviate rheumatism, gout and water retention. Nursing mothers should avoid artichoke – it makes breast milk taste bitter and slows down the production of milk.

RECIPES *Roman-style artichoke (page 101), artichoke-leaf wine (page 128), artichoke-leaf tincture (page 130).*

## JERUSALEM ARTICHOKE

★ VITAMINS A, C, TRACE ELEMENTS, INULIN

● **DIGESTIVE SYSTEM** Constipation, dyspepsia, gastritis.

Jerusalem artichoke is a nutritious vegetable that is often overlooked in cooking – it is recommended for people with diabetes. To retain its nutritional value, grate the Jerusalem artichoke in salads, steam or boil lightly; keep the cooking water for use in soups.

## AVOCADO

★ VITAMINS A, B, C, FOLIC ACID, ESSENTIAL AMINO ACIDS

Avocado, a fruit that is widely used as a vegetable, inhibits certain types of bacteria in the intestine and helps to regulate cholesterol (studies suggest that it may lower blood cholesterol levels).
Mashed avocado flesh can be applied to the skin as a treatment for ageing or dryness, or made into a beauty mask by combining with egg white, egg yolk or honey.

RECIPES *avocado dressing (page 95), avocado tartar (page 101).*

## FENNEL

★ VITAMINS A, B COMPLEX, PHOSPHORUS, POTASSIUM, SULPHUR, ESSENTIAL OILS

● **DIGESTIVE SYSTEM** Abdominal cramp and colic, nausea.

● **NERVOUS SYSTEM, MIND AND EMOTIONS** Headache.

● **WOMEN'S HEALTH** Period pain.

Fennel stimulates appetite, facilitates digestion and promotes the secretion of bile. It is best eaten raw in salads (it goes very well with radicchio) but is also excellent cooked. If fennel is eaten in combination with pulses, it facilitates their digestion and prevents the formation of digestive gases. An infusion of fennel seeds has the same medicinal effects as eating the bulb. Fennel can be eaten by breast-feeding mothers to stimulate the baby's appetite and to prevent colic and digestive problems.

RECIPES *fennel and radicchio salad (page 97), fennel with wine (page 110), fennel infusion (page 123), corn-hair and fennel-seed decoction (page 125), fennel-seed decoction (page 126).*

## SEAWEED

★ VITAMIN C, CALCIUM, IRON, MAGNESIUM, PHOSPHORUS, POTASSIUM, SODIUM

● **BLOOD AND CIRCULATION** Atherosclerosis, high blood pressure.

Seaweed has bactericidal and anti-cancer properties, it boosts the immune system, heals ulcers, reduces levels of cholesterol in the blood, lowers blood pressure, thins the blood and helps to prevent stroke and other cardiovascular diseases.

### SALSIFY

★ **CARBOHYDRATE, INULIN**

● **BONES AND JOINTS** Arthritis (rheumatoid), gout.

● **DIGESTIVE SYSTEM** Diabetes.

● **SKIN, HAIR AND NAILS** Eczema.

Salsify belongs to the daisy family and has a long root similar to that of a parsnip. Salsify is often overlooked in cooking. It has detoxifying properties and is good for liver and kidney function. When peeling salsify, plunge it in cold water with the juice of half a lemon (or 2 tablespoons of vinegar) to prevent it turning black. The juice is a natural remedy for verrucae – apply it directly to the skin.

*RECIPES salsify (page 110).*

### PUMPKIN

★ **FOLIC ACID, ANTIOXIDANTS, CAROTENE**

● **DIGESTIVE SYSTEM** Diabetes, dysentery, dyspepsia.

● **KIDNEYS AND BLADDER** Cystitis.

● **NERVOUS SYSTEM, MIND AND EMOTIONS** Insomnia.

Pumpkins are low in calories, high in water, calming and cooling. The juice is a good laxative, and the flesh can be applied to the skin to calm inflammation, burns and abscesses. Pumpkin seeds, peeled and cooked in water or milk, can ease insomnia and cystitis. The roasted seeds are a good source of essential fatty acids, magnesium, phosphorus, zinc and potassium.

*RECIPES baked pumpkin strudel (page 107), pumpkin in syrup (page 112).*

### AUBERGINE

★ **VITAMINS A, B, C, CALCIUM, COPPER, MAGNESIUM, MANGANESE, PHOSPHORUS, POTASSIUM, ZINC, BIOFLAVONOIDS**

● **DIGESTIVE SYSTEM** Constipation.

Aubergine is a low-calorie vegetable that is widely used in Mediterranean, Indian and oriental cuisine. It has laxative properties, it calms the mind and gently stimulates liver and pancreas function. The unripe aubergine is slightly toxic. Aubergine should always be cooked before eating – sprinkling salt on slices of aubergine 1 hour before cooking can reduce the water content and the amount of fat that is absorbed during cooking. Aubergine leaves are cooling and anti-inflammatory, they can be applied to burns, abscesses and eczema.

*RECIPES pepper and aubergine salad (page 95), smoked salmon with aubergine sauce (page 103).*

### MUSHROOM

★ **COPPER, IODINE, MANGANESE, POTASSIUM, SELENIUM, ZINC, PROTEIN**

Mushrooms have stimulant properties and can help to strengthen the immune system. They are a useful source of protein in a meat-free diet. Mushrooms harvested from the wild should be identified as edible and cooked thoroughly before eating (they should not be added raw to salads). Some varieties are highly toxic.

*RECIPES buckwheat pancakes with field mushrooms (page 104).*

## PULSES

### BEAN (RED KIDNEY, HARICOT, FLAGEOLET, BORLOTTI)

★ **CALCIUM, IRON, MAGNESIUM, PHOSPHORUS, POTASSIUM, CARBOHYDRATE, FIBRE, PROTEIN**

● **DIGESTIVE SYSTEM** Diabetes.

Beans are good for people with diabetes or weak liver function, but should be eaten in moderation by gout and rheumatism sufferers. Germinated beans are particularly tasty and nutritious. Beans are easier to digest if they are cooked and eaten with aromatic herbs such as garlic, thyme and bay leaves. Red kidney beans contain a substance that can upset the stomach – boiling them vigorously for 15 minutes renders this substance harmless.

*RECIPES mediterranean bean salad (page 96), spicy spinach, prunes and beans (page 107), beans with carrots and onions (page 110).*

### BROAD BEAN

★ **CALCIUM, IRON, MAGNESIUM, PHOSPHORUS, POTASSIUM, CARBOHYDRATE, PROTEIN**

● **DIGESTIVE SYSTEM** Diarrhoea, dysentery.

Broad beans are good for the kidneys and bladder. An infusion of broad bean flowers (steep a handful of flowers in 150 ml of boiling water for 10 minutes) eases pain from kidney stones and sciatica.

*RECIPES broad bean soup (page 92).*

### LENTIL

★ **FOLIC ACID, CALCIUM, IRON, POTASSIUM, PROTEIN, CARBOHYDRATE**

● **BLOOD AND CIRCULATION** Atherosclerosis, high blood pressure.

● **DIGESTIVE SYSTEM** Diabetes, constipation.

Lentils are nutritious, digestible, regulate colon function and should be eaten frequently as part of a healthy diet. They are recommended for pregnant women and people on a cholesterol-lowering diet.

Lentils and other pulses may help to inhibit cancerous growth.
RECIPES *lentil soup (page 95), lamb with spinach and lentils (page 105).*

### PEA

★ **VITAMIN C, FOLIC ACID, IRON, PHOSPHORUS, CARBOHYDRATE, FIBRE, PROTEIN**

Peas are an energy-providing food that has tonic properties and helps to regulate bowel function.
RECIPES *peas with bacon pieces (page 110).*

### CHICKPEA

★ **CALCIUM, IRON, MAGNESIUM, PHOSPHORUS, POTASSIUM, SILICA, CARBOHYDRATE, PROTEIN**

● **DIGESTIVE SYSTEM** Intestinal parasites.

Chickpeas are a staple food in many Mediterranean and North African countries. They are nutritious, easy to digest and have antiseptic and diuretic properties. They are good for inflammation of the urinary tract and for poor digestion.
RECIPES *chickpea broth (page 92).*

### SOYA

★ **VITAMINS A, B COMPLEX, FOLIC ACID, CALCIUM, MAGNESIUM, CARBOHYDRATE, FIBRE, LECITHIN, PROTEIN**

Soya in the form of miso, tofu, beans and bean sprouts is a staple food in the East. Most soya is now genetically modified. Soya bean sprouts are anti-inflammatory, can reduce stomach acidity and relieve rheumatism.

## CEREALS

### BUCKWHEAT

★ **VITAMIN A, PROTEIN, SELENIUM, CARBOHYDRATE, IMPORTANT AMINO ACIDS AND RUTIN**

Buckwheat contains rutin – a substance that protects the heart – and is free of gluten, a protein that is insoluble in water and can be difficult to eliminate. It is a useful alternative to wheat for people who suffer from celiac disease or are gluten-intolerant. Buckwheat flour can be used instead of wheat flour during illnesses characterized by mucus production (gluten has a glue-like quality and acts in a similar way to mucus).
RECIPES *buckwheat with leek sauce (page 103), buckwheat pancakes with field mushrooms (page 104).*

### CORN

★ **VITAMINS A, B, E, IRON, MAGNESIUM, PHOSPHORUS, POTASSIUM, CARBOHYDRATE, FIBRE, POLYUNSATURATED FAT AND OTHER FATTY ACIDS**

Corn should be eaten from the cob or as coarse-ground polenta. Other forms of corn are depleted of nutrients by milling and processing. Corn is suitable for people with gluten intolerance. It is said to be a gentle moderator of the thyroid gland. Cold-pressed corn oil is rich in polyunsaturated fat (mostly oleic acid) and helps to reduce high cholesterol levels. It is good in salad dressings but is rapidly damaged by heat and loses its therapeutic value when used in cooking and frying. Organic corn oil is difficult to find.

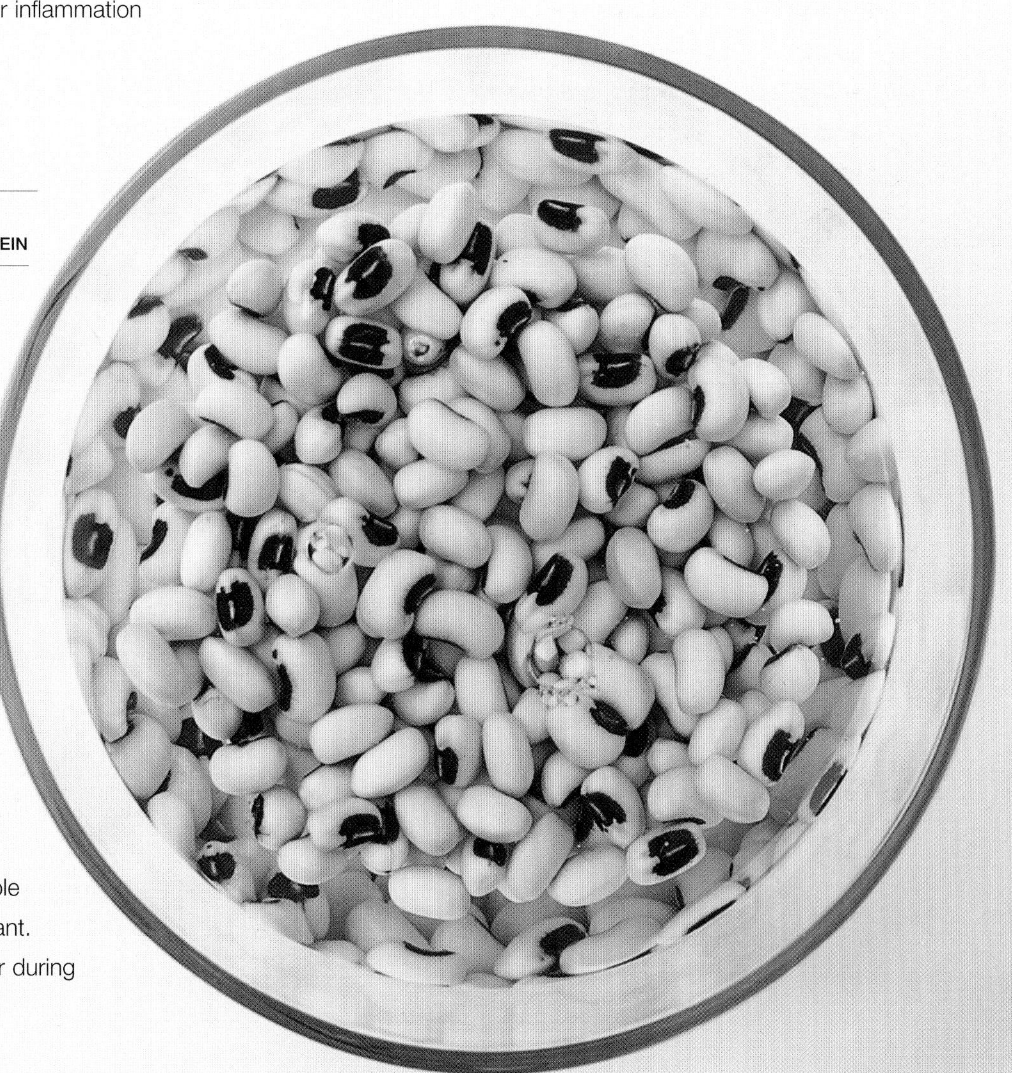

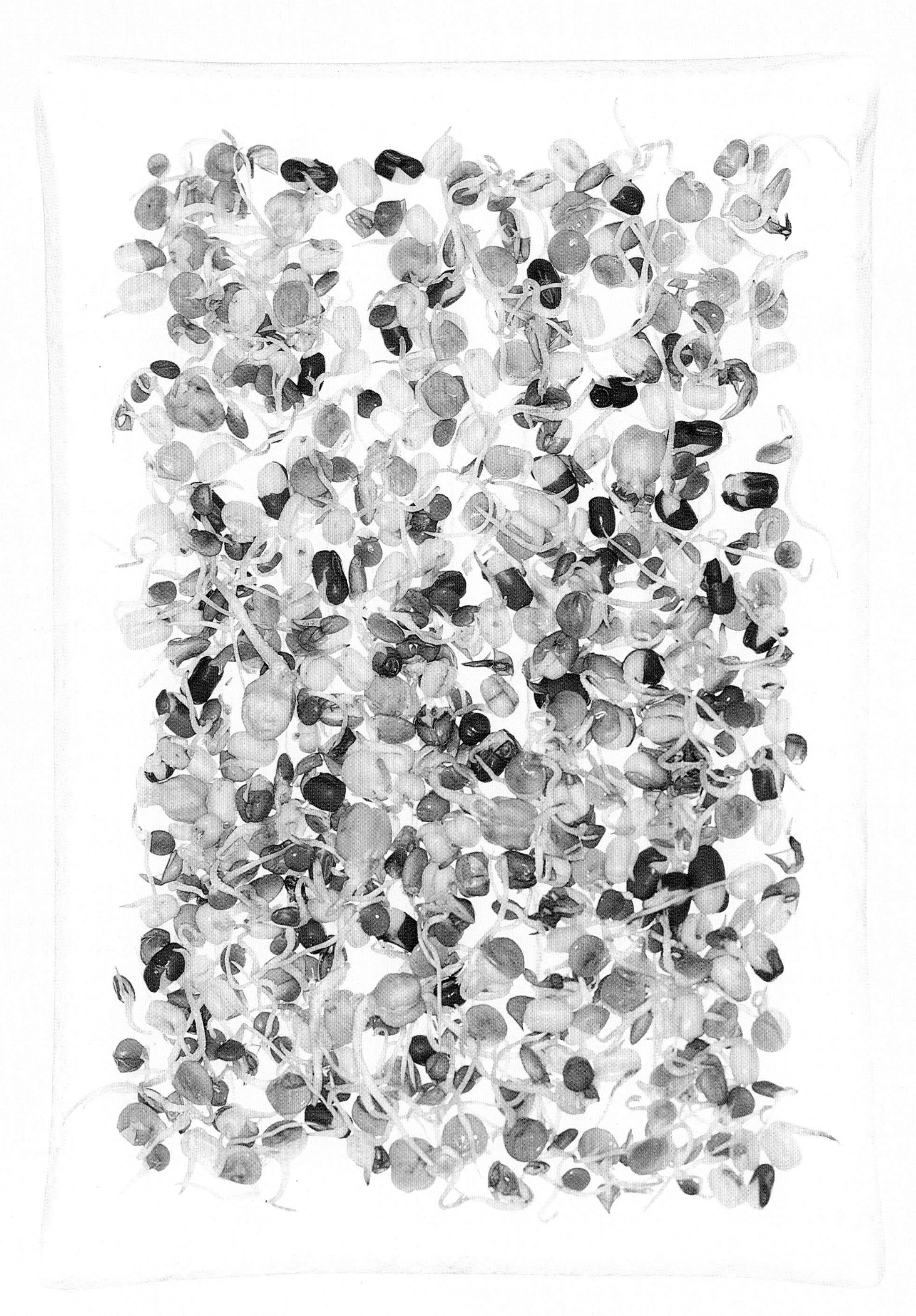

RECIPES *polenta with basil tomato sauce (page 105), corn-hair and fennel-seed decoction (page 125)*

### MILLET

★ **IRON, MAGNESIUM, PHOSPHORUS, SILICA, CARBOHYDRATE, FIBRE, PROTEIN**

Millet is a useful cereal for people who need to follow a gluten-free diet. It also eases fatigue, has a balancing effect upon the nervous system and is recommended during pregnancy and recovery from illness. Millet increases in volume when cooked in water – because it is very filling, is a useful part of a weight-reducing diet.

RECIPES *chicken, millet, barley and celeriac pilaff (page 107).*

### BARLEY

★ **VITAMINS B, E, CALCIUM, COPPER, IODINE, IRON, MAGNESIUM, POTASSIUM, CARBOHYDRATE, FIBRE, L-TRYPTOPHAN**

● **DIGESTIVE SYSTEM** Diarrhoea, dyspepsia.

● **NERVOUS SYSTEM, MIND AND EMOTIONS** Mild insomnia.

● **WOMEN'S HEALTH** Premenstrual syndrome.

Barley is good for the digestive and nervous systems, and contains L-tryptophan, an amino acid that is useful in the treatment of mild insomnia and premenstrual syndrome. It also lowers blood sugar and contains hordenine, a substance with cardio-tonic and anti-diarrhoeic properties. A variety of enzymes that can relieve dyspepsia and hyperacidity can be found in germinated barley. However, because cooking destroys these enzymes, the best way to benefit from the medicinal properties of this cereal is to drink barley water made from germinated barley (page 127). The whole barley grain – germinated if possible – should be eaten for maximum nutritional and health benefits (the polished grain is of little therapeutic value).

RECIPES *barley and fruit porridge (page 75), chickpea broth (page 92), chicken, millet, barley and celeriac pilaff (page 107), barley infusion (page 124), barley water (page 127).*

### OAT

★ **FOLIC ACID, CALCIUM, IRON, MAGNESIUM, PHOSPHORUS, POTASSIUM, SODIUM, CARBOHYDRATE, FATTY ACIDS, FIBRE, PROTEIN**

● **DIGESTIVE SYSTEM** Diabetes.

● **NERVOUS SYSTEM, MIND AND EMOTIONS** Depression, insomnia, mental fatigue.

Oats are nutritious and help to lower levels of cholesterol in the body. They have diuretic properties, stimulate thyroid function and are helpful for people who have diabetes. A tincture of oats (*Avena sativa*) is often prescribed by herbalists and homeopaths for insomnia, mild depression and mental fatigue.

RECIPES *barley and fruit porridge (page 75).*

### RICE

★ **VITAMINS A, B COMPLEX, MINERALS AND TRACE ELEMENTS, CARBOHYDRATE, FIBRE, PROTEIN**

● **DIGESTIVE SYSTEM** Diarrhoea, diabetes, diverticulitis.

Rice is an energy-providing food that helps lower blood pressure and has astringent properties. The water in which rice is cooked (rice water) is a remedy for mild diarrhoea: in Vietnam, a cup of rice is soaked in a mixture of water and honey, strained and stir-fried in a wok without oil; then, when the rice has coloured, 2 litres of water are added and the rice is simmered until overcooked. The resulting water is drunk as a diarrhoea remedy. The same recipe can be used as an energy-providing drink for convalescents. Rice is suitable for people on a gluten-free diet. Because polished white rice has lost most of its important ingredients it is preferable to eat organically-produced brown rice. Macrobiotic diets based on brown rice are not recommended for children or menopausal women as they may lead to calcium and iron deficiency.

RECIPES *nettle risotto (page 103), stuffed peppers (page 104), rice with cucumber balls (page 109).*

### WHEAT

★ **VITAMINS A, B, E, CARBOHYDRATE, FIBRE, PROTEIN**

Wheat is the staple food of the West. Unfortunately, extensive processing and genetic modification have meant that wheat is largely stripped of its nutritious and healing potential. Wheat that is allowed to germinate has increased vitamin and protein content. Wheat bran contains enzymes that facilitate digestion and ease dyspepsia and hyperacidity.

RECIPES *taboule (page 100).*

### RYE

★ **CALCIUM, IRON, POTASSIUM, SULPHUR, CARBOHYDRATE, FIBRE**

● **BLOOD AND CIRCULATION** Arteriosclerosis, high blood pressure.

Rye contains a substance that reduces blood viscosity and helps to maintain healthy heart function. The rate of cardiovascular problems is low in populations where rye is eaten as a staple food.

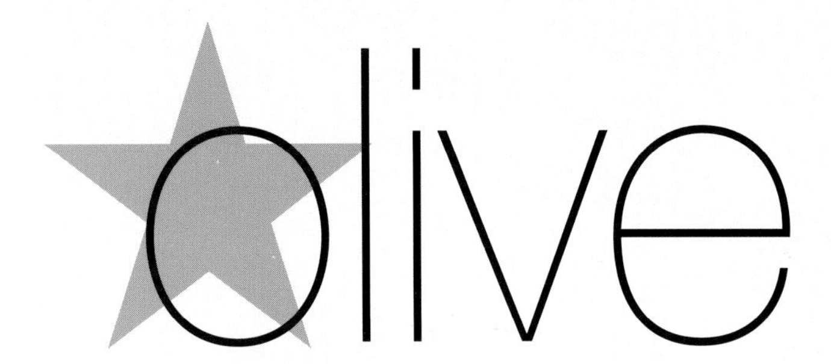


**OLIVES FORM A MAJOR PART OF THE MEDITERRANEAN DIET AND, IN CONJUNCTION WITH A LOW INTAKE OF ANIMAL FAT, ARE THOUGHT TO BE IMPORTANT IN REGULATING BLOOD CHOLESTEROL LEVELS AND REDUCING THE RISK OF CARDIOVASCULAR DISEASE.**

## The properties of olives

There are numerous references to olive trees in the Bible and it is thought that olives were cultivated in Syria around 6000 years ago. Today, major olive producers include Italy, Greece, France, Spain, Portugal, Turkey, Israel, Australia, Africa and many Middle Eastern countries.

Olives contain vitamins A and E, phosphorus, potassium, magnesium, manganese, antioxidants, oleic and linoleic acid. Black olives are easier to digest and have a higher vitamin and antioxidant content than green olives. Only the black olive is edible in its natural state; green olives are washed repeatedly in brine to remove their bitter taste.

Research has demonstrated that people who follow a Mediterranean diet – which is rich in olives and olive oil, and low in animal fat – have a low incidence of cardiovascular disease compared to people who eat a high proportion of animal fat. Studies show that the high oleic acid content in olive oil helps to regulate the balance between high-density lipoprotein (the "good" type of cholesterol) and low-density lipoprotein (the "bad" type of cholesterol) in the blood. This prevents fatty deposits being laid down in the arteries and reduces the risk of atherosclerosis and other types of cardiovascular disease.

Olives are also good for diabetes, constipation and gallstones. A remedy for constipation and gallstones is 2 tablespoons of cold-pressed olive oil taken every morning on an empty stomach (an equal amount of lemon juice can be added). The leaves of the olive tree can be used as a remedy for high blood pressure, atherosclerosis, bladder stones, diabetes and angina: bring 50 g dried leaves (or 80 g fresh leaves) and 1 litre of water to the boil. Cover and allow to infuse for 10 minutes and then strain. Drink 150 ml of this decoction three or four times a day. Olive oil has been used as a skin treatment for centuries; it is thought to be invaluable in relieving psoriasis, dry skin and eczema.

## Choosing olive oil

Olive oil is traditionally obtained by crushing olives in a stone mill. However, modern extraction techniques have superseded traditional ones and centrifugal or chemical methods are now the most widely used.

The best olive oil to buy is first cold-pressed extra virgin oil. Although the taste and colour may vary from one country to another, or from year to year, this oil is the most nutritious. Try to avoid buying semi-fine or refined olive oil. Check that olive oil falls into one of the following categories:

- Extra virgin olive oil: this is obtained from the first cold pressing of the olives; it is low in acidity (below 1 per cent) and is perfect for medicinal purposes and use in salads.
- Fine virgin olive oil: this is obtained from the second pressing of the olives. Although it has a higher acidity, the taste and medicinal qualities are good.

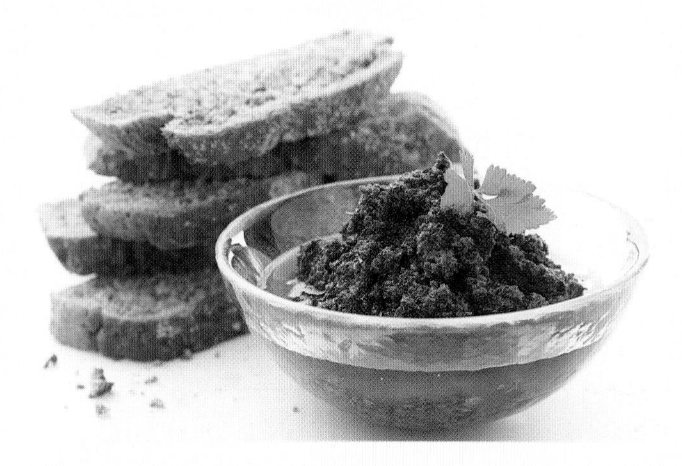

## STAR FOOD PROFILE

- **BLOOD AND CIRCULATION** Angina, atherosclerosis, high blood pressure.
- **DIGESTIVE SYSTEM** Constipation, diabetes, gallstones.
- **KIDNEYS AND BLADDER** Bladder stones.
- **SKIN, HAIR AND NAILS** Dermatitis and eczema.

# black olive tapenade

200 g black olives, stoned
2 or 3 cloves garlic, peeled
150 g capers
100 g anchovy fillet, soaked in milk for 10 minutes
1 tsp Dijon mustard
2 tbsp olive oil

Blend the ingredients to a thick paste in a food processor. Serve on toast or with salads or pasta.

# aromatic olive oil

Use in vinaigrette and marinades or to brush food prior to cooking.

6 sprigs of thyme
1 or 2 sprigs of rosemary
1 sprig of sweet marjoram
1 tsp black peppercorns
3 cloves garlic, peeled and left whole
2 shallots, left whole
6 bay leaves
1 litre olive oil

Seal all ingredients in a pickling jar. Leave for 1 month (page 120).

# green olives and lemon

400 g green olives in brine
Lemons preserved in salt (page 45)
Several small sprigs of thyme
Cold-pressed olive oil (see recipe for amount)
50 ml dry white wine

Drain the olives, setting aside half the brine. In a pickling jar, arrange the olives and lemons in alternate layers. Add the sprigs of thyme. Mix the brine with an equal amount of olive oil and the wine. Pour this over the olives and lemons so that they are covered. Tightly seal the jar and leave for 2 or 3 weeks before using as a starter or with salad.

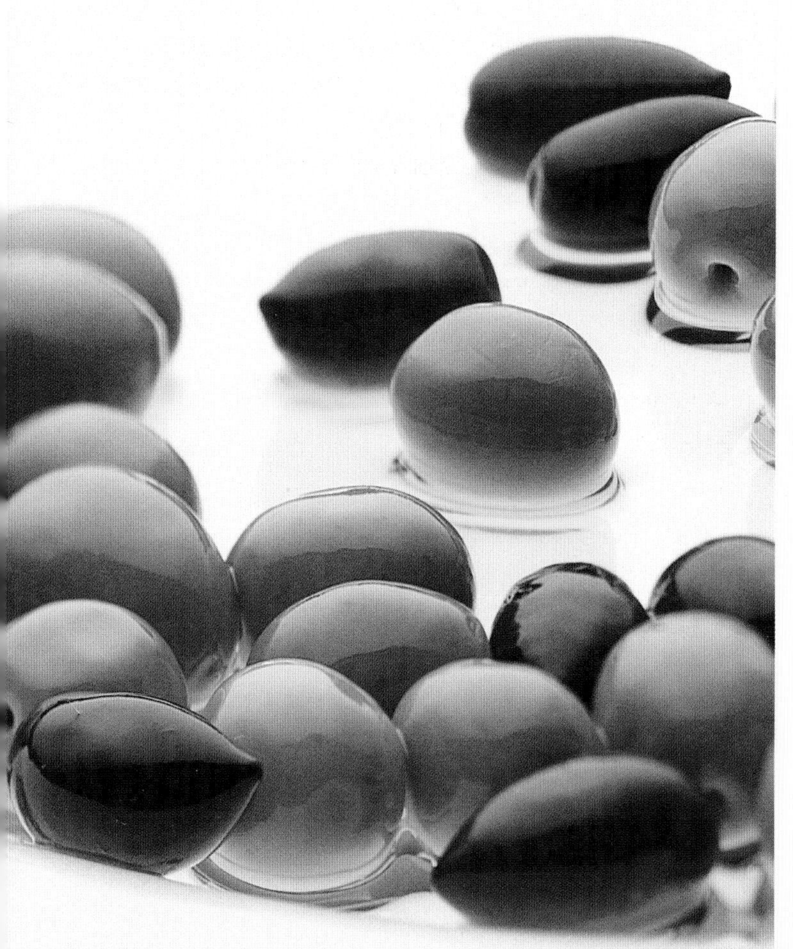

# fruits and nuts

## EXOTIC FRUIT

### COCONUT

★ NATURAL SUGAR, PALMITIC AND OLEIC ACIDS, PROTEIN

Coconut is an excellent protein-based, between-meal snack. It has slight diuretic and laxative properties. The milk can be used to treat stomach ulcers and gastritis.

### DATE

★ VITAMINS A, B, D, CALCIUM, MAGNESIUM, POTASSIUM, NATURAL SUGAR

● BLOOD AND CIRCULATION Anaemia.

● RESPIRATORY SYSTEM Bronchitis.

● NERVOUS SYSTEM, MIND AND EMOTIONS Mental fatigue.

Dates may help to prevent cancer. They are a traditional remedy for tuberculosis. In North Africa, respiratory problems are treated with powdered or boiled date stones.

RECIPE *banana and date salad (page 112).*

### FIG

★ VITAMINS A, B, C, FOLIC ACID, CALCIUM, COPPER, IRON, MANGANESE, POTASSIUM, ZINC, NATURAL SUGAR

● DIGESTIVE SYSTEM Constipation, dyspepsia, gastritis, gingivitis.

● RESPIRATORY SYSTEM Bronchitis.

● IMMUNE SYSTEM Sore throat.

Figs are laxative and slightly diuretic. For constipation, cook 4–5 fresh figs in milk with 2 dates and a few raisins – eat for breakfast. For respiratory problems, boil 120 g fresh figs in 1 litre water for 15 minutes, strain and drink. This mixture can also be used as a gargle for sore throats or gingivitis. Figs are good for pregnant women, people recovering from illness and elderly people.

RECIPES *fresh figs with raspberry cheese (page 115)*

### BANANA

★ VITAMINS A, B, FOLIC ACID, E, IODINE, IRON, MAGNESIUM, POTASSIUM, ZINC, CARBOHYDRATE, TRYPTOPHAN

Bananas have antacid and mild antibacterial properties. Consult your doctor about eating bananas if you suffer from diabetes.

RECIPE *banana and date salad (page 112).*

### GUAVA

★ VITAMIN C, POTASSIUM, SULPHUR, CAROTENE, NATURAL SUGAR

● DIGESTIVE SYSTEM Dyspepsia.

Guava has astringent properties and is good for digestion. However, the unripe fruit is difficult to digest and the seeds should not be eaten by people with intestinal problems.

### KUMQUAT

★ VITAMIN C, CITRUS FLAVONOIDS, NATURAL SUGAR

Kumquats have the same properties as oranges (page 39).

RECIPES *radish and kumquat salad (page 96).*

### LYCHEE

★ VITAMINS B, C, MAGNESIUM, PHOSPHORUS, POTASSIUM, BIOFLAVONOIDS, NATURAL SUGAR

Lychees stimulate digestion and are slightly astringent. For abdominal pain, drink a decoction of lychee seeds.

RECIPES *lychee fruit salad (page 112), lychee-seed decoction (page 126).*

### MANGO

★ VITAMINS A, B, C, PHOSPHORUS, SULPHUR, CAROTENES, NATURAL SUGAR

● DIGESTIVE SYSTEM Colitis, diarrhoea, ulcerative colitis.

Mango has an astringent effect on the gut which means that it promotes contractions and enhances digestive processes.

### PINEAPPLE

★ VITAMINS A, B, C, CITRIC, FOLIC AND MALIC ACIDS, MAGNESIUM, POTASSIUM, BROMELAIN, NATURAL SUGAR

● BONES AND JOINTS Arthritis (rheumatism), gout.

● BLOOD AND CIRCULATION Arteriosclerosis.

● DIGESTIVE SYSTEM Dyspepsia.

Pineapple contains bromelain enzymes that reduce inflammation,

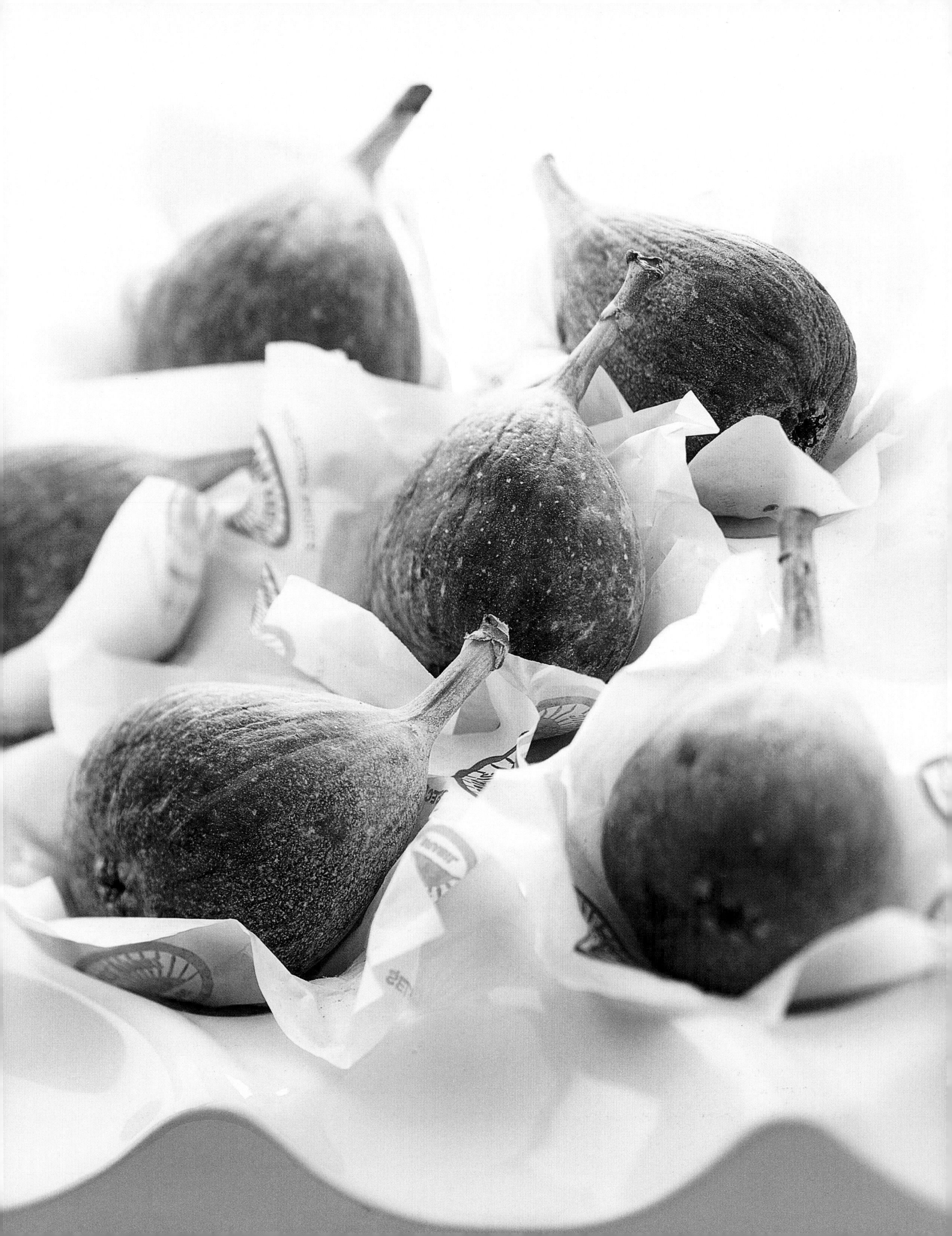

aid digestion and help to break down proteins. Bromelain is used to make various medicines, including anti-inflammatory drugs; it is most concentrated in the core of the pineapple.

RECIPES *pineapple and cucumber salad (page 99).*

### PAPAYA

★ **VITAMINS A, B, C, POTASSIUM, NATURAL SUGAR, PAPAIN**

Papaya contains papain, an enzyme that aids the digestive process by facilitating the breakdown of protein. Papaya is useful for reducing fever.

RECIPES *baked papaya with ginger (page 115).*

# SOFT FRUIT AND BERRIES

### APRICOT

★ **VITAMINS A, B, C, IRON, MAGNESIUM, MANGANESE, PHOSPHORUS, POTASSIUM, NATURAL SUGAR**

● **BLOOD AND CIRCULATION** Anaemia.

● **NERVOUS SYSTEM, MIND AND EMOTIONS** Mental fatigue, mild anxiety, insomnia.

Apricots have a balancing effect on the nervous system. Both fresh and dried apricots are beneficial for pregnant women, people recovering from illness and elderly people.

RECIPES *poached apricots with cardamom (page 115), apricot, lime and mint juice (page 117).*

### GRAPE AND RAISIN

★ **VITAMINS A, B, C, CALCIUM, IODINE, MANGANESE, POTASSIUM, SODIUM, BIOFLAVONOIDS, NATURAL SUGAR**

● **BONES AND JOINTS** Arthritis (rheumatoid), gout.

● **SKIN, HAIR AND NAILS** Dermatitis and eczema.

Grapes are diuretic, detoxifying and laxative. They promote the elimination of uric acid and enhance liver function and bile flow. Black grapes are rich in bioflavonoids, particularly quercetin, which is good for the heart and circulation. Raisins are recommended as a snack for children, pregnant women, convalescents and elderly people. A cold-pressing of grape pips (grape seed oil) is rich in polyunsaturated fatty acids and good for cardiovascular health.

RECIPES *autumn fruit compote (page 114).*

### GOOSEBERRY

★ **VITAMINS A, B, C, IRON, PHOSPHORUS, POTASSIUM, MALIC AND CITRIC ACIDS, NATURAL SUGAR**

● **BONES AND JOINTS** Arthritis (rheumatoid), gout.

Gooseberries are laxative and diuretic. They stimulate liver function and ease inflammation of the digestive and urinary tracts.

### PEACH

★ **VITAMINS A, B, C, COPPER, MAGNESIUM, PHOSPHORUS, POTASSIUM, ZINC, NATURAL SUGAR**

● **DIGESTIVE SYSTEM** Dyspepsia.

● **KIDNEYS AND BLADDER** Bladder stones.

Peaches are diuretic and laxative. Peach blossom is traditionally used to make an infusion or syrup that has calming and laxative properties (suitable for children). An infusion of peach leaves has an even stronger purgative effect. Fresh peach juice may be applied to the skin as a beauty treatment.

RECIPES *peach syrup (page 130).*

### PLUM AND PRUNE

★ **CALCIUM, IRON, MAGNESIUM, PHOSPHORUS, POTASSIUM, FIBRE, NATURAL SUGAR**

● **BONES AND JOINTS** Gout, rheumatism.

● **BLOOD AND CIRCULATION** Atherosclerosis.

● **DIGESTIVE SYSTEM** Constipation.

Both plums and prunes are a good source of fibre – prunes are well known for their laxative effects. Prunes also aid liver function, help to lower levels of cholesterol in the blood and have anti-cancer properties.

RECIPES *spicy spinach, prunes and beans (page 107).*

### MELON (ALL TYPES)

★ **VITAMINS A, B, C, NATURAL SUGAR, WATER**

● **BONES AND JOINTS** Gout, rheumatism.

● **DIGESTIVE SYSTEM** Constipation, dyspepsia, irritable bowel syndrome.

Melon is cooling, laxative and diuretic. Applied topically, crushed melon flesh eases the pain of mild burns, including sunburn. A beauty lotion for dry skin can be made with equal amounts of distilled water, milk and melon juice.

RECIPES *minted melon (page 112), watermelon and summer fruits (page 112).*

### BLACKCURRANT

★ **VITAMIN C, CALCIUM, MAGNESIUM, PHOSPHORUS, POTASSIUM, NATURAL SUGAR**

- **BONES AND JOINTS** Gout, rheumatism.
- **IMMUNE SYSTEM** Sore throat.

Blackcurrants promote vitality and speed recovery after illness. They may aid bone remineralization after fractures. The leaves have the same properties as the berries and are also diuretic.

*RECIPES blackcurrant wine (page 127).*

### REDCURRANT

★ **VITAMINS A, B, C, CALCIUM, IRON, PHOSPHORUS, POTASSIUM, CITRIC ACID, PECTIN, NATURAL SUGAR**

- **BONES AND JOINTS** Arthritis (rheumatoid), gout.
- **DIGESTIVE SYSTEM** Constipation.
- **KIDNEYS AND BLADDER** Cystitis.

Redcurrants are laxative, diuretic and depurative. They ease inflammation of the digestive tract, mild fever and liver problems. Redcurrants are very acidic and should not be eaten in excess.

*RECIPES red- and whitecurrants with raspberry coulis (page 113), redcurrant, blackberry and blueberry juice (page 118).*

### BLACKBERRY

★ **VITAMINS A , B, C, E, CALCIUM, PHOSPHORUS, POTASSIUM, NATURAL SUGAR, PECTIN, TANNIN, ESSENTIAL OIL**

- **DIGESTIVE SYSTEM** Diarrhoea.
- **IMMUNE SYSTEM** Sore throat.

Blackberries are astringent, laxative, tonic and depurative. The syrup is a good remedy for diarrhoea in babies, respiratory infections and sore throats. An infusion of the leaves is a traditional gargle for acute sore throat.

*RECIPES watermelon and summer fruits (page 112), fruit salad with lemon balm (page 113), redcurrant, blackberry and blueberry juice (page 118), blackberry syrup (page 131).*

### CHERRY

★ **VITAMINS A, B, C, CALCIUM, MAGNESIUM, PHOSPHORUS, POTASSIUM, ELLAGIC ACID, NATURAL SUGAR**

- **BONES AND JOINTS** Arthritis (rheumatoid), gout, rheumatism.
- **BLOOD AND CIRCULATION** Atherosclerosis, arteriosclerosis.
- **KIDNEYS AND BLADDER** Bladder stone, cystitis.

Cherries are diuretic, laxative, depurative; they stimulate the immune system and help to prevent infection. Cherry-stem decoction can be used to treat cystitis, rheumatism and oedema.

*RECIPES cherry-stem decoction (page 125), cherry-stem and apple decoction (page 126), cherry-leaf wine (page 128).*

### STRAWBERRY

★ **VITAMINS A, B AND C, IRON, MAGNESIUM, PHOSPHORUS, SILICA, SULPHUR, NATURAL SUGAR, SALICYLIC ACID**

- **BONES AND JOINTS** Gout.
- **BLOOD AND CIRCULATION** High blood pressure.
- **DIGESTIVE SYSTEM** Colitis, constipation, diarrhoea.
- **KIDNEYS AND BLADDER** Cystitis.

Strawberries are tonic, laxative and antibacterial. They enhance liver and gallbladder function. Strawberries may cause an allergic response (in the form of a rash) or exacerbate allergic dermatitis. The leaves and roots can be made into a medicinal decoction.

*RECIPES carrot and strawberry salad (page 95), fruit salad with lemon balm (page 113), strawberry and raspberry juice (page 118), strawberry-leaf decoction (page 126).*

### RASPBERRY

★ **VITAMINS A, B, C, IRON, MAGNESIUM, POTASSIUM, CITRIC, MALIC AND SALICYLIC ACIDS, NATURAL SUGAR**

- **BONES AND JOINTS** Gout.
- **DIGESTIVE SYSTEM** Indigestion, vomiting.
- **SKIN, HAIR AND NAILS** Eczema.

Raspberries are slightly diuretic and laxative. They are good for frequent urination. Raspberry leaf infusion can facilitate labour.

*RECIPES red- and whitecurrants with raspberry coulis (page 113), apple and raspberry juice (page 117), cherry and raspberry juice (page 118), strawberry and raspberry juice (page 118), raspberry vinegar (page 120).*

## CITRUS FRUIT

### ORANGE

★ **VITAMINS B, C, CALCIUM, COPPER, MANGANESE, PHOSPHORUS, POTASSIUM, ZINC, BIOFLAVONOIDS, NATURAL SUGAR, PECTIN**

- **DIGESTIVE SYSTEM** Dyspepsia.

Oranges have tonic, diuretic and laxative properties. They stimulate the immune system, liver function and appetite.

*continues on page 43*

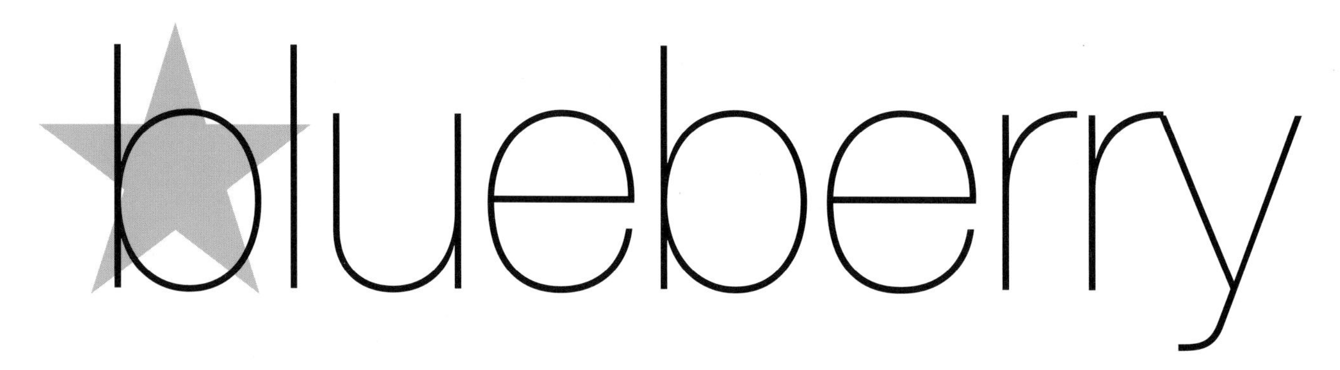

# blueberry

**BLUEBERRIES HAVE ANTI-CANCER AND ANTIBACTERIAL PROPERTIES. THEY ARE GOOD FOR THE HEALTH OF THE EYES, INTESTINES, CIRCULATORY SYSTEM AND URINARY TRACT.**

## The properties of blueberry

Blueberries are part of the *Vaccinium* species, which also includes cranberries and bilberries. They are small, purple berries that are commonly found in western and central Europe and North America. Thought to have been used in European folk medicine since the 16th century, blueberries have excellent antioxidant properties which make them useful for preventing cancer and other degenerative diseases. In fact, when compared to other fruits, blueberries are among the top sources of antioxidants.

Blueberries have a powerful antibacterial action in the intestine – especially upon coli bacteria – they promote the healing of gastric ulcers, and the leaves of the blueberry plant contain tannin, which has strong anti-diarrhoeal properties.

Blood circulation is enhanced by substances found in blueberries, such as vitamin C, bioflavonoids, anthocyanosides, glycosides and delphininol. Blueberries may help to lower blood sugar, decrease the chances of blood clots forming and enhance the health of blood capillaries.

Blueberries can improve eyesight. This is thought to be due to compounds in the berries that enhance the health of capillaries in the eye.

Cranberries (*Vaccinium macrocarpon*) are a close relative of blueberries and are native to North America. They are a well-known and popular treatment for urinary-tract infections, such as cystitis (an inflammation of the bladder resulting in frequent, urgent and often painful urination). Drinking the fresh juice of either blueberries or cranberries can help to prevent urinary-tract infections.

## Blueberries in the diet

Since blueberries are excellent antioxidants, they are important in the diet to promote long-term health and to prevent age-related physical changes and chronic diseases. In particular, people with cardiovascular problems, mild diabetes, eye problems, urinary tract or intestinal infections should eat blueberries regularly. Blueberries make wonderful pies, syrups and jam and are much enjoyed by children. They can be made into liqueurs or preserves for adults or the berries can be added to fruit salad or simply eaten as a snack on their own.

## Medicinal preparations

In addition to eating blueberries, the berries and leaves can be made into medicinal preparations. Blueberry decoction is useful for diarrhoea, colitis and poor night vision. It can be used as a mouthwash for sore throats and ulcers, and as a face wash for eczema. To make, boil 75 g blueberries in 1 litre of water until the volume of water has halved. Strain and use as appropriate.

Blueberry and strawberry leaf decoction is good for mild diabetes, intestinal problems, arteriosclerosis, rheumatism and arthritis and can be drunk throughout the day. Boil 20 g each of blueberry and strawberry leaves in 1 litre of water for 3 minutes. Leave to infuse for 10 minutes, strain and drink. To make a tincture of blueberries, add 100 g fresh blueberries, a handful of blueberry leaves and the zest of one lemon to 700 ml vodka. Leave in a cool, dark place for 3 weeks and then press and strain the mixture and store in a tightly sealed bottle. Take 20–30 drops of this tincture in a glass of water every day for diarrhoea, intestinal problems, circulatory problems and mild diabetes. It can also be used as a gargle for sore throats.

**STAR FOOD PROFILE**

- **BONES AND JOINTS** Arthritis (rheumatoid), rheumatism.
- **BLOOD AND CIRCULATION** Atherosclerosis, arteriosclerosis, Raynaud's disease.
- **DIGESTIVE SYSTEM** Abdominal cramp and colic, colitis, diarrhoea, gastroenteritis, intestinal infections, ulcerative colitis.
- **KIDNEYS AND BLADDER** Cystitis and urethritis.
- **IMMUNE SYSTEM** Sore throat.

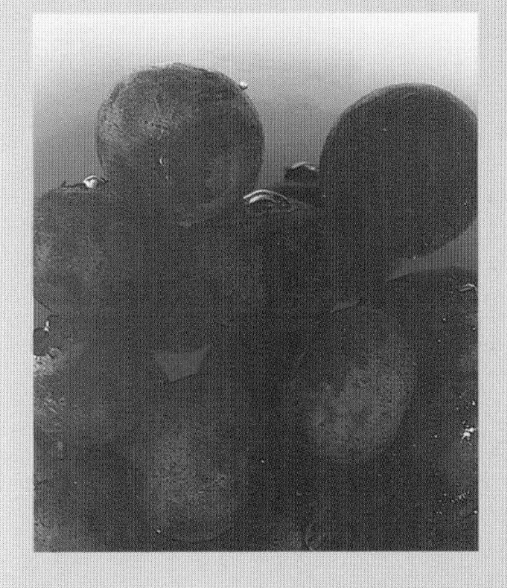

# blueberry vinegar

Use in dressings or take a teaspoon, diluted in water, every morning.

300 g blueberries
700 ml white wine vinegar or cider vinegar

Put the blueberries in a hermetically-sealable pickling jar. Pour over the white-wine or cider vinegar and seal the jar tightly. Leave to macerate in a cool, dark place for 2 weeks. Strain and bottle the vinegar.

# blueberries and cottage cheese

200 g cottage cheese
3 tbsp caster sugar
3 tbsp live yoghurt
200 g fresh blueberries
1 apple, peeled and grated
Lemon juice to taste
To garnish: a few raspberries

Beat the cottage cheese with the sugar and yoghurt. Stir in the blueberries, apple and lemon juice. Garnish with raspberries. Chill and serve.

# blueberry syrup

This can be added to water for children or to white wine for adults.

1 kg blueberries
300 ml water
Sugar

In a stainless steel saucepan bring the blueberries and water to the boil. Strain them through muslin. Allow the juice to ferment at room temperature for 24 hours. Weigh the juice and add an equal amount of sugar. Dissolve the sugar in the juice, bring to the boil, simmer for 1 minute and allow to cool. Store the syrup in sterilized bottles in the refrigerator.

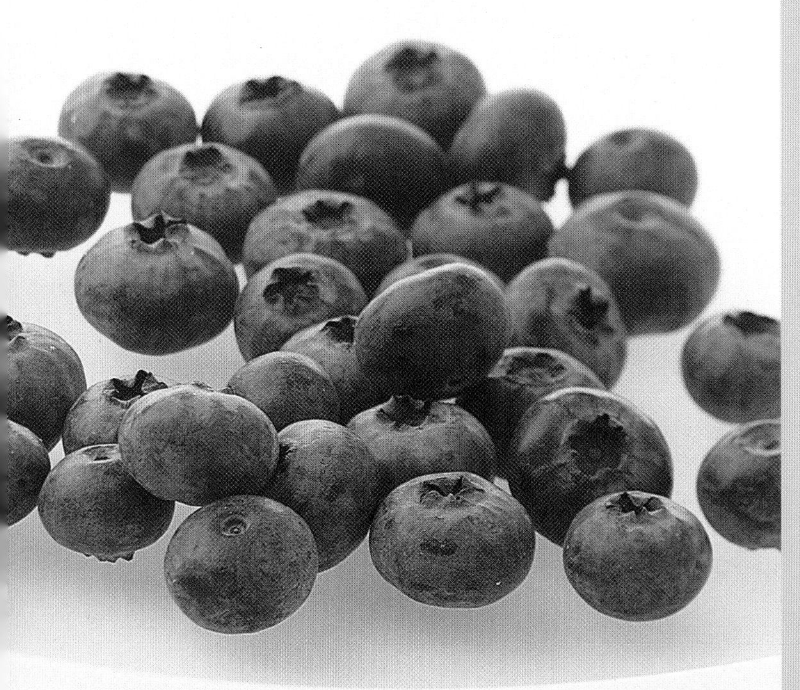

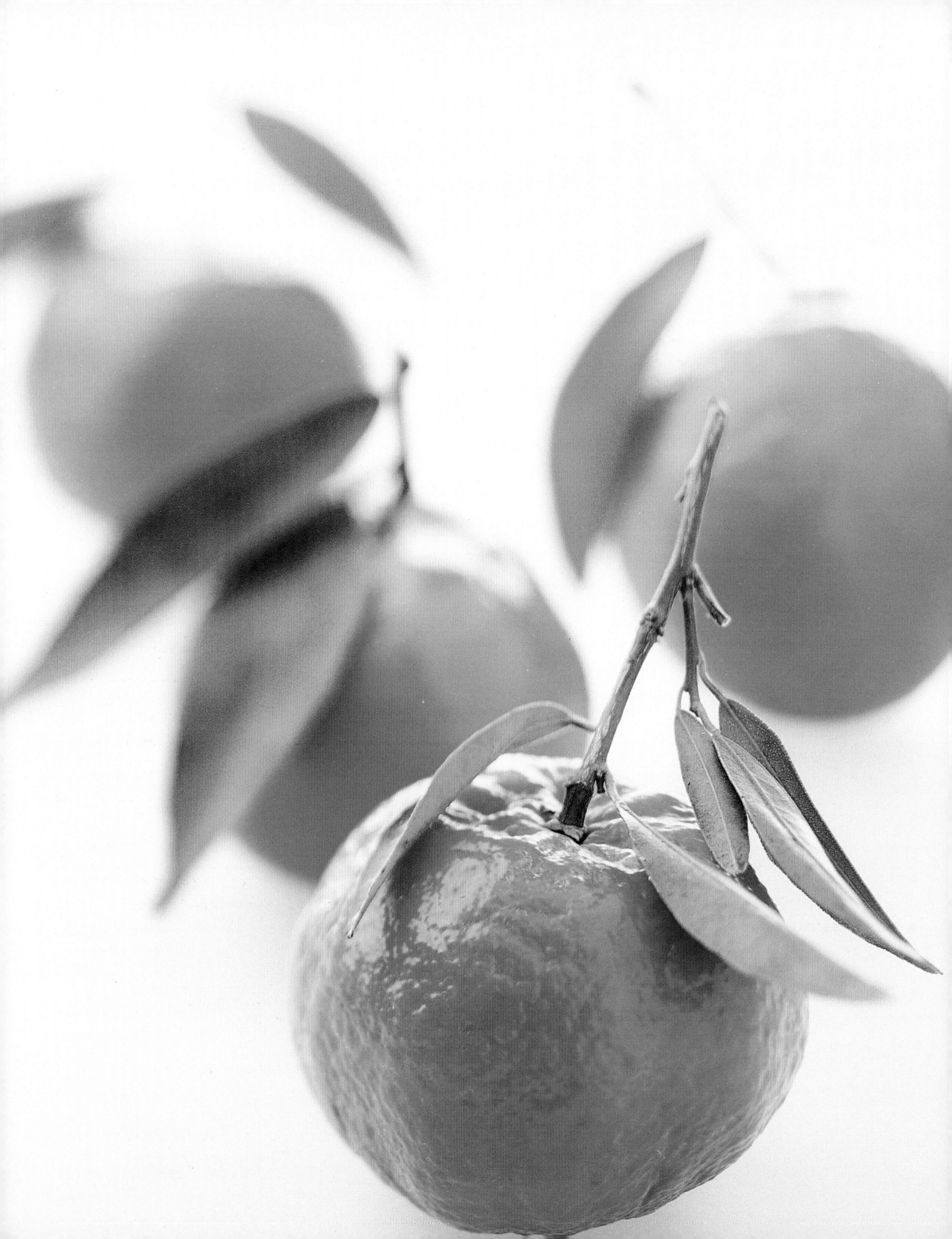

Oranges also help to lower levels of cholesterol in the blood and they are rich in antioxidants. Eating whole oranges is preferable to drinking concentrated juice.

RECIPES *radish and kumquat salad (page 96), orange-zest infusion (page 123).*

### MANDARIN AND TANGERINE

★ VITAMINS B, C, CALCIUM, COPPER, MANGANESE, PHOSPHORUS, POTASSIUM, ZINC, BIOFLAVONOIDS, NATURAL SUGAR, PECTIN

Mandarin and tangerine have similar properties to orange. Mandarin rind contains an essential oil that acts as a sedative and, in Chinese medicine, an infusion of dried tangerine peel is used for poor digestion, abdominal distension and irritability.

### GRAPEFRUIT

★ VITAMINS B, C, COPPER, MAGNESIUM, POTASSIUM, ANTIOXIDANTS, BIOFLAVONOIDS, ESSENTIAL OIL, NATURAL SUGAR, PECTIN

● BONES AND JOINTS Arthritis (rheumatoid).

● DIGESTIVE SYSTEM Dyspepsia, obesity.

Grapefruit has strong antioxidant and cholesterol-lowering properties. It contains an astringent essential oil, stimulates appetite and liver function, aids detoxification, and is slightly diuretic. Grapefruit is recommended for circulatory problems and obesity. It has a negative interaction with a variety of prescribed drugs – consult your doctor if in doubt.

## OTHER FRUIT

### APPLE

★ MAGNESIUM, MANGANESE, PHOSPHORUS, POTASSIUM, SULPHUR, NATURAL SUGAR, PECTIN, MALIC ACID

● BONES AND JOINTS Arthritis (rheumatoid), gout, rheumatism.

● DIGESTIVE SYSTEM Constipation, diarrhoea, dyspepsia, peptic ulcers.

Apples are gently diuretic, they aid the elimination of uric acid and lower levels of cholesterol in the blood. Traditionally, raw apples are eaten to ease constipation and cooked apples are eaten as a remedy for diarrhoea. Apple blossom infusion can ease coughs and sore throats.

RECIPES *autumn fruit compote (page 114), apple and raspberry juice (page 117), cherry and apple juice (page 118), pear and apple infusion (page 124), cherry-stem and apple decoction (page 126).*

### PEAR

★ COPPER, IODINE, MAGNESIUM, PHOSPHORUS, SULPHUR, ZINC, NATURAL SUGAR, PECTIN

● BONES AND JOINTS Arthritis (rheumatoid), gout, rheumatism.

● DIGESTIVE SYSTEM Diarrhoea.

Pears are laxative, diuretic, astringent and calming. They aid uric acid elimination and prevent bacteria proliferating in the intestines. They are good for pregnant women, elderly people and convalescents. An infusion of pear tree leaves can ease urinary problems.

RECIPES *autumn fruit compote (page 114), pears with herbs (page 114), pear and apple infusion (page 124).*

### PHYSALIS

★ VITAMIN C, PHYSALIN

● BONES AND JOINTS Arthritis (rheumatoid), gout.

● KIDNEYS AND BLADDER Bladder stones.

Physalis contains physalin, which is diuretic and facilitates the elimination of urea. The jam is good for kidney or bladder inflammation.

RECIPES *physalis jam (page 122), physalis-berry decoction (page 126).*

### PERSIMMON

★ VITAMINS A, B, C, COPPER, IODINE, MAGNESIUM, PHOSPHORUS, SULPHUR, ZINC, NATURAL SUGAR, PECTIN

● DIGESTIVE SYSTEM Crohn's disease.

Persimmon is a nutritious fruit that prevents the proliferation of bacteria in the intestines. It has laxative and astringent properties.

### POMEGRANATE

★ VITAMINS A, B, C, TRACE ELEMENTS, NATURAL SUGAR

● BLOOD AND CIRCULATION High blood pressure.

● DIGESTIVE SYSTEM Constipation.

Pomegranate is considered to be a tonic for the heart, kidneys and bladder. The juice is recommended for people with bladder disorders or tapeworm.

### QUINCE

★ VITAMINS A, B, C, CALCIUM, COPPER, IRON, MAGNESIUM, PHOSPHORUS, NATURAL SUGAR, PECTIN, TANNIN

● DIGESTIVE SYSTEM Diarrhoea.

Quince has astringent properties and enhances digestion and liver function.

RECIPES *quince liqueur (page 129).*

*continues on page 47*

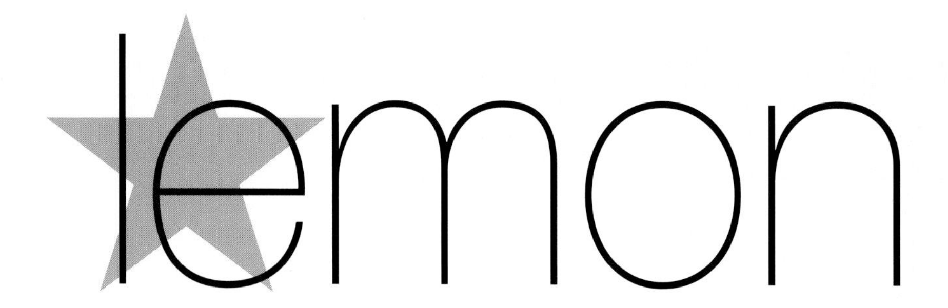

# lemon

**LEMON IS A NATURAL DISINFECTANT. IT IS RICH IN VITAMIN C AND CITRUS FLAVONOIDS THAT HAVE A POWERFUL ANTIOXIDANT FUNCTION. LEMON IS GOOD FOR STRENGTHENING THE IMMUNE SYSTEM AND PREVENTING INFECTION AND DISEASE.**

## The properties of lemon

The lemon tree *(Citrus limon)* is a small evergreen indigenous to the forests of northern India. It bears bright yellow segmented fruit that, together with lime, orange and grapefruit, belong to the citrus family (page 39).

Although there is some doubt about their origin and distribution, it is thought that lemon trees were introduced to Europe by Arabs, probably around the 11th century. In the past, lemons were the mainstay of prevention and treatment for scurvy, a disease that results from a deficiency of vitamin C. Lemons were traditionally taken on long sea voyages and the juice given to sailors in order to prevent scurvy. Today, lemons are widely produced in the US, Spain, Portugal, Italy and, to a lesser extent, southern France.

Lemons are rich in citrus flavonoids that, alongside vitamin C, have an important antioxidant function. Citrus flavonoids are phytochemicals (biologically active plant compounds) that can assist the healing of wounds, strengthen the walls of blood capillaries and prevent diseases such as arteriosclerosis. Vitamin C also helps to fight infection, strengthen the immune system, make collagen (the main protein found in connective tissue), keep the skin and joints healthy and prevent cancer. Other substances found in lemon are citric and malic acid, vitamins A and B, glucose, fructose, potassium, phosphorus, silica, manganese and copper.

Pectin is another important component of lemon. It is concentrated in the skin around the segments and can help to lower levels of unhealthy cholesterol in the blood.

## Lemon as a cure

Lemons can be used to treat a range of ailments. They are a natural booster of the immune system; they can help to reduce mild fever, lower blood pressure, reduce gastric acidity, promote liver function and increase the fluidity of blood. They also have diuretic properties.

Specific illnesses that can be treated with lemon are rheumatism, arthritis, high blood cholesterol, dyspepsia, colds and influenza. As well as using lemons in recipes, try to use the juice freely as a flavouring in cooking, as a dressing for salads and fish, and in cold drinks and teas.

Lemon juice is a natural disinfectant and antiseptic – prior to the development of modern antiseptics, it was used in hospitals for this purpose. The juice can be applied directly to the skin – it is an astringent and a bactericide – and it is a useful ingredient in home-made beauty masks. Lemon juice can be used as a skin toner, an anti-aging treatment and to reduce or eliminate freckles.

A fragrant essential oil is found in the outer skin of the lemon and this can be extracted under pressure. This essential oil has excellent antibacterial properties and is available from health food shops, aromatherapy suppliers and some pharmacies. It can be used to treat colds, sore throats, gingivitis or mouth ulcers. Take four drops in a teaspoon of honey for colds and sore throats. For gingivitis or mouth ulcers, use one drop of essential oil on a toothbrush with a small amount of toothpaste. This will disinfect the teeth and mouth. Lemon essential oil is also antiparasitic.

## STAR FOOD PROFILE

- **BONES AND JOINTS** Arthritis (rheumatoid), rheumatism.
- **BLOOD AND CIRCULATION** Atherosclerosis, palpitations.
- **DIGESTIVE SYSTEM** Dyspepsia.
- **IMMUNE SYSTEM** Colds, influenza, sore throat.

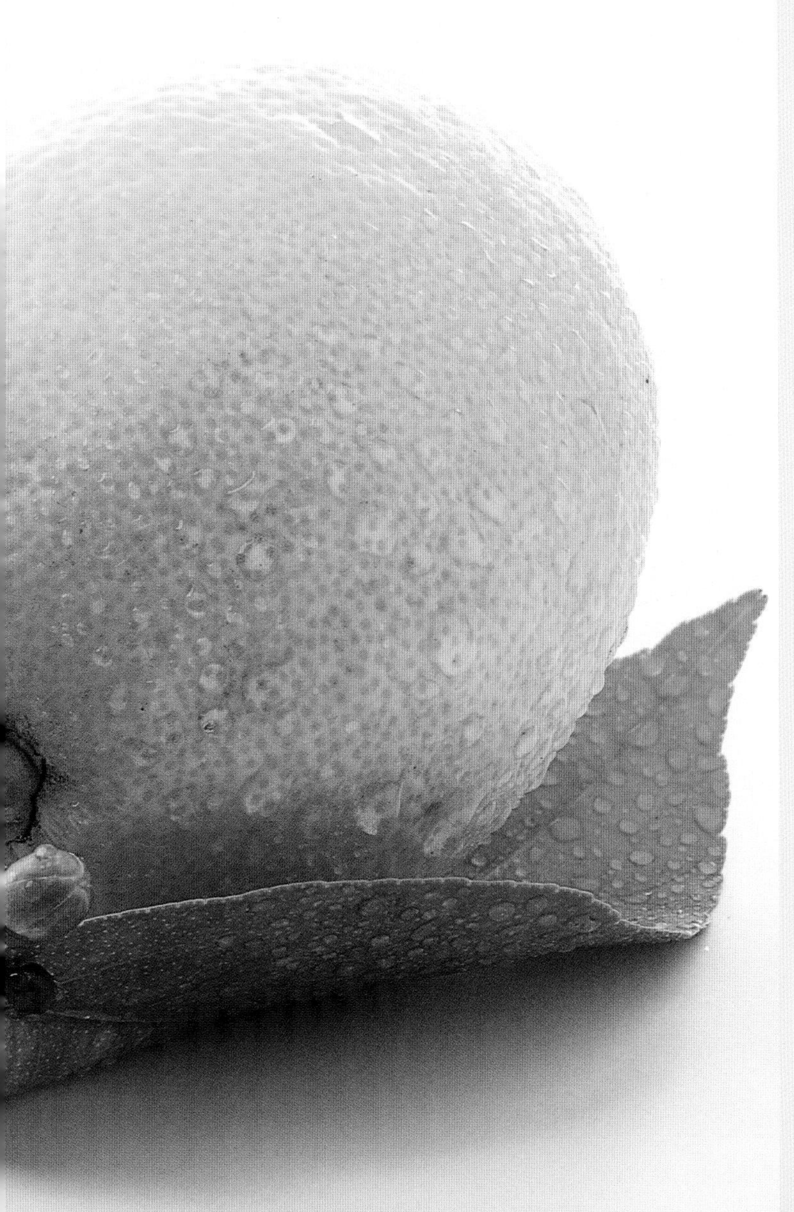

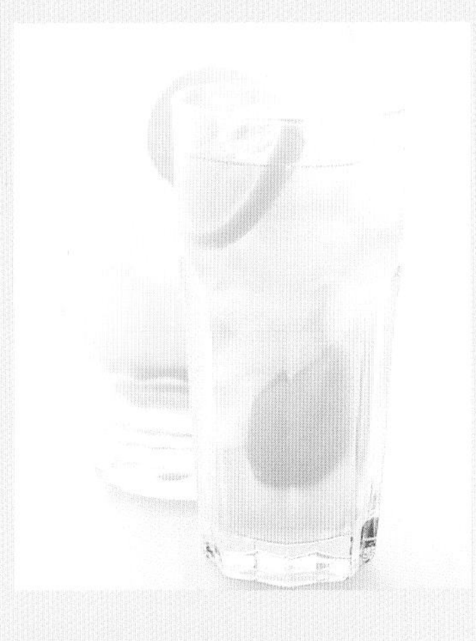

# lemonade

2 lemons, wiped and sliced
60 g brown sugar
1 litre water

Mix the lemons with the sugar and water. Leave to macerate for 12 hours in the refrigerator, stirring intermittently to dissolve the sugar, and then drink cold.

# lemon preserved in salt

Use in salads or stews. The lemon juice can also be used, sparingly, as a seasoning.

3 lemons, wiped and quartered
Salt

In a small, hermetically-sealable pickling jar, put a 1 cm-deep layer of salt. Place one layer of lemon quarters on top and cover with salt. Continue until the last layer of lemon is covered in salt and then tightly seal the jar and store in a cool, dark place for 1 month. After a month, wash the lemon quarters under cold, running water and use.

# lemon in oil

Lemons will keep for months if they are covered in oil – use them in salads or with meat or fish dishes. The oil can be used in dressings.

6 lemons, wiped and sliced or quartered
3 tbsp salt
Olive oil
1 bay leaf

Place the lemons in a bowl and sprinkle them with the salt. Toss and then refrigerate for 24 hours. Drain the juice from the lemons, then leave in a colander for 2 hours, or press the lemon gently to remove as much juice as possible. Wipe the salt off the lemons and place in a hermetically-sealable pickling jar. Cover the lemons with the olive oil – press them down to make sure they are covered – and add the bay leaf.

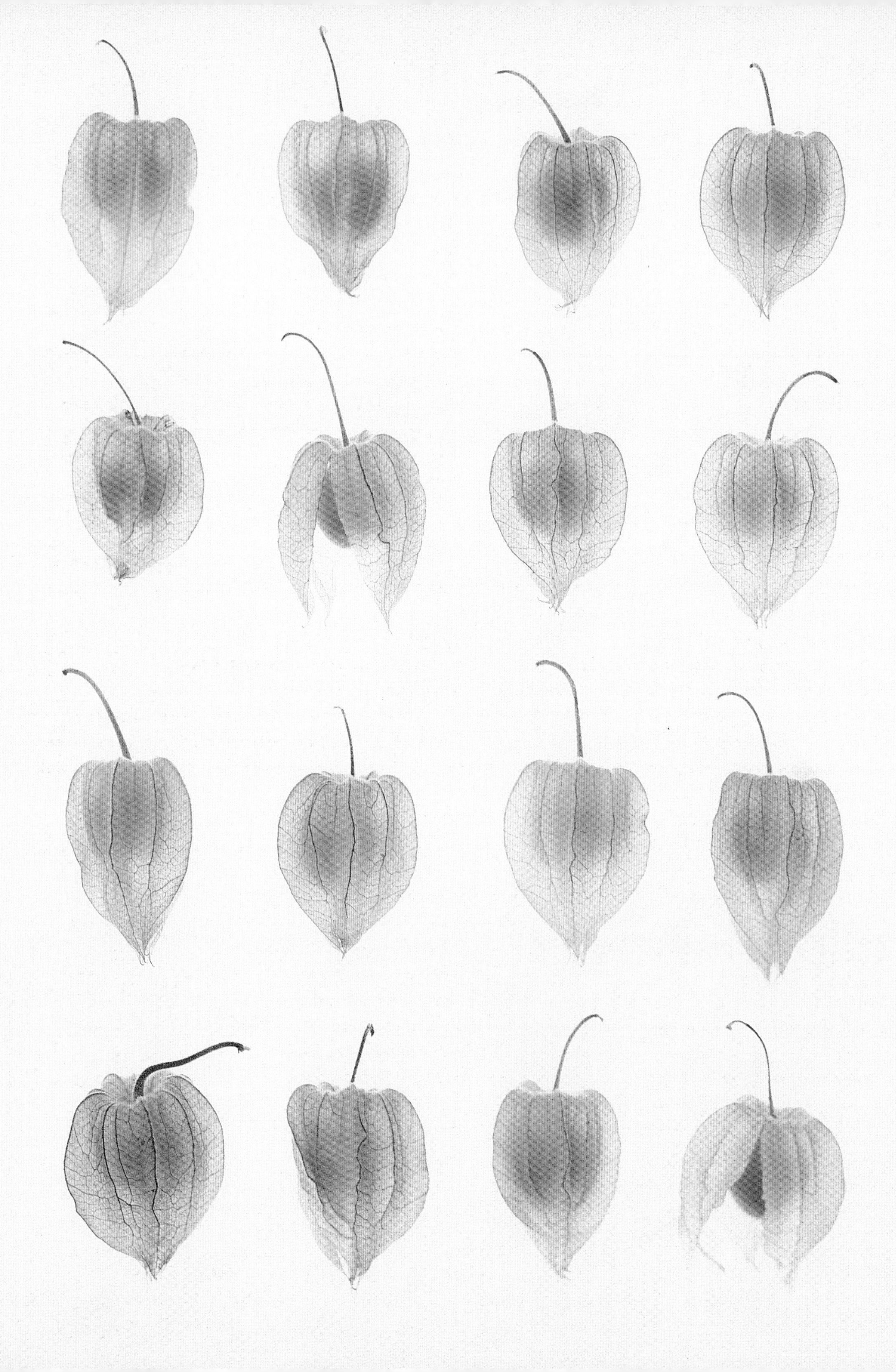

### RHUBARB

★ **VITAMINS B, C, IRON, MAGNESIUM**

● **DIGESTIVE SYSTEM** Constipation.

Rhubarb has tonic, laxative and anti-parasitic properties. It facilitates bile flow and prevents the proliferation of bacteria in the gut. The root may be used in powder or tincture form as a laxative. Rhubarb should be avoided by people suffering from hyperacidity, gout, kidney stones or gallstones. The leaves are poisonous.

*RECIPES rhubarb and ginger tart (page 113).*

# NUTS

### HAZELNUT

★ **CALCIUM, PHOSPHORUS, COPPER, IRON, MAGNESIUM, POTASSIUM, SULPHUR, POLYUNSATURATED FATTY ACIDS**

Hazelnuts are excellent energy-providing snacks that are also rich in fibre. They are recommended for people who are prone to kidney or gall bladder stones. They may also help get rid of intestinal worms – treatment consists of 1 tablespoon of cold-pressed hazelnut oil every morning on an empty stomach for 15 days. Cold-pressed hazelnut oil can also be used externally. It is particularly recommended for oily skin owing to its regulatory effect on sebum secretion. It can be helpful in the treatment of acne, dermatitis and seborrhoeic eczema. An infusion of hazelnut leaves makes an excellent astringent fluid that can be applied to the skin for the treatment of varicose veins. Cover 30 g of dried leaves with 1 litre of boiling water and infuse for 12 hours – strain and use as a skin wash two or three times a day. A fluid extract from the leaves (available commercially) can be taken internally for the same condition.

*RECIPES green beans with dijon mustard (page 111).*

### ALMOND

★ **VITAMINS A, B, CALCIUM, MAGNESIUM, PHOSPHORUS, POTASSIUM, OLEIC ACID**

● **DIGESTIVE SYSTEM** Irritable bowel syndrome.

Almonds are an energy-providing and nutritious snack. They have a balancing effect upon the nervous system and are useful for digestive problems. Almond milk relieves intestinal spasm and inflammation in cases of irritable bowel syndrome; sweet almond oil is a mild laxative suitable for children. Externally, almond paste and oil can be used for eczema, rashes, and as an ingredient in beauty masks. Bitter almonds are toxic and should be avoided.

*RECIPES almond milk (page 77)*

### CHESTNUT

★ **VITAMINS B, C, IRON, MAGNESIUM, POTASSIUM, ZINC**

● **BLOOD AND CIRCULATION** Anaemia.

● **DIGESTIVE SYSTEM** Dyspepsia.

Chestnuts are good for convalescents, elderly people and those prone to varicose veins and haemorrhoids. A handful of the leaves infused for 10 minutes in 1 litre of water is a good expectorant.

*RECIPES brussels sprouts with chestnuts (page 110).*

### PINE NUT

★ **VITAMINS A, B, CALCIUM, MAGNESIUM, PHOSPHORUS, POTASSIUM, ZINC, OLEIC ACID**

Pine nuts are energy-providing and nutritious; they have laxative properties and can help to ease digestive problems.

### PEANUT

★ **VITAMINS B, E, TRACE ELEMENTS AND AMYLASE**

● **DIGESTIVE SYSTEM** Dyspepsia.

Peanuts contain amylase, an enzyme that eases dyspepsia and hyperacidity. Some people are allergic to peanuts: the symptoms include vomiting and diarrhoea. In severe cases the allergy is fatal.

### WALNUT

★ **VITAMINS A, B, C, COPPER, IRON, MAGNESIUM, POTASSIUM, SELENIUM, ZINC, LINOLEIC AND OLEIC ACID**

● **DIGESTIVE SYSTEM** Diarrhoea.

Walnuts have astringent and cholesterol-lowering properties and are good for getting rid of intestinal parasites and for alleviating heart and circulatory problems. Walnut oil can be applied to skin affected by dermatitis or eczema.

*RECIPES garlic and walnut sauce (page 55).*

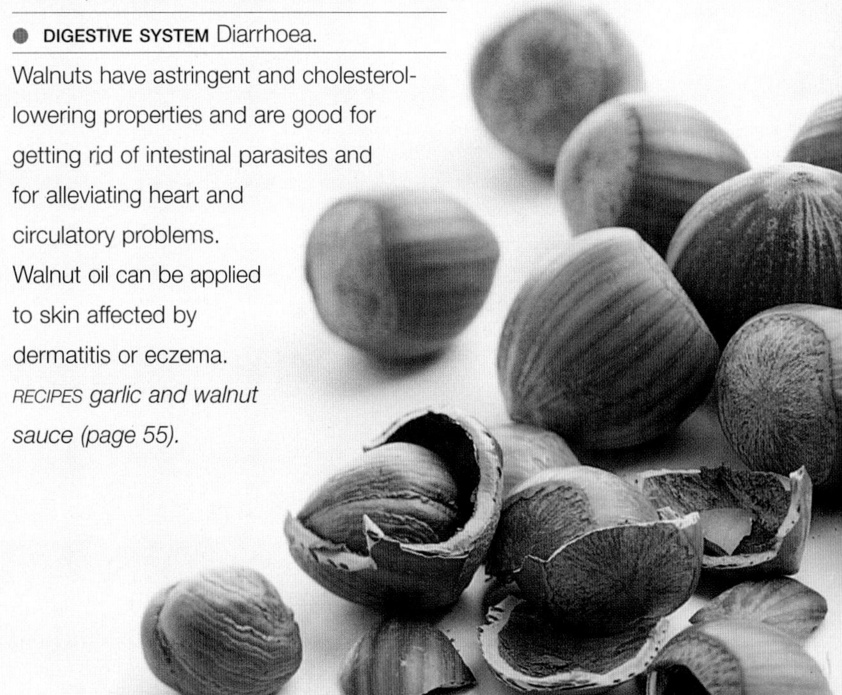

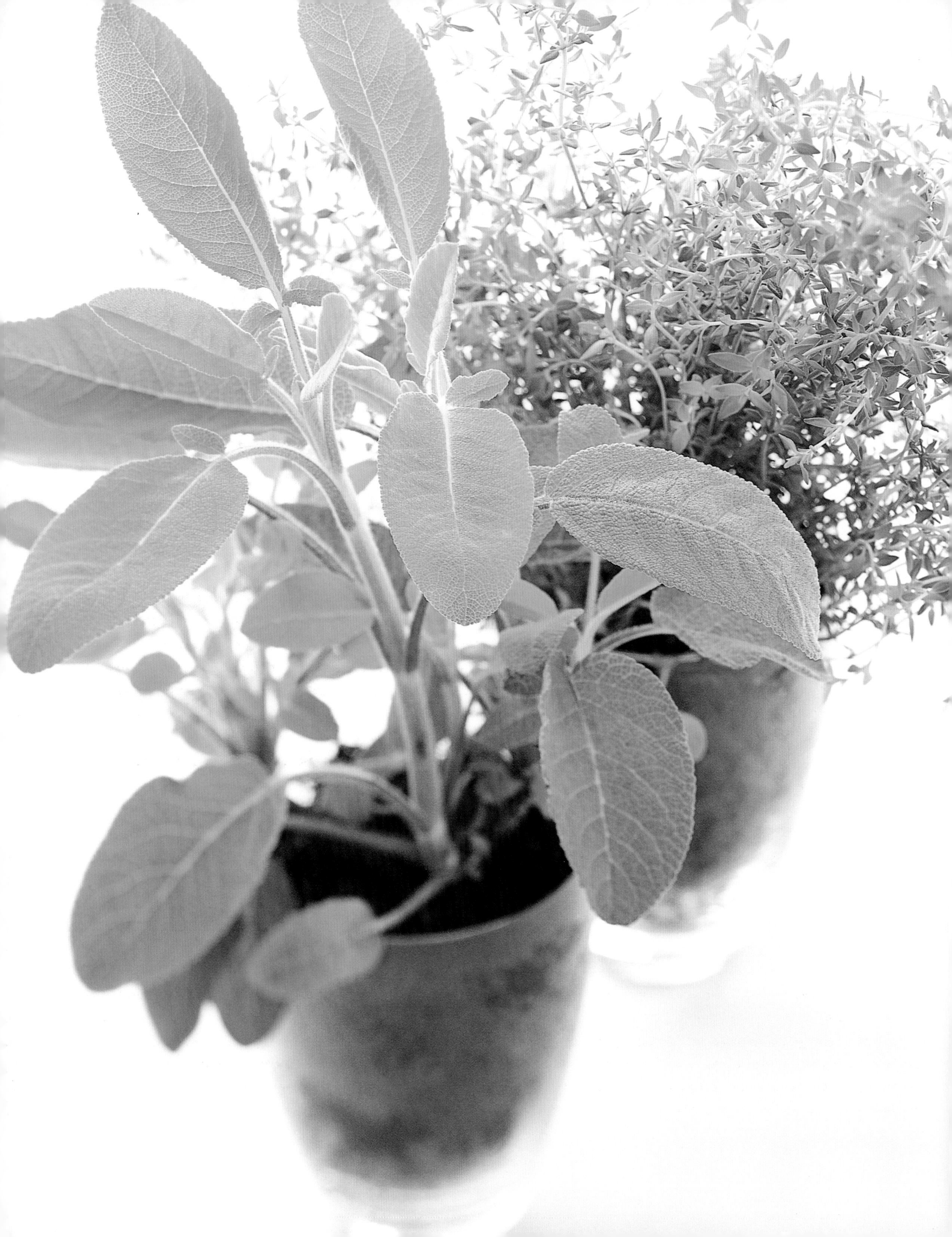

# herbs, spices and condiments

## HERBS

### PARSLEY

★ VITAMINS A, B, C, CALCIUM, IRON, ESSENTIAL OIL

● BLOOD AND CIRCULATION Anaemia.

● DIGESTIVE SYSTEM Dyspepsia, flatulence.

Parsley has diuretic, depurative, tonic and laxative properties. It stimulates appetite and liver function, regulates bile flow and is a good antiseptic for the lungs. Parsley is best eaten raw in salads or chopped and sprinkled generously over casseroles, meat, fish and other main-course dishes. It can also be used in broths or in raw juice cocktails. Freshly chopped parsley can be rubbed into the skin as an anti-ageing treatment or as a remedy for insect bites and stings. An infusion of parsley seeds can be used to treat urine retention and digestive problems such as dyspepsia.

RECIPES *parsley, onion and lemon salad (page 99), taboule (page 100), potatoes with herb sauce (page 111).*

### MINT

★ ESSENTIAL OIL

● BLOOD AND CIRCULATION Palpitations.

● DIGESTIVE SYSTEM Colic, colitis, intestinal parasites, irritable bowel syndrome, nausea and vomiting (including morning sickness).

● RESPIRATORY SYSTEM Asthma, bronchitis.

● NERVOUS SYSTEM, MIND AND EMOTIONS Mental fatigue, migraine, neuralgia.

Mint is a nervous-system stimulant (an infusion of mint taken in the evening may prevent sleep). Mint essential oil is a powerful antispasmodic, analgesic, anti-inflammatory and antiseptic agent for the intestines; it may also help to expel intestinal worms.

RECIPES *taboule (page 100), minted melon (page 112), fresh mint sorbet (page 113), mint syrup (page 131).*

### BASIL

★ ESSENTIAL OIL

● BONES AND JOINTS Gout.

● DIGESTIVE SYSTEM Abdominal cramp, colic, intestinal infections.

● NERVOUS SYSTEM, MIND AND EMOTIONS Anxiety, insomnia, mental fatigue, migraine.

Basil is a popular herb in Mediterranean countries. It contains a powerful essential oil that has antispasmodic and antiseptic properties; it acts as a tonic for the nervous system and helps to ease digestive complaints, including intestinal infections. Basil can be used in soups, sauces, medicinal drinks, such as basil liqueur, or raw in salads. Fresh basil leaves can be preserved by freezing or storing in oil. To preserve basil in oil, choose leaves from the top part of the plant, rinse gently in cold water and allow to dry on kitchen paper. Sprinkle the leaves with salt, wait 30 minutes, gently wipe the salt off, place the leaves in a sterilized jar or bottle and fill with cold-pressed olive oil. Keep the jar tightly closed and store in the refrigerator.

RECIPES *polenta with basil tomato sauce (page 105), pasta twists with pesto (page 104), basil liqueur (page 129).*

### MARJORAM AND OREGANO

★ ESSENTIAL OIL

● DIGESTIVE SYSTEM Abdominal pain, distention and wind.

● RESPIRATORY SYSTEM Bronchitis, colds, influenza.

Marjoram and oregano are two distinct plants, but for culinary and medicinal purposes they are interchangeable. Both are potent bactericides, expectorants and digestive-system stimulants. They are good natural remedies for ear, nose, throat and lung infections. The essential oils of these herbs can be applied to the skin as a treatment for rheumatism and skin infections. They should be diluted with a base oil, such as almond, before they are applied to the skin.

RECIPES *marjoram infusion (page 123).*

## ROSEMARY

★ **ESSENTIAL OIL**

- **BONES AND JOINTS** Gout.
- **DIGESTIVE SYSTEM** Colitis, diarrhoea, flatulence, intestinal infections, irritable bowel syndrome.
- **RESPIRATORY SYSTEM** Asthma.
- **NERVOUS SYSTEM, MIND AND EMOTIONS** Headache, neuralgia.
- **IMMUNE SYSTEM** Colds, influenza.

Rosemary contains a potent essential oil that is diuretic, promotes perspiration, stimulates the production and flow of bile, improves digestion and acts as an antiseptic for the lungs and the digestive system. It can be diluted with a base oil, such as almond, then massaged into the skin to ease muscular cramps or rheumatism.

RECIPES *carrots with rosemary (page 21).*

## THYME

★ **ESSENTIAL OIL**

- **BONES AND JOINTS** Rheumatism.
- **DIGESTIVE SYSTEM** Intestinal infections and parasites.
- **RESPIRATORY SYSTEM** Bronchitis, cough.
- **KIDNEYS AND BLADDER** Cystitis.
- **IMMUNE SYSTEM** Colds, influenza.

Thyme has powerful antibacterial properties. It is a general stimulant and acts as an antiseptic for the throat, lungs and digestive system. Thyme may improve poor circulation.

RECIPES *amazingly aromatic vinegar (page 122).*

## TARRAGON

★ **ESSENTIAL OIL**

- **DIGESTIVE SYSTEM** Colic, intestinal parasites.
- **WOMEN'S HEALTH** Period pain.

Tarragon is a general stimulant, it is antispasmodic and improves digestive function. The infused oil can be applied to the skin to treat rheumatism, muscular spasms and cramps. Fill a jar with tarragon leaves, cover with olive oil and leave for two weeks.

RECIPES *tarragon vinegar (page 122), amazingly aromatic vinegar (page 122).*

## SAGE

★ **ESSENTIAL OIL**

- **WOMEN'S HEALTH** Irregular or painful periods, menopausal symptoms.

There are more than 200 species of sage but the one most commonly used in cooking is *Salvia officinalis*. Sage is a general stimulant and a digestive-system tonic. It is good for hypotension, excessive perspiration and fatigue.

RECIPES *garlic and sage soup (page 55).*

## BAY

★ **ESSENTIAL OIL**

- **DIGESTIVE SYSTEM** Dyspepsia, flatulence.
- **WOMEN'S HEALTH** Period pain.

Bay leaves have antiseptic, stimulant and antispasmodic properties. They can be used in casseroles and soups or made into an infusion for indigestion and bloated stomach, or as a gargle for mouth and throat infections (add 3–4 leaves to a cup of boiling water, cover, infuse for 10 minutes and then strain).

RECIPES *orange-zest infusion (page 123).*

## CHIVE AND SPRING ONION

★ **VITAMINS A, B, C, CALCIUM, MAGNESIUM, PHOSPHORUS, POTASSIUM, SULPHUR COMPOUNDS, BIOFLAVONOIDS, ESSENTIAL OIL**

- **BONES AND JOINTS** Arthritis (rheumatoid), gout, rheumatism.
- **BLOOD AND CIRCULATION** Arteriosclerosis.
- **DIGESTIVE SYSTEM** Diabetes, diarrhoea, intestinal infections and parasites.
- **WOMEN'S HEALTH** Period pain.

Chives and spring onions are antibacterial, antiviral, antifungal and diuretic; they prevent tumour and blood-clot formation and help to lower levels of cholesterol in the body. Chives and spring onions also prevent water retention, promote the elimination of urea and the expectoration of mucus and are good for the digestive and circulatory systems. Both chives and spring onions may be eaten raw, chopped and sprinkled over main courses and salads, or made into raw juice cocktails. A broth containing chives or spring onions (especially combined with garlic, clove and ginger) can alleviate colds and influenza as well as digestive problems, such as diarrhoea. The fresh juice can be applied to insect stings, warts and boils.

RECIPES *chive and ginger broth (page 94), leek and chive mimosa with polenta (page 105).*

## CORIANDER

★ **VITAMIN B, FOLIC ACID, ESSENTIAL OIL**

- **DIGESTIVE SYSTEM** Abdominal pain, dyspepsia, flatulence, indigestion, irritable bowel syndrome.

Coriander is an aromatic herb that has antibiotic properties and helps to treat a range of digestive problems. It is widely used in Asian and North African cooking. The leaves can be chopped and sprinkled on salads, main dishes and soups. The seeds contain a greater concentration of active ingredients than the leaves and can be made into medicinal drinks.

RECIPES *coriander dressing (page 95), coriander-seed infusion (page 125), coriander-seed tincture (page 130).*

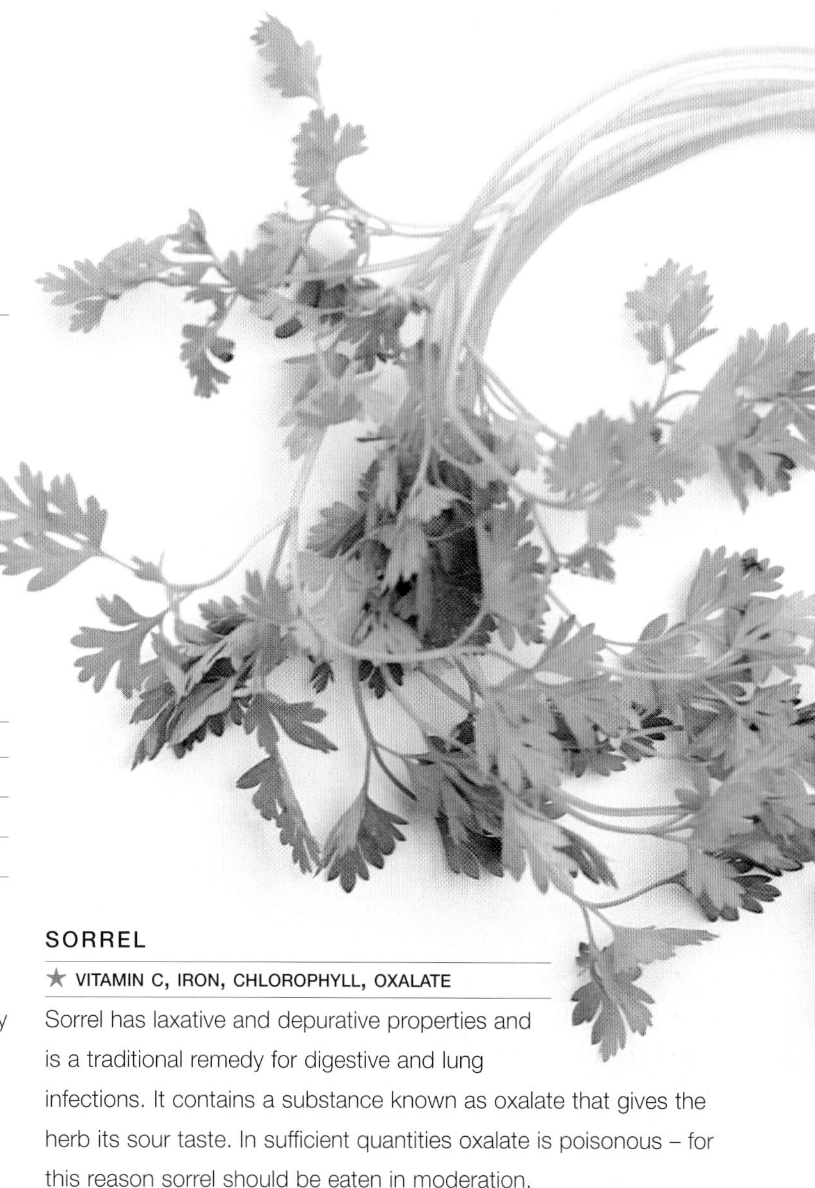

## CHERVIL

★ **VITAMINS A, B, C, IRON, ESSENTIAL OIL**

- **BONES AND JOINTS** Gout.
- **BLOOD AND CIRCULATION** Anaemia.
- **RESPIRATORY SYSTEM** Bronchitis.

Chervil has diuretic, tonic and laxative properties. It stimulates appetite and liver function and regulates the flow of bile. It is also a good antiseptic for the lungs and helps to get rid of phlegm in the chest. Chervil can be eaten raw in salad or sprinkled generously over casseroles, fish, meat and main course dishes. It can also be used in broths or raw juice cocktails. Freshly chopped chervil can also be rubbed on the skin to treat insect bites or stings.

RECIPES *herbal broth (page 92), parsley, onion and lemon salad (page 99), potatoes with herb sauce (page 111).*

## BORAGE

★ **GAMMA-LINOLENIC ACID (GLA)**

- **RESPIRATORY SYSTEM** Bronchitis.

Borage has depurative, diuretic and laxative properties and promotes the elimination of toxins. Borage seeds contain gamma-linolenic acid (GLA), an essential fatty acid that helps the body to make prostaglandins. Prostaglandins are hormone-like substances that have numerous health benefits, such as keeping the blood thin, lowering blood pressure, maintaining water balance and regulating blood sugar. Another good, but less abundant source of GLA is evening primrose oil. Borage oil can be applied to the skin as a treatment for mature skin and dry, scaly eczema. Young borage leaves are excellent raw in salads, especially with dandelion and watercress. They can also be added to soups or included in a variety of raw juice cocktails.

RECIPES *borage leaves in vinegar (page 122).*

## SORREL

★ **VITAMIN C, IRON, CHLOROPHYLL, OXALATE**

Sorrel has laxative and depurative properties and is a traditional remedy for digestive and lung infections. It contains a substance known as oxalate that gives the herb its sour taste. In sufficient quantities oxalate is poisonous – for this reason sorrel should be eaten in moderation.

RECIPES *herbal broth (page 92).*

## SAVORY

★ **ESSENTIAL OIL**

- **DIGESTIVE SYSTEM** Diarrhoea, flatulence.
- **RESPIRATORY SYSTEM** Asthma, bronchitis.

Two species of savory are commonly used in cooking: summer savory (usually grown in the garden), and winter savory (usually found in the wild). Savory is a nervous system stimulant and a tonic. It is particularly effective for poor digestion.

## CAMOMILE

★ **COMPLEX CHEMICALS SUCH AS NOBILINE AND CHAMAZULENE, ESSENTIAL OIL**

- **DIGESTIVE SYSTEM** Colic, diarrhoea, indigestion, irritable bowel syndrome.
- **NERVOUS SYSTEM, MIND AND EMOTIONS** Insomnia, migraine, neuralgia.
- **WOMEN'S HEALTH** Period pain.

Camomile contains nobiline, which is a bitter tonic, and chamazulene, a potent anti-inflammatory agent. An infusion of camomile is widely recommended for its calming properties and its ability to improve digestion and ease digestive problems. Camomile infusion stimulates liver function and regulates the flow of bile. It can be used externally as a douche for thrush, a wash for inflamed skin, mild burns, sunburn, dermatitis and eczema, and as an eyewash for conjunctivitis. Camomile flowers mixed with white wine is an excellent bitter aperitif.

*RECIPES lemon-balm and camomile infusion (page 124), elder and camomile infusion (page 124), camomile and citrus wine (page 129), camomile aperitif (page 129).*

### ELDER

★ ESSENTIAL OIL

Elderflowers promote perspiration (useful for colds and influenza) and help to advance skin eruptions in chicken pox, German measles and scarlet fever. They are diuretic, promote detoxification and stimulate bile flow. Elderberries ease constipation, headache and mild neuralgia. The bark, which is diuretic, is useful for rheumatism, arthritis, nephritis (inflammation of the kidneys) and bladder stones. All parts of the elder plant have anti-inflammatory properties.

*RECIPES elder and camomile infusion (page 124), elderberry syrup (page 131).*

### LINDEN (LIME TREE)

★ ESSENTIAL OIL

Linden- or lime-tree blossom has antispasmodic, sedative and slight hypnotic properties. It also induces sweating. Research suggests that lime flowers may reduce the viscosity and rate of coagulation of the blood. This may help to prevent cardiovascular problems. An infusion of lime blossom has a delicate fragrance and is a good remedy for insomnia in children as well as adults (steep a small handful of the blossom in 300 ml water for 5 minutes).

*RECIPES pears with herbs (page 114).*

### LEMON BALM (MELISSA)

★ ESSENTIAL OIL

● DIGESTIVE SYSTEM Indigestion.

● NERVOUS SYSTEM, MIND AND EMOTIONS Anxiety, insomnia, migraine, neuralgia.

Lemon balm contains a potent essential oil that has tonic and antispasmodic properties. Although rarely used in cooking, lemon balm is often included in herbal liqueurs such as Chartreuse, Benedictine and Eau de Melissa des Carmes. Lemon balm can help to relieve spasms (muscular, digestive or asthmatic).

*RECIPES lemon-balm and camomile infusion (page 124), sparkling lemon-balm infusion (page 125).*

### DILL

★ ESSENTIAL OIL

● DIGESTIVE SYSTEM Abdominal cramp, colic.

● WOMEN'S HEALTH Irregular periods, period pain.

Dill is a type of wild fennel that is often used in fish recipes or in pickling vinegar. Both the leaves and the seeds can be used. Dill is recommended for lactating mothers as its aromatic compounds pass into breast milk and enhance the flavour.

*RECIPES lentil soup (page 95), dill-seed decoction (page 126), amazingly aromatic vinegar (page 122).*

## SPICES AND SEEDS

### CHILLI

★ VITAMIN C, TRACE ELEMENTS, ESSENTIAL OIL CONTAINING UP TO 1 % CAPSAICIN

● DIGESTIVE SYSTEM Diarrhoea, dyspepsia, flatulence.

● IMMUNE SYSTEM Colds.

There may be over 50 species of chilli of varying shapes and sizes. The colour of a chilli – green, yellow, red or purple – indicates its stage of maturity. An essential oil in chillies contains capsaicin, which is thought to be good for the heart and circulation. Chillies are recommended for digestive problems and circulatory problems such as chilblains. Excessive consumption of chillies should be avoided as it may cause chronic inflammation of the stomach and intestines.

*RECIPES cardamom hot sauce (page 111).*

### CARDAMOM

★ ESSENTIAL OIL

● DIGESTIVE SYSTEM Diarrhoea.

Cardamom seeds are strongly aromatic and are widely used in Indian cooking to flavour curries, sweets and desserts. They

*continues on page 56*

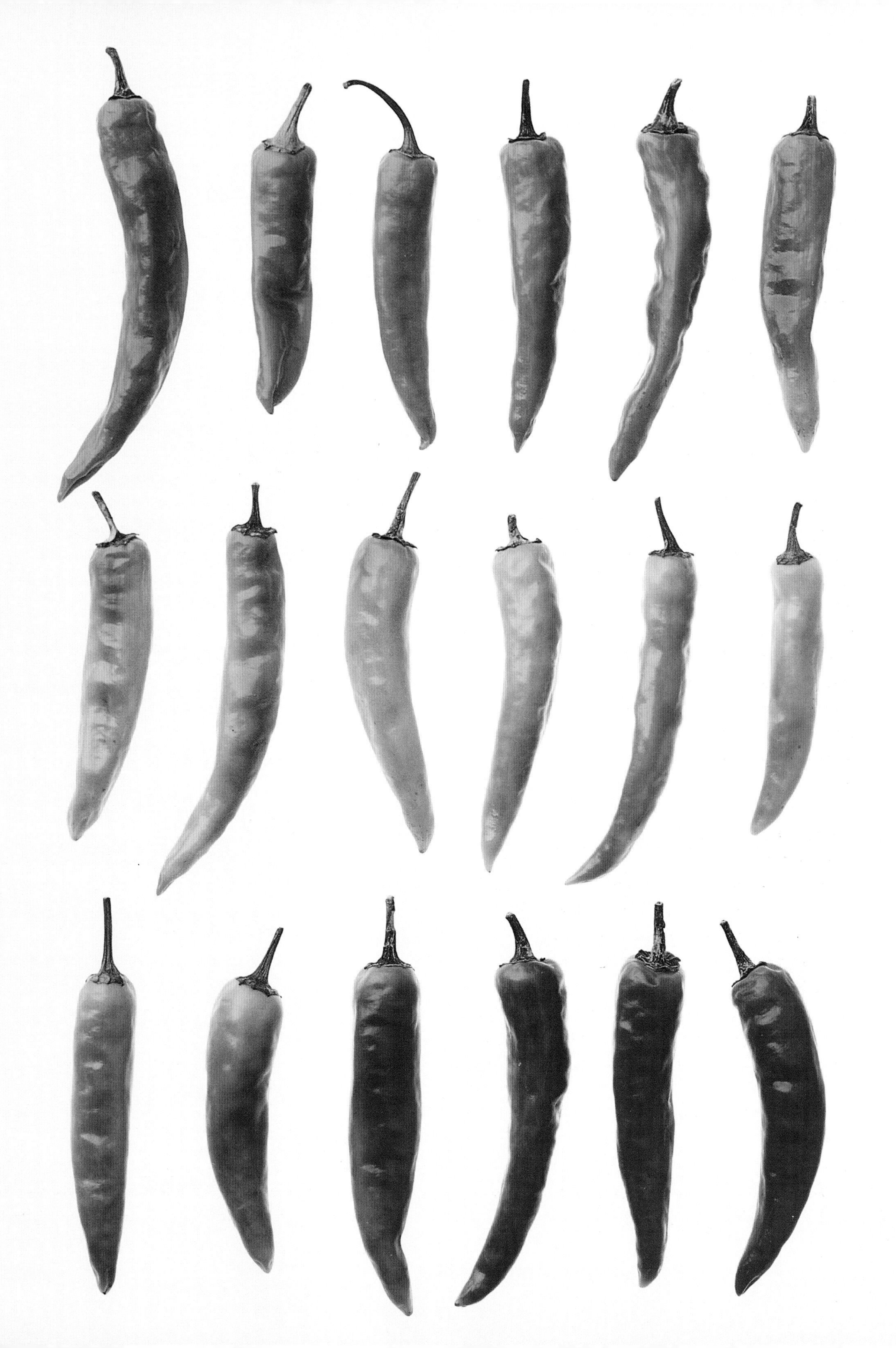

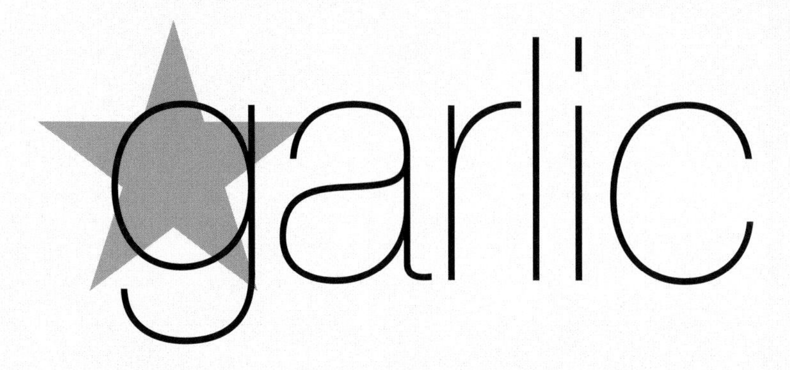


**GARLIC IS AN ANTI-COAGULANT AND HELPS TO REDUCE CHOLESTEROL LEVELS IN THE BLOOD. IT ALSO HAS ANTI-BACTERIAL AND ANTI-FUNGAL PROPERTIES.**

### The history of garlic

Garlic is part of the Liliacaea family, which also includes onions, shallots, leeks, chives and spring onions. It is native to central Asia, and its cultivation began in China, Mesopotamia (modern Turkey, Iran and Iraq) and Egypt thousands of years ago. Garlic has a long reputation as a health-giving food used both to prevent and to cure illness. In Egypt, as early as 2600 BCE, workers building the pyramids were given garlic to keep them strong. Ancient Greek soldiers ate it to improve their strength and increase their resistance to infection. In Europe, garlic has long been used to protect against disease – 16th-century monks took it to ward off the plague and its use was widespread during the cholera epidemics of the 19th century.

### The properties of garlic

The principal active ingredients in garlic are a volatile oil called allicin, released when the cloves are crushed, and several sulphur compounds, released when garlic is steamed or boiled.

Recent scientific research has shown that allicin is a powerful anti-coagulant. It inhibits blood-clotting and helps to break down existing clots, allowing the blood to flow more freely thus reducing blood pressure. Garlic inhibits the production of cholesterol in the liver and increases the rate at which dietary cholesterol is expelled from the body. As a result, it is extremely useful for those who suffer from high cholesterol levels, thrombosis (obstructive blood clots), heart disease and other circulatory problems.

Allicin has potent anti-bacterial and anti-fungal properties, and raw garlic is effective in relieving the symptoms of colds and respiratory infections, such as nasal congestion. It is also useful in combating digestive system infections and controlling the balance of bacteria in the gut, as well as helping to repel parasites, such as intestinal worms. Boiling a head of garlic in milk and drinking the resulting decoction every morning is a traditional remedy for intestinal parasites.

Recent research has suggested that diallyl sulfide, a component of garlic, may help to prevent the growth of some malignant tumours.

### Garlic as a cure

A traditional European folk custom involved placing a head of garlic in a small bag and tying it around a child's neck as a protection against colds or flu. Fixing the bag around the abdomen was thought to protect against worms. Scientists have now discovered that some of the sulphur compounds found in garlic can indeed be absorbed through the skin.

For maximum therapeutic value, at least two raw garlic cloves should be eaten every day. For many people, however, this is unpalatable: odourless garlic supplements can provide a useful additional source of this important food. If you are worried about bad breath, try chewing cardamom seeds, parsley leaves or a few roasted coffee beans to help disguise the smell.

Garlic can also be used to great effect in tinctures, drinks, soups and sauces. To make a garlic tincture, soak 50 g of garlic in 250 ml of strong vodka; leave it to macerate in a sealed opaque bottle for two weeks. Strain the mixture, pressing the garlic with the back of a spoon to extract all the remaining liquid. Add up to 15 drops to a small amount of water and take twice a day to reduce high blood pressure and high cholesterol, to combat colds and chronic bronchitis or as an antiseptic for the digestive system. Keep the tincture in an airtight bottle, away from light, and it will last for up to two years.

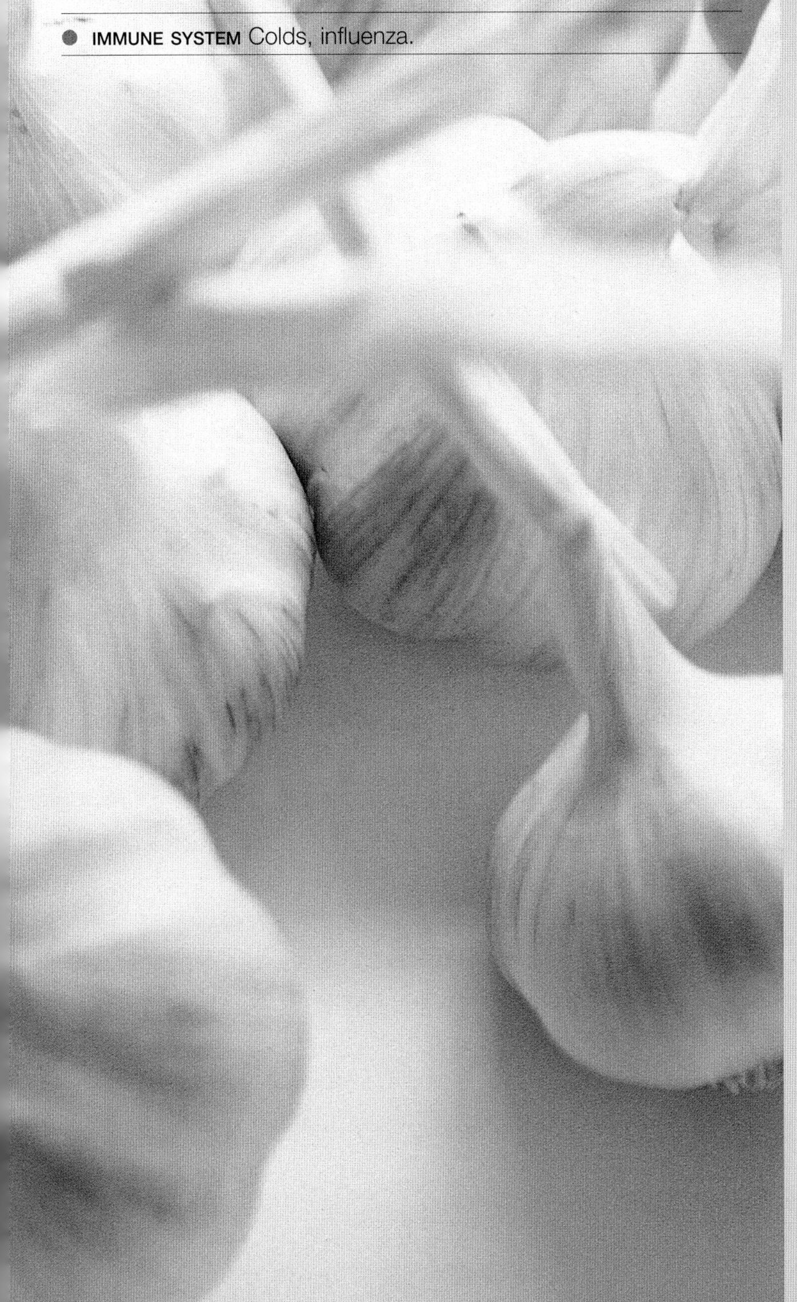

**STAR FOOD PROFILE**

- **BLOOD AND CIRCULATION** Atherosclerosis, high blood pressure, thrombosis.
- **DIGESTIVE SYSTEM** Gastroenteritis, intestinal parasites, ulcerative colitis.
- **IMMUNE SYSTEM** Colds, influenza.

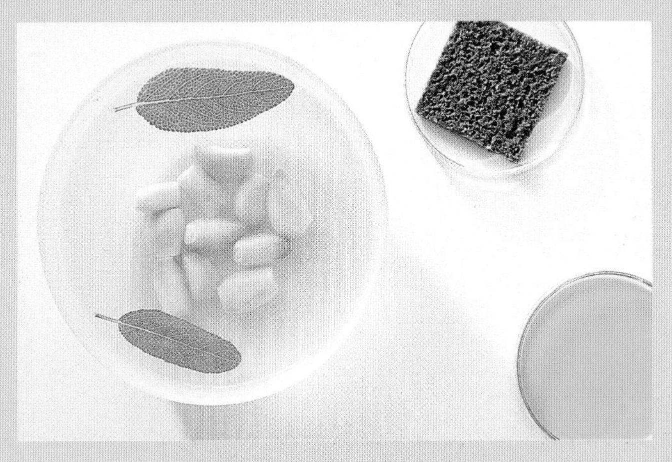

# garlic and sage soup

4 or 5 garlic bulbs, peeled
2 litres water
Approximately 10 sage leaves
Salt and pepper
3 or 4 thick slices of rye bread
150 ml cold-pressed olive oil
To garnish: fresh parsley or chervil, finely chopped

Peel the cloves from the bulbs of garlic and boil in the water for 20 minutes. Add the sage and season with salt and pepper. Leave to infuse for a few minutes. Place the rye bread in a large dish, and pour the olive oil over the bread. Pour the garlic and sage soup over the bread. Sprinkle with the parsley or chervil and serve immediately.

# garlic, carrot and spinach cocktail

4 medium-sized carrots, peeled and chopped
120 g fresh spinach leaves
2 cloves of garlic, peeled
Crushed ice
Salt and pepper

Process all the ingredients in a juicer and mix with some crushed ice. Add salt and pepper to taste. Serve immediately.

# garlic and walnut sauce

50 g garlic cloves, peeled
75 g shelled walnuts
250 ml walnut oil
Salt and pepper
1 tbsp parsley, finely chopped
Iced water (optional)

Process all the ingredients in a blender, adding iced water if necessary.

stimulate the appetite and aid digestion. They contain an essential oil that is an effective breath freshener: after eating an excessive amount of garlic chewing cardamom seeds will both freshen the breath and prevent heartburn.

RECIPES *cardamom hot sauce (page 111), poached apricots with cardamom (page 115).*

## CINNAMON

★ **ESSENTIAL OIL**

● **IMMUNE SYSTEM** Colds, influenza.

Cinnamon is a bactericide that improves the function of the respiratory and cardiovascular systems. It is also antispasmodic and stimulates digestion. Chinese herbalists use cinnamon to promote vitality, warm the body and treat colds and influenza.

RECIPES *cinnamon wine (page 127).*

## CLOVES

★ **ESSENTIAL OIL**

● **DIGESTIVE SYSTEM** Diarrhoea.

● **IMMUNE SYSTEM** Colds, influenza.

Clove essential oil acts as a powerful antiseptic. Cloves are good for intestinal infections – travellers used to chew them in order to prevent both intestinal infections and hepatitis. They also have a slight anaesthetic action. Clove oil can be used externally to treat infected wounds, dental pain and mouth ulcers.

## GINGER

★ **ESSENTIAL OIL**

● **DIGESTIVE SYSTEM** Nausea and vomiting.

● **IMMUNE SYSTEM** Colds, influenza.

● **WOMEN'S HEALTH** Morning sickness.

Ginger is one of the most widely used spices in Asia. It stimulates the appetite, has antiseptic and tonic properties and alleviates nausea, particularly morning sickness. Combined in a broth with spring onions, garlic and cloves, it promotes sweating and eases cold symptoms. Ginger can also be used as a massage oil for rheumatism or to improve blood circulation in muscles. Mix together 3 ml ginger essential oil, 1 ml rosemary essential oil, 1 ml juniper-berry essential oil and 100 ml vegetable oil.

RECIPES *honey and ginger grilled salmon (page 63), chive and ginger broth (page 94), rhubarb and ginger tart (page 113), baked papaya with ginger (page 115), ginger infusion (page 125).*

## CUMIN

★ **ESSENTIAL OIL**

● **DIGESTIVE SYSTEM** Flatulence.

Cumin seeds are rich in an essential oil that has sedative and carminative properties. They can help to treat poor digestion and are recommended for lactating mothers.

RECIPES *cumin-seed decoction (page 126).*

## SAFFRON

★ **BITTER COMPOUNDS, ESSENTIAL OIL**

● **DIGESTIVE SYSTEM** Dyspepsia.

● **WOMEN'S HEALTH** Period pain.

Saffron has calming and antispasmodic properties. It can be used to treat bronchial spasms. It can also be applied to sore and inflamed gums as a painkiller.

## HORSERADISH

★ **VITAMIN C, CALCIUM, IRON, MAGNESIUM, PHOSPHORUS, POTASSIUM, SULPHUR, ESSENTIAL OIL**

● **BONES AND JOINTS** Arthritis (rheumatoid), gout, rheumatism.

● **RESPIRATORY SYSTEM** Bronchitis, colds, coughs.

Horseradish has antispasmodic properties, promotes the flow of bile and is good for sinus problems.

RECIPES *horseradish sauce (page 111).*

## ANISE

★ **ESSENTIAL OIL**

● **DIGESTIVE SYSTEM** Colic, distention and wind, dyspepsia, flatulence, nausea and vomiting.

● **NERVOUS SYSTEM, MIND AND EMOTIONS** Migraine.

● **WOMEN'S HEALTH** Period pain, irregular periods.

Aniseed (the seeds of the anise plant) and star anise (the fruit) have the same properties. They both contain a potent essential oil that is strongly antispasmodic and acts as a stimulant to the heart, respiratory and digestive systems. Anise is slightly diuretic and helps to promote bile flow and digestion. It is recommended for lactating mothers.

RECIPES *pears with herbs (page 114), anisette (page 129), aniseed tincture (page 130).*

## JUNIPER BERRIES

★ **ESSENTIAL OIL**

● **BONES AND JOINTS** Gout, rheumatism.

● **DIGESTIVE SYSTEM** Intestinal infections.

● **KIDNEYS AND BLADDER** Cystitis.

Juniper berries have tonic, antiseptic, depurative and diuretic qualities. They help to eliminate uric acid and toxins from the body and contain a powerful antibacterial essential oil. In France and neighbouring countries, houses and stables are traditionally fumigated by burning juniper twigs and leaves – their disinfectant action helps to eliminate parasites and insects. Juniper berries are good for poor digestion and chest infections; they are also recommended for diabetes because they stimulate the pancreas (the organ that produces insulin). To treat acne, eczema and slow healing wounds: boil 50 g juniper berries and twigs in 1 litre of water for 10 minutes; strain and use the cooled water as a skin wash.

RECIPES *pickled turnips (page 120), juniper-berry wine (page 128).*

## NUTMEG

★ **ESSENTIAL OIL**

● **DIGESTIVE SYSTEM** Diarrhoea.

Nutmeg contains a potent essential oil that is poisonous in large doses, but beneficial in small amounts. It is a good general antiseptic for the digestive system, has analgesic properties and stimulates the brain and nervous system. Nutmeg is recommended for bad breath, poor digestion and other digestive ailments. The diluted essential oil can be applied to the skin for rheumatism and neuralgia (dilute with a base oil such as almond).

## VANILLA

★ **ESSENTIAL OIL**

Vanilla is a mild excitant and a tonic. It also stimulates the digestive system. Vanilla essential oil has antiseptic qualities.

## COCOA

★ **IRON, MAGNESIUM, THEOBROMINE, VEGETABLE FAT**

Cocoa contains theobromine, a substance that has a similar effect to caffeine, but is less toxic, does not raise blood pressure, accumulate in the body or result in addiction. Good-quality cocoa is slightly diuretic and helps to eliminate toxins from the body. In some cases, cocoa may trigger migraines. Good brands of chocolate contain at least 60 per cent cocoa.

## SUNFLOWER SEED

★ **LINOLEIC, STEARIC AND PALMITIC ACIDS, POLYUNSATURATED OILS**

● **DIGESTIVE SYSTEM** Constipation.

Sunflower seeds are a useful part of a low-cholesterol diet. They are delicious toasted and provide essential fatty acids.

## FENNEL SEED

★ **ESSENTIAL OILS**

● **BONES AND JOINTS** Gout.

● **DIGESTIVE SYSTEM** Abdominal pain, colic, nausea and vomiting (including morning sickness).

Fennel seeds are gently tonic and diuretic. They have an oestrogen-like effect and can help to regulate menstruation. The main medicinal use of fennel seeds is for digestive problems, such as poor appetite and digestion, bloating, nausea and flatulence. The seeds also promote urination and the elimination of uric acid.

RECIPES *fennel-seed decoction (page 126).*

# CONDIMENTS, HONEY AND WINE

## PEPPERCORNS

★ TRACE ELEMENTS (INCLUDING CHROMIUM), COMPLEX ESSENTIAL OIL (PIPERIN)

● DIGESTIVE SYSTEM Diarrhoea, dyspepsia.

● IMMUNE SYSTEM Colds, sore throat.

Peppercorns are good for digestive problems and circulatory problems, such as chilblains. They stimulate the heart and peripheral circulation, although excessive consumption of pepper may aggravate any inflammation of the stomach and intestines.

## VINEGAR

★ POTASSIUM, PHOSPHORUS, TRACE ELEMENTS SUCH AS COPPER AND ZINC

● BONES AND JOINTS Arthritis (rheumatoid), gout, rheumatism.

● IMMUNE SYSTEM Sore throat.

Vinegar is helpful for a variety of conditions. A gargle made of honey, vinegar and water may help to ease sore throats. Vinegar is also a traditional toner and disinfectant for the skin. Because it acts as a solvent it is able to take up the active ingredients of the medicinal plants that are preserved in it. Home-made aromatic vinegar can be added to salads or used in cooking, thereby increasing the medicinal value of other foods. Excessive consumption of vinegar should be avoided as it may upset the stomach and cause digestive problems, such as gastritis.

RECIPES *pickled turnips (page 120), pickled beetroot (page 120), pickled cauliflower (page 120), blackberry vinegar (page 120), raspberry vinegar (page 120), borage leaves in vinegar (page 122), tarragon vinegar (page 122), shallot vinegar (page 122), herb vinegar (page 122), amazingly aromatic vinegar (page 122).*

## MUSTARD

★ ESSENTIAL OIL, FERMENTING AGENTS

● DIGESTIVE SYSTEM Constipation.

The white mustard seed is used as a condiment and the black seed is commonly used by herbalists. Mustard causes a sensation of heat in the stomach and stimulates the digestion.

RECIPES *table mustard (page 122).*

## HONEY

★ AROMATIC SUBSTANCES, FRUCTOSE, GLUCOSE, POLLEN

● DIGESTIVE SYSTEM Diarrhoea.

● RESPIRATORY SYSTEM Asthma, bronchitis.

● IMMUNE SYSTEM Sore throat.

Honey is a natural antibiotic that works both internally and externally. It eases respiratory infections, calms the nerves, induces sleep and disinfects wounds and sores. As well as being an effective treatment for diarrhoea, it also has laxative properties. A few drops of lemon juice mixed with a teaspoon of honey is an excellent sore throat remedy.

RECIPES *honey and ginger grilled salmon (page 63), peach syrup (page 130).*

## POLLEN

★ VITAMINS B, D, E, MAGNESIUM, POTASSIUM, TRACE ELEMENTS, ESSENTIAL AMINO ACIDS

Pollen is an easily assimilated natural food supplement that is recommended for anyone suffering from low energy levels. One tablespoon a day is the standard recommended dose, although some specialists recommend more.

## ROYAL JELLY

★ VITAMINS B COMPLEX, C, AMINO ACIDS

● BLOOD AND CIRCULATION Anaemia.

● NERVOUS SYSTEM, MIND AND EMOTIONS Depression, mental fatigue.

Royal jelly is a white substance produced by bees to feed to the larvae of potential queen bees. It is a powerful tonic that is particularly recommended for children and elderly people.

## WINE

★ BIOFLAVONOIDS, TANNINS

● BLOOD AND CIRCULATION High blood pressure.

Small amounts of wine (no more than 2 glasses a day) are recommended for enhancing the health of the cardiovascular system. Red wine, in particular, has been found to reduce the incidence of heart disease, particularly among those suffering from high cholesterol and high blood pressure.

RECIPES *blackcurrant wine (page 127), cinnamon wine (page 127), artichoke-leaf wine (page 128), cherry-leaf wine (page 128), juniper-berry wine (page 128), camomile and citrus wine (page 129), camomile aperitif (page 129).*

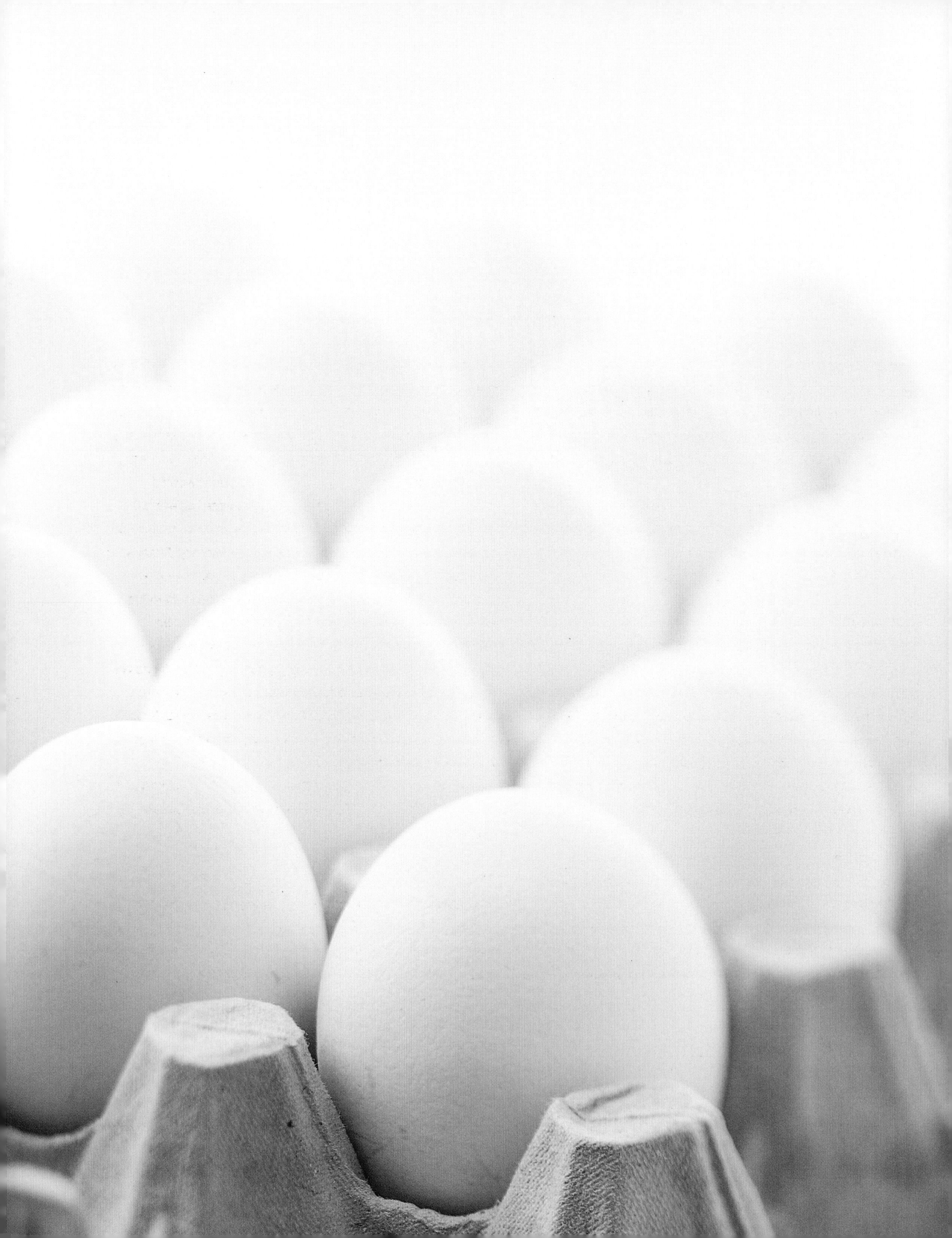

# meat, fish and dairy produce

### POULTRY AND GAME

★ **VITAMIN B COMPLEX, IRON, TRACE ELEMENTS, ZINC, PROTEIN**

The main advantage of poultry and game is that they are usually leaner than other types of meat. Red meat, for example, contains a large amount of hidden fat – this can have an adverse effect on cholesterol levels and increase the risk of fatty deposits building up in the arteries. Reducing your intake of red meat and eating game and poultry instead can reduce the risk of cardiovascular disease.

RECIPES *chicken breasts with celeriac mash (page 106), chicken, millet, barley and celeriac pilaff (page 107).*

### RED MEAT

★ **VITAMIN B COMPLEX (ESPECIALLY B12), IRON, SELENIUM, ZINC, ESSENTIAL AMINO ACIDS AND PROTEIN**

Red meat should be eaten in moderation because of its high fat content. Lean cuts of lamb, pork and beef should be selected and visible fat trimmed off. Modern food production methods mean that there may be traces of antibiotics and hormones in meat. As with all food, use organic produce where possible.

RECIPES *lamb with spinach and lentils (page 105).*

### SHELLFISH

★ **IODINE, IRON, SELENIUM, ZINC AND OTHER TRACE ELEMENTS AND PROTEIN**

Shellfish provide energy and are a good source of the antioxidant minerals zinc and selenium. They help to boost the immune system and are a low-fat source of protein. It is a good idea to eat shellfish on a regular basis as an alternative to meat.

### MILK, CHEESE, BUTTER, YOGHURT

★ **VITAMINS A, B, D, CALCIUM, ALL ESSENTIAL AMINO ACIDS, PROTEIN**

Although milk and milk products are good sources of protein and calcium, they are also difficult to digest. This is because during the sterilization process milk is subjected to intense heat that destroys its natural ferments. These ferments help the digestion of lactose – the sugar found in milk. Without the aid of these bacteria, lactose intolerance becomes more likely. Symptoms of lactose intolerance include diarrhoea, bloating, abdominal pain and wind. Milk can also exacerbate eczema and respiratory problems involving mucus. If you suspect that you suffer from lactose intolerance, eliminate milk and milk products from your diet for two weeks and see if your symptoms diminish in frequency or intensity. Cheese, butter and cream should be consumed only in small quantities because they are rich in saturated fat and can contribute to the build up of fatty deposits in the arteries. Avoid these foods altogether if you are overweight or have high cholesterol levels (or switch to low-fat products). Live yoghurt is good for the health of the digestive tract and retains the natural bacteria that help to digest lactose. Dairy products can be made more digestible by mixing them with live yoghurt. For example, mix cottage cheese with 2–3 tablespoons of live yoghurt.

RECIPES *cottage cheese with watercress (page 101), halibut steak and nettle butter (page 107), fresh figs with raspberry cheese (page 115).*

### EGG

★ **VITAMINS B, D, CALCIUM, CHROMIUM, IODINE, IRON, SELENIUM, ZINC, CHOLESTEROL, PROTEIN**

Eggs are a good source of protein but they should be avoided by people with high cholesterol levels. Choose organically produced free-range eggs.

RECIPES *buckwheat with leek sauce (page 103), leek and chive mimosa with polenta (page 105).*

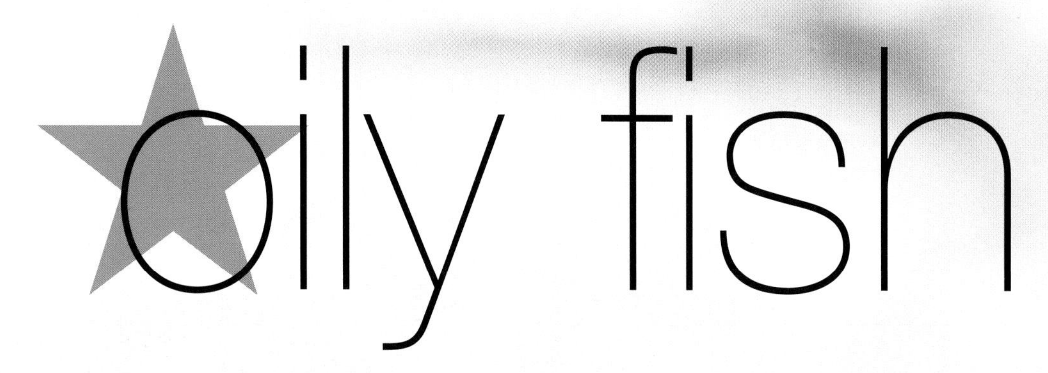

# oily fish

**OILY FISH, SUCH AS MACKEREL, SALMON, HERRING AND TUNA, ARE RICH IN POLYUNSATURATED FATS KNOWN AS OMEGA-3 FATTY ACIDS. A SUBSTANTIAL BODY OF RESEARCH HAS LINKED DIETS RICH IN OMEGA-3 FATTY ACIDS WITH A LOW INCIDENCE OF CARDIOVASCULAR DISEASE.**

## The properties of oily fish

Both freshwater and saltwater oily fish are an important part of a nutritious, medicinal diet. Most nutrition experts suggest that they should be eaten frequently, particularly as an alternative to red meat. Oily fish are rich in vitamin D and omega-3 fatty acids which makes them good for the health of the cardiovascular system. Research shows that the incidence of cardiovascular disease is lowest in populations that eat a diet high in omega-3 fatty acids – the Eskimo population, whose diet is dominated by oily fish, is an excellent example of this.

## Preventing illness

Oily fish can help to reduce some major health problems, such as high blood pressure, atherosclerosis and arteriosclerosis. It is estimated that regular consumption of fish and fish oil can reduce the risk of heart attack by approximately one third. Oily fish have an anti-inflammatory action that makes them useful for health problems, such as ulcerative colitis and rheumatoid arthritis, that are characterized by inflammation. Oily fish are also recommended for eczema, psoriasis, multiple sclerosis and they may help to protect the body from cancer. Research suggests that omega-3 fatty acids may counteract certain types of allergies and assist brain development in children.

An important role of omega-3 fatty acids is the creation of prostaglandins. Prostaglandins are hormone-like substances that have numerous health benefits, such as keeping the blood thin, lowering blood pressure, maintaining water balance and regulating blood sugar.

## Including fish in the diet

Omega-3 fatty acids are found in a range of fish and shellfish but the most abundant sources are mackerel, herring, anchovies, trout, salmon, sardine, whitebait, pilchards and red tuna. People who have had a heart attack or who suffer from chronic cardiovascular illness are advised to eat 30 g of these types of oily fish every day. Those who are in reasonable health and do not have cardiovascular disease are advised to eat oily fish twice weekly in order to maintain long-term health.

It is easy to confuse fish oil and omega-3 fatty acids with cod liver oil. Many people take cod liver oil in supplement form during the winter months (care should be taken as overdosing on this may damage your health). Although cod liver oil is an excellent source of the fat-soluble vitamins A and D, it is a poor source of omega-3 fatty acids. The best source of omega-3 fatty acids is fresh oily fish; if this is not available, canned sardine or mackerel is a good alternative.

### STAR FOOD PROFILE

- **BONES AND JOINTS** Arthritis (rheumatoid).
- **BLOOD AND CIRCULATION** Atherosclerosis, arteriosclerosis, high blood pressure.
- **DIGESTIVE SYSTEM** Ulcerative colitis.
- **SKIN, HAIR AND NAILS** Eczema, psoriasis.

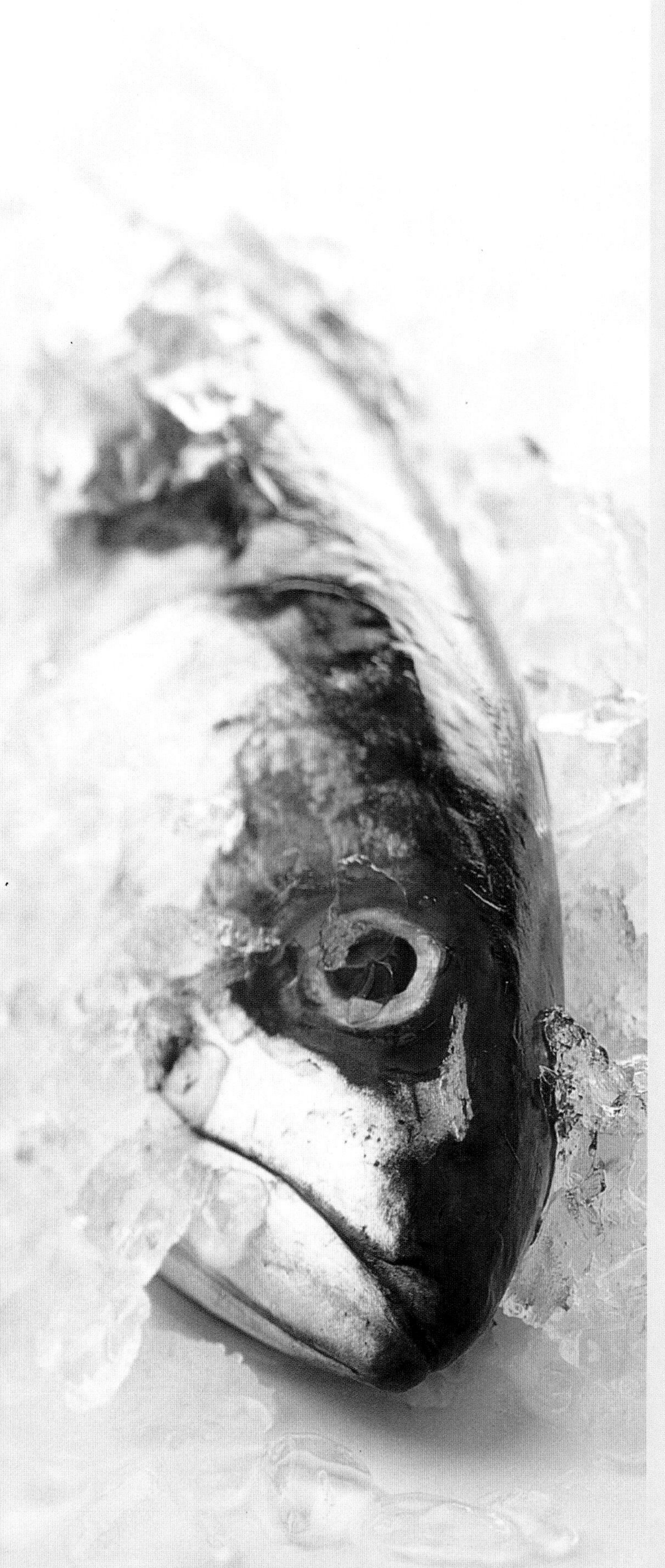

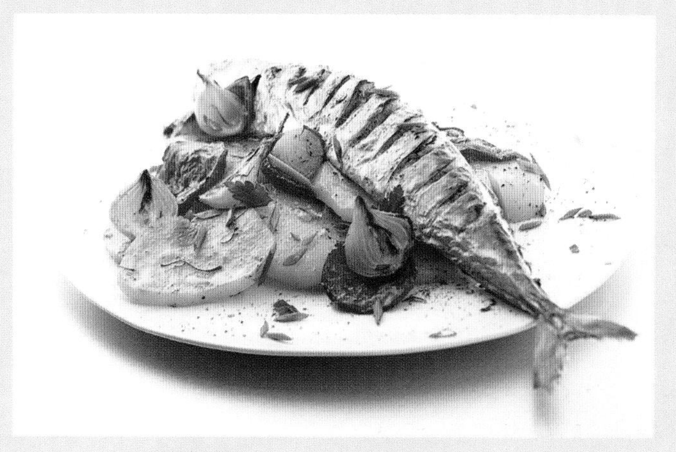

# cotriade of mackerel

3 potatoes, sliced
2 medium tomatoes, sliced
150 g small onions, halved
2 cloves
2 cloves of garlic
1 bouquet garni
Pinch of saffron
Salt and pepper
150 ml dry white wine
300 ml water
1 kg mackerel, cleaned and gutted
To garnish: 2 tbsp parsley or chives, chopped

Spread the potatoes on the bottom of a large, well-oiled ovenproof dish. Add the other ingredients, except the parsley or chives. Put the dish in a preheated oven at 200ºC/gas mark 6 for 20 minutes or until the fish is cooked. Serve hot or warm sprinkled with parsley or chives.

# honey and ginger grilled salmon

800 g salmon fillet
5-cm piece of ginger root, peeled and grated
2 cloves of garlic
3 tbsp soy sauce
½ tsp Chinese five spice powder
2 tbsp clear honey
2 spring onions, chopped

In a large bowl, combine all of the ingredients. Mix well, cover with cling film and refrigerate for 30 minutes. Remove the salmon from the marinade (keep the marinade) and pat dry. Grill or pan fry for 5 minutes on either side, brushing with the marinade during cooking.

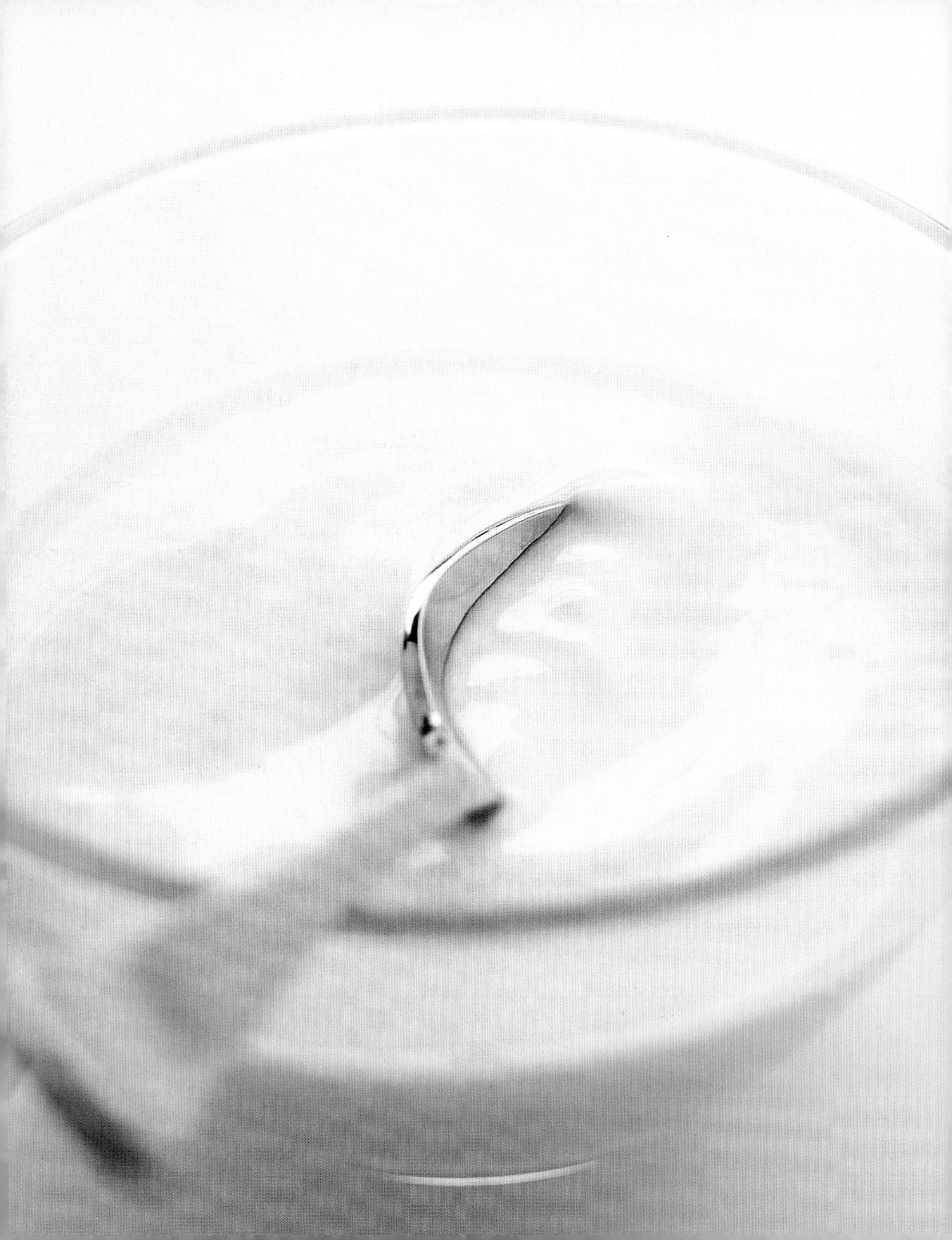

chapter two

# foods for common ailments

When the body is fighting disease it needs all the help it can get – informed dietary choices can provide this help. To guide you through these choices, the following pages list over 100 ailments, organized by the body system that they affect. Symptom profiles, lists of beneficial foods and foods to avoid, menu suggestions to ensure the healthy function of each body system and page references to useful recipes are all designed to help you to help your body combat illness and glow with health.

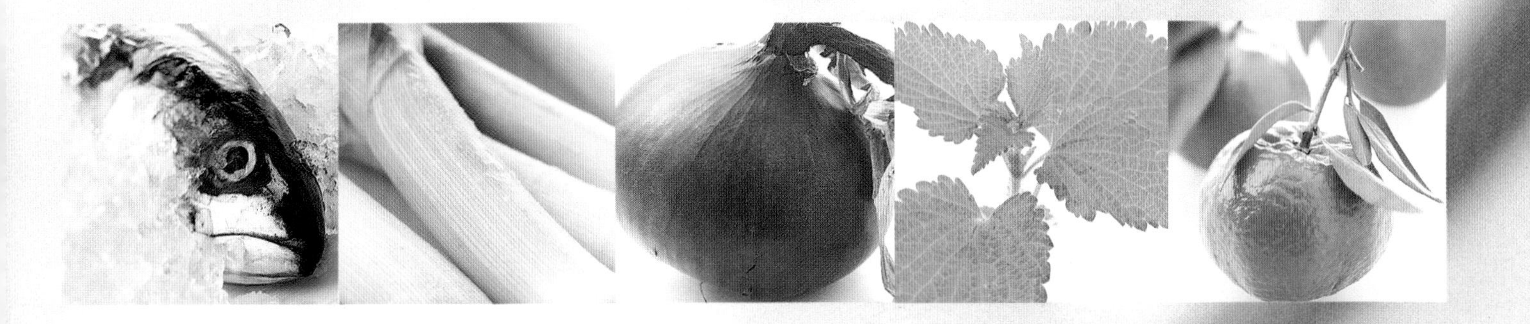

# bones and joints

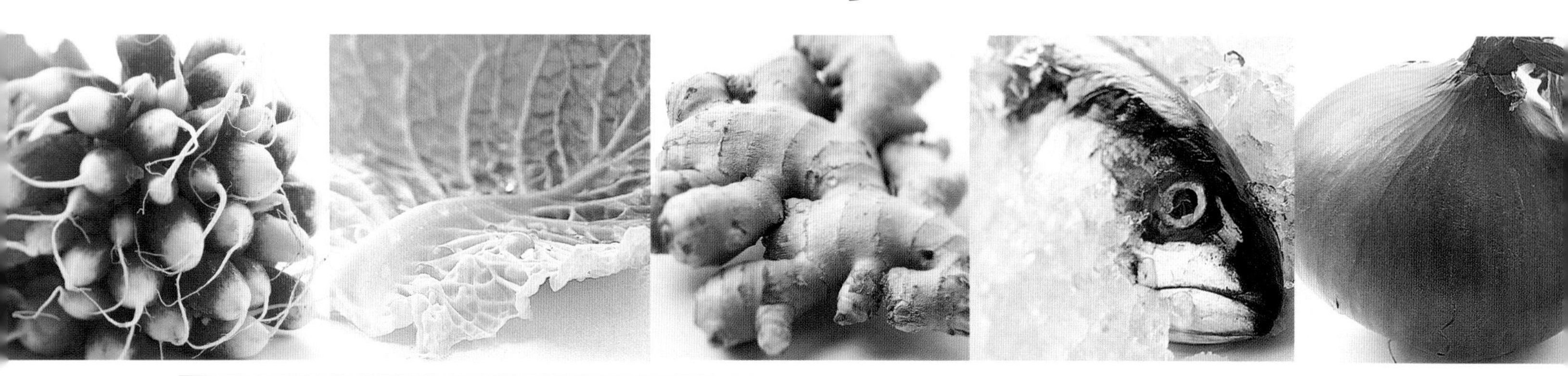

**STAR FOODS FOR BONES AND JOINTS: ARTICHOKE, CABBAGE, CHEESE, CUCUMBER, DANDELION, FISH OIL, GINGER, GREEN BEAN, LEEK, MILK, NETTLE, OILY FISH, ONION, RADISH.**

Our muscles, bones and joints suffer constantly from small traumas during everyday use. The musculo-skeletal system also changes gradually over the years, which may result in pain, stiffness, inflammation or some restriction of movement.

Good circulation and the elimination of uric acid are important factors in retaining maximum mobility and staying free of aches and pains. To protect your bones and joints, a constitutional approach is best: avoid alcohol, acid-forming foods and too much red meat; increase your intake of foods that are rich in minerals (such as green beans), foods that promote detoxification (artichokes, dandelion, radishes) and foods that are diuretic (cucumber, leeks, onions). Calcium and vitamin D help to strengthen the bones – calcium-rich foods include cheese, milk and fresh vegetables, and oily fish is a good source of vitamin D. Juices and infusions are useful for both bone mineralization and the elimination of waste. If you suffer from chronic arthritis or rheumatism, you should follow a strict detox programme (such as the one outlined on pages 134–37) at regular intervals.

Regular gentle exercise helps you to stay mobile. Excess weight can have an adverse effect on weight-bearing joints, such as the hips, knees and the lower part of the spine. If you experience pain or discomfort in these joints, you may need to consider losing weight by following a low-calorie diet.

(N.B. To make a medicinal infusion, steep 1 tablespoon of the dried ingredient in a cup of boiling water for 10 minutes.)

## ARTHRITIS (RHEUMATOID)

**PAIN, INFLAMMATION AND SWELLING IN ANY OF THE JOINTS WITH OVERALL ACHING OR STIFFNESS. ARTHRITIS IS A CHRONIC, HEREDITARY ILLNESS INVOLVING AN AUTO-IMMUNE REACTION.**

**! ALLERGIES TO DAIRY, WHEAT, FAT OR OTHER FOOD CAN SOMETIMES EXACERBATE OR EVEN TRIGGER AN ATTACK. IF YOU SUSPECT THAT THIS IS THE CASE, ELIMINATE A FOOD FROM YOUR DIET FOR 2–3 WEEKS, RE-INTRODUCE IT GRADUALLY AND MONITOR SYMPTOMS.**

✓ Apple, artichoke, asparagus, banana, blackcurrant, blueberry, cabbage, cauliflower, celery, cherry, chicory, chive and spring onion, corn, cucumber, dandelion, fennel, garlic, gooseberry, grapefruit, grape and raisin, green bean, horseradish, juniper berry, lamb's lettuce, leek, lemon, lettuce, melon, millet, nettle, oily fish, onion, parsnip, pear, pepper, pineapple, potato, prune, radish, redcurrant, salsify, tarragon, thyme, tomato, vinegar, watercress. Ginger has analgesic properties and promotes circulation – massage painful joints with a combination of ginger, rosemary and juniper-berry essential oils mixed with vegetable oil (page 56).

✗ Alcohol, coffee, cooked fat and oil, dairy products, dried beans and lentils, game and poultry, peanuts, processed food, red meat, refined oils, sorrel, sugar, tea, white flour.

RECIPES *carrot, cabbage and sweet pepper juice (page 21), chick-pea broth (page 92), broccoli and green bean juice (page 119), pear and apple infusion (page 124), cherry-stem decoction (page 125), cherry-stem and apple decoction (page 126), strawberry-leaf decoction (page 126), cherry-leaf wine (page 128).*

## ANKYLOSING SPONDYLITIS

**PROGRESSIVE, CHRONIC INFLAMMATION OF THE SPINE CAUSING FLARE-UPS OF PAIN AND STIFFNESS. MOST COMMON AMONG YOUNG MEN.**

✓ To relieve pain, rub some olive oil infused with bay leaves, juniper berries, camomile and rosemary flowers on the affected area of the back. Take infusions of blackcurrant leaves or strawberry root and leaves. *SEE ALSO* Arthritis (rheumatoid).

✗ *SEE* Arthritis (rheumatoid).

*RECIPES strawberry-leaf decoction (page 126), artichoke-leaf wine (page 128).*

## BURSITIS

**INFLAMMATION OF A FLUID-FILLED SAC (BURSA) THAT PROTECTS A JOINT FROM FRICTION. SYMPTOMS INCLUDE PAIN, SWELLING AND RESTRICTION OF MOVEMENT IN AFFECTED JOINTS, TYPICALLY THE SHOULDER, WRIST, ELBOW, KNEE AND FINGERS.**

✓ Drink pear- or blackcurrant-leaf infusion. Apply a poultice of fresh cabbage leaves to the affected joints two or three times a day to reduce inflammation. *SEE ALSO* general advice on the care of muscles and joints.

*RECIPES pear and apple infusion (page 124).*

## CARPAL TUNNEL SYNDROME

**COMPRESSION OF A NERVE THAT TRAVELS THROUGH THE WRIST. SYMPTOMS INCLUDE PAIN THAT SHOOTS UP THE ARM, AND NUMB, TINGLING OR BURNING SENSATIONS IN THE HAND AND FINGERS. MAY BE HORMONAL (IT CAN OCCUR SPONTANEOUSLY DURING PREGNANCY), OR CAUSED BY A REPETITIVE STRAIN INJURY.**

✓ Frequent application of a poultice of cabbage leaves or a mixture of green clay, cabbage leaves (processed in a blender) and mashed cucumber may help to reduce pain and inflammation in the wrist. *SEE ALSO* general advice on the care of bones and joints and Bursitis.

## SUGGESTED MENUS FOR INFLAMED JOINTS AND OTHER PAINFUL JOINT CONDITIONS

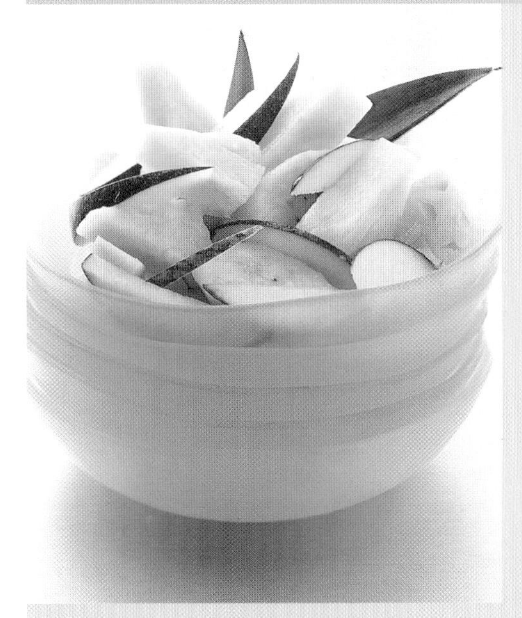

The following menus are designed for people suffering from arthritis, rheumatism, joint pain and inflammation, fibrositis or polymyalgia rheumatica, and include foods that have anti-inflammatory properties. Arthritis sufferers whose condition is exacerbated by an allergy to alcohol, dairy products or wheat should avoid the foods marked with an asterisk.

### MENU 1

**BREAKFAST**

A bowl of sugar-free porridge with skimmed milk*, yoghurt* and a small glass of juice made from green beans, cabbage or other vegetables; or a fruit juice combination such as pineapple, apple and strawberry.

**SNACKS**

Dried fruit, especially raisins or apricots, and dandelion or roast-chicory coffee.

**LUNCH**

Chickpea or leek and potato soup with brown bread*; a mixed salad of lamb's lettuce, green beans and radishes with olive oil and lemon juice; poached salmon with potatoes; a pear or an apple.

**DINNER**

Steamed vegetables with ginger and garlic and a small amount of rice or noodles; an infusion of dandelion or blackcurrant leaves or a small glass of artichoke-leaf wine*.

### MENU 2

**BREAKFAST**

A bowl of cottage cheese* mixed with two or three tablespoons of yoghurt*, a glass of fruit juice (grape, apple or cherry) and a slice of melon or a banana.

**SNACKS**

Dried fruit, especially blackcurrants or raisins, and dandelion or roast-chicory coffee.

**LUNCH**

Pasta with vegetables, smoked salmon and brown bread*; a piece of fruit.

**DINNER**

A mixed salad with brown bread*; an infusion of camomile or blackcurrant leaves or a small glass of artichoke-leaf wine*.

## CHRONIC BACK PAIN

! MAY REQUIRE OSTEOPATHIC OR CHIROPRACTIC TREATMENT.

✓ *SEE* Arthritis (rheumatoid) and Osteoarthritis.

## CRAMPS (MUSCULAR)

A SUDDEN MUSCULAR SPASM CAUSING TEMPORARY PAIN AND DISCOMFORT – MAY BE DUE TO A CIRCULATORY PROBLEM.

✓ Tarragon is well known for its anti-spasmodic action. Eat plenty of magnesium-rich foods, such as whole-grain cereals, nuts, seeds, seafood and green vegetables. *SEE ALSO* general advice in Heart and Circulation.

## FIBROSITIS

MUSCULAR STIFFNESS IN AREAS SUCH AS THE BACK, NECK AND SHOULDERS CAUSED BY DEPOSITS OF LACTIC AND URIC ACID AROUND THE MUSCLE FIBRES.

✓ Massage some olive oil infused with rosemary and juniper or bay berries into the affected area. *SEE ALSO* Arthritis (rheumatoid), Gout and Ankylosing spondylitis.

## GOUT

SUDDEN ATTACK OF SEVERE PAIN, SWELLING AND INFLAMMATION, OFTEN IN THE BIG TOES, ANKLES, KNEES OR ELBOWS, OWING TO A BUILD-UP OF URIC ACID CRYSTALS IN THE JOINTS. RECURRENT ATTACKS MAY BE FREQUENT.

✓ Basil, celery, chervil, nettle, raisin, raspberry, rosemary, strawberry. Apply a poultice of fresh cabbage leaves to affected joints to reduce pain and inflammation. *SEE ALSO* Arthritis (rheumatoid).

✗ Tea, coffee, rhubarb.

*RECIPES apple and raspberry juice (page 117), dandelion infusion (page 123), strawberry-leaf decoction (page 126), artichoke-leaf tincture (page 130).*

## OSTEOARTHRITIS

A CHRONIC, DEGENERATIVE CONDITION AFFECTING MOSTLY WEIGHT-BEARING JOINTS, COMMON IN THOSE AGED 40 AND OVER.

✓ Apple, asparagus, blackcurrant, cabbage, celery, chervil, bean, dandelion, ginger, leek, olive, radish, salsify, yoghurt. Drink fresh vegetable or fruit juice every day and increase the amount of oily fish, fish oil and shellfish in your diet. *SEE ALSO* general advice on Bones and Joints.

## OSTEOPOROSIS

LITERALLY "POROUS BONE" – A GRADUAL LOSS OF CALCIUM CAUSES BONES TO BECOME WEAK, BRITTLE AND PRONE TO FRACTURE. OSTEOPOROSIS IS COMMON IN POSTMENOPAUSAL WOMEN WHO HAVE LOW OESTROGEN LEVELS (THIS HORMONE REGULATES THE UPTAKE OF CALCIUM).

! A CALCIUM- AND MAGNESIUM-RICH DIET MUST BE SUPPORTED BY REGULAR LOW-INTENSITY EXERCISE AND EXPOSURE TO SUNLIGHT.

✓ Cottage cheese, fish oil, fresh fruit, goat's cheese, all green, leafy vegetables, hard cheese such as Parmesan, oily fish, soya, tofu, yoghurt.

## POLYMYALGIA RHEUMATICA

INFLAMMATION OF CONNECTIVE TISSUE AROUND A GROUP OF MUSCLES CAUSING PAIN, STIFFNESS AND MILD FEVER.

✓ *SEE* Anaemia, Arthritis (rheumatoid) and Fibrositis.

## RESTLESS LEGS SYNDROME

BURNING, ACHING SENSATION IN THE LEGS CAUSING RESTLESSNESS AND TWITCHING. THE SUFFERER BECOMES IRRITABLE AND FIDGETY.

! MAY BE ASSOCIATED WITH IRON AND VITAMIN-B DEFICIENCY.

✓ Take infusions of camomile, elderberry, ginger, lemon balm, limeflower, rosemary. Use ginger, chillies and rosemary regularly in cooking. *SEE ALSO* general advice in Heart and Circulation.

✗ Tea, coffee.

*RECIPES lemon-balm and camomile infusion (page 124), elder and camomile infusion (page 124), ginger infusion (page 125).*

## RHEUMATISM

ANY DISEASE THAT IS CHARACTERIZED BY INFLAMMATION IN THE MUSCLES AND JOINTS, PARTICULARLY RHEUMATOID ARTHRITIS.

✓ *SEE* Arthritis (rheumatoid) and Fibrositis.

## TENDINITIS

INFLAMMATION OF A TENDON (THE FIBROUS TISSUE THAT CONNECTS MUSCLES AND BONES).

✓ *SEE* Bursitis.

## TENOSYNOVITIS

INFLAMMATION OF A TENDON AND THE PROTECTIVE SHEATH THAT SURROUNDS IT.

✓ *SEE* Bursitis.

# heart and circulation

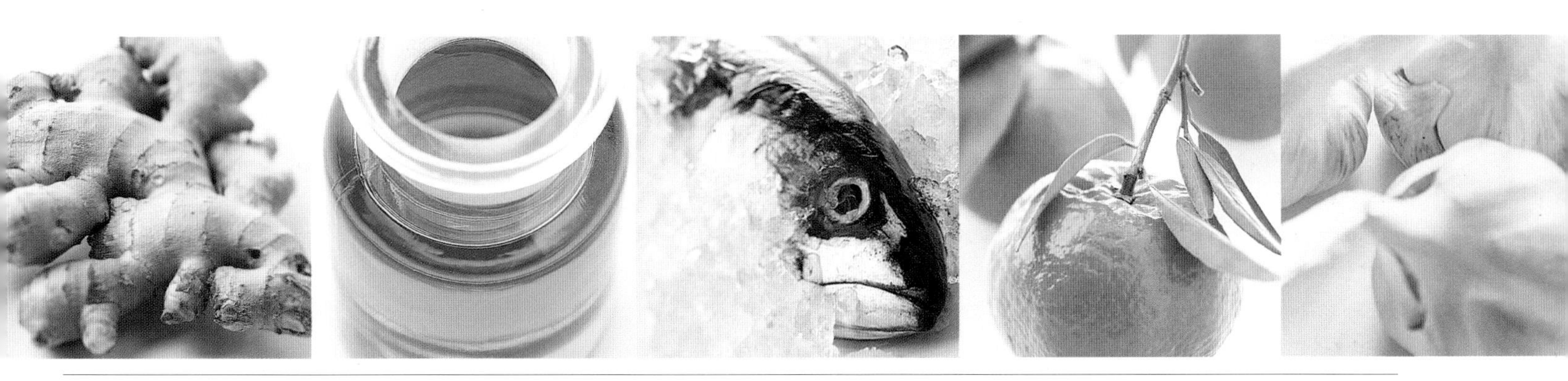

STAR FOODS FOR HEART AND CIRCULATION: BARLEY, BUCKWHEAT, CHICORY, CLOVE, GARLIC, GINGER, GREEN BEAN, LEEK, LEMON, LETTUCE, LIME, OAT, OILY FISH, OLIVE OIL, OLIVE, ONION, ORANGE, PARSLEY, PARSNIP, POTATO, PULSES, ROSEMARY, SHALLOT AND SPINACH.

Diet plays a fundamental role in the health of the heart and blood vessels. A good diet can help to keep the cardiovascular system working efficiently throughout life whereas a bad diet is a major risk factor for hypertension, atherosclerosis, heart attack and stroke. The Western diet, which tends to be high in saturated fat, sugar and salt encourages the development of fatty deposits, known as atheroma, in the arteries. The arteries narrow and problems such as blood clots and heart attacks become more likely.

If you have suffered a heart attack, the most effective way to avoid a second attack is to follow a diet that protects your cardiovascular system. Increase your intake of oily fish and fibre-rich foods; eat more potassium-rich vegetables, garlic, ginger, green vegetables and fruit, as these may help to lower your blood pressure. Bioflavonoids, found in yellow, orange, red and green vegetables and fruit, are antioxidants that help to reduce the formation of fatty deposits and clots in the arteries. Reduce your consumption of red or fatty meat (especially pork), full-fat dairy products, eggs, sugar, salt and alcohol. Eliminate fried and fast foods from your diet. Take regular, low intensity exercise, such as swimming, cycling, walking or jogging, three times a week for at least one hour at a time. If you are overweight, start following a low-calorie diet. If you smoke, it is vital that you make every effort to give up. (N.B. To make a medicinal infusion, steep 1 tablespoon of the dried ingredient in a cup of boiling water for 10 minutes.)

## ANAEMIA

A DEFICIENCY OF IRON IN THE BLOOD, COMMONLY CAUSED BY A LACK OF IRON-RICH FOODS IN THE DIET OR BY A LOSS OF BLOOD, OFTEN THROUGH HEAVY MENSTRUATION. PERNICIOUS ANAEMIA IS CAUSED BY AN INABILITY TO ABSORB VITAMIN B12

✓ Iron-rich foods: apricot (dried), beetroot, blackberry, blackcurrant, broccoli, carrot, chervil, chestnut, dandelion, fresh fruit and vegetable juices, green bean, lamb's lettuce, nettle, parsley, prune, royal jelly, spinach, watercress. Vitamin B-rich foods: lean red meat, molasses, yeast extract. Drink plenty of fresh fruit and vegetable juices including blackberry, black cherry, grape, lettuce, spinach, fennel. If you are a vegetarian, it may be helpful to take a daily vitamin B12 supplement (this should be available from most health shops).

RECIPES *nettle soup (page 94), cabbage, carrot and celery juice (page 119), green bean and garlic juice (page 119), broccoli and green bean juice (page 119), celery and red onion juice (page 119), fennel infusion (page 123), fennel-seed decoction (page 126), blackcurrant wine (page 127).*

## ANGINA

TEMPORARY SENSATIONS OF PRESSURE OR PAIN IN THE CENTRE OF THE CHEST RESULTING FROM POOR BLOOD SUPPLY TO THE HEART. USUALLY CAUSED BY BLOCKED AND NARROWED ARTERIES. ATTACKS ARE TRIGGERED BY STRESS AND EXERTION.

! DO NOT STOP TAKING MEDICATION PRESCRIBED BY YOUR DOCTOR.

**SEVERE CHEST PAIN THAT IS NOT ALLEVIATED BY REST SHOULD BE TREATED AS A MEDICAL EMERGENCY.**

✓ Eat a small portion of oily fish every day. Increase your intake of magnesium-rich food, such as whole-grain cereal products, nuts and seeds. Drink infusions of olive leaves and limeflower. *SEE ALSO* Atherosclerosis, Arteriosclerosis, High blood pressure and Stress (page 83).

✗ Fatty red meat, full-fat dairy products (such as butter, high-fat cheese and double cream), egg, sugary foods, salt and alcohol. Avoid fried and fast foods.

*RECIPES garlic tincture (page 54), green bean and garlic juice (page 119), broccoli and green bean juice (page 119), celery and red onion juice (page 119), lemon-balm and camomile infusion (page 124), ginger infusion (page 125).*

## ARTERIOSCLEROSIS

**THE HARDENING OF ARTERIES IN OLD AGE, A CONDITION OFTEN ACCELERATED OR AGGRAVATED BY A DIET THAT CONTAINS AN EXCESS OF ALCOHOL, FAT, SALT AND SUGAR.**

**! DO NOT STOP TAKING MEDICATION PRESCRIBED BY YOUR DOCTOR.**

✓ Apricot, artichoke leaf, asparagus, black radish, blueberry, camomile, celery, chicory, dandelion, fish, garlic, grape, lamb's lettuce, lettuce, limeflower, onion, orange, parsley, pineapple, potato, pumpkin, raspberry, rosemary, rye, saffron, spring onion and chive, strawberry. *SEE ALSO* Atherosclerosis.

✗ Alcohol, fast and processed foods, fatty red meat, fried or oily foods, full-fat dairy products, salt, sugar.

*RECIPES garlic tincture (page 54), strawberry-leaf decoction (page 126), artichoke-leaf wine (page 128).*

## ATHEROSCLEROSIS

**THE CLOGGING UP OF ARTERIES BY FATTY DEPOSITS KNOWN AS ATHEROMAS. THIS CONDITION IS DIRECTLY LINKED TO AN EXCESS OF FAT AND SUGAR IN THE DIET.**

**! DO NOT STOP TAKING MEDICATION PRESCRIBED BY YOUR DOCTOR.**

✓ Apricot, blackcurrant, blueberry, celery, cherry, fig, garlic, germinated barley, ginger, grape, lemon, oat, olive, pineapple, prune, sage, seaweed. Eat oily fish as often as possible and plenty of yellow, orange, red and green, leafy vegetables. Take artichoke, blackcurrant (leaves and fruit) and strawberry-leaf infusions or decoctions. Drink blueberry juice.

✗ Fatty red meat, full-fat dairy products, fried or oily foods, fast and processed foods, foods that are high in sugar.

*RECIPES cabbage, carrot and blueberry juice (page 25), cabbage, carrot and celery juice (page 119), ginger infusion (page 125), strawberry-leaf decoction (page 126), barley water (page 127).*

## SUGGESTED MENUS FOR HIGH BLOOD PRESSURE

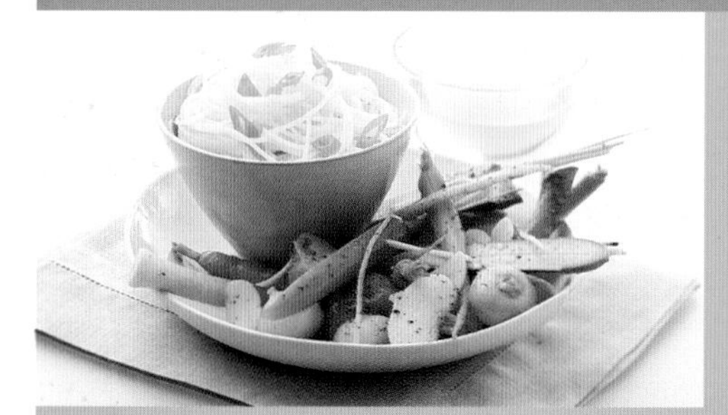

The following menus are designed to promote weight loss and should ease symptoms associated with stress and high blood pressure, such as digestive problems and water retention. The menus are also recommended for anyone with a heart or circulatory condition. If you are not trying to lose weight, simply increase the amount of food in each meal.

**MENU 1**

**BREAKFAST**
A bowl of sugar-free cereal with skimmed milk; yoghurt; a small glass of lettuce, cucumber and garlic juice or pineapple, apple and strawberry juice.

**SNACKS**
Any dried fruit; dandelion coffee substitute.

**LUNCH**
Lentil soup with brown bread; a salad of fennel, radicchio and olives with olive oil and lemon juice dressing; fish with potatoes; a piece of fruit.

**DINNER**
Steamed vegetables with ginger and garlic on a small bed of noodles (left); a small glass of artichoke-leaf wine (page 128).

**MENU 2**

**BREAKFAST**
A bowl of porridge; grape or apple juice.

**SNACKS**
Any dried fruit; dandelion coffee substitute.

**LUNCH**
Leek and potato soup; cottage cheese, smoked salmon and brown bread; a piece of fruit.

**DINNER**
A mixed salad with brown bread; an infusion of camomile or blackcurrant leaves.

### CHILBLAINS

**PAINFUL, ITCHY SWELLINGS OF THE SKIN CAUSED BY EXPOSURE TO COLD AND POOR CIRCULATION.**

✓ To improve circulation: blackcurrant, blackberry, blueberry, cabbage, carrot, chervil, garlic, ginger, redcurrant. Consume a lot of warm food and drinks. Drink blackberry-leaf infusion. SEE ALSO Anaemia.

RECIPES *ginger infusion (page 125).*

### HIGH BLOOD PRESSURE

**HIGH BLOOD PRESSURE (HYPERTENSION) OCCURS WHEN THERE IS RESISTANCE IN THE BLOOD VESSELS TO THE FLOW OF BLOOD. IT IS OFTEN SYMPTOMLESS OR ASSOCIATED WITH HIGH CHOLESTEROL AND ARTERIOSCLEROSIS. RISK FACTORS INCLUDE CHRONIC STRESS, AGE, POOR DIET AND EXCESSIVE ALCOHOL CONSUMPTION. HIGH BLOOD PRESSURE GREATLY INCREASES THE PATIENT'S RISK OF SUFFERING A STROKE OR HEART ATTACK.**

**! DO NOT STOP TAKING MEDICATION PRESCRIBED BY YOUR DOCTOR.**

✓ Artichoke, asparagus, broccoli, celery, dandelion, garlic, grape, leek, lettuce, oat, oily fish, olive and olive oil, olive-leaf infusion, onion, pomegranate, potassium-rich vegetables, red wine, rice, rye, sunflower seeds and oil, tomato. Increase your intake of magnesium-rich food, such as whole-grain cereal products, nuts and seeds. In many cases, overcoming obesity is the most effective way of lowering high blood pressure – follow a low-calorie, dairy-free, wheat-free diet for as long as necessary. Combine this diet with regular low-intensity, prolonged exercise. Drink grape juice and infusions of artichoke and olive leaf. SEE ALSO Atherosclerosis.

✗ High-fat foods, including dairy products, and wheat.

RECIPES *cabbage, carrot and blueberry juice (page 25), garlic tincture (page 54), celery and tomato juice (page 118), green bean and garlic juice (page 119), celery and red onion juice (page 119), cucumber and lettuce heart juice (page 119), lettuce and basil juice (page 119), dandelion infusion (page 123).*

### HYPERLIPIDAEMIA

**AN EXCESSIVE AMOUNT OF FAT IN THE BLOOD. OFTEN LINKED TO HEAVY ALCOHOL CONSUMPTION, SMOKING, LACK OF EXERCISE AND A DIET THAT IS HIGH IN FAT.**

**! DO NOT STOP TAKING MEDICATION PRESCRIBED BY YOUR DOCTOR.**

✓ Celeriac, dandelion, fig, garlic, germinated barley, nuts, oat, oily fish, onion, papaya. Drink infusions of artichoke and olive leaf. Include plenty of olive oil in your diet. SEE ALSO Atherosclerosis and Arteriosclerosis.

✗ Avoid fatty foods, except oily fish.

RECIPES *garlic tincture (page 54), artichoke-leaf wine (page 128).*

### PALPITATIONS/ARRHYTHMIA

**AN IRREGULAR HEARTBEAT, WHICH MAY BE CAUSED BY CONGENITAL FACTORS, OR MAY BE THE RESULT OF EXERTION, STRESS OR HEART DISEASE.**

**! DO NOT STOP TAKING MEDICATION PRESCRIBED BY YOUR DOCTOR.**

✓ Buckwheat, chicory, clove, garlic, germinated barley, green bean, leek, lemon, lemon balm, lettuce, limeflower, mint, parsley, parsnip, passion fruit, oat, olive leaf (in infusion) and oil, onion, rosemary, shallot, tarragon, valerian.

✗ Alcohol, coffee, tea, tobacco.

RECIPES *green bean and garlic juice (page 119), celery and red onion juice ( page 119), lettuce and basil juice (page 119), lemon-balm and camomile infusion (page 124), barley water (page 127).*

### RAYNAUD'S DISEASE

**INADEQUATE CIRCULATION IN THE HANDS OR FEET DUE TO ARTERIAL SPASM CAUSES FINGERS OR TOES TO TURN WHITE OR BLUE AND STING ON EXPOSURE TO COLD. THE CHEEKS, EARS AND NOSE MAY ALSO BE AFFECTED.**

✓ Blackberry, blackcurrant, black pepper, blueberry, cabbage, carrot, cayenne pepper, chervil, cinnamon, garlic, ginger, redcurrant. Consume a lot of warm food and drinks. Increase your intake of magnesium-rich food, such as whole-grain cereal products, nuts and seeds. Drink blackberry leaf infusion. SEE ALSO Anaemia.

RECIPES *ginger infusion (page 125).*

### THROMBOSIS

**FORMATION OF A BLOOD CLOT WITHIN A BLOOD VESSEL OR INSIDE THE HEART, OFTEN IMPEDING THE FLOW OF BLOOD.**

**! DO NOT STOP TAKING MEDICATION PRESCRIBED BY YOUR DOCTOR.**

✓ Borage oil, buckwheat, camomile, fenugreek, garlic, lemon, limeflower, oily fish, olive oil, orange, pineapple, pumpkin, raspberry, strawberry, tarragon. Eat oily fish on a regular basis.

✗ Alcohol, tobacco.

RECIPES *garlic tincture (page 54), strawberry and raspberry juice (page 118), green bean and garlic juice (page 119), celery and red onion juice (page 119), strawberry-leaf decoction (page 126).*

# digestive system

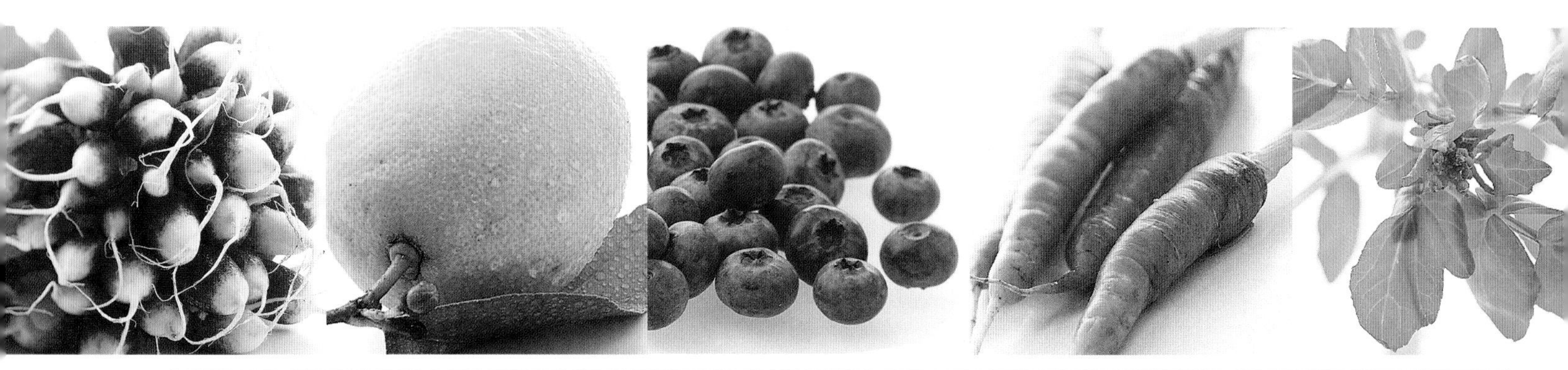

**STAR FOODS FOR THE DIGESTIVE SYSTEM: ALL BITTER GREENS, ARTICHOKE, BASIL, BLACKCURRANT, BLACK RADISH, BLUEBERRY, CARROT, CHERVIL, CHICORY, COURGETTE, DANDELION, FENNEL, FIG, GARLIC, GERMINATED BARLEY, GINGER, GRAPEFRUIT, JUNIPER BERRY, LEMON, LETTUCE, OLIVE OIL, PAPAYA, PARSLEY, PINEAPPLE, NUTMEG, QUINCE, RADISH, ROSEMARY, THYME, WATERCRESS.**

The digestive system includes the mouth, oesophagus, stomach, liver, pancreas, gallbladder and intestines. A diet that consists largely of convenience foods and is high in sugar and fat – as well as alcohol, fizzy drinks, spicy snacks and tobacco – puts the digestive tract under constant strain. The digestive system is also notoriously sensitive to stress and emotional conditions. If you often experience minor digestive problems, or suffer from a chronic condition, you should try to reduce your stress levels as much as possible.

Many digestive problems can be alleviated by eliminating alcohol, coffee, spicy or salty snacks, fatty food (such as cream, cheese and butter) and junk food from your diet. Eating less, but at regular intervals, can also help. Increase your food intake in the morning, eat moderately at lunchtime and lightly in the evening. Some people feel better if they eat five small meals a day.

Two or three times a year, go on a wheat- and dairy-free diet for two to three weeks at a time, or follow the detox program outlined on pages 134–37. Fibre encourages food to pass quickly though the gut so try to increase the amount you include in your diet by eating plenty of fresh vegetables (don't just rely on cereals as a source of fibre). When cooking, use plenty of herbs, such as basil, garlic, ginger, juniper, rosemary and thyme – these are naturally antibacterial and promote digestion. Cabbage, carrots, courgettes, lettuce, fennel, blueberries, figs, papaya and pineapple are beneficial to both the stomach and the intestines; germinated barley is good for dyspepsia. Efficient liver function is important for healthy digestion – bitter greens, artichokes, blackcurrant berries and leaves, black radishes, chervil, chicory, dandelion, grapefruit, lemon, olive oil, parsley, quince and watercress all help the liver to function efficiently. They also promote the flow and emulsification of bile.

(N.B. To make a medicinal infusion, steep 1 tablespoon of the dried ingredient in a cup of boiling water for 10 minutes.)

## ABDOMINAL PAIN

**SUDDEN ACUTE ABDOMINAL PAIN, WHICH MAY BE ACCOMPANIED BY SWELLING OF THE ABDOMEN, DIARRHOEA OR VOMITING.**

**! MAY RAPIDLY TURN INTO A MEDICAL EMERGENCY – SEE A DOCTOR AS SOON AS POSSIBLE. USE SELF-HELP MEASURES ONLY WHEN POTENTIALLY SERIOUS CONDITIONS HAVE BEEN RULED OUT.**

## ABDOMINAL CRAMP

**DISCOMFORT IN THE ABDOMEN MAY BE DUE TO TRAPPED WIND, CONSTIPATION OR IRRITABLE BOWEL SYNDROME.**

✓ Infusions of aniseed, basil, bay leaf, camomile, coriander, cumin seed, dill, fennel seed, ginger, lemon balm, lychee seed, marjoram, mint, oregano, tarragon. Blueberry, cucumber, carrot and garlic may alleviate intestinal fermentation and inflammation. *SEE ALSO* general advice on the care of the digestive system and Distention and Wind.

*RECIPES cabbage, carrot and blueberry juice (page 25), blueberry decoction (page 40), cucumber and lettuce heart juice (page 119), fennel infusion (page 123), lemon-balm and camomile infusion (page 124), lychee-seed decoction (page 126), dill-seed decoction (page 126), fennel-seed decoction (page 126), cumin-seed decoction (page 126), camomile and citrus wine (page 129), anisette (page 129), basil liqueur (page 129).*

## BLOATING

SEE ABDOMINAL PAIN, DISTENTION AND WIND.

## CHOLECYSTITIS

AN ACUTE OR CHRONIC INFLAMMATION OF THE GALLBLADDER, OWING TO A BLOCKAGE (USUALLY BY GALLSTONES) OR AN INFECTION, CAUSING PAIN IN THE UPPER RIGHT ABDOMEN AND/OR BETWEEN THE SHOULDERS. THE CONDITION IS OFTEN ACCOMPANIED BY INDIGESTION AND NAUSEA AFTER EATING FATTY FOOD.

! ACUTE PAIN MAY RAPIDLY TURN INTO A MEDICAL EMERGENCY – SEE A DOCTOR AS SOON AS POSSIBLE. USE SELF-HELP MEASURES ONLY WHEN POTENTIALLY SERIOUS CONDITIONS HAVE BEEN RULED OUT.

✓ Bitter greens, dandelion, fresh fruit and vegetables, hazelnut. Try to use plenty of rosemary in your cooking. Every morning drink some olive oil mixed with lemon juice (see page 34) followed by a glass of black radish and carrot juice (see below). Artichoke-leaf, lemon, lemon-peel or rosemary infusions or fresh cherry juice may also provide some relief.

✗ Biscuits and other refined carbohydrates, fatty foods, rhubarb.

*RECIPES cherry and raspberry juice (page 118), cherry and apple juice (page 118), black radish and carrot juice (page 119), dandelion infusion (page 123), artichoke-leaf wine (page 128), lemon liqueur (page 129), artichoke-leaf tincture (page 130).*

## COLIC

SEE ABDOMINAL CRAMP, CONSTIPATION, INDIGESTION.

## SUGGESTED MENUS TO AID DIGESTION

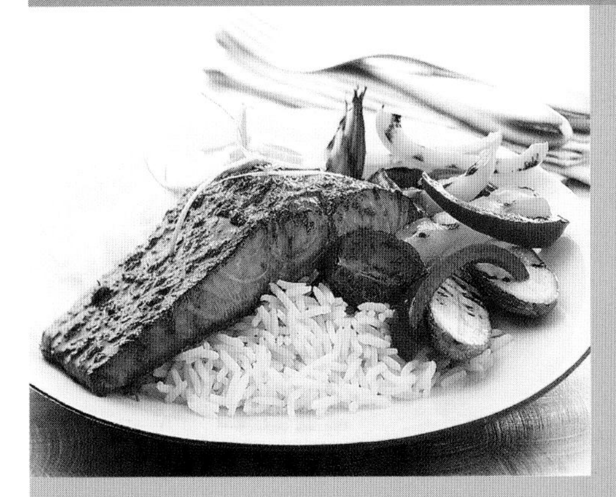

The following menus are helpful for anyone suffering from minor problems, such as constipation, distention and wind, that are caused by a weak or sluggish digestive sytem.

### MENU 1

**BREAKFAST**

A bowl of porridge; yoghurt; a small glass of juice made of carrot, cabbage and green or red pepper; or a fruit juice combination such as blackcurrant, blueberry and blackberry or pineapple, apple and strawberry.

**SNACKS**

Dried fruit, especially blueberries, pineapple or papaya; dandelion or roast-chicory coffee substitute; fennel, ginger and basil infusion or lemon-balm infusion.

**LUNCH**

Fish or chicken with potatoes and herb sauce (page 111) or buckwheat with leek sauce (page 103) or tabouleh (page 100) with a grilled lamb chop and a carrot and orange salad; rhubarb and ginger tart (page 113).

**DINNER**

Broad-bean soup or herbal broth (page 92) cooked with barley; fresh fruit salad; a camomile infusion; a small glass of basil liqueur (page 129) or a teaspoon of anisette (page 129) in a glass of water.

### MENU 2

**BREAKFAST**

A bowl of rice or corn flakes with soya milk or an autumn fruit compote; fruit juice (grape, apple or blueberry); half a grapefruit, a banana or a kiwi fruit.

**SNACKS**

Dried fruit, especially raisins, papaya, pineapple or blueberries; dandelion or roast-chicory coffee substitute; fennel, ginger or cumin-seed infusion.

**LUNCH**

Honey and ginger grilled salmon (page 63) with steamed vegetables; pumpkin in syrup (page 112).

**DINNER**

Roman-style artichoke (page 101) or lentil soup (page 95); pears with herbs (page 114); a small glass of camomile and citrus wine (page 129).

## COLITIS

**SEE ABDOMINAL PAIN, IRRITABLE BOWEL SYNDROME, ULCERATIVE COLITIS.**

## CONSTIPATION

**SLOW INTESTINAL TRANSIT CAUSING IRREGULAR BOWEL MOVEMENTS.**

**! STRONG LAXATIVES SHOULD BE AVOIDED. A HIGH-FIBRE DIET AND AN INCREASED INTAKE OF RAW FRUIT AND VEGETABLES OFTEN HELPS TO RELIEVE THIS CONDITION.**

✓ All green leafy vegetables, apple, asparagus, Brussels sprout, chervil, coconut, cooked rhubarb, cucumber, elderberry, fig, grapefruit, hazelnut, Jerusalem artichoke, kumquat, leek, live yoghurt, melon, mustard, olive, orange, peach, pea, persimmon, pomegranate, prune, raspberry, raw apple, redcurrant, sorrel, strawberry, turnip, tomato, watermelon. Drink plenty of water and fresh apple, melon, prune or tomato juice – mix the juice with yoghurt if desired. Every morning drink some olive oil mixed with lemon juice (page 34) and eat some figs boiled in milk (page 36).

✗ Guava seeds. If the condition worsens when you eat foods that contain wheat, you should suspect a wheat allergy and eliminate it from your diet.

RECIPES *almond milk (page 77), rhubarb and ginger tart (page 113), apple and raspberry juice (page 117), prune juice (page 118), celery and tomato juice (page 118), cucumber and lettuce heart juice (page 119), elderberry syrup (page 131).*

## CROHN'S DISEASE

**A RECURRENT INFLAMMATION OF THE INTESTINE WHICH MAY NECESSITATE SURGERY. SYMPTOMS – WHICH ARE NOT ALWAYS PRESENT, EVEN IN SERIOUS CASES – INCLUDE CRAMPING PAIN, DIARRHOEA, WEIGHT LOSS, ANAEMIA AND SOMETIMES JOINT PAIN.**

**! DO NOT STOP TAKING MEDICATION PRESCRIBED BY YOUR DOCTOR.**

✓ Almond, blueberry, cabbage, carrot, courgette, fig, ginger, grapefruit, mint, peach, pumpkin, pollen, quince, tarragon. Aniseed or mint infusion or fennel tea may also provide some relief. SEE ALSO general advice on the care of the digestive system.

✗ Guava seeds and all dairy products except live yoghurt.

RECIPES *cabbage, carrot and blueberry juice (page 25), almond milk (page 77), cabbage, carrot and celery juice (page 119), fennel infusion (page 123), coriander-seed infusion (page 125), anisette (page 129), quince liqueur (page 129).*

## DIABETES MELLITUS

**A CHRONIC CONDITION IN WHICH AN ABSENCE OR INSUFFICIENCY OF INSULIN LEADS TO PROBLEMS IN THE METABOLISM OF SUGAR. AS A RESULT, SUGAR BUILDS UP IN THE BLOOD AND URINE.**

**! DO NOT STOP TAKING MEDICATION PRESCRIBED BY YOUR DOCTOR. YOUR DOCTOR MAY REFER YOU TO A REGISTERED DIETICIAN.**

✓ Artichoke, bean, blueberry, brown bread and pasta, brown flour, cabbage, chive and spring onion, fresh fruit, garlic, Jerusalem artichoke, nut, oat, olive, onion, potato, pulses, pumpkin, salsify, shallot, rice, unrefined cereals. Drink fresh blueberry, cabbage, celery or citrus-fruit juice and blueberry, blueberry-leaf or juniper infusion.

✗ Excessive amounts of animal fat. Consult your doctor before eating bananas.

RECIPES *blueberry tincture (page 40), cabbage, carrot and celery juice (page 119), beetroot and celery juice (page 119), juniper-berry wine (page 128).*

## DIARRHOEA

**THE PASSING OF FREQUENT LIQUID STOOLS CAUSED BY PARASITES, BACTERIAL OR VIRAL ACTIVITY, FOOD INTOLERANCE, STRESS OR DRUGS.**

**! DIARRHOEA CAN CAUSE RAPID DEHYDRATION. SEE YOUR DOCTOR IF THE ATTACK IS PROLONGED.**

✓ Barley, blackberry, blueberry, boiled carrot, boiled rice, broad bean, cabbage, camomile, cardamom, chilli, chive, clove, cooked apple, honey, lychee, nettle, nutmeg, onion, pear, peppercorns, pepper, quince, rice water, rosemary, savory, strawberry, walnut. Drink fresh blackberry, blueberry or carrot juice and fennel-seed or rice-water infusion.

RECIPES *blueberry decoction (page 40), blueberry tincture (page 40), fennel infusion (page 123), fennel-seed decoction (page 126), quince liqueur (page 129), blackberry syrup (page 131).*

## DISTENTION AND WIND

**ABDOMINAL BLOATING, DISCOMFORT OR PAIN CAUSED BY FERMENTATION OF FOOD, EXCESS YEAST, BACTERIAL ACTIVITY OR STRESS.**

✓ Anise, blackberry, blueberry, carrot, chilli, garlic, lettuce, marjoram, oregano, pepper, savory. Use plenty of bay leaf, clove, coriander, cumin seed, fennel, juniper and rosemary in your cooking. Drink fresh blackberry, blueberry or lettuce and garlic juice and aniseed, camomile, cumin-seed, dill-seed or fennel-seed infusion.

✗ Alcohol, fermented foods and foods that may ferment, such as bread, flour-based foods, pulses and sugary foods.
RECIPES *bay-leaf infusion (page 50), lettuce and basil juice (page 119), dill-seed decoction (page 126), fennel-seed decoction (page 126), cumin-seed decoction (page 126).*

## DIVERTICULITIS

**SMALL POUCHES IN THE LARGE INTESTINE WHICH BECOME INFLAMED, CAUSING PAIN, WIND, DIARRHOEA OR CONSTIPATION.**

✓ High-fibre foods: apple, bean, blackberry, blueberry, brown bread, brown rice, Brussels sprout, cabbage, chestnut, chickpea, dried fruit, grapefruit, green vegetables, Jerusalem artichoke, lentil, melon, orange, parsnip, pea, porridge, potato, turnip, watermelon. As some of these foods may increase the production of gas, use plenty of fresh herbs and garlic in your cooking.

✗ Guava seeds.
RECIPES *cabbage, carrot and blueberry juice (page 25), garlic and sage soup (page 55), cucumber and lettuce heart juice (page 119), fennel infusion (page 123), lemon-balm and camomile infusion (page 124), dill-seed decoction (page 126), fennel-seed decoction (page 126), cumin-seed decoction (page 126), anisette (page 129).*

## DYSENTERY

**SEE ABDOMINAL PAIN, DIARRHOEA.**

✗ Pumpkin.

## DYSPEPSIA AND HEARTBURN

**INDIGESTION AND A BURNING SENSATION IN THE CHEST, OFTEN TRIGGERED BY RICH OR SWEET FOOD, OVEREATING, ALCOHOL OR STRESS.**

✓ Anise, apple, banana, barley, bay leaf, carrot, chestnut, chilli, coriander, courgette, fennel, fig, grapefruit, guava (seeded), Jerusalem artichoke, lemon, lettuce, melon, orange, peach, peanut, peppercorns, pepper, persimmon, pineapple, potato, pumpkin, quince, radish, rocket, saffron.

✗ Alcohol, coffee, fatty food, tea. Do not eat late at night.
RECIPES *lemon-balm and camomile infusion (page 124), coriander-seed infusion (page 125), fennel-seed decoction (page 126), anisette (page 129), aniseed tincture (page 130).*

## FLATULENCE

**SEE DISTENTION AND WIND.**

## FOOD POISONING

**SEE GASTROENTERITIS, INDIGESTION, NAUSEA AND VOMITING.**

## GALLSTONES

**SEE CHOLECYSTITIS (PAGE 73).**

## GASTRITIS

**A GENERAL INFLAMMATION OF THE LINING OF THE STOMACH, CAUSING SYMPTOMS SIMILAR TO THOSE OF INDIGESTION.**

✓ A 20-hour fast, drinking only barley water or rice water (see Rice; page 33) may reduce the symptoms considerably. Follow this with a diet of bland foods such as: banana, barley, cabbage, carrot, courgette, fennel, fig, Jerusalem artichoke, potato, pumpkin, quince, rice, watermelon. Drink fresh carrot, cabbage or courgette juice, and aniseed, dill-seed, fennel-seed or mint infusions. *SEE ALSO* general advice on the care of the digestive system, Dyspepsia and Indigestion.

### BARLEY AND FRUIT PORRIDGE

This recipe by Hanne Glasse, which was first published in 1747, can help to boost a sluggish digestive system.

50 g germinated barley
1 litre water (or equal parts of water and milk)
25 g raisins
25 g dried blackcurrants or blueberries
Pinch of ground nutmeg
2 tbsp brown sugar
50 ml white wine or a little brandy
2 egg yolks (optional)

In a large saucepan, boil the barley in the water with the raisins, blackcurrants or blueberries and nutmeg until the barley is tender. Remove from the heat and stir in the brown sugar and white wine. Return to the heat, bring to the boil and cook over a low heat for a further 2 minutes. Add the egg yolks at this stage if desired, but remove from the heat before stirring them in. The end result should resemble rice pudding.

RECIPES *cabbage, carrot and celery juice (page 119), lettuce and basil juice (page 119), coriander-seed infusion (page 125), dill-seed decoction (page 126), fennel-seed decoction (page 126).*

### GASTROENTERITIS

AN INFLAMMATION OF THE DIGESTIVE TRACT CAUSED BY MICRO- ORGANISMS AND RESULTING IN NAUSEA, VOMITING, DIARRHOEA, ABDOMINAL PAIN AND FEVER.

! DO NOT EAT ANYTHING FOR 24 HOURS. DRINK SMALL AMOUNTS OF FLUIDS FREQUENTLY. GINGER, FENNEL OR MINT TEA OR AN INFUSION OF THYME, JUNIPER OR BASIL MAY HELP.

✓ When you feel you can start eating again, eat very lightly, preferably food cooked with garlic and basil, juniper, marjoram, mint, rosemary or thyme to reduce the infection. Also eat: blueberry, boiled carrot, chickpea, chive and spring onion, courgette, lamb's lettuce, pumpkin, quince, persimmon, watercress.

RECIPES *garlic and sage soup (page 55), almond milk (see opposite page), herbal broth (page 92), ginger infusion (page 125), fennel-seed decoction (page 126), barley water (page 127), basil liqueur (page 129).*

### GINGIVITIS

INFECTED OR BLEEDING GUMS, OFTEN CAUSED BY BACTERIAL ACTIVITY AND OCCASIONALLY BY VITAMIN DEFICIENCY.

! ALWAYS BRUSH TEETH AND GUMS THOROUGHLY.

✓ Chew lemon peel, cloves, fresh or dried blueberries or figs. Add a tablespoon of salt and a drop or two of lemon essential oil to a strong thyme infusion to make a mouth wash. A strong sage infusion with a teaspoon of lemon juice added also makes a good mouth wash, as does fig water (see Fig; page 36).

✗ sugary food.

### HALITOSIS (BAD BREATH)

BAD BREATH IS OFTEN CAUSED BY YEAST OR BACTERIAL ACTIVITY IN THE MOUTH OF BY VARIOUS DIGESTIVE PROBLEMS.

✓ Nutmeg and an infusion of cardamom seeds. SEE ALSO Gingivitis.

### HANGOVER

DELAYED EFFECTS OF DRINKING AN EXCESSIVE AMOUNT OF ALCOHOL, INCLUDING FATIGUE, HEADACHE, NAUSEA, INDIGESTION.

✓ Drink plenty of water and infusions throughout the day. SEE ALSO Indigestion.

RECIPES *garlic and sage soup (page 55), dandelion infusion (page 123), fennel infusion (page 123), ginger infusion (page 125).*

### HEPATITIS (A, B OR C)

CHRONIC OR ACUTE INFECTION OF THE LIVER CAUSED BY A VIRUS. SYMPTOMS INCLUDE FATIGUE, INDIGESTION, JAUNDICE AND LOSS OF APPETITE.

! IT IS IMPERATIVE TO FOLLOW MEDICAL ADVICE.

✓ Bitter greens, apple, artichoke, asparagus, black radish, blueberry, cabbage, celery, chard, chervil, chicory, dandelion, grapefruit, green bean, horseradish, lemon, olive and olive oil, parsley. Drink fresh lettuce juice, mint tea or some olive oil mixed with lemon juice (page 34) .

✗ Alcohol, fatty food, meat, tobacco.

RECIPES *dandelion infusion (page 123).*

### INDIGESTION

A VARIETY OF SYMPTOMS, WHICH MAY INCLUDE NAUSEA, VOMITING, HEARTBURN AND BELCHING. INDIGESTION IS OFTEN CAUSED BY EXCESSIVE CONSUMPTION OF FATTY FOOD OR ALCOHOL.

✓ Drink water or take a decoction, infusion or tincture (see below). Eat as little as possible until symptoms have cleared.

RECIPES *garlic and sage soup (page 55), herbal broth (page 92), fennel infusion (page 123), lemon-balm and camomile infusion (page 124), coriander-seed infusion (page 125), ginger infusion (page 125), fennel-seed decoction (page 126), aniseed tincture (page 130).*

### INTESTINAL INFECTIONS AND PARASITES

SEE GASTROENTERITIS

### IRRITABLE BOWEL SYNDROME

ABDOMINAL CRAMPS AND SPASMS, AND ALTERNATING OR IRREGULAR BOUTS OF CONSTIPATION AND DIARRHOEA. OFTEN ASSOCIATED WITH STRESS, PSYCHOLOGICAL PROBLEMS AND CHANGE OF ROUTINE.

! AVOID ALL DAIRY PRODUCTS AND WHEAT FOR 2 WEEKS. A WEEK OR TWO LATER REINTRODUCE WHEAT, THEN DAIRY INTO YOUR DIET – IF EITHER CAUSES A SUDDEN RETURN OR AGGRAVATION OF THE CONDITION, ELIMINATE IT FROM YOUR DIET FOR GOOD.

✓ Almond milk, barley, blueberry, camomile, carrot, coriander, courgette, germinated pulses, ginger, melon, mint, persimmon, potato, quince, pumpkin, rice, rosemary, tarragon. Drink parsley-seed or mint infusion.

✗ Dairy products and wheat (if they exacerbate symptoms).

RECIPES *almond milk (see below), fennel infusion (page 123), dill-seed decoction (page 126), fennel-seed decoction (page 126), anisette (page 129), basil liqueur (page 129).*

### NAUSEA AND VOMITING

**MAY BE A SYMPTOM OF INDIGESTION OR GASTROENTERITIS, BUT OCCASIONALLY INDICATES A SERIOUS DISORDER.**

**! SEE A DOCTOR IF SYMPTOMS ARE PROLONGED. SEE A DOCTOR IMMEDIATELY IF YOU ARE IN PAIN, WORRIED ABOUT THE CAUSE OF VOMITING, OR IF THERE IS BLOOD IN THE VOMIT.**

✓ Infusions of anise, fennel, ginger, mint. SEE ALSO Cholecystitis, Gastritis, Hangover, Indigestion and Migraine (page 82–3).

RECIPES *ginger infusion (page 125), fennel-seed decoction (page 126), basil liqueur (page 129).*

### OBESITY

**EXCESSIVE BODY WEIGHT WHICH IMPAIRS MOVEMENT AND MAY LEAD TO SERIOUS HEALTH DISORDERS. OBESITY IS OFTEN DUE TO OVEREATING COMBINED WITH A LACK OF EXERCISE. OTHER CAUSES MAY BE A SLOW METABOLISM OR A MALFUNCTIONING THYROID GLAND.**

**! IT IS NOT POSSIBLE TO REDUCE WEIGHT WITHOUT DECREASING CALORIE INTAKE (EATING LESS) AND INCREASING THE RATE AT WHICH CALORIES ARE USED (EXERCISING MORE).**

✓ Eat plenty of foods that are both low-calorie and high-volume, such as green vegetables, potato and pulses.

✗ Dairy products, wheat (if they cause an allergy). SEE ALSO the detox programme (pages 134–37).

### PEPTIC ULCERS

**INCLUDES GASTRIC AND DUODENAL ULCERS; A SMALL AREA OF THE LINING OF THE STOMACH OR DUODENUM BECOMES INFLAMED, THEN ERODED. SYMPTOMS OF PEPTIC ULCERS INCLUDE A BURNING, GNAWING PAIN IN THE UPPER ABDOMEN OR CHEST, INDIGESTION, NAUSEA AND VOMITING.**

**! DO NOT STOP TAKING MEDICATION PRESCRIBED BY YOUR DOCTOR. SEVERE PAIN AND VOMITING BRIGHT RED BLOOD INDICATE THAT THE ULCER HAS BECOME PERFORATED – SEE A DOCTOR IMMEDIATELY. GIVE UP SMOKING.**

✓ Apple, banana, cabbage, carrot, fennel, fig, lettuce, potato, quince, rice barley. Eat small meals. Drink a potato-juice remedy (page 18) mixed with fresh carrot juice.

✗ Acidic, fatty or spicy foods, alcohol, coffee, tea.

RECIPES *cabbage, carrot and blueberry juice (page 25), fennel infusion (page 123), coriander-seed infusion (page 125), fennel-seed decoction (page 126), aniseed tincture (page 130).*

### ULCERATIVE COLITIS

**CHRONIC INFLAMMATION AND ULCERATION OF THE LOWER PART OF THE COLON CAUSING ABDOMINAL PAIN, AND DIARRHOEA WITH BLOOD AND MUCUS.**

**! DO NOT STOP TAKING MEDICATION PRESCRIBED BY YOUR DOCTOR.**

✓ Barley, beetroot, blackberry, blueberry, broad bean, cabbage, carrot, cauliflower, cereals, cooked apple, courgette, cucumber, dandelion, fresh fruit and vegetables, garlic, gooseberry, lamb's lettuce, lettuce, lychee, mango, nettle, oily fish, pear, persimmon, potato, quince, rosemary, strawberry. Eat high-fibre foods and reduce your meat intake. SEE ALSO Anaemia (page 69).

✗ Alcohol, dairy products, guava seeds, tobacco.

RECIPES *almond milk (left), cabbage, carrot and blueberry juice (page 25), mango juice (page 118), fennel infusion (page 123), lemon-balm and camomile infusion (page 124), elder and camomile infusion (page 124), fennel-seed decoction (page 126).*

### ALMOND MILK

Almond milk is helpful for people suffering from constipation, Crohn's disease, gastroenteritis, irritable bowel syndrome and ulcerative colitis. It also acts as a mild laxative for children and is also good for coughs and bronchial inflammation (page 78).

- 100 g almonds
- 1 tbsp water
- 50 g clear honey
- 1 litre water
- 2 tbsp orange-blossom water

Blend the almonds and the tablespoon of water in a food processor until you have a paste. Add the honey and then dilute the paste with the litre of water. Filter and add the orange-blossom water. Take 3 tablespoons 3 times a day.

# respiratory system

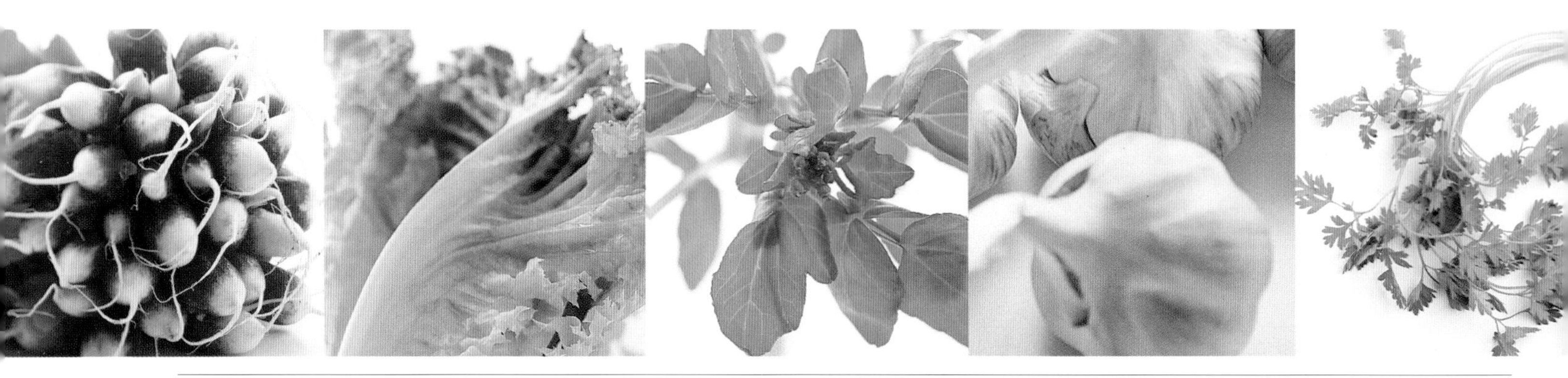

STAR FOODS FOR THE RESPIRATORY SYSTEM: BASIL, CHERVIL, CHIVE AND SPRING ONION, GARLIC, GINGER, LAMB'S LETTUCE, LETTUCE, MARJORAM, MINT, PARSLEY, RED AND BLACK RADISH, ROSEMARY, SAVORY, THYME, WATERCRESS.

Common problems that affect the lungs include irritation and inflammation accompanied by excess mucus. Some mucus is normal and healthy as it helps to keep the lungs lubricated. However, when the lungs are exposed to allergens, bacteria, viruses or pollutants, mucus production increases.

One of the most damaging pollutants to which the lungs are exposed is tobacco smoke. If you have respiratory problems and you smoke, it is imperative that you stop. Exercise is also very important – long walks in the open-air are ideal. Avoid mucus-forming foods, such as wheat and dairy products, and use herbs, such as basil, chives, garlic, ginger, marjoram, mint, rosemary, savory and thyme in cooking. Drink plenty of fresh juices – they are rich in zinc and vitamin C which boosts the immune system, making the lungs less prone to infection. (N.B. To make a medicinal infusion, steep 1 tablespoon of the dried ingredient in a cup of boiling water for 10 minutes.)

## ASTHMA

AN INFLAMMATION AND CONTRACTION OF THE BRONCHI, CAUSING BREATHLESSNESS, WHEEZING, TIGHT CHEST AND COUGHING. ASTHMA MAY BE HEREDITARY. TRIGGERS INCLUDE ALLERGIES, STRESS, EXERCISE AND EXPOSURE TO COLD AIR.

! DO NOT STOP TAKING MEDICATION PRESCRIBED BY YOUR DOCTOR.

✓ Blackcurrant, cabbage, carrot, chervil, grapefruit, honey, horseradish, lettuce, mint, radish, rosemary, savory, sorrel, watercress. Drink chervil, carrot, cabbage, lemon, watercress and apple juices and infusions of mint, thyme (with lemon juice) and rosemary. During an attack, eat a lump of sugar infused with three drops of fennel essential oil.

✗ Dairy products.

*RECIPES carrot, apple and ginger juice (page 118), cabbage, carrot and celery juice (page 119), lemon-balm and camomile infusion (page 124), ginger infusion (page 125), lettuce-seed decoction (page 126), strawberry-leaf decoction (page 126).*

## BRONCHITIS

AN INFLAMMATION OF THE LINING OF THE BRONCHI, RESULTING IN COUGHING, SPUTUM PRODUCTION AND BREATHLESSNESS. MAY BE ACUTE (CAUSED BY VIRUSES AND BACTERIA) OR CHRONIC (DUE TO RECURRENT INFECTIONS, SMOKING OR POLLUTION).

✓ Blackcurrants, borage, carrot, chervil, fig, garlic, grape, honey, horseradish, lettuce, mint, quince, radish, sage, savory, thyme, watercress. Drink infusions of rosemary and borage. SEE ALSO general advice on the care of the respiratory system.

✗ Dairy products, wheat.

*RECIPES almond milk (page 77), carrot, apple and ginger juice (page 118), marjoram infusion (page 123), lemon-balm and camomile infusion (page 124), ginger infusion (page 125), lettuce-seed decoction (page 126), leek syrup (page 130).*

## COUGH

A SYMPTOM OF AN INFECTION, INFLAMMATION OR IRRITATION OF THE

THROAT, USUALLY ASSOCIATED WITH A COLD, FLU, BRONCHITIS OR SORE THROAT. SEE ALSO IMMUNE SYSTEM.

! IF THE COUGH IS PERSISTENT, OR IF MUCUS IS SPECKLED WITH BLOOD, SEE A DOCTOR IMMEDIATELY.

✓ *SEE* Asthma, Bronchitis and Sore throat (page 85).

## HAY FEVER (ALLERGIC RHINITIS)

AN ALLERGIC REACTION TO POLLEN FROM TREES, FLOWERS OR GRASS, CAUSING SNEEZING, RUNNY NOSE AND ITCHING OF THE EYES, NOSE AND THROAT.

✓ *SEE* general advice on the respiratory system and Asthma.
RECIPES *marjoram infusion (page 123), lemon-balm and camomile infusion (page 124), elder and camomile infusion (page 124).*

## PLEURISY

SEVERE ONE-SIDED CHEST PAIN CAUSED BY AN INFLAMMATION OF THE MEMBRANES SURROUNDING THE LUNGS AS A RESULT OF AN UNDERLYING ILLNESS. PAIN IS WORSE ON BREATHING/COUGHING.

✓ Cabbage, carrot, cherry, chervil, fig, garlic, leek, onion, radish, saffron, watercress. *SEE ALSO* Asthma, Bronchitis.
RECIPES *cabbage, carrot and celery juice (page 119), marjoram infusion (page 123), lemon-balm and camomile infusion (page 124), elder and camomile infusion (page 124), cherry-stem decoction (page 125), lettuce-seed decoction (page 126).*

## PNEUMONIA

AN INFLAMMATION OF THE LUNGS, CAUSED BY A VIRUS OR BACTERIA. SYMPTOMS INCLUDE BREATHLESSNESS, A COUGH THAT MAY PRODUCE BLOODY SPUTUM, HIGH FEVER AND CHEST PAIN. SEVERE CASES LEAD TO COMPLICATIONS AND MAY BE LIFE THREATENING.

! DO NOT STOP TAKING MEDICATION PRESCRIBED BY YOUR DOCTOR.

✓ Foods rich in vitamin C and zinc plus blackberry, borage, carrot, chervil, clove, fig, garlic, juniper berry, lamb's lettuce, leek, nettle, onion, rosemary, savory, thyme. *SEE ALSO* Asthma, Bronchitis.
RECIPES *cherry and apple juice (page 118), cabbage, carrot and celery juice (page 119), green bean and garlic juice (page 119), celery and red onion juice (page 119), lettuce and basil juice (page 119), marjoram infusion (page 123), lemon-balm and camomile infusion (page 124), elder and camomile infusion (page 124), cherry-stem decoction (page 125).*

## SORE THROAT AND TONSILLITIS

SEE SORE THROAT (PAGE 85).

## WHOOPING COUGH

A HIGHLY CONTAGIOUS BACTERIAL INFECTION, CAUSING SEVERE SPASMODIC COUGH. OCCURS PRIMARILY IN INFANTS.

! ANTIBIOTIC TREATMENT IS REQUIRED IMMEDIATELY.

✓ Take a mixture of lemon juice and honey. *SEE ALSO* Asthma, Bronchitis and Immune system.
RECIPES *almond milk (page 77), marjoram infusion (page 123), lemon-balm and camomile infusion (page 124), elder and camomile infusion (page 124), leek syrup (page 130), black radish syrup (page 130).*

### SUGGESTED MENU FOR CHRONIC LUNG DISORDERS

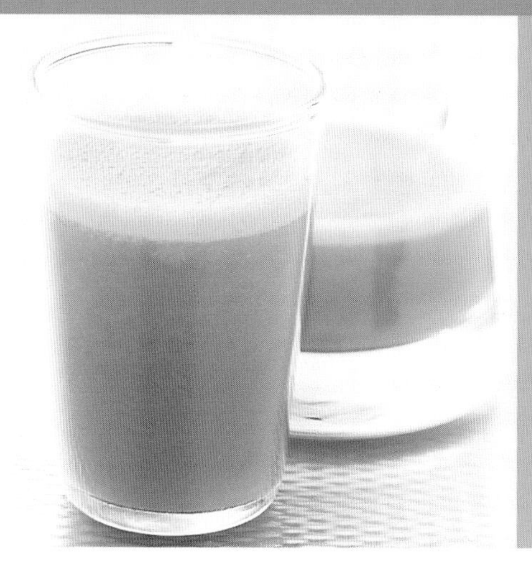

The following menu is designed for someone suffering from a chronic lung disorder such as asthma or bronchitis.

**BREAKFAST**
A bowl of rice cereal with soya milk; a small glass of carrot juice; a cup of coffee; grapefruit or kiwi fruit.

**SNACKS**
Dried fruit, especially raisins and figs; fresh fruit, such as orange, kiwi, papaya and pineapple; ginger infusion.

**LUNCH**
Black radish salad and grilled fish with mustard or horseradish sauce; melon with fresh mint.

**DINNER**
Lentil soup (page 95) with rye bread; avocado tartar (page 101); lettuce-seed, marjoram or lemon-balm infusion.

# kidneys and bladder

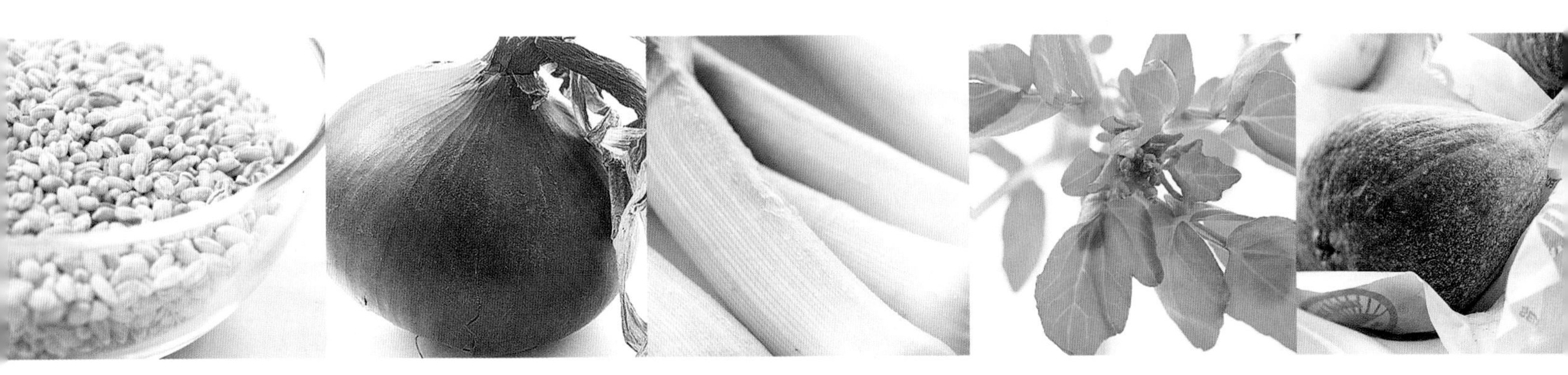

STAR FOODS FOR THE KIDNEYS AND BLADDER: BARLEY, BLACKCURRANT, BLUEBERRY, CABBAGE, CELERY, CRANBERRY, CUCUMBER, DANDELION, FIG, FRESH FRUIT, GRAPE, LEEK, ONION, UNPROCESSED CEREALS, WATERCRESS, WHEATGERM.

The kidneys' role in the body is to filter waste products from the blood. The waste is then eliminated from the body via the bladder and urethra in the form of urine. The body produces approximately one litre of urine daily and the bladder is emptied, on average, four to six times a day. The appearance of your urine provides a rough indication of whether you are drinking enough: a dark orange or amber colour is a sign that you need to increase your fluid intake. Changes in urinary habits or function that warrant medical attention include: cloudy or discoloured urine, unexplained changes in urinary output, and pain or discomfort on urination. A problem that becomes common in men over the age of 50 is enlarged prostate gland (page 89). This typically causes a hesitant, weak or trickling flow of urine from the urethra.

You can enhance your kidney function by drinking more water, fruit juices and herbal infusions, and regularly eating foods from the above list. Reduce your intake of coffee, tea and alcohol. Alcohol suppresses the production of antidiuretic hormone in the body, with the result that urine output by the kidneys increases dramatically. Foods that are rich in fibre and magnesium, such as fresh fruit, unprocessed cereals and wheatgerm, are beneficial to the kidneys and bladder. It is also important to prevent kidney, bladder and urethral infections by keeping your immune system healthy (pages 84–85).

(N.B. To make a medicinal infusion, steep 1 tablespoon of the dried ingredient in a cup of boiling water for 10 minutes.)

## BLADDER OR KIDNEY STONES

SMALL HARD MASSES OF CALCIUM AND OTHER SALTS OCCURRING ANYWHERE IN THE URINARY TRACT. STONES MAY LODGE IN THE BLADDER CAUSING FREQUENT, PAINFUL URINATION AND BLOOD IN THE URINE; THEY MAY OCCUR IN THE URINE-COLLECTING DUCT OF THE KIDNEYS CAUSING SEVERE PAIN; OR THEY MAY REMAIN IN THE KIDNEYS CAUSING MILD PAIN. KIDNEY OR BLADDER STONES MAY NECESSITATE SURGERY OR ANOTHER MEDICAL PROCEDURE.

! DRINK AT LEAST 6–8 GLASSES OF WATER PER DAY AND 1 DURING THE NIGHT.

✓ Almond, artichoke, bean, blackberry, blackcurrant, broad bean, cabbage, celery, cherry, chickpea, chicory, dandelion, grape, green bean, lamb's lettuce, leek, lettuce, melon, nettle, olive, onion, peach, physalis, radish, redcurrant, strawberry, tomato, watercress. Drink olive-leaf infusion and blackcurrant, grape, cranberry, cherry and watercress juices.

✗ Animal protein, chocolate, coffee, gooseberry, peanut, rhubarb, sorrel, spinach, tea.

RECIPES *broad bean-flower infusion (page 30), chickpea broth (page 92), cabbage, carrot and celery juice (page 119), celery and red onion juice (page 119), cucumber and lettuce heart juice (page 119), physalis jam (page 122), dandelion infusion (page 123), pear and apple infusion (page 124), corn-hair and fennel-seed decoction (page 125), physalis-berry decoction (page 126), strawberry-leaf decoction (page 126), barley water (page 127), juniper-berry wine (page 128).*

## CYSTITIS AND URETHRITIS

**INFLAMMATION OF THE BLADDER AND URETHRA CAUSED BY AN INFECTION. SYMPTOMS INCLUDE PAIN IN THE LOWER ABDOMEN, FREQUENT, URGENT AND PAINFUL URINATION AND BLOOD IN THE URINE. CYSTITIS IS MOST COMMON IN WOMEN.**

✓ Artichoke, blueberry, cherry, cranberry, cucumber, dandelion, juniper berry, melon, pumpkin, redcurrant, strawberry, thyme, watermelon. Drink plenty of water and watercress, blackcurrant, blueberry, cranberry and grape juices.

✗ Asparagus.

RECIPES *cabbage, carrot and blueberry juice (page 25), chickpea broth (page 92), cherry and raspberry juice (page 118), cherry and apple juice (page 118), cabbage, carrot and celery juice (page 119), celery and red onion juice (page 119), cucumber and lettuce heart juice (page 119), physalis jam (page 122), corn-hair and fennel-seed decoction (page 125), physalis-berry decoction (page 126), strawberry-leaf decoction (page 126), barley water (page 127).*

## ENLARGED PROSTATE GLAND

**THE GLAND GROWS TO THE POINT WHERE IT NARROWS THE URETHRA AND IMPEDES THE FLOW OF URINE. SEE MEN'S HEALTH.**

## IRRITABLE BLADDER

**A FREQUENT URGE TO PASS URINE. SEE CYSTITIS AND URETHRITIS.**

## PYELONEPHRITIS

**AN INFECTION OF THE KIDNEYS (ACUTE OR CHRONIC) CAUSING PAIN IN THE BACK AND LOWER ABDOMEN, FEVER AND PAINFUL URINATION.**

**! ANTIBIOTICS ARE URGENTLY REQUIRED.**

✓ Almond, artichoke, bean, blackberry, blackcurrant, borage, broad bean, cabbage, celery, cherry, chickpea, chicory, cucumber, dandelion, garlic, grape, leek, lettuce, melon, onion, peach, physalis, radish, redcurrant, strawberry, watercress, watermelon. Drink plenty of water and onion, cabbage, celery, cucumber, watercress, grape, cranberry, cherry and blueberry juices.

RECIPES *cabbage, carrot and blueberry juice (page 25), chickpea broth (page 92), cherry and apple juice (page 118), celery and red onion juice (page 119), cucumber and lettuce heart juice (page 119), physalis jam (page 122), corn-hair and fennel-seed decoction (page 125), physalis-berry decoction (page 126), strawberry-leaf decoction (page 126), barley water (page 127).*

## SUGGESTED MENUS FOR KIDNEY AND BLADDER PROBLEMS

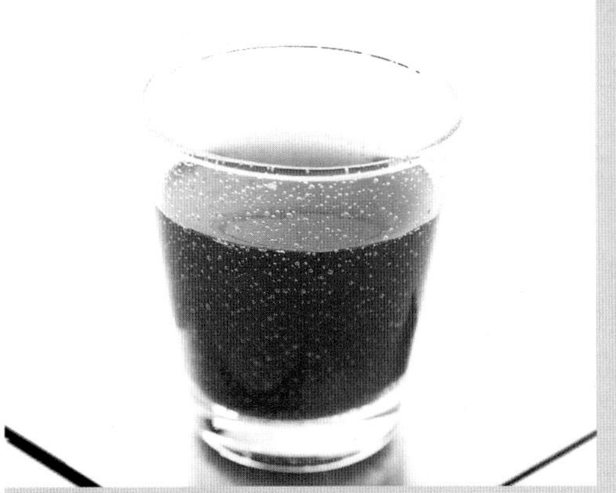

The following menus are designed to enhance the health of the urinary tract for people who are suffering from problems such as kidney or bladder stones. The emphasis is on drinking plenty of fluids and eating foods that have diuretic and anti-inflammatory properties such as chickpea, leek and onion.

### MENU 1

**BREAKFAST**

A bowl of cereal or porridge; a small glass of celery and carrot juice; a cup of herbal tea; grapefruit or kiwi fruit.

**SNACKS**

Dried fruit, such as fig, or fresh fruit rich in vitamin C, such as orange; dandelion or ginger infusion; cranberry juice.

**LUNCH**

Courgette cake (page 103) and grilled fish with rice and cucumber; barley water (page 127); melon with fresh mint.

**DINNER**

Buckwheat with leek sauce (page 103); blueberries and cottage cheese (page 41); lettuce-seed or thyme infusion; juniper decoction.

### MENU 2

**BREAKFAST**

A boiled egg with rye bread; a juice (celery and onion, or green bean, lettuce and garlic); live yoghurt; a cup of herbal tea.

**SNACKS**

Dried fruit, especially raisin and fig; fresh fruit, such as blackcurrant, blueberry and pear; barley water (page 127).

**LUNCH**

Onions in cider (page 109) with a slice of roast meat, bread and a little table mustard; a cucumber salad; a piece of fruit.

**DINNER**

Chickpea broth (page 92) with bread; barley water (page 127); thyme or camomile infusion.

# nervous system, mind and emotions

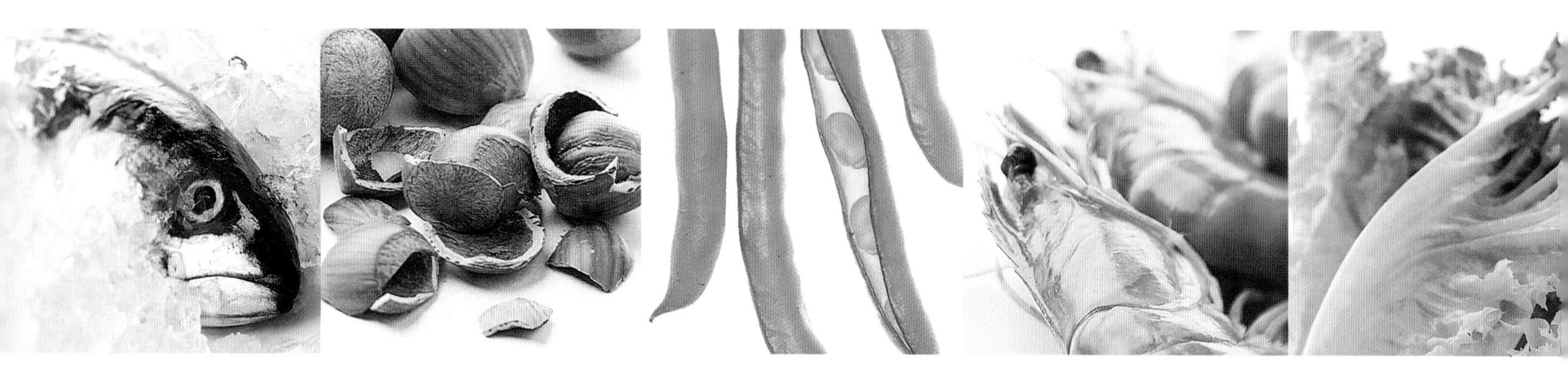

STAR FOODS FOR THE NERVOUS SYSTEM: APPLE, APRICOT, ASPARAGUS, AVOCADO, BANANA, BEETROOT, CABBAGE, CAMOMILE, CELERY, DILL SEED, FISH, GREEN VEGETABLES, LETTUCE, NUTS, OAT, PEACH, PULSES, PUMPKIN, QUINCE, POTATO, SHELLFISH, UNREFINED CEREALS.

Good stress management, relaxation, meditation and open-air exercise combined with small dietary changes can alleviate many symptoms of common nervous system disorders. Foods that have a calming effect on the nervous system are those that are rich in vitamin B, folic acid, magnesium, potassium, zinc, selenium and manganese. Try to eat plenty of fish, green vegetables, nuts, potatoes, pulses and unrefined cereals. Increase your intake of proteins and cut down on alcohol, coffee and tea. Drink infusions of camomile, lemon verbena, lemon balm, limeflower, olive-tree leaf, orange blossom or valerian. Bear in mind that problems such as irritability and poor concentration – as well as headaches and dizziness – may be caused by mild hypoglycaemia, in which case you should eat regular carbohydrate-based meals or snacks. (N.B. To make a medicinal infusion, steep 1 tablespoon of the dried ingredient in a cup of boiling water for 10 minutes.)

## ANXIETY

PSYCHOLOGICAL SYMPTOMS SUCH AS FEAR ARE ASSOCIATED WITH TENSION, SWEATING, PALPITATIONS, INSOMNIA AND LOSS OF APPETITE.

✓ Almond, apple, apricot, aubergine, basil, bean, beetroot, celery, lemon balm, lettuce, peach, pulses, quince. Drink fresh apple, apricot, cucumber, lettuce or peach juices and aniseed, basil, camomile, lemon-balm, lettuce-seed, limeflower, rosemary or thyme infusions. Eat more carbohydrates. Eating sugary snacks may reduce anxiety – this should be an occasional measure only.

✗ Coffee, cola drinks, tea.

RECIPES *lemon-balm and camomile infusion (page 124), sparkling lemon-balm infusion (page 125), lettuce-seed decoction (page 126), camomile and citrus wine (page 129), asparagus syrup (page 131).*

## DEPRESSION

A NEGATIVE MENTAL STATE ASSOCIATED WITH A BROAD SPECTRUM OF PHYSICAL SYMPTOMS.

✓ Oats, walnuts, fresh fruit and vegetables that are rich in vitamin B complex. SEE ALSO Anxiety.

✗ Alcohol.

## HEADACHES AND MIGRAINE

OFTEN CAUSED BY LOCAL MUSCLE TENSION OR STRESS; MIGRAINES ARE SEVERE, PROLONGED HEADACHES THAT MAY BE TRIGGERED BY CERTAIN FOODS, HORMONAL FLUCTUATIONS OR HYPOGLYCAEMIA.

✓ Almond, anise, basil, broad bean, cabbage, camomile, cherry, chive, fennel, ginger, lemon balm, mint, oily fish, onion, peach, rosemary, white meat. Eat plenty of fresh fruit and vegetables. Drink fresh apple, apricot and lettuce juices or aniseed, basil, camomile, fennel-seed, lemon-balm or mint infusions. SEE ALSO Anxiety.

✗ Alcohol, coffee, cheese, chocolate, food with additives ("E" numbers), ice-cream, monosodium glutamate, sweeteners, tea.

RECIPES *ginger infusion (page 125), anisette (page 129), basil liqueur (page 129), aniseed tincture (page 130).*

## INSOMNIA

**A PATTERN OF PERSISTENT SHORT SLEEPING, EITHER WITH DIFFICULTY FALLING ASLEEP OR FREQUENTLY INTERRUPTED SLEEP.**

✓ Aubergine, basil, barley, camomile, corn, courgette, fennel, lettuce, lime blossom, marjoram, onion, pumpkin. Eat a carbohydrate snack 20 minutes before you go to bed. SEE ALSO Anxiety.

✗ Coffee, cola drinks, tea.

RECIPES *lime-blossom infusion (page 52), mango juice (page 118), marjoram infusion (page 123), lemon-balm and camomile infusion (page 124), sparkling lemon-balm infusion (page 125), camomile and citrus wine (page 129), camomile aperitif (page 129), asparagus syrup (page 131).*

## IRRITABILITY AND STRESS

**SYMPTOMS SUCH AS ANXIETY, POOR CONCENTRATION AND INSOMNIA ARE OFTEN COMBINED WITH PHYSICAL SYMPTOMS SUCH AS DIGESTIVE DISTURBANCES AND SOMETIMES HIGH BLOOD PRESSURE.**

✓ SEE Anxiety, Insomnia, Heart and Circulation, Digestive System.

## MENTAL FATIGUE

**LACK OF MENTAL FOCUS AND POOR CONCENTRATION AND MEMORY.**

✓ Fruit and vegetables (especially apricots and carrots), mint, royal jelly, shellfish, foods rich in vitamin B (green vegetables and unrefined cereals), zinc and selenium. Drink apricot, cherry and grape juices and basil and mint infusions. SEE ALSO Anxiety, Insomnia.

✗ Excessive amounts of coffee and alcohol.

## MULTIPLE SCLEROSIS

**CHRONIC DEGENERATIVE DISORDER OF THE NERVOUS SYSTEM.**

**! DO NOT STOP TAKING MEDICATION PRESCRIBED BY YOUR DOCTOR.**

✓ Buckwheat, corn, fresh fruit and vegetables, millet, pulses. Eat more oily fish and cold-pressed vegetable oils, such as sunflower seed and olive oil. Drink fresh apple, apricot, cabbage, grape or lettuce juices or aniseed, basil, camomile, fennel-seed, lemon-balm or mint infusions. Take evening primrose oil daily.

✗ Dairy products, gluten, meat.

RECIPES *ginger infusion (page 125).*

## NEURALGIA

**SEE HEADACHES AND MIGRAINE.**

## VERTIGO

**DIZZINESS AND LOSS OF BALANCE, SOMETIMES WITH NAUSEA.**

**! MAY INDICATE A SERIOUS PROBLEM – CONSULT YOUR DOCTOR.**

✓ Basil, fennel, lemon balm, orange, mint, sage, thyme. SEE ALSO general advice on the care of the nervous system.

## SUGGESTED MENU FOR STRESS-RELATED SYMPTOMS

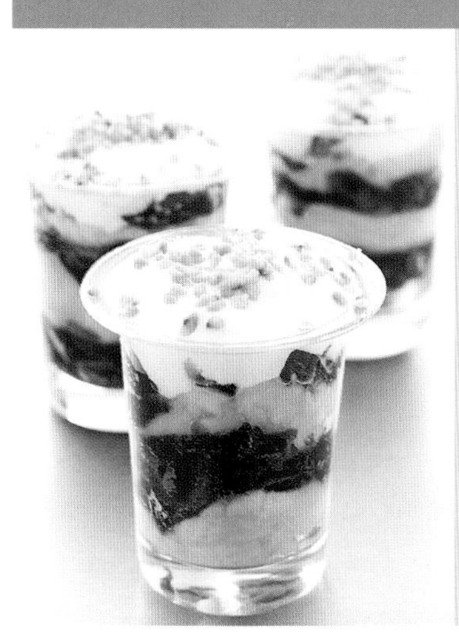

The following menu is designed for someone suffering from mild anxiety, depression, poor concentration, headaches or mild insomnia.

**MENU**

**BREAKFAST**

A bowl of porridge; a small glass of carrot juice; herbal infusions such as lemon balm or camomile; a banana.

**SNACKS**

Dried fruit, such as raisins or figs; fresh fruit rich in vitamin C, such as orange; nuts; herbal infusions.

**LUNCH**

Grilled meat, beans with carrots and onions (page 110), rice with cucumber balls (page 109) or grated celeriac and carrot salad (page 98); fruit salad with lemon balm (page 113).

**DINNER**

Grilled salmon with aubergine sauce (page 103); banana and date salad (page 112); lettuce-seed, camomile or lemon-balm infusion.

# immune system

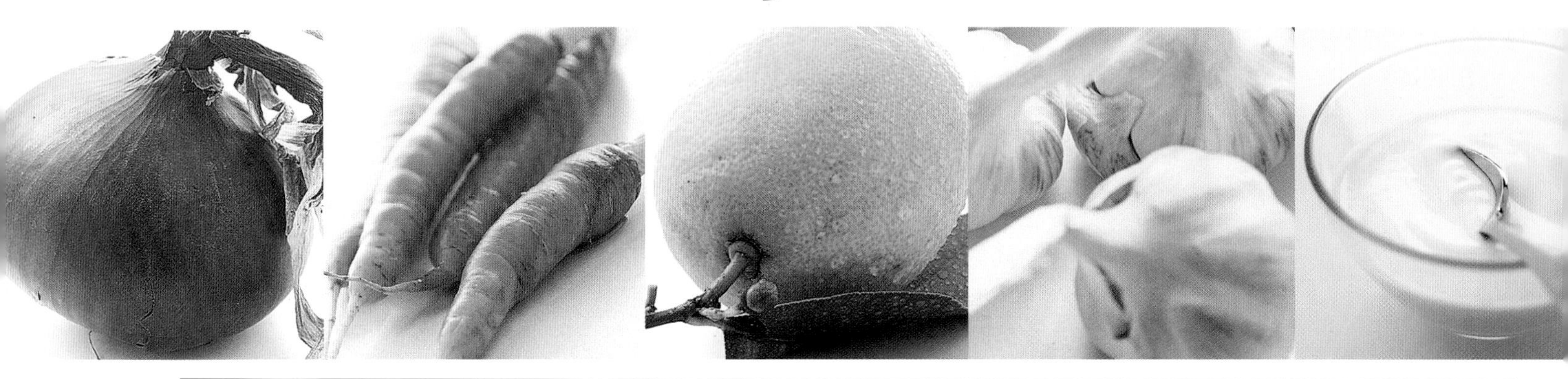

**STAR FOODS FOR THE IMMUNE SYSTEM: APPLE, ARTICHOKE, BASIL, BLACKBERRY, BLACKCURRANT, BLUEBERRY, CABBAGE, CAMOMILE, CARROT, CHERRY, CHIVE, CINNAMON, CLOVE, CUCUMBER, CUMIN, DANDELION, ELDER, GARLIC, GREEN BEAN, LEMON, LEMON BALM, LEEK, LIVE YOGHURT, MINT, OILY FISH, PEAR, PULSES, RASPBERRY, RED ONION, REDCURRANT, SHELLFISH, THYME, UNREFINED CEREALS, WATERCRESS, WATERMELON.**

The immune system protects the body from infection due to bacteria, viruses and other microbes. Allergies occur when the immune system over-reacts to a substance. Regular physical exercise and a healthy diet strengthen the immune system – poor nutrition, alcohol, drugs and stress weaken it.

To boost your immune system, try to cut down on your intake of alcohol and animal fat and eliminate from your diet any foods that you suspect may be causing an allergy – the most common culprits are citrus fruit, corn, eggs, milk and cheese, nuts, pork, processed tomatoes, shellfish, wheat, and food containing monosodium glutamate or any "E numbers".

Three categories of foods strengthen the immune system:
1) anti-infective: basil, blackberries, blueberries, cinnamon, cloves, cumin, garlic, juniper, lemon, thyme and live yoghurt, which is rich in lactobacilli.
2) anti-inflammatory: apple, artichoke, blackcurrants, cabbage, camomile, cherries, cucumber, elder, lemon balm, mint, oily fish, pears, raspberries, redcurrants, watercress, watermelon.
3) diuretic and depurative: artichoke, chives, dandelion, green beans, leeks, onions.

Green vegetables are rich in vitamins, beta-carotene, minerals and trace elements, all of which play an important part in maintaining a healthy immune system. Red, green and yellow vegetables and fruit contain powerful antioxidants that help prevent the deterioration of the immune system. Oily fish contains an oil that has important anti-inflammatory properties. Fresh raw fruit and vegetables are the best source of vitamin C; and pulses, shellfish and unrefined cereal provide a good supply of zinc, an important immuno-stimulant.
(N.B. To make a medicinal infusion, steep 1 tablespoon of the dried ingredient in a cup of boiling water for 10 minutes.)

## CANDIDA

**A LOW-LEVEL INFECTION CAUSED BY THE PROLIFERATION OF *CANDIDA ALBICAN*. THIS OCCURS WHEN THE BALANCE OF THE INTESTINAL FLORA IS DISTURBED AFTER TAKING ANTIBIOTICS OR IMMUNO-SUPPRESSANTS.**

✓ Blueberry, garlic, live yoghurt, pickled turnip; infusions of cumin seed, thyme, fennel and aniseed. Follow the detox programme on pages 134–37. *SEE ALSO* general advice on the care of the immune system and the digestive system.

RECIPES *fennel infusion (page 123), marjoram infusion (page 123).*

## COMMON COLD

**A VIRAL INFECTION CAUSING WATERY DISCHARGE FROM THE NOSE, SLIGHT FEVER, SORE THROAT AND COUGH. RECURRENT COLDS ARE USUALLY A SIGN OF A WEAK IMMUNE SYSTEM.**

✓ Basil, blackberry, blueberry, chilli, chive, cinnamon, clove, cumin, garlic, ginger, juniper, lemon, live yoghurt, onion, orange, peppercorns, rosemary, shellfish, spring onion, thyme, unrefined cereal. Eat plenty of fresh, raw fruit and vegetables, especially those that are red, green or yellow in colour. Drink fresh blackberry, carrot, lemon or orange juice.

RECIPES *garlic and sage soup (page 55), chive and ginger broth (page 94), elder and camomile infusion (page 124).*

### INFLUENZA

SEE COMMON COLD.

### LARYNGITIS

SEE SORE THROAT.

### POST-VIRAL FATIGUE

CHRONIC ILLNESS CHARACTERIZED BY LOW ENERGY LEVELS AND POOR CONCENTRATION. USUALLY FOLLOWS A VIRAL ILLNESS.

✓ Fresh apricot, beetroot, blueberry, cabbage, carrot, cherry or grape juices and basil, mint or thyme infusions. *SEE ALSO* Anaemia (page 69), Mental fatigue (page 83), general advice on the care of the immune system and detoxification (pages 134–37).

RECIPES *garlic tincture (page 54).*

### SINUSITIS

AN INFLAMMATION OF THE SINUSES, CAUSED BY RECURRENT COLDS OR FOLLOWING AN UPPER RESPIRATORY TRACT INFECTION. CHRONIC SINUSITIS IS USUALLY CAUSED BY AN ALLERGY. SEE COMMON COLD.

### SORE THROAT

A COMMON SYMPTOM RESULTING FROM COLDS, LARYNGITIS, PHARYNGITIS OR TONSILLITIS.

✓ Bay leaf, blackberry, blackcurrant, blueberry, borage, carrot, celery, chervil, clove, fig, garlic, honey, juniper berry, lamb's lettuce, leek, lemon, onion, peppercorns, nettle, rosemary, savory, thyme, vinegar. *SEE ALSO* general advice on the care of the immune system and the respiratory system.

RECIPES *almond milk (page 77), marjoram infusion (page 123), leek syrup (page 130), black radish syrup (page 130).*

### TONSILLITIS

AN ACUTE INFLAMMATION OF THE TONSILS, MOST FREQUENT IN CHILDREN.

✓ A thyme infusion with honey and lemon juice may help to soothe the pain. *SEE ALSO* Common cold, Influenza, Sore throat.

RECIPES *redcurrant, blackberry and blueberry juice (page 118), leek syrup (page 130), black radish syrup (page 130).*

## SUGGESTED MENUS FOR THE IMMUNE SYSTEM

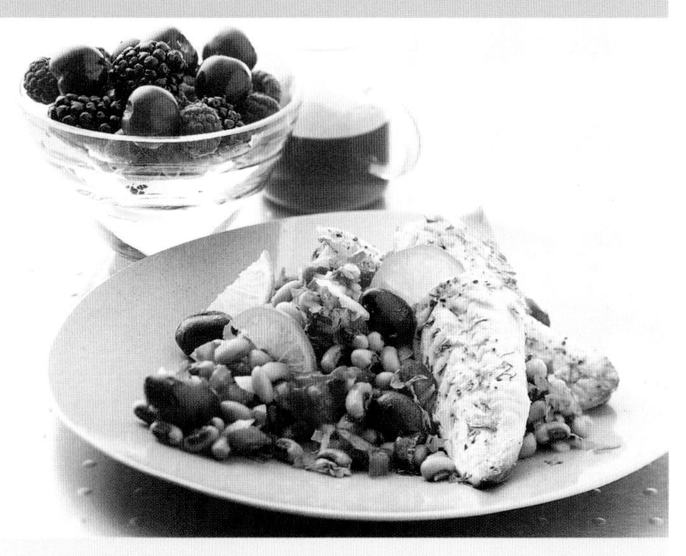

The following menus are designed to enhance the health of the immune system and prevent illness.

#### MENU 1

**BREAKFAST**

Live yoghurt with kiwi fruit; a small glass of carrot juice; a cup of dandelion root coffee or a herbal infusion such as lemon balm or camomile.

**SNACKS**

Fresh fruit rich in vitamin C; nuts; herbal infusions.

**LUNCH**

Grated celeriac and carrot salad (page 98); dandelion, bacon and potato cakes (page 106); lychee fruit salad (page 112).

**DINNER**

Spinach with green beans; camomile or lemon-balm infusion.

#### MENU 2

**BREAKFAST**

A boiled egg with wholemeal bread; a glass of carrot juice.

**SNACKS**

Dried fruit or nuts; dandelion infusion.

**LUNCH**

Mediterranean bean salad (page 96); boiled fish; fruit salad.

**DINNER**

Watercress or nettle soup (page 94); cottage cheese with blueberries (page 41); elderflower and camomile infusion.

# skin, hair and nails

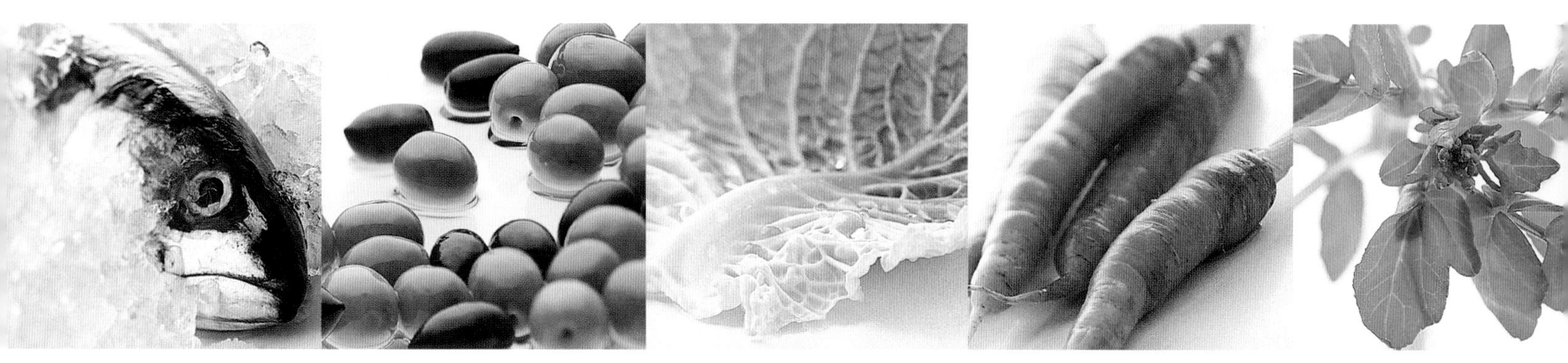

**STAR FOODS FOR SKIN, HAIR AND NAILS: ALL RED, YELLOW OR GREEN FRUIT AND VEGETABLES, CABBAGE, CAMOMILE, CARROT, CHERVIL, DANDELION, OILY FISH, OLIVE, SHELLFISH, WATERCRESS.**

To improve or control a skin condition, try following a detox programme such as the one outlined on pages 134–37. It is important to identify any foods to which you may be allergic and to eliminate them from your diet. If you smoke, make an effort to give up. You should also treat the skin externally by applying skin washes and poultices to eliminate inflammation and bacterial activity (see specific skin problems).

The following foods promote healthy skin, hair and nails:
1) dandelion is a general detoxifier;
2) carrots and all red, yellow or green fruit and vegetables are rich in beta-carotene and antioxidants;
3) green, leafy vegetables contain vitamins and minerals that are beneficial for the skin;
4) camomile infusion can help to relieve stress (which may exacerbate skin problems), it can also be used as a skin wash;
5) shellfish and oily fish contain essential fatty acids and minerals.
(N.B. To make a medicinal infusion, steep 1 tablespoon of the dried ingredient in a cup of boiling water for 10 minutes.)

## ACNE

**A SKIN CONDITION CHARACTERIZED BY INFLAMED SPOTS ON THE FACE, NECK OR BACK, USUALLY RELATED TO HORMONAL FLUCTUATIONS.**

✓ Foods that are rich in zinc and vitamin A. Apply cabbage leaves or juice, carrot juice or a lettuce-seed decoction to very inflamed spots and use a camomile infusion as a face wash.

✗ Cheese, chocolate, food that is rich in iodine (such as shellfish and kelp), refined carbohydrate.

RECIPES *cabbage, carrot and blueberry juice (page 25), juniper-berry water (apply externally, see page 57), black radish and carrot juice (page 119).*

## BOILS AND CARBUNCLES

**SEE ACNE.**

## DANDRUFF

**A FLAKY SCALP, SOMETIMES CAUSED BY A YEAST INFECTION.**

✓ Rinse your hair with a thyme or rosemary infusion. SEE ALSO general advice on the care of the Skin, Hair and Nails.

## DERMATITIS AND ECZEMA

**AN INFLAMMATION OF THE SKIN WHICH IS OFTEN CHRONIC. SORES MAY BE DRY AND ITCHY OR WEEPING.**

✓ Artichoke, carrot, chervil, cucumber, dandelion, all green vegetables, grape, melon, oily fish, raspberry, salsify. An application of olive or walnut oil is effective in relieving dry skin. A camomile or thyme infusion can be used as a skin wash to reduce inflammation and prevent bacterial activity.

✗ Alcohol and spicy food. Reduce your intake of dairy products, meat, processed food and any other suspected allergens.

RECIPES *cabbage, carrot and blueberry juice (page 25), juniper-berry water (apply externally, see page 57), black radish and carrot juice (page 119), dandelion infusion (page 123).*

### FUNGAL INFECTIONS

AN IRRITATION OF THE SKIN BETWEEN THE TOES OR FINGERS, AROUND THE GROIN OR ON THE SCALP.

✓ Use a thyme infusion to bathe or wash the affected area. *SEE ALSO* general care of the Immune System.

### PSORIASIS

A HEREDITARY CONDITION CAUSING AN EXCESSIVE PRODUCTION OF NEW SKIN CELLS. THIS RESULTS IN SORE, SCALY PATCHES ON THE SKIN.

! STRESS IS KNOWN TO AGGRAVATE AND EVEN TRIGGER PSORIASIS.

✓ Eat plenty of oily fish and increase your exposure to sunlight. *SEE ALSO* Irritability and Stress (page 83).

✗ Animal fat and dairy products.

### ROSACEA

A CHRONIC INFLAMMATION OF THE FACE CAUSING RED AREAS TO APPEAR ON THE CHEEKS, NOSE, FOREHEAD AND CHIN.

! THE CONDITION IS EXACERBATED BY ALCOHOL AND STRESS.

✓ Try following a dairy-free diet. Use a camomile infusion as an anti-inflammatory face wash. A thyme infusion or cabbage or lettuce leaves applied to the affected area can also help to reduce the inflammation.

✗ Alcohol and spicy food.

RECIPES *cabbage, carrot and blueberry juice (page 25), black radish and carrot juice (page 119).*

### URTICARIA (HIVES)

RAISED RED, ITCHY PATCHES CAUSE BY AN ALLERGIC REACTION AND AGGRAVATED BY STRESS.

! THIS CONDITION MAY BE A REACTION TO A PRESCRIPTION DRUG – CONSULT YOUR DOCTOR. HIVES CAN BE DANGEROUS IF THE MOUTH, LIPS AND TONGUE ARE AFFECTED.

✓ Artichoke, carrot, cucumber, dandelion, green vegetables (especially nettle and watercress), radish, watermelon. Drink camomile or lemon-balm infusions. Use a mixture of equal amounts of camomile and peppermint infusion as a skin wash.

✗ Try to identify and eliminate the cause of the allergy (for example strawberries or shellfish). Avoid alcohol, animal fat, dairy products, eggs, stimulants and wheat for a few days.

RECIPES *lemon-balm and camomile infusion (page 124), sparkling lemon-balm infusion (page 125).*

# women's health

For specific conditions affecting women's health, see below. For lactating mothers, fennel is recommended, as it is thought to stimulate the baby's appetite and prevent colic and digestive problems; dill enhances the flavour of breast milk.
(N.B. To make a medicinal infusion, steep 1 tablespoon of the dried ingredient in a cup of boiling water for 10 minutes.)

### AMENORRHOEA

ABSENCE OF OR IRREGULAR PERIODS. MAY BE CAUSED BY HORMONAL IMBALANCE, STRESS, OVER-EXERCISE, RAPID WEIGHT LOSS OR ANOREXIA.

✓ Anise, dill, dried fruit, fennel, green, leafy vegetables, liver, parsley, red meat, sage, yeast extract. Drink fresh apricot, broccoli or spinach juice and aniseed, fennel-seed or sage infusion.

RECIPES *apricot, lime and mint juice (page 117), broccoli and green bean juice (page 119), fennel infusion (page 123), carrot-seed infusion (page 124), coriander-seed infusion (page 125), corn-hair and fennel-seed decoction (page 125), dill-seed decoction (page 126), fennel-seed decoction (page 126), anisette (page 129), aniseed tincture (page 130), coriander-seed tincture (page 130).*

### CYSTITIS

SEE KIDNEYS AND BLADDER.

### DIGESTIVE PROBLEMS DURING PREGNANCY

PROBLEMS SUCH AS HEARTBURN, SLUGGISH DIGESTION, HYPER-ACIDITY AND INDIGESTION ARE COMMON DURING PREGNANCY.

✓ Apple, banana, carrot, courgette, fig, germinated barley, ginger, papaya, peach, pineapple, potato. Eat small, frequent meals. Drink apple, carrot, peach or pineapple juice; and basil, camomile, fennel-seed or lemon-balm infusion. *SEE ALSO* constipation (page 74).

✗ Avoid fatty and processed foods.

RECIPES *fennel infusion (page 123), lemon-balm and camomile infusion (page 124), sparkling lemon-balm infusion (page 125), ginger infusion (page 125), corn-hair and fennel-seed decoction (page 125), fennel-seed decoction (page 126), barley water (page 127).*

## ENDOMETRIOSIS

**INFLAMMATION RESULTING FROM FRAGMENTS OF THE ENDOMETRIUM MIGRATING IN THE PELVIS AND AROUND THE INTESTINES CAUSING PAINFUL PERIODS AND SHARP PAIN IN THE PELVIS DURING INTERCOURSE. SEE PREMENSTRUAL SYNDROME AND PAINFUL PERIODS.**

## FLUID RETENTION

**SOME WOMEN SUFFER FROM FLUID RETENTION PRIOR TO MENSTRUATION OR DURING PREGNANCY.**

✓ Drink barley infusion. Leek and onion are good diuretics.

RECIPES *barley infusion (page 124)*

## IRREGULAR PERIODS

**SEE AMENORRHOEA.**

## MENOPAUSAL SYMPTOMS

**THE HORMONAL CHANGES ASSOCIATED WITH THE MENOPAUSE (CESSATION OF PERIODS AROUND THE AGE OF 50) GIVE RISE TO A RANGE OF SYMPTOMS INCLUDING HOT FLUSHES AND MOOD SWINGS.**

✓ Foods rich in calcium and manganese: avocado, cottage cheese, chestnut, date, fig, green vegetables, live yoghurt, nut, soya, tea, tofu, unrefined cereals. Foods rich in boron: almond, raisin, prune, soya. Food rich in B vitamins (pages 138–39). Drink fresh cabbage, cherry, grape, grapefruit and watercress juice and aniseed, camomile, cumin-seed, lemon-balm and sage infusion and live yoghurt drinks.

RECIPES *cabbage, carrot and blueberry juice (page 25), cherry and raspberry juice (page 118), cherry and apple juice (page 118), lemon-balm and camomile infusion (page 124), sparkling lemon-balm infusion (page 125), cumin-seed decoction (page 126), anisette (page 129), aniseed tincture (page 130).*

## MORNING SICKNESS

**NAUSEA, AND SOMETIMES VOMITING, IS A COMMON SYMPTOM IN THE FIRST TRIMESTER OF PREGNANCY.**

✓ Eat small, frequent meals and increase your intake of carbohydrate (bean, bread, chestnut, pasta and rice). Drinking fennel, ginger or peppermint infusions or a eating a small amount of crystallized ginger can help alleviate nausea.

RECIPES *fennel infusion (page 123), ginger infusion (page 125).*

## PERIOD PAIN

**PAIN IN THE LOWER ABDOMEN JUST BEFORE AND DURING PERIODS.**

✓ Aniseed, dill and sage have hormone-like properties – drink as infusions. The following are powerful antispasmodics and analgesics and are excellent as infusions for abdominal cramps and pain: bay leaf, camomile, chive and spring onion, coriander seed, fennel, mint, onion and shallot, rosemary, saffron, tarragon.

RECIPES *tarragon-infused oil (apply externally, see page 50), raspberry-leaf infusion (page 123), lemon-balm and camomile infusion (page 124), coriander-seed infusion (page 125), dill-seed decoction (page 126).*

## PREGNANCY (GENERAL WELL-BEING)

**GOOD NUTRITION IS IMPORTANT FOR THE HEALTH OF BOTH MOTHER AND BABY DURING PREGNANCY.**

✓ Foods that are rich in iron and folic acid (these include dried fruit and dark-green, leafy vegetables such as watercress, spinach and broccoli) should be eaten on a daily basis, plus beetroot, blackberry, celery, fennel root, germinated pulses, live yoghurt, red meat, unrefined cereals. Drink one and a half litres of mineral water every day and fresh apple, apricot, beetroot, cabbage, grape, green bean, lettuce or watercress juice and camomile, fennel, lime-blossom flower and mint infusion.

✗ Alcohol and fast or processed food. Do not smoke.

RECIPES *cabbage, carrot and blueberry juice (page 25), apple and raspberry juice (page 117), apricot, lime and mint juice (page 117), cherry and apple juice (page 118), green bean and garlic juice (page 119), beetroot and celery juice (page 119), lettuce and basil juice (page 119), fennel infusion (page 123), raspberry-leaf infusion (page 123), lemon-balm and camomile infusion (page 124), ginger infusion (page 125), fennel-seed decoction (page 126).*

## PREMENSTRUAL SYNDROME (PMS)

**A VARIETY OF PHYSICAL AND EMOTIONAL SYMPTOMS OCCURRING A FEW DAYS BEFORE A PERIOD IS DUE. SYMPTOMS INCLUDE CONSTIPATION, FATIGUE, FLUID RETENTION, IRRITABILITY, LOWER ABDOMINAL PAIN AND DISTENSION, AND MOOD SWINGS.**

✓ Increase your intake of fruit and vegetables rich in vitamin B6, calcium, magnesium, manganese and zinc (pages 140–41). Eat small, frequent meals rich in carbohydrates (bean, bread, chestnut, pasta and rice) and root vegetables. Aniseed, dill and sage have hormone-like properties – drink as infusions; tarragon and mint are powerful anti-spasmodics and analgesics and are excellent as infusions for abdominal cramps. Barley contains an amino acid that may help to relieve PMS. SEE ALSO general advice on the care of the Nervous System, and Irritability and Stress (page 83).

✗ Fatty or salty foods, stimulants such as coffee, cola drinks and tea. Reduce your consumption of dairy products.

RECIPES *celery and red onion juice (page 119), cucumber and lettuce heart juice (page 119), lettuce and basil juice (page 119), lemon-balm and camomile infusion (page 124), sparkling lemon-balm infusion (page 125).*

### THRUSH

A VAGINAL INFECTION RESULTING IN SORENESS AND DISCHARGE. SEE CANDIDA (PAGE 84). DOUCHE WITH CAMOMILE AND THYME INFUSION.

# men's health

### ENLARGED PROSTATE

A COMMON CONDITION IN MEN OVER 45. DIFFICULTY URINATING IN THE MORNING IS AN EARLY SYMPTOM OF AN ENLARGED PROSTRATE.

✓ Bread, chicken, corn, dried fig, egg, fish, green vegetables, live yoghurt, nettle, nut, pumpkin seed, pumpkin seed oil, soya, tofu and foods rich in zinc (page 141). The following remedy may alleviate the condition: mix equal amounts of almond, brazil nut, cucumber seed, linseed, peanut, pumpkin seed, sesame seed, soya bean and walnut. Make into a paste using a food processor. Take 2 tablespoons daily.

### PROSTATITIS

SEE ENLARGED PROSTATE AND GENERAL ADVICE ON THE CARE OF THE IMMUNE SYSTEM.

✓ Infusions of juniper berries or blueberries.

# children's health

Most of the advice given in this part of the book also applies to children, with the exception of alcohol-based preparations.

### ANXIETY, FEAR, NIGHTMARES

✓ Infusions of camomile, lemon balm or linden in the evening.

RECIPES *lemon-balm and camomile infusion (page 124), sparkling lemon-balm infusion (page 125).*

### CHICKENPOX

SEE MEASLES.

### CONSTIPATION

SEE DIGESTIVE SYSTEM.

✓ For infants, use puréed boiled carrot or cooked apple.

RECIPES *peach syrup (page 130).*

### DIARRHOEA

SEE DIGESTIVE SYSTEM.

✓ Blueberry, boiled carrot and rice water (see Rice; page 33) are the safest dietary remedies for children.

### MEASLES

A HIGHLY CONTAGIOUS VIRAL INFECTION CHARACTERIZED BY FEVER AND A SKIN RASH.

✓ Blackberry, celery, cherry, cucumber, onion and thyme help reduce fever and fight infection. Camomile tea can be used as a skin wash to calm down itching and irritation. Olive oil mixed with 3 per cent of lavender essential oil is also helpful for skin rashes.

RECIPES *cabbage, carrot and blueberry juice (page 25), black radish and carrot juice (page 119), cherry-stem decoction (page 125), cherry-stem and apple decoction (page 126).*

### WHOOPING COUGH

SEE RESPIRATORY SYSTEM.

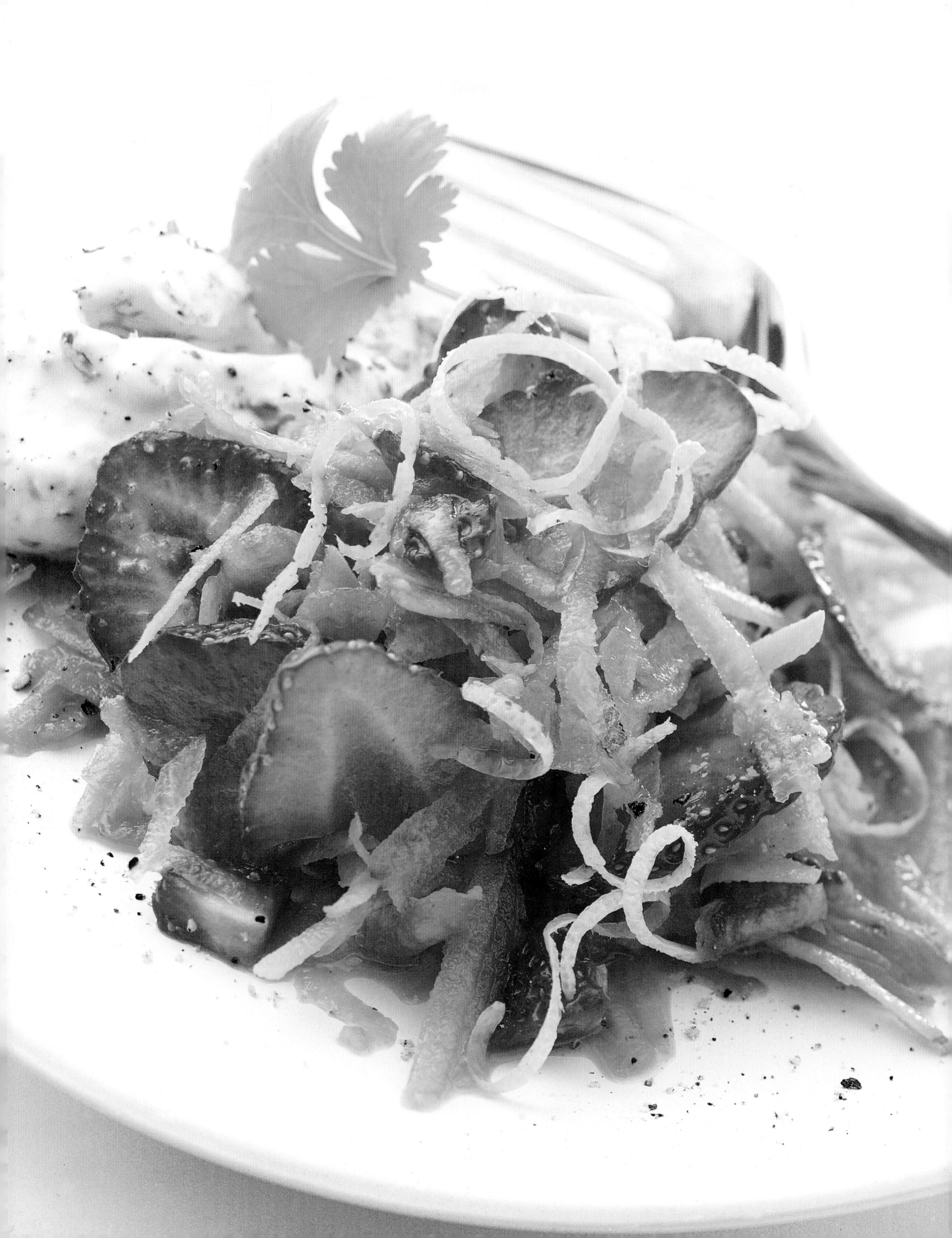

chapter three

# healing recipes

Incorporating medicinal foods into our diet is a perfect opportunity for creative and delicious cooking. The recipes on the following pages range from quick and unusual dishes that boost good health to recipes for medicinal drinks, tinctures and syrups that target specific ailments (bear in mind that some of the wines and liqueurs need to be prepared in advance). To find ways of using a particular medicinal food, start with the food – by looking in Chapter One of the book where you will find references to the recipes in this section. To find a dish or a remedy that will alleviate a particular ailment, start with the ailment – by looking under the appropriate body system in Chapter Two where beneficial recipes are recommended. Or simply browse through the recipes to devise your own health-giving menu.

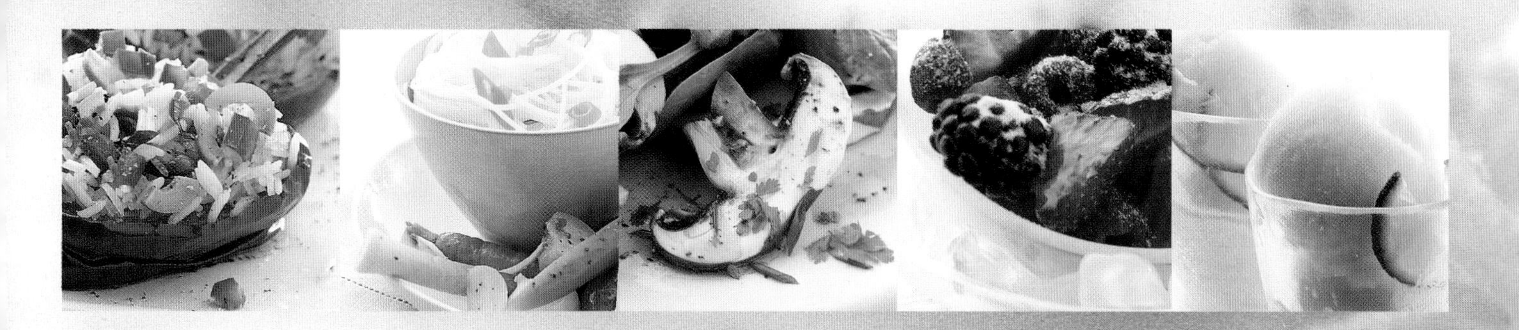

# soups and salads

The following recipes serve 4 people unless otherwise stated. Where possible, harvest your own ingredients or use fresh, organic produce. Take care to wash ingredients thoroughly.

## SOUPS

### croutons

1 clove of garlic
4 thick slices of bread (1 day old at least)
Olive oil

Rub the garlic on the bread, then dice the bread and fry lightly in olive oil. Leave to drain on kitchen paper for a few minutes.

### broad bean soup *(right)*

1½ kg fresh or dried broad beans
2 tbsp olive oil
1 red onion, finely chopped
50 g fresh chervil, parsley or rocket, chopped
2 litres cold water
Salt and pepper to taste.

If you choose to use dried broad beans, soak them according to the instructions on the packet. In a saucepan, heat the olive oil and add the onion. Cover and sweat slowly for 10 minutes over a gentle heat. Add the broad beans, chervil, parsley or rocket and water. Bring to the boil and simmer until the beans are cooked. Blend the soup in a food processor, add salt and pepper and serve hot with croutons (see recipe above).

### herbal broth

50 g sorrel leaves, finely chopped
25 g lettuce leaves, finely chopped
25 g Swiss chard leaves, finely chopped
25 g fresh chervil, finely chopped
25 g leeks, chopped
Salt to taste
1½ litres water
1 tbsp olive oil

Blend all the ingredients in a food processor. Transfer the mixture to a saucepan. Bring to the boil, and then simmer for 20 minutes or until cooked.

### borscht

½ medium green or white cabbage
½ medium red cabbage
2 medium red beetroots, peeled
1½ litres stock (meat or vegetable)
1 parsnip, peeled and cut in two
1 large carrot, peeled and cut in two
A few cumin seeds
3 tbsp tomato purée
2 tbsp red wine vinegar
Salt and pepper to taste
To garnish: soured cream or yoghurt

Chop the cabbage and one of the beetroots into thin strips. In a large saucepan, bring the stock to the boil and add the cabbage, beetroot strips, parsnip, carrot, cumin and tomato purée. Cover and simmer for approximately 1 hour, topping up with stock if necessary. Remove the parsnip and carrot from the broth (if they have not already disintegrated), mash with a fork and return to the saucepan. Using a juicer, extract the juice from the remaining beetroot. Add the juice, vinegar, salt and pepper to the broth. Garnish with a little soured cream or yoghurt and serve.

### chickpea broth

Boiling chickpeas and barley together produces a medicinal decoction that has diuretic properties and can be drunk as a treatment for cystitis and oedema. Simply drain off the cooking water after 30 minutes and store in the refrigerator. Top up the pan with water and continue cooking. The finished broth is bland in taste and excellent for babies or people recovering from illness.

100 g chickpeas, soaked and allowed to germinate (this may take up to 48 hours)
150 g pot barley
1 litre water
Salt and pepper to taste
50 g fresh parsley, chopped

Boil the chickpeas and the barley in the water for 60 minutes or until thoroughly cooked. Season with salt and pepper. Add the parsley and leave to infuse for 10 minutes. Blend in a food processor and serve.

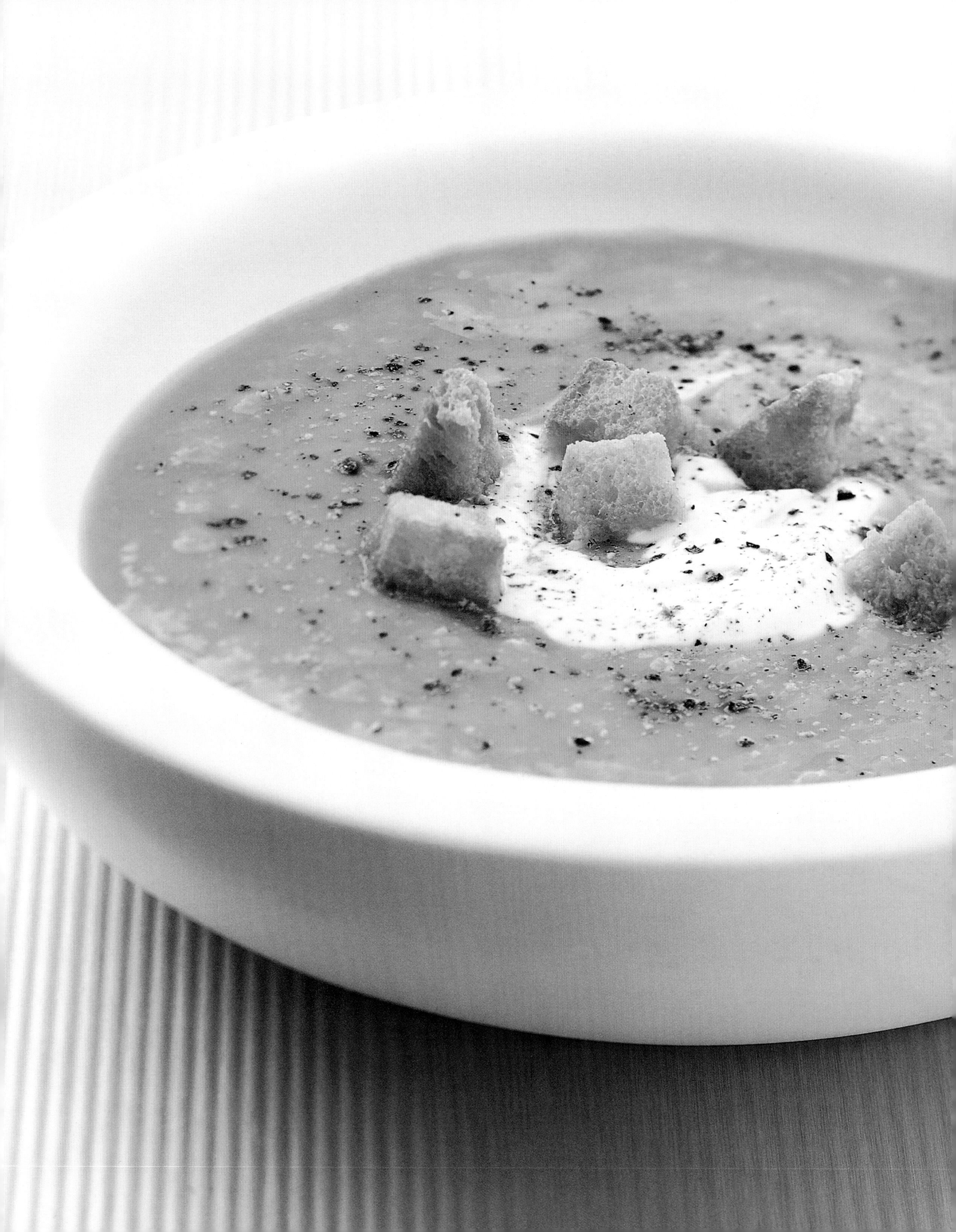

# chive and ginger broth *(below)*

1 bunch of chives or 8 spring onions, trimmed
1 clove
5-cm piece of root ginger, peeled and sliced
2 cloves of garlic
5 black peppercorns
Small root of Chinese angelica, chopped
1 litre water

Boil all the ingredients in the water for 15 minutes and serve hot. Chicken pieces can be added to this broth – put the raw pieces in the broth and simmer for 30 minutes. Serve.

# nettle soup

Harvest fresh, young nettle tops from nettles growing away from busy paths and polluted areas.

500 g potatoes, peeled and chopped
300 g nettle tops (leaves and stems)
Salt and pepper to taste
75 ml olive oil
2 tbsp fresh chervil or parsley, finely chopped

In a large pan, cover the potatoes with cold water. Bring to the boil and then simmer for about 20 minutes or until cooked. Add the nettles and simmer for 5-8 minutes. Season with salt and pepper. In a food processor, blend the soup, then stir in the olive oil and chervil or parsley. Serve hot with croutons (see page 92).

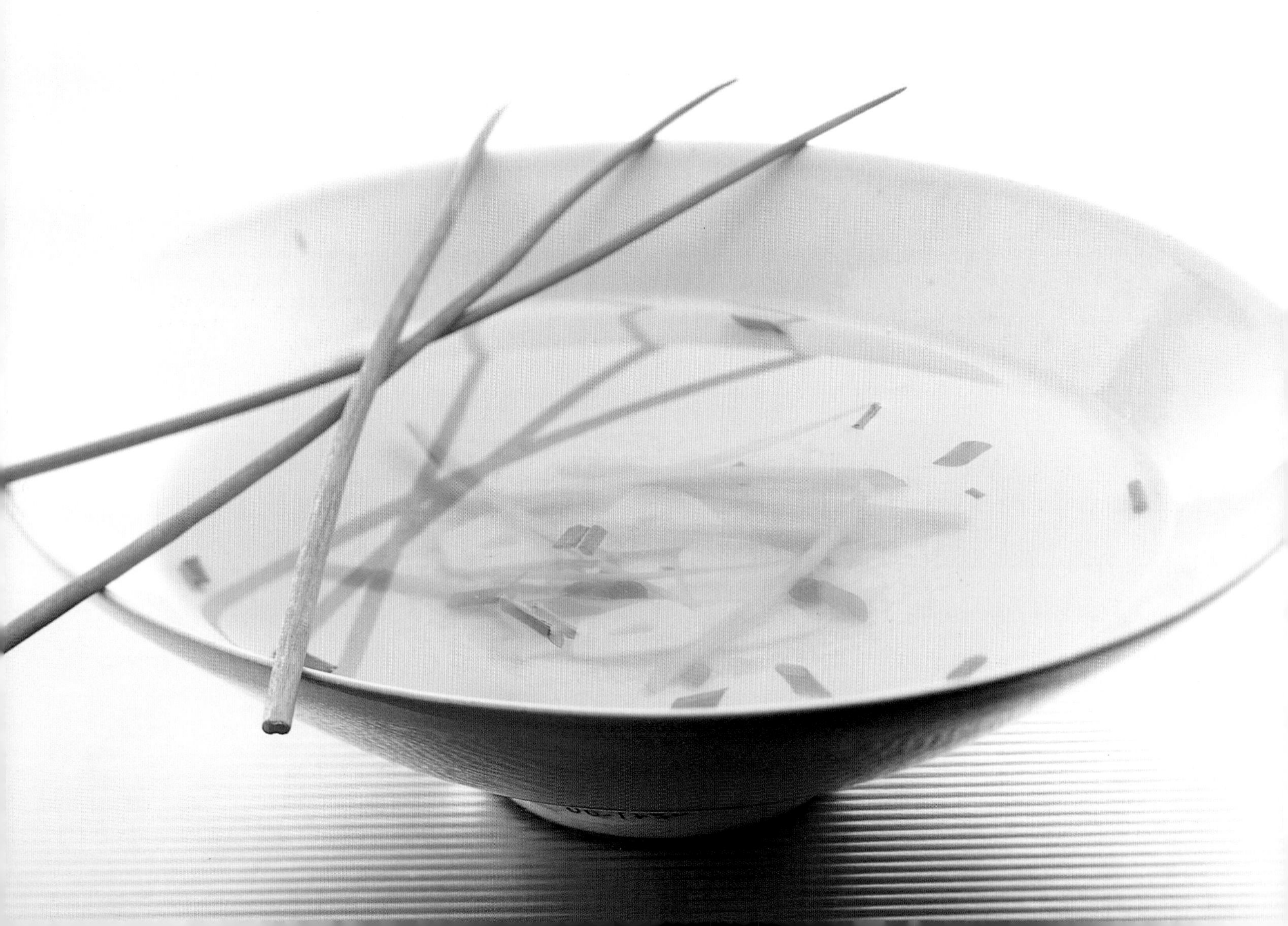

## lentil soup

You can use germinated lentils for this recipe. Buy whole lentils that are green on the outside and red inside rather than split red lentils. Soak them in cold water for 24 hours, then strain, rinse with cold water and place in a flat dish. Cover the lentils with a wet cloth and leave them in a well-ventilated place for a further 24 hours to allow the shoots to grow. Leave the lentils for 48 hours for even longer shoots.

400 g germinated lentils or non-germinated split red lentils
Chicken or vegetable stock (enough to cover the lentils)
3 red onions, chopped
2 tomatoes, chopped
4 cloves of garlic, crushed
2 tbsp dill
Black pepper to taste
To garnish: soured cream, cottage cheese or yoghurt

Steam the lentils for 20 minutes and then cover with chicken or vegetable stock and simmer for a further 20 minutes. Meanwhile, steam the onions, tomatoes and garlic for 5 minutes and then blend in a food processor. Add the onion mixture to the simmering lentils, together with the dill and pepper. Simmer for a further 5 minutes; Garnish with a little soured cream, cottage cheese or yoghurt and serve immediately.

# SALADS

## vinaigrette dressing

1 or 2 cloves of garlic (or to taste)
2 tbsp lemon juice
4 tbsp olive oil
1 tsp Dijon mustard (optional)
Salt and pepper to taste

Crush the garlic, mix with the lemon juice and then stir in the olive oil and mustard (if using). Season with salt and pepper and then pour the dressing over the salad. Vinaigrette can be made very quickly by blending the ingredients in a food processor.

## avocado dressing

2 avocados, peeled and stoned
1 clove of garlic (optional)
Lemon juice to taste
1 tbsp Dijon mustard
1 tbsp fresh parsley, finely chopped
Salt and pepper to taste

Blend the ingredients in a food processor and use as an alternative to mayonnaise or vinaigrette.

## pepper and aubergine salad

1 green pepper, halved
1 red pepper, halved
1 yellow pepper, halved
500 g aubergine, chopped into small pieces
Juice of ½ lemon
2 shallots, finely chopped
250 g tomatoes, quartered
Vinaigrette dressing
2 tbsp fresh basil or mint, finely chopped

Under a preheated grill, char the peppers. When the skin has turned black put the peppers in a plastic bag and seal it. When cool enough to handle, rub off the skin and slice the peppers thinly. Lightly cook the aubergine in salted, boiling water with the lemon juice until tender. Drain the aubergine and mix with the peppers, shallots and tomatoes. Toss in the vinaigrette and sprinkle with the basil or mint. Chill in the refrigerator for 2 hours before serving.

## carrot and strawberry salad

This salad goes well with coriander dressing.

3 tbsp olive oil
Juice of 1 small lemon
500 g carrot, peeled and grated
300 g strawberries, chopped
To garnish: 3 strawberries
Thin strips of lemon zest

Mix the olive oil and lemon juice in a bowl. Add the carrots and strawberries. Garnish with the 3 strawberries and the lemon zest. This salad will improve if it is refrigerated for 3 hours.

## coriander dressing

1 tbsp coriander, finely chopped
300 ml live natural yoghurt
Salt and pepper to taste

Mix the coriander with the yoghurt, and season with salt and pepper.

# mediterranean bean salad *(below)*

200 g dried haricot, borlotti or black-eye beans
Pinch of ground cinnamon
1 onion, finely chopped
2 tomatoes, chopped
50 g black olives
1 clove
Salt and pepper to taste
4 tbsp olive oil
1 tbsp fresh mint leaves, chopped

Soak the beans according to the instructions on the packet, then put them in cold water, bring to the boil and simmer for about 2 hours with the cinnamon. Drain the beans and mix them with the other ingredients, except the mint leaves. Finally, sprinkle the mint leaves on top of the salad and refrigerate for as long as possible (up to 12 hours). Serve with garlic bread.

# radish and kumquat salad *(below right)*

Large bunch of radishes, tops removed
2 oranges
12 kumquats
Lemon juice to taste
Pinch of salt
Sugar or clear honey (optional)

Slice the radishes and oranges and mix in a salad bowl. Slice the kumquats in half lengthways and add to bowl. Sprinkle on the lemon juice and salt. Refrigerate and toss before serving. If desired, add sugar or honey to taste.

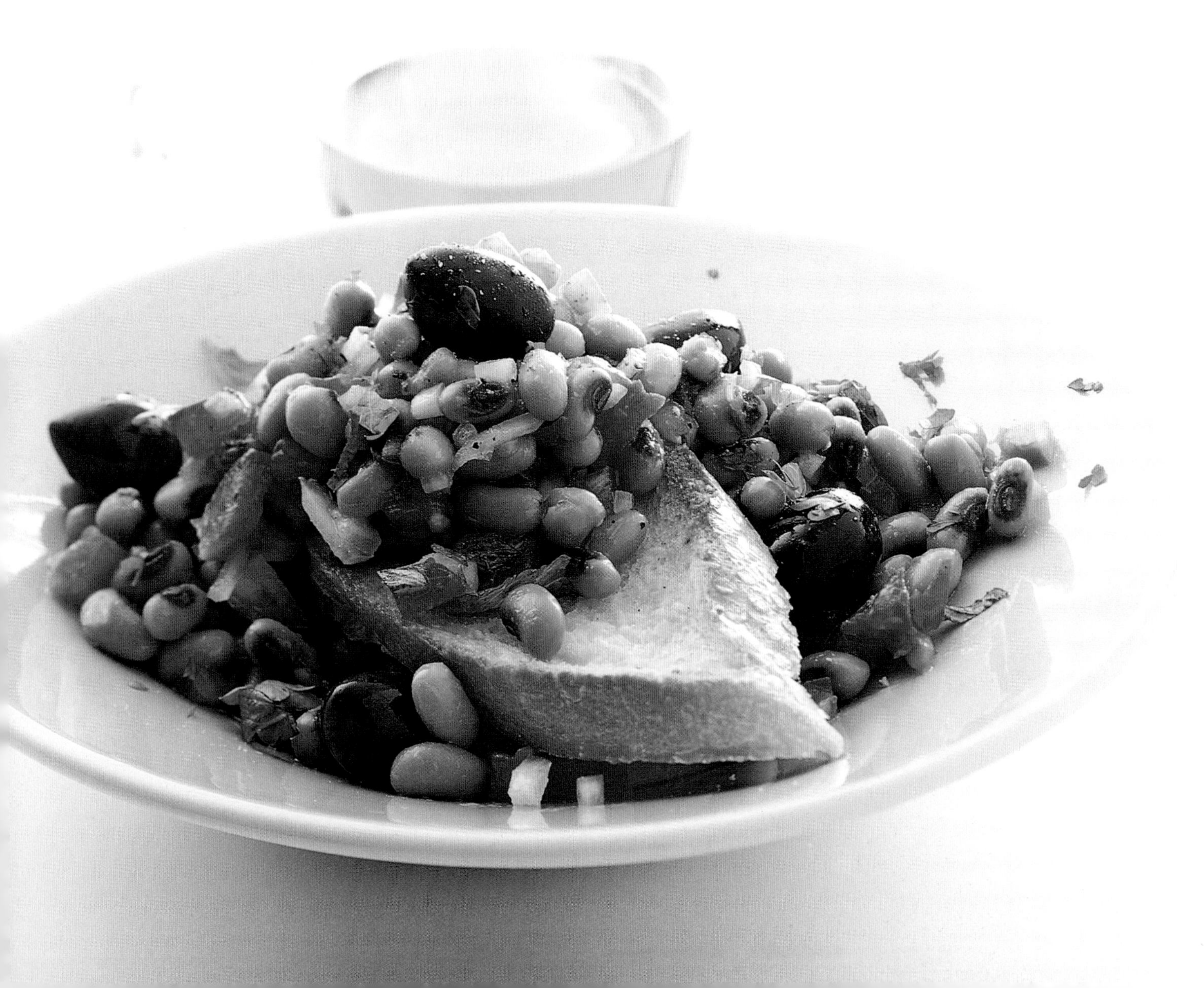

# fennel and radicchio salad

2 fennel bulbs, finely chopped
Radicchio leaves (roughly equal in quantity to the fennel)
4 tbsp vinaigrette (made from one-third vinegar or lemon juice and two-thirds olive oil)

Mix the fennel and radicchio leaves in a large salad bowl. Sprinkle with vinaigrette immediately prior to serving.

# green bean salad

500 g green beans
30 g hazelnuts, chopped
3 tbsp vinaigrette (page 95)
½ lettuce
2 tbsp fresh parsley or chervil, chopped

In boiling, salted water cook the green beans until al dente. When they are ready, plunge them into cold water, then drain. Roast the hazelnuts in a frying pan without oil. Toss the beans in the vinaigrette and place them on a bed of lettuce. Sprinkle the hazelnuts, together with the parsley or chervil, over the beans. Serve.

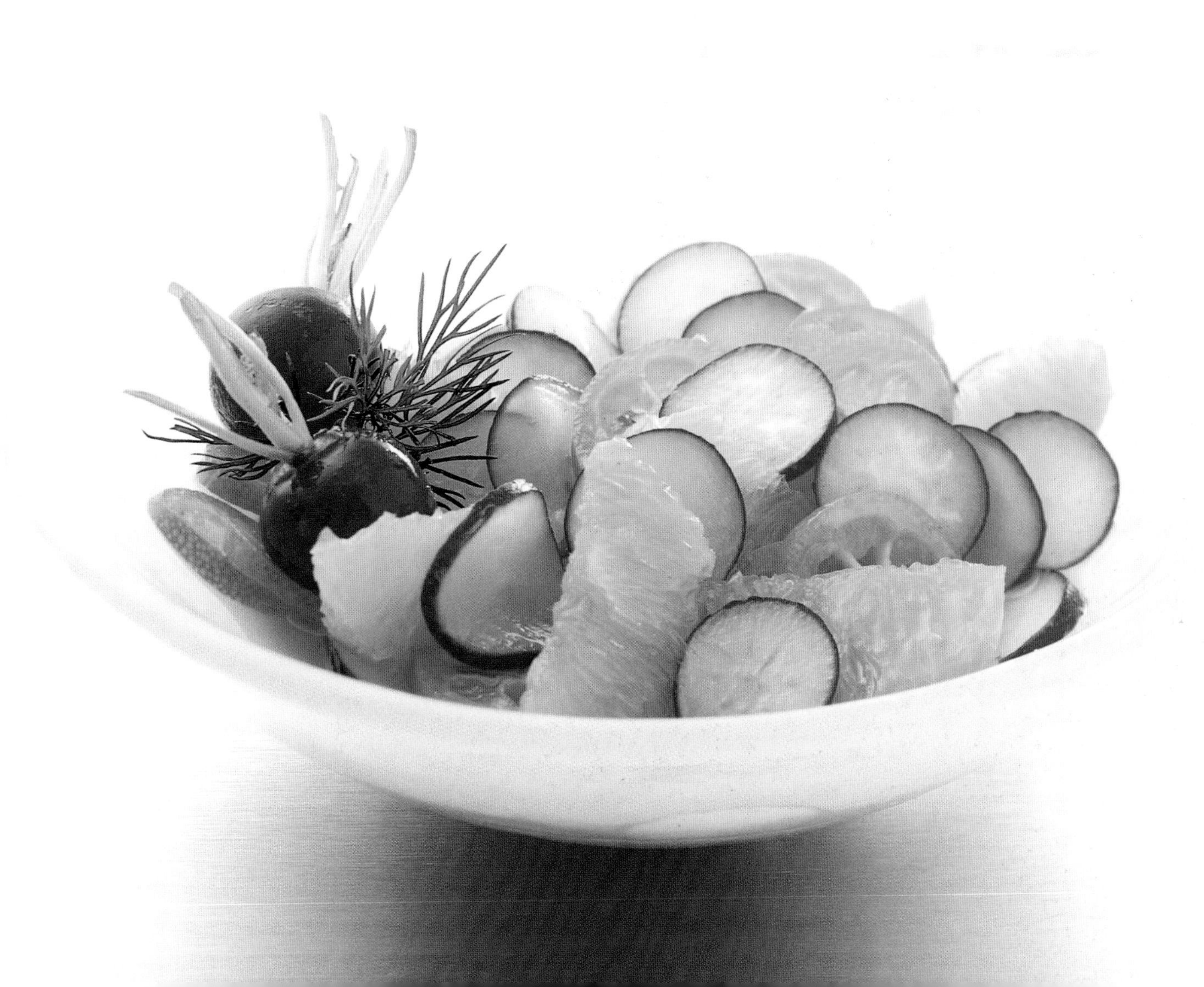

# grated celeriac and carrot salad

300 g celeriac, peeled and grated or cut into julienne strips
300 g carrots, peeled and grated or cut into julienne strips
A few tbsp avocado dressing (page 95)
To garnish: 2 tbsp fresh chervil or parsley, finely chopped

In boiling, salted water blanch the celeriac for 5 seconds and drain. Mix together the celeriac and raw carrot and toss in the avocado dressing (use just enough to coat the vegetables). Refrigerate for 2 hours, garnish with the chervil or parsley and serve.

# young turnip salad *(below)*

This salad goes well with thin slices of smoked fish.

1 kg young turnips, peeled
½ litre chicken or vegetable stock
3 tbsp fresh chives, finely chopped
3 tbsp fresh tarragon, finely chopped
3 tbsp fresh chervil, finely chopped
2 tbsp olive oil
1 tbsp lemon juice

In boiling, salted water blanch the turnips for 2 minutes. Drain and then cook further in the stock for 10–15 minutes. Drain and allow to cool. Place the turnips in a serving dish and sprinkle over the chives, tarragon and chervil. Mix the olive oil and lemon juice together and pour over the turnips. Gently toss the salad and serve warm.

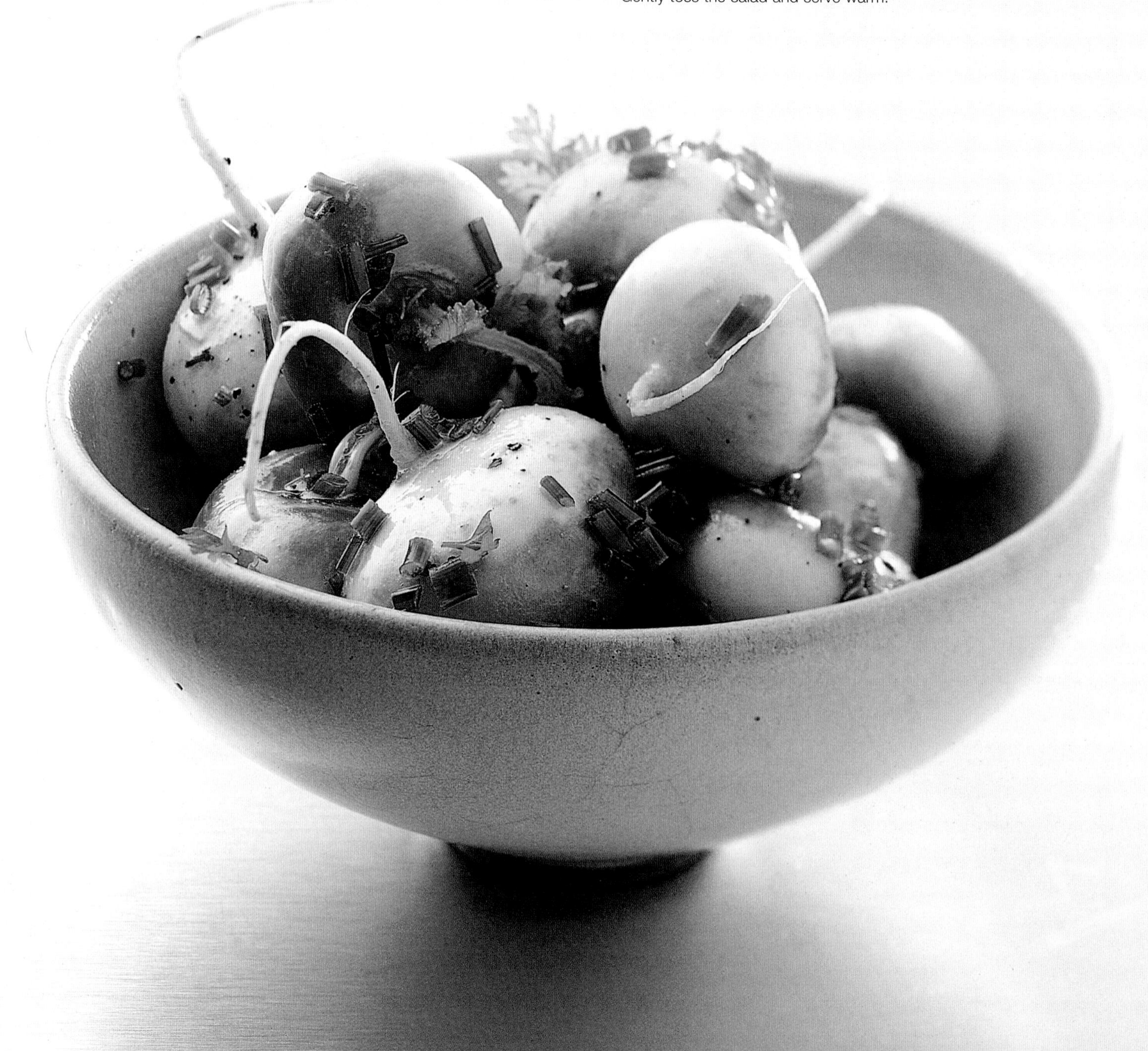

# escarole salad

1 escarole (or any type of salad leaf)
A few radishes, tops removed
100 g black olives, stoned
A few anchovies (optional)
3 tomatoes, quartered
1 shallot, finely chopped
2 tbsp fresh chives, finely chopped
2 tbsp fresh tarragon, finely chopped
4 tbsp vinaigrette dressing (page 95)
150 g hard goat's cheese, feta cheese or mozzarella

In a bowl, put the escarole, radishes, olives, anchovies (if using), tomatoes, shallot, chives and tarragon. Add the vinaigrette, toss gently and sprinkle over the cheese. Refrigerate for 30 minutes before serving.

# pineapple and cucumber salad

300 g cucumber, peeled and thinly sliced
Salt
300 g fresh pineapple, diced
2 tbsp light mayonnaise or single cream mixed with lemon juice (optional)
To decorate: A few borage leaves in vinegar (page 122), fresh borage flowers or mint leaves

Put the cucumber into a colander, sprinkle with salt to extract the juice and leave for 45 minutes. Rinse away the salt and squeeze the water from the cucumber. In a bowl, mix the cucumber slices and diced pineapple and refrigerate for 2 hours. Before serving, drain away any excess water, toss in the mayonnaise or cream if desired, and decorate with the borage or mint.

# warm asparagus salad

1 kg fresh thick asparagus, trimmed (remove woody ends)
Salt and pepper
6 tbsp olive oil
2 tbsp fresh chervil (optional), finely chopped
A few capers
Parmesan cheese shavings
Balsamic vinegar

In a roasting tin, place the asparagus in a single layer (avoid overcrowding) and season well. Pour over the olive oil and roast in a preheated oven at 200ºC/gas mark 6 for about 20 minutes or until tender. Carefully place the cooked asparagus on a warm serving dish and sprinkle with the chervil (if using), capers, Parmesan cheese and a little balsamic vinegar. Serve warm.

# parsley, onion and lemon salad

Serve as a side dish with grilled fish.

2 tbsp olive oil
1 bunch parsley or chervil, finely chopped
1 large red onion, thinly sliced
2 lemons, peeled and diced
Salt and pepper

Mix all the ingredients in a bowl. Chill before serving. Serve on a bed of lettuce leaves.

# black radish salad

1 or 2 black radish (depending on size), peeled and sliced
Salt
150 g Gruyere or a cheese of your choice, finely diced
3 tbsp vinaigrette dressing (page 95)
2 tbsp fresh parsley, finely chopped
1 shallot, finely chopped

Put the radish in a colander, sprinkle with salt to extract the juice and leave for 45 minutes. Rinse the salt off and press down gently on the radish to squeeze out excess water. Mix the radish with some chunks of cheese in a salad bowl and add the vinaigrette. Sprinkle over the parsley and shallot, and lightly toss all the ingredients. Serve on a bed of lettuce leaves.

# cucumber salad

1 large cucumber, peeled and thinly sliced
Salt
2 tbsp fresh chervil or flat-leaf parsley, finely chopped
1 shallot, finely chopped
100 g cooked ham or turkey, diced
4 tbsp vinaigrette dressing (page 95)
Salt and pepper to taste

Put the cucumber into a colander, sprinkle with salt to extract the juice and leave for 45 minutes. Rinse the salt off and, in a bowl, mix with the chervil or flat-leaf parsley, shallot and cooked ham or turkey. Toss in vinaigrette, add salt and pepper and refrigerate before serving.

# starters, main courses and accompaniments

The following recipes serve 4 people unless otherwise stated. Where possible, harvest your own ingredients or use fresh, organic produce. Take care to wash ingredients thoroughly.

## STARTERS

### tabouleh *(below)*

This dish can be served as a starter or a main course. To serve as a main course, double the amount of bulgar wheat in the recipe and add olives, preserved lemon slices (page 45), diced cucumber and a few chopped hard-boiled eggs.

120 g bulgar wheat (or couscous)
Salt and pepper to taste
10 tablespoons olive oil
Juice of 1 lemon
300 g parsley, finely chopped
100 g mint, finely chopped
3 medium shallots or spring onions, chopped
To garnish: 2 tomatoes, diced

Soak the bulgar wheat or couscous in warm water for about 15 minutes (or as indicated on the packet). In a sieve, drain well, pressing the grains to remove any excess water. Put the bulgar wheat or couscous in a bowl and add the salt, pepper, olive oil and lemon juice. Allow the wheat to absorb the dressing, then add the parsley, mint and shallots or spring onions. Refrigerate for 24 hours and then garnish with the tomatoes and serve on a bed of lettuce leaves.

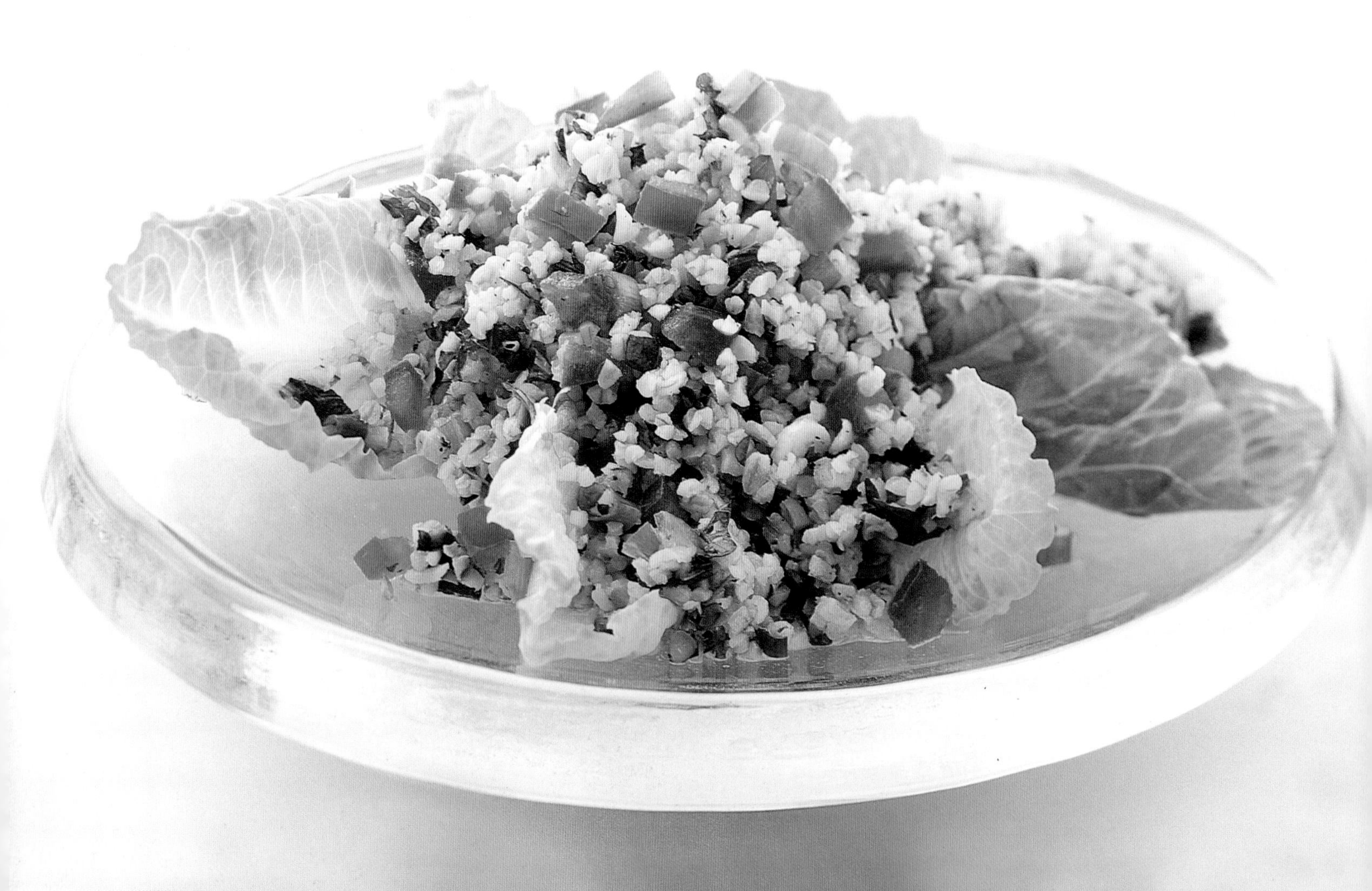

# roman-style artichoke

This dish is excellent served cold a day after making.

50 g parsley, finely chopped
1 tbsp mint leaves, finely chopped
1 clove of garlic, crushed
Salt and pepper to taste
2 tbsp olive oil
4 medium or 8 small globe artichokes
250 ml olive oil
Juice of ½ lemon

Mix the parsley and mint with the garlic, salt, pepper and 2 tablespoons of olive oil. Rinse the artichokes in water. Remove the outer, damaged leaves and the middle leaves. Trim the stalks off each choke (the centre) and remove the chokes using a curved, serrated grapefruit knife. Spoon the herb mixture into the middle of each artichoke and press the remaining leaves around the mixture. In a large casserole dish, cover the artichokes with salted water and 250 ml of olive oil. Bring slowly to the boil, then transfer the casserole dish to a preheated oven at 180°C/gas mark 4 for about 35 minutes or until cooked. Add the lemon juice and serve hot.

# avocado tartar *(right)*

This can be served as a dip with carrot sticks or on toast.

2 avocados, peeled and stoned
2 shallots, finely chopped
1 tbsp chervil, finely chopped
1 tbsp tarragon, finely chopped
Juice of ½ lemon
Salt and pepper to taste

Put the ingredients in a blender and whizz. Refrigerate before serving.

# cottage cheese with watercress

Serve as a starter, or as a snack on toast.

1 bunch watercress
1 tbsp vinegar
250 g low-fat cottage cheese
Salt and pepper to taste
1 tbsp parsley and shallots (optional), finely chopped

Wash the watercress in a bowl of cold water with the vinegar. Dry the watercress, chop finely and combine with the cottage cheese. Season with salt and pepper, and a mixture of the parsley and shallots if desired. Serve.

# green olive tapenade

Serve on toast, with eggs or as a sauce for pasta.

1 clove of garlic, peeled
1 tbsp tarragon, finely chopped
1 tbsp parsley, finely chopped
1 or 2 anchovies, soaked in milk for 10 minutes
3 tbsp olive oil
Juice of ½ small lemon
100 g small green olives, stoned and finely chopped
Salt and pepper to taste

In a food processor blend the garlic, tarragon, parsley, anchovies, olive oil and lemon juice. Add the olives to the herb and oil mixture and season with salt and pepper. Serve.

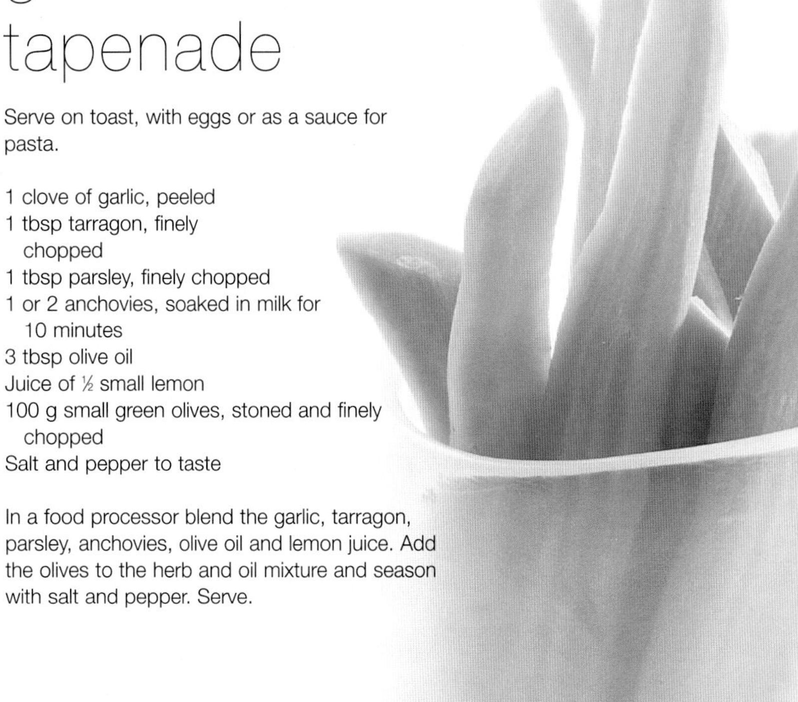

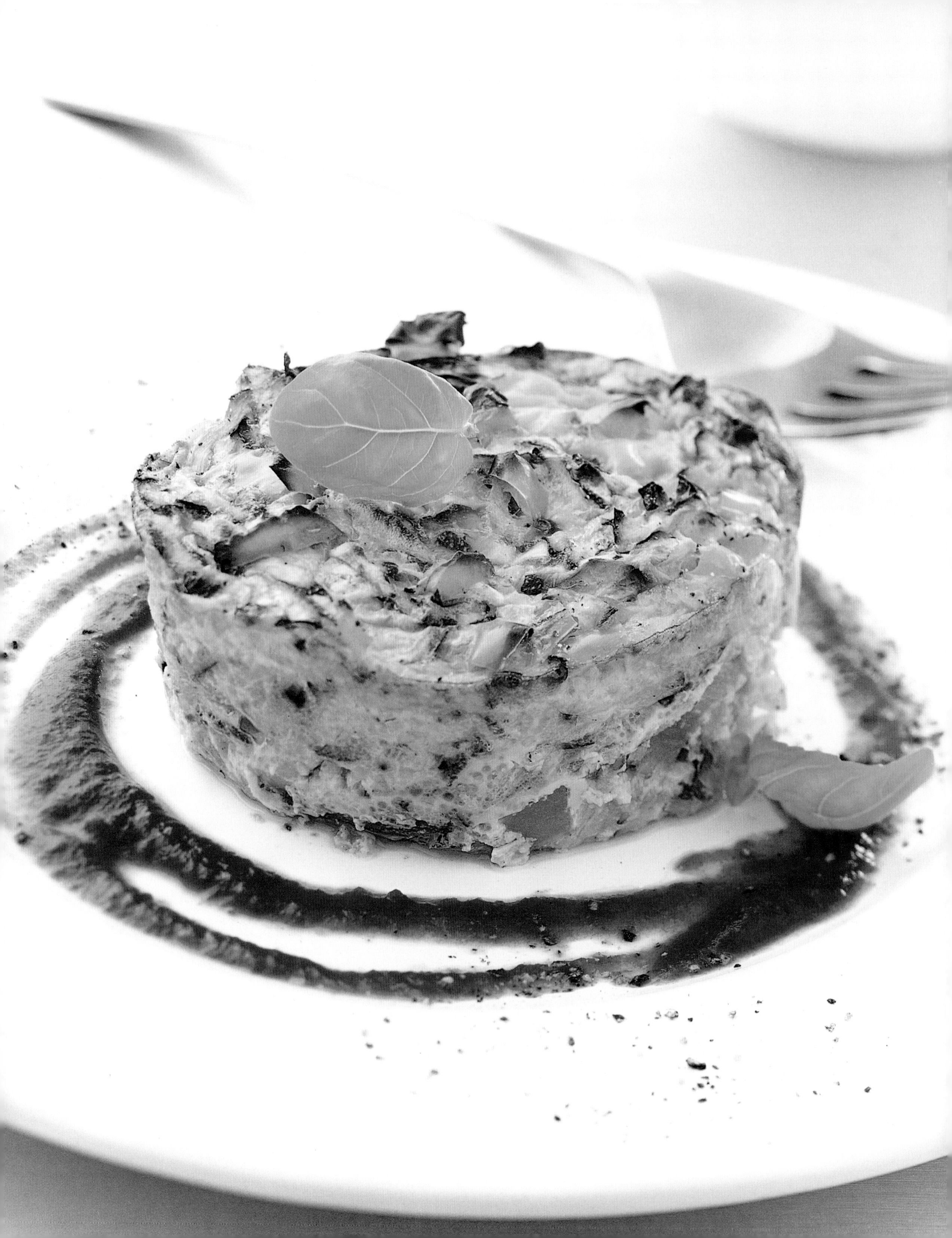

# courgette cake *(left)*

800 g courgettes, roughly chopped
1 egg
3 tbsp cottage cheese or ricotta cheese
Salt and pepper
1 yellow pepper, finely diced

Boil the courgettes for approximately 4 minutes. In a food processor, blend them with the egg, cottage cheese or ricotta, and salt and pepper to taste. Stir in the diced pepper. Divide the mixture between 4 individual dishes and place in a roasting tin, half-filled with hot water. Bake in a preheated oven at 170°C/gas mark 3 for 25 minutes. Serve hot with tomato coulis (see recipe below).

# tomato coulis

Serve with courgette cake (see recipe above).

4 ripe beef tomatoes, quartered
Pinch of sugar
1 tsp tomato purée
4 tbsp olive oil
Salt and pepper to taste

In a food processor, blend the ingredients to an emulsion. Sieve to remove skin and seeds and use as required. Serve as a starter or as an accompaniment to grilled meat.

# MAIN COURSES

# nettle risotto

See page 94 for instructions on harvesting nettles. If nettles are out of season, use young spinach leaves instead.

2 medium onions, sliced
2 tbsp olive oil
400 g risotto rice
150 ml dry white wine
1 litre vegetable or chicken stock, kept hot
200 g nettle tops
Salt and pepper
115 g Parmesan cheese, freshly grated
To garnish: 2 tbsp chervil or parsley, finely chopped

In a heavy-based saucepan, gently sweat the onions in the olive oil for about 10 minutes. Stir in the rice to coat with oil and cook for about 2 minutes. Pour in the wine and cook until the rice has absorbed all the liquid. Add the vegetable or chicken stock, a ladleful at a time, allowing the rice to absorb it all before adding more. Continue until the rice is cooked, but still retaining bite – the risotto should be loose and creamy. Meanwhile, steam the nettles until thoroughly wilted. Squeeze lightly and chop roughly. Stir into the risotto and heat through for 2 minutes. Season well and serve immediately, sprinkled with Parmesan and chervil or parsley.

# buckwheat with leek sauce

Buckwheat comes either green or roasted. Green buckwheat has a much improved flavour if it is dry-roasted first. Cook it on its own in a pan, stirring all the time until there is a nutty, toasted aroma.

500 g dry-roasted green buckwheat
1 litre water
4 large leeks, chopped
3 eggs, beaten
Salt and pepper

For the sauce:
Half the cooked leeks (see recipe)
150 ml single cream, soya milk, cottage cheese or yoghurt
3 tbsp chervil or parsley, chopped
Lemon juice

In a wide, heavy-based saucepan, bring the dry-roasted buckwheat and water to the boil. Simmer, covered, for 15–20 minutes or until the buckwheat is cooked. The buckwheat will absorb all the liquid and be light and fluffy in texture. Steam the leeks for 10 minutes or until cooked and divide in half. Combine one half of the leeks with the buckwheat and eggs. Season well and pour into a greased, ovenproof dish. Bake in a preheated oven at 180°C/gas mark 4 for 20 minutes or until browned. Meanwhile, blend the remaining half of the leeks with the cream, soya milk, cottage cheese or yoghurt, and the chervil or parsley. Add lemon juice to taste. Re-heat (carefully if using single cream or yoghurt) and serve with the baked buckwheat and leek.

# grilled salmon with aubergine sauce

3 large aubergines
6 tbsp olive oil
Salt and pepper to taste
2 tbsp basil, finely chopped
4 salmon fillets

Using a fork, prick the aubergines all over and cook under a preheated grill, set to maximum, turning them until the skins are completely charred. When cool enough to handle, peel. Put into a sieve and, using a saucer or a small plate, press out as much juice as possible. Pound the flesh in a mortar and slowly beat in the olive oil as if making mayonnaise. Alternatively, use a food processor and drizzle oil through the feeder. Season with salt and pepper. Add the basil. Under a preheated grill set to maximum, grill the salmon for 5 minutes on either side. Serve with a dollop of the aubergine sauce.

# stuffed peppers *(below)*

225 ml salted water
115 g basmati rice, rinsed
2 green peppers
2 red peppers
1 large tomato, chopped
1 tbsp tarragon, chopped
100 g green and/or black olives, stoned and chopped
1 clove of garlic, crushed
1 tsp oil or butter
Salt and pepper to taste

In a medium saucepan, bring the salted water to the boil. Add the rice and cook, covered, over a low heat for about 20 minutes or until the water is fully absorbed. Slice the tops off the peppers, remove the core and seeds and set aside. Stir the remaining ingredients into the cooked rice. Fill the peppers with the rice mixture and replace the tops. Put into an oiled, ovenproof dish and cover. Bake in a preheated oven at 180ºC/gas mark 4 for about 35–40 minutes or until cooked. Serve.

# buckwheat pancakes with field mushrooms

For the stuffing:
2 tbsp vegetable oil
1 large onion, finely chopped
2 large cloves of garlic, crushed
1 tsp paprika
675 g field mushrooms, cut into 1-cm chunks
1 red pepper, deseeded and cut into 1-cm chunks
150 ml red wine
4 large sage leaves, roughly chopped
3 tbsp parsley, finely chopped
Salt and pepper

For the pancakes:
225 g buckwheat flour
1 tsp salt
1 large egg
½ litre water
Oil to fry

In a large frying pan, heat the oil and cook the onion and garlic over a low heat for about 10 minutes or until soft. Add the paprika and mushroom chunks and stir. Add the pepper chunks and wine and cook for a further 10 minutes until all the moisture has evaporated. Stir through the herbs and season to taste. Keep warm while you make the pancakes. To make the batter, put the flour and salt into a large bowl and make a well in the middle. Put the egg into the well and beat together. Gradually add the water. Refrigerate for at least 30 minutes, overnight if desired. Pour a small ladleful of batter into a hot, lightly oiled frying pan and cook on each side over a moderate heat for about 3–4 minutes or until lightly browned. Stack on a plate and keep warm. Place a little mushroom stuffing in the middle of each pancake, roll up and serve.

# pasta twists with pesto

For the pesto:
5 cloves of garlic
15 large basil leaves (more for a stronger flavour)
50 g pine nuts
Salt and pepper to taste
100 g Parmesan cheese, grated
100 ml olive oil

500 g fusilli pasta twists

Using a pestle and mortar, crush the garlic, basil and pine nuts (or use a blender). Add the salt, pepper, Parmesan and olive oil to make an emulsion. Bring a large pan of salted water to the boil. Add the pasta and return to the boil. Cook uncovered for about 12 minutes or until al dente. Do not drain the pasta completely as a little cooking water will help the pesto to coat the pasta. Toss generously in pesto and serve immediately.

# leek and chive mimosa with polenta

4 leeks, coarse outer leaves removed
4 eggs, hard-boiled
2 tbsp olive oil
2 tbsp chives, chervil, parsley or tarragon, chopped
To garnish: 4 lemon wedges

For the polenta:
250 g instant polenta
200 ml soya cream
1–2 tablespoons hot chilli sauce, or to taste
200 g Parmesan cheese or a strong cheddar, grated
Salt and pepper

Cut the leeks lengthways, rinse well under cold, running water and then boil in salted water (or steam) until tender. While the leeks are cooking, separate the yolks and the whites of the eggs, and mash separately with a fork. Boil the polenta according to the instructions on the packet and then stir through the cream, chilli sauce and cheese. Season well. To assemble: spoon the polenta onto a warmed serving dish and arrange the leeks on top. Sprinkle over the mashed egg whites and yolks. Keep warm. In a small frying pan, heat the olive oil, add the chives or other herbs, fry for about 30 seconds and pour over the leeks. Garnish with lemon wedges and serve immediately.

# lamb with spinach and lentils

As a vegetarian alternative, the spinach and lentil mixture can be served with boiled rice instead of lamb.

225 g brown lentils, soaked overnight
1 large clove of garlic
500 g fresh spinach, cut into thin strips
1 tbsp vegetable oil
½ tsp ground coriander
½ tsp ground cumin
Salt and pepper to taste
4 tbsp olive oil
2 tbsp coriander leaves, finely chopped
2 tbsp plain yoghurt (optional)
2 lamb fillets, trimmed
Oil to fry

In a large saucepan of boiling water, cook the lentils with the garlic for about 15 minutes or until soft but not mushy. Pan-fry the spinach quickly in the vegetable oil until all excess moisture has evaporated. Add the spinach, coriander, cumin, seasoning and olive oil to the lentils. Just before serving, stir through the coriander and plain yoghurt ( if using). In a very hot frying pan, fry the lamb fillets quickly on all sides, turning them over with a wooden spoon, for about 12 minutes or until they are well browned and crisp on the outside. (For well-done fillets, cook on the top shelf of a preheated oven at 230ºC/gas mark 8 for a further 10 minutes.) Slice the fillets thickly and serve on a bed of the spinach and lentil mixture.

# polenta with basil tomato sauce *(above)*

For the sauce:
1 medium onion, chopped
2 tbsp olive oil
500 g tomatoes
1 handful of basil leaves, chopped
Salt and pepper

For the polenta:
1½ litres water
1 tsp salt
375 g pre-cooked polenta
100 g butter
200 g Parmesan cheese, grated

Using a heavy-based saucepan, gently sweat the onion in the olive oil over a low heat. Peel the tomatoes (plunging them in boiling water helps the skin to come away) and add to the onions. Season to taste and simmer for 30–40 minutes. When the sauce is thick and pulpy, add the basil and remove from the heat. Using a heavy-based saucepan, bring the water and salt to the boil, stir in the polenta and cook over a low heat for about 10 minutes, stirring all the time. Stir in the butter and Parmesan cheese and transfer to a rectangular, shallow dish. Spread level with a spatula and allow to set solid. Cut into slices, reheat in the oven or microwave, or by grilling, and serve with a generous portion of basil tomato sauce.

# chicken breasts with celeriac mash *(below)*

4 skinless chicken breasts
Pepper
4 lettuce, large spinach or sorrel leaves
8 slices smoked streaky bacon
Oil to fry

For the mash:
1 celeriac, peeled and cut into chunks
Same weight of potatoes, peeled and cut into chunks
A little hot milk, olive oil or butter
Salt and pepper

Make a slit the length of the chicken breasts and open like a book. Grind pepper into the opening and cover with a lettuce, spinach or sorrel leaf. Close up the breasts and wrap each one in two pieces of bacon. Secure with a toothpick. Refrigerate until ready to use. In two large saucepans, boil the celeriac and potatoes separately until cooked. Drain and transfer into one large pan. Cover with a clean folded tea towel to absorb any steam. Mash the vegetables together, beat in a little hot milk, olive oil or butter to make a creamy consistency and season to taste. Keep warm. In a frying pan, heat the oil and cook the chicken breasts for about 12 minutes or until they are brown on all sides and the juices run clear. Serve with the celeriac mash.

# dandelion, bacon and potato cakes

Pancetta or smoked ham can be used instead of bacon. If using smoked ham, add just before serving. Dandelion, bacon and potato cakes are delicious served with green bean salad (page 97).

115 g smoked, streaky bacon, chopped and rind removed
1 tbsp vegetable oil
500 g young dandelion leaves (or destalked watercress, or lettuce)
2 cloves of garlic
2 tbsp white wine vinegar
500 g potatoes, boiled and mashed
2 tbsp flour
1 large egg
Oil to fry

In a large, heavy-based frying pan, fry the bacon in the oil. When cooked, remove and set aside. Add the dandelion leaves, watercress or lettuce and the garlic to the pan. Soften over a low heat for about 12 minutes or until cooked. Remove the garlic, add the vinegar and continue cooking until the liquid has evaporated and the mixture is quite dry. Mix the leaf mixture into the mashed potato together with the bacon. Beat in the flour and egg thoroughly. With floured hands, make into 4 large or 8 small equal patties and fry in hot oil until they are golden brown on both sides. Serve piping hot.

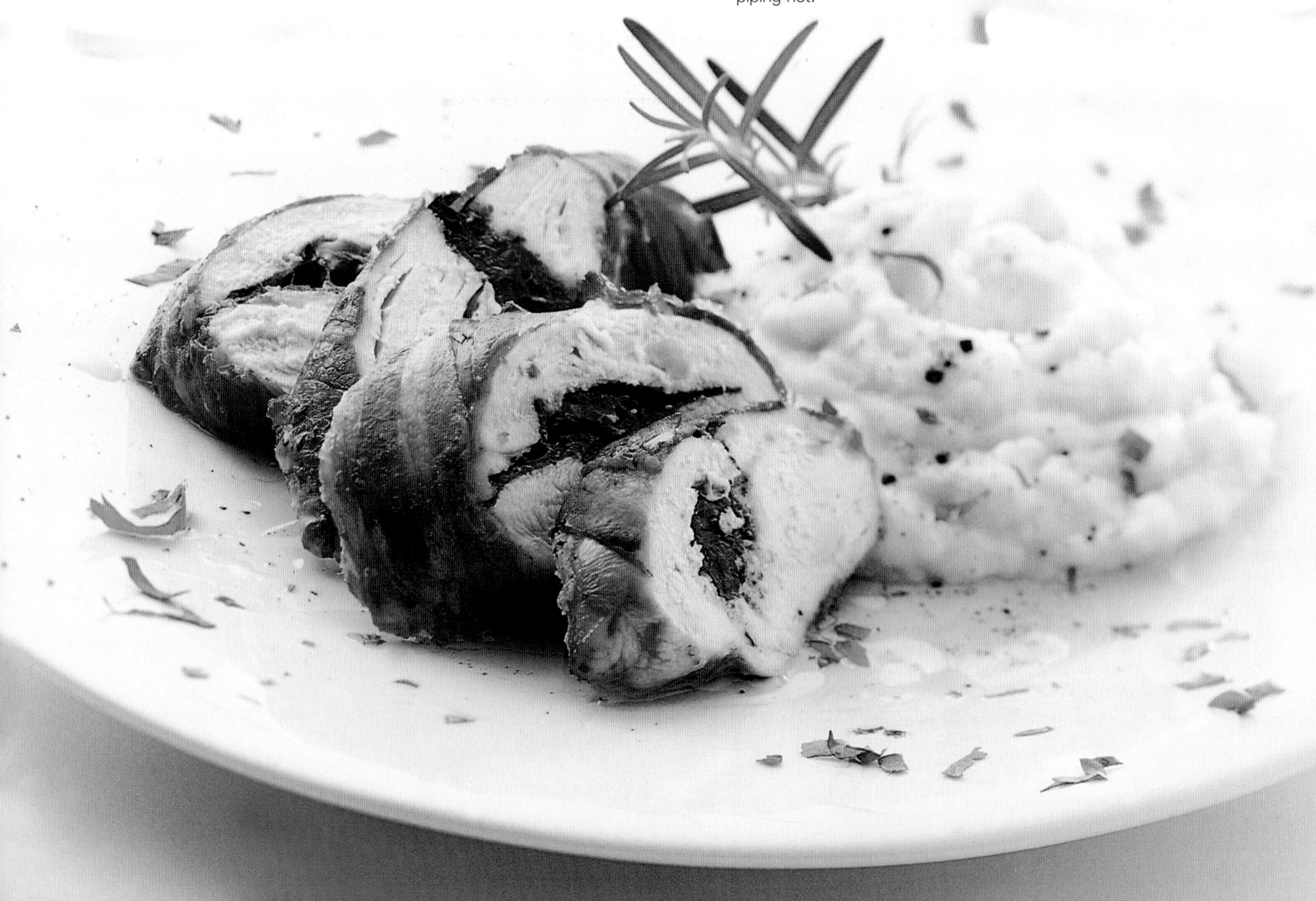

# baked pumpkin strudel

3 tbsp olive oil
2 red onions, finely chopped
800 g pumpkin or squash flesh, cut into small chunks
2 cloves of garlic, crushed
1 bay leaf
Sprig of fresh thyme
Salt and pepper to taste
1 x 400 g packet fresh filo pastry
Plenty of olive oil to brush
1 egg, beaten
115 g Parmesan cheese, freshly grated
55 g wholemeal breadcrumbs

In a 25-cm wide pan, heat the oil, add the onion and cook for 10 minutes or until soft. Add the pumpkin or squash, garlic, bay leaf, thyme and seasoning. Cover and cook over a low heat, allowing the ingredients to cook gently in their own juices. If the pumpkin starts to stick, stir in a little water. Allow to cool slightly. Lay out 4 overlapping sheets of filo pastry and brush quickly with oil. Cover with another 4 sheets and brush with oil. Repeat once more to make three layers. Spoon over the pumpkin mixture to within 5 cm of the edges and roll up into a sausage. Tuck the ends under. Slip a baking sheet underneath, brush with beaten egg and sprinkle over a mixture of Parmesan and breadcrumbs. Bake in a preheated oven at 200ºC/gas mark 6 for about 20 minutes or until the pastry and breadcrumb mixture is golden brown. Serve immediately.

# chicken, millet, barley and celeriac pilaff

To make a seafood pilaff use a mixture of prawns, squid and mussels instead of chicken

4 chicken breasts, skinned
8 tbsp olive oil
1 large clove of garlic, crushed
Salt and pepper to taste
200 g millet
500 g celeriac, peeled and finely diced
200 g barley, soaked overnight
150 ml pesto (page 104)
Pepper
To garnish: 8 large basil leaves

Marinate the chicken in the oil, garlic and seasoning for at least 2 hours. Cook the millet in twice its own volume of boiling water for about 10 minutes or until al dente. Meanwhile, steam the celeriac with the barley for 15 minutes or until both are cooked. Combine the celeriac, millet and barley, with plenty of pesto and pepper. Keep warm. In a frying pan, cook the chicken with the marinade juices for about 6 minutes on each side. When cool enough to handle, tear into strips and fork through the millet mixture. Tear the basil leaves and sprinkle over the top to garnish. Serve.

# spicy spinach, prunes and beans

Cinnamon, chopped almonds, raisins and chopped parsley can be added to the couscous if desired. Alternatively, basmati rice can be used instead of couscous.

1 tbsp oil
1 red onion, chopped
125 g black-eye beans (or other beans), soaked overnight
½ tsp ground turmeric
1 tsp ground cinnamon
Black pepper to taste
350 ml water
125 g no-soak prunes
1 kg young spinach leaves, picked over
225 g couscous

In a large saucepan, heat the oil and sweat the onion over a low heat for 10 minutes or until soft. Drain the beans and add to the pan along with the turmeric, cinnamon and pepper. Cover with the water and simmer with the lid on. When the beans are three-quarters cooked (after about 30 minutes), add the prunes. Add the spinach, in batches, to the stew and cook for a further 10 minutes. Cook the couscous according to the instructions on the packet and serve with the stew.

# halibut steak and nettle butter

If nettles are out of season, use fresh sorrel leaves.

150 g young nettle leaves
150 g unsalted butter, softened
Salt and pepper
4 tbsp white wine
4 tbsp salted water or fish stock
1 bay leaf
Juice of ½ lemon
4 halibut steaks
To garnish: black pepper
Butter

Steam the nettles for about 8 minutes or until wilted. Squeeze dry. Blend the nettles and butter in a food processor and season to taste. Spread onto greaseproof paper and roll into a log. Refrigerate. Cut into discs when hard. In a large shallow pan bring the wine and salted water or fish stock to the boil, add the bay leaf and lemon juice. Add the halibut and simmer for 5 minutes on each side. Garnish with black pepper and a disc of butter.

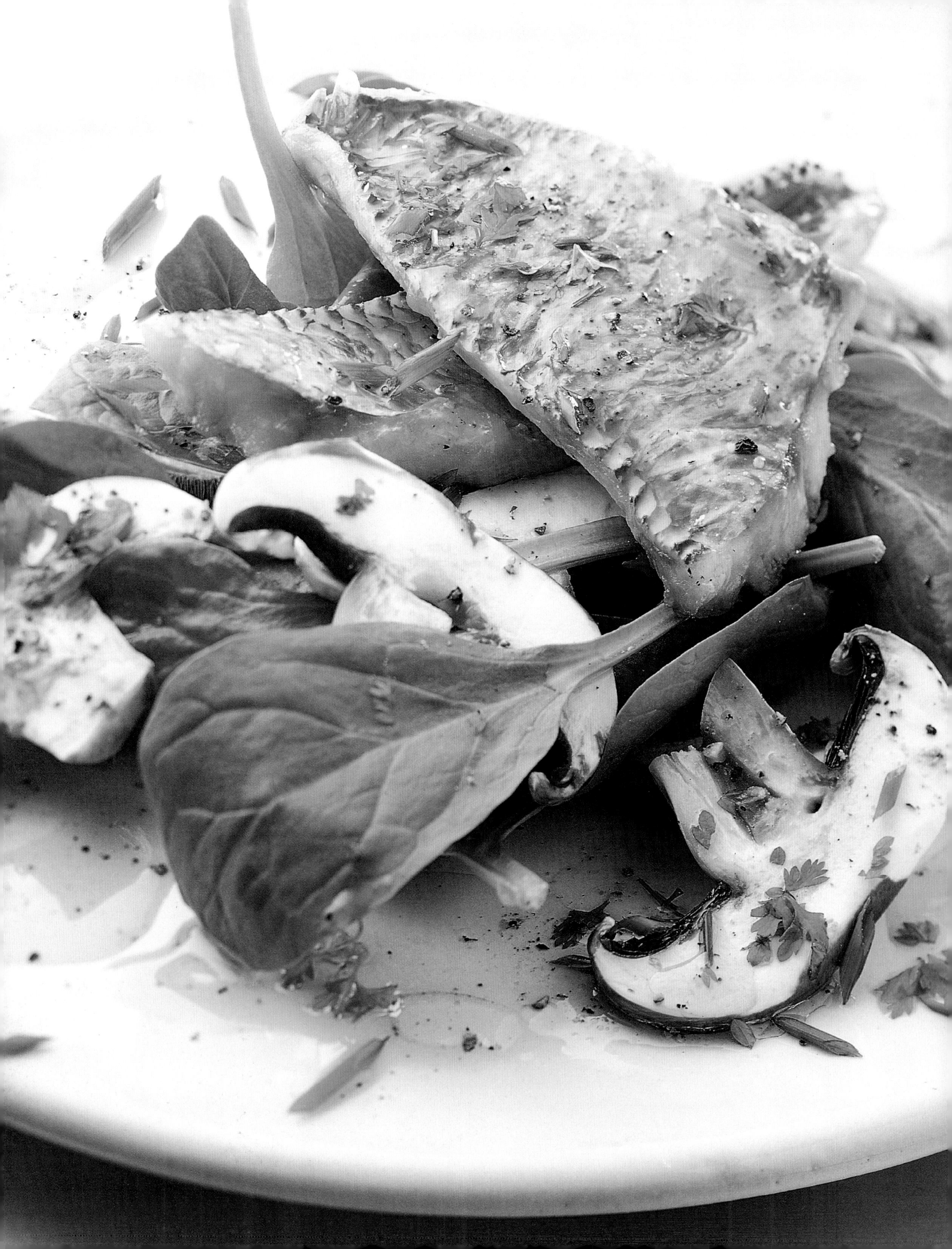

## red mullet with raw spinach salad *(left)*

1 ½ kg young spinach leaves, picked over
6 medium mushrooms, sliced
A few rocket leaves (optional)
Salt and pepper to taste
3 tbsp vinaigrette (page 95)
3 tbsp oil
8 red mullet fillets
To garnish: chervil and chives, chopped

Remove the stems from the spinach, place the leaves in a serving dish and add the mushrooms, rocket (if desired), salt and pepper. Toss in the vinaigrette. In a frying pan, heat the oil and rapidly sauté the mullet for 5 minutes on each side or until cooked. Place the mullet on the salad. Garnish with the chervil and chives and serve.

# ACCOMPANIMENTS

## onions in cider *(below right)*

4 tbsp oil
10 medium onions
25 ml dry cider
1 sprig of rosemary
2 bay leaves
Salt and pepper to taste

In a large frying pan, heat the oil and slowly fry the whole onions until they are golden brown all over. Add the cider, rosemary, bay leaves, salt and pepper, then cover and simmer gently until the onions are well cooked (they should retain their shape). Remove the onions and reduce the sauce by boiling rapidly to a syrupy consistency. Cover the onions with the sauce. Serve with cooked courgettes.

## steamed shallots

Serve as a main dish accompaniment or use to thicken sauces.

300 g shallots, peeled
½ tsp ground cinnamon

Steam the shallots, then blend in a food processor with the cinnamon and serve.

## rice with cucumber balls

500 ml salted water
250 g brown rice, rinsed
1 cucumber
1 shallot, finely chopped
30 g butter
To garnish: 1 tbsp coriander or parsley, finely chopped

In a large saucepan, bring the salted water to the boil. Add the rice and cook, covered, over a low heat for 20 minutes or until ready. Cut the cucumber in half lengthways and, using a melon baller, make as many balls as possible. Blanch the balls in boiling water for 2 minutes, then drain and rinse in cold water. In a frying pan, cook the shallot and cucumber in the butter over a low heat. As soon as they start to colour, add the rice, then garnish with a sprinkle of the coriander or parsley and serve.

## potato and watercress mash

500 g potatoes, peeled and chopped
300 g watercress, damaged stalks removed
1 tbsp butter or single cream
Large pinch of nutmeg
Salt and pepper to taste

Cook the potatoes in boiling, salted water. Drain and return to a low heat to drive off excess moisture. In a food processor, blend the watercress with the butter or cream. Add to the potato, and use a masher to make a smooth pureé. Stir in the nutmeg and salt and pepper. Serve.

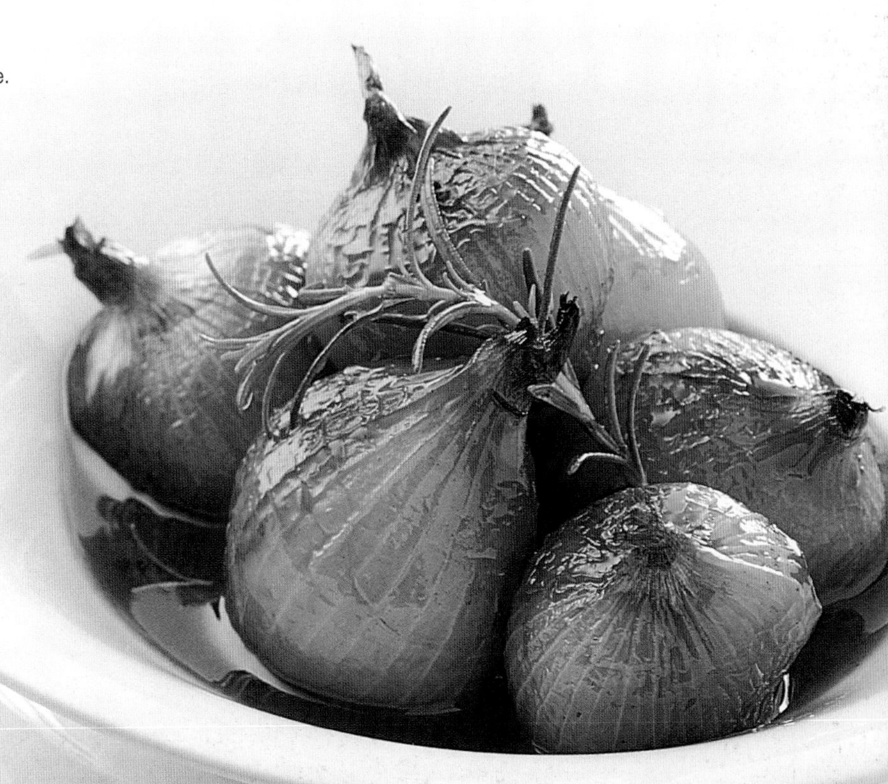

# celery with wine and herbs

1 large head of celery (or 2 small ones)
75 ml white wine
75 ml water
4 tbsp olive oil
2 tbsp parsley, finely chopped
2 tbsp tarragon, finely chopped
Salt and pepper to taste
Lemon juice

Carefully wash the celery and remove the root, leaves and stringy parts of the stalks. Cut into small pieces and cook in boiling, salted water for 4–6 minutes. Drain (the cooking water can be kept and used in a soup) and place in an ovenproof dish. Boil the wine and water for 1 minute, then pour over the celery in the ovenproof dish. Add the olive oil and cook for 20 minutes at 170ºC/gas mark 3. Add the parsley, tarragon and seasoning. Add a few drops of lemon juice and serve hot.

# peas with bacon pieces

100 g lardons or chopped lean bacon, rind removed
500 g fresh or frozen peas or 500 g can pease pudding
150 ml vegetable stock
Rocket, finely chopped
Black pepper to taste

In a frying pan, sauté the lardons or bacon until golden. Drain away the fat and set aside. In a food processor, blend the peas, if using, with the vegetable stock. Transfer the pea mixture or pease pudding to the frying pan and heat. Mix the lardons or bacon with the pea mixture or pease pudding. Transfer to a serving dish. Sprinkle over the rocket and pepper.

# salsify

Salsify will keep well in the refrigerator for a few days and is an interesting accompaniment to main courses. Canned salsify can be used instead of fresh; just sauté before serving.

1½ litres cold water
1 tbsp plain flour
3 tbsp vinegar
10 g salt
1 kg fresh salsify
Olive oil
To garnish: 1 tbsp parsley, finely chopped

In a large pan, mix the water, flour, vinegar and salt. Bring to the boil, stirring well. Plunge the salsify into the boiling water, then cover and simmer for 20 minutes or until cooked. (Cool and store the salsify in its cooking water in the refrigerator.) Before serving, lightly sauté in olive oil and garnish with the parsley.

# brussels sprouts with chestnuts

600 g chestnuts
1 litre meat or vegetable stock
750 g Brussels sprouts, damaged outer leaves removed
100 g chopped bacon, lardons or pancetta, rind removed
1 tbsp vegetable oil
Salt and pepper

Using a sharp knife, make an incision in each chestnut. Place the chestnuts in a pan and cover with cold water. Bring to the boil for 2 minutes, drain and peel the outer and inner skin. Cook the peeled chestnuts in the meat or vegetable stock for 30 minutes. Cook the Brussels sprouts for about 15 minutes in salted, boiling water (the sprouts should remain firm). Using a frying pan, sauté the bacon, lardons or pancetta in the oil. When cooked, drain the fat and add the sprouts and chestnuts to the pan. Mix by shaking the pan, heat through for 4 minutes. Season to taste and serve immediately.

# beans with carrots and onions

This is an excellent accompaniment to sausages or red meat.

200 g onions, sliced
200 g carrots, diced
3 cloves of garlic
150 ml olive oil or 30 g butter
1 kg dried beans (flageolet, red kidney or borlotti beans), soaked overnight
Bouquet garni (made with a bay leaf, 2 or 3 sprigs of thyme, 2 or 3 sprigs of parsley and 1 clove)
Salt and pepper to taste

In a large saucepan, cook the onions, carrots and garlic in the olive oil or butter over a low heat for approximately 10 minutes or until the onions are soft. Stir frequently. Add the drained beans and cook for 3 minutes, then cover with water and bring to the boil. Add the bouquet garni, cover and simmer for 1½ hours or until the beans are cooked. Add salt and pepper after 45 minutes. Serve hot.

# fennel with wine

This dish goes very well with smoked fish or cold meat.

800 g fennel, bruised outer layer and tops removed
300 ml white wine
2 bay leaves
1 cinnamon stick or ½ tsp ground cinnamon
A few crushed black peppercorns
30 g pistachio nuts, shelled
2 anchovy fillets (optional)
1 tsp sugar
Pinch of nutmeg

3 tbsp olive oil
1 tbsp vinegar
½ lemon, juice and grated zest

Cut the fennel into quarters and slice thinly. Put the white wine, bay leaves, cinnamon, peppercorns and fennel in a saucepan, and cover with water. Bring to the boil, then cover and simmer until the fennel is cooked but still firm. Strain the fennel and put into a deep dish. Blend the pistachio, anchovy (if using), sugar, nutmeg, olive oil, vinegar and lemon in a food processor and spoon the sauce over the fennel. Cover with cling film and refrigerate for 24 hours. Serve at room temperature.

# potatoes with herb sauce

For the sauce:
1 tbsp white wine
Small bunch (5 or 6 sprigs) of parsley, finely chopped
Small bunch (5 or 6 sprigs) of chervil, finely chopped
2 tbsp tarragon leaves, finely chopped
4 anchovy fillets (optional), finely chopped
1 egg, hard-boiled and finely chopped
2 small shallots, finely chopped
Pinch of black pepper
3 tbsp olive oil
1 tbsp white wine vinegar

16 small new or salad potatoes, boiled
2 tsp fresh capers (replace with preserved capers if necessary)

To make the sauce: boil the white wine briefly, in order to allow the alcohol to evaporate, then mix all of the ingredients together. Slice the boiled potatoes while hot and place them in a serving dish. Warm the sauce over a gentle heat and then pour on the potatoes. Sprinkle over the capers and toss very gently. Serve warm.

# green beans with dijon mustard *(right)*

1 kg green beans
150 g single cream or yoghurt
Juice of 1 small lemon
1 tbsp Dijon mustard
100 g toasted hazelnuts, chopped
Salt and pepper to taste

Using a steamer, cook the green beans until al dente. Rinse in cold water and then drain. Mix the cream or yoghurt, lemon juice and mustard in a bowl, then add the beans and toss lightly. Sprinkle over the toasted hazelnuts, season and refrigerate before serving.

# cardamom hot sauce

Use this sauce to add flavour to soups or stews.

4 cardamom pods
4 dried chillies
1 bulb of garlic, peeled
1 tsp black peppercorns
1 tsp caraway seeds
Bunch of coriander leaves (stems removed), rinsed

In a food processor, blend all of the ingredients and use as desired.

# horseradish sauce

Adjust the ingredients according to taste. Use as a condiment.

20 g shallots, finely chopped
Pinch of ground black pepper
50 g salt
200 g mustard powder
1 dried red chilli, ground
60 g fresh horseradish root, grated
1 tsp grated nutmeg
125 ml vinegar
50 ml dry white wine
Vegetable stock (optional)

In a food processor, blend all the ingredients into a smooth paste. If the mixture is too dry, add a little vegetable stock. To reduce the strength and sharpness, boil the blended ingredients for 5 minutes. Refrigerate.

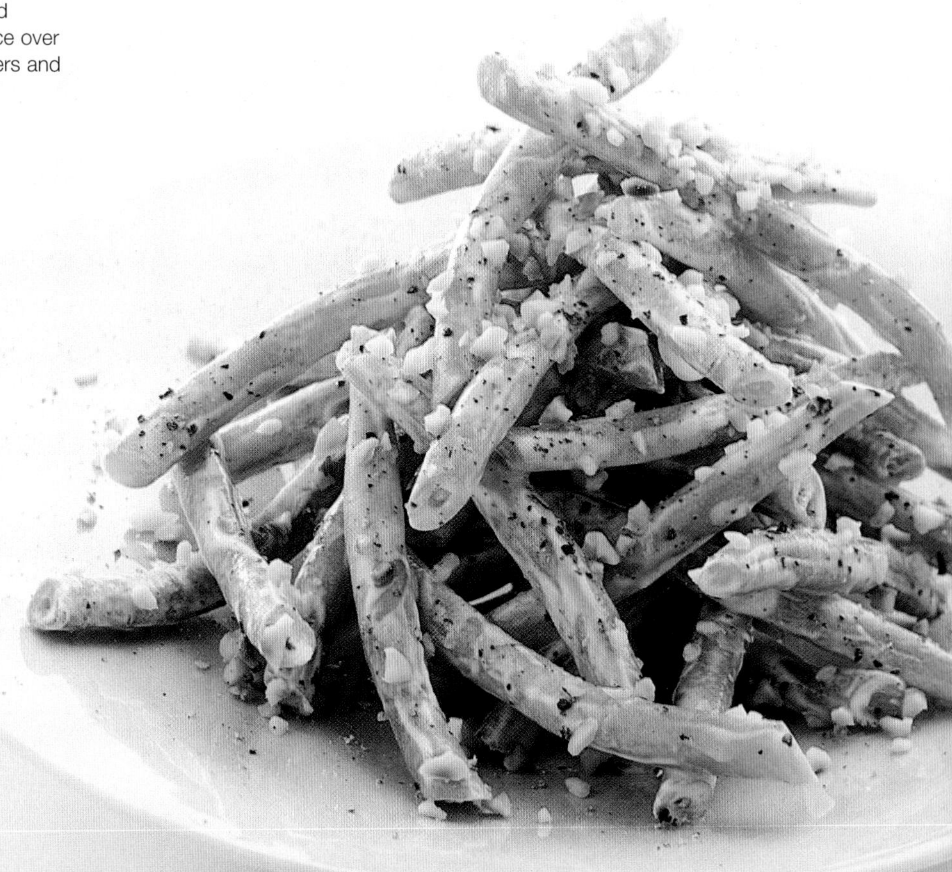

# desserts

The following recipes serve 4 people unless otherwise stated. Where possible, harvest your own ingredients or use fresh, organic produce. Take care to wash thoroughly, peel or de-seed fruit where necessary.

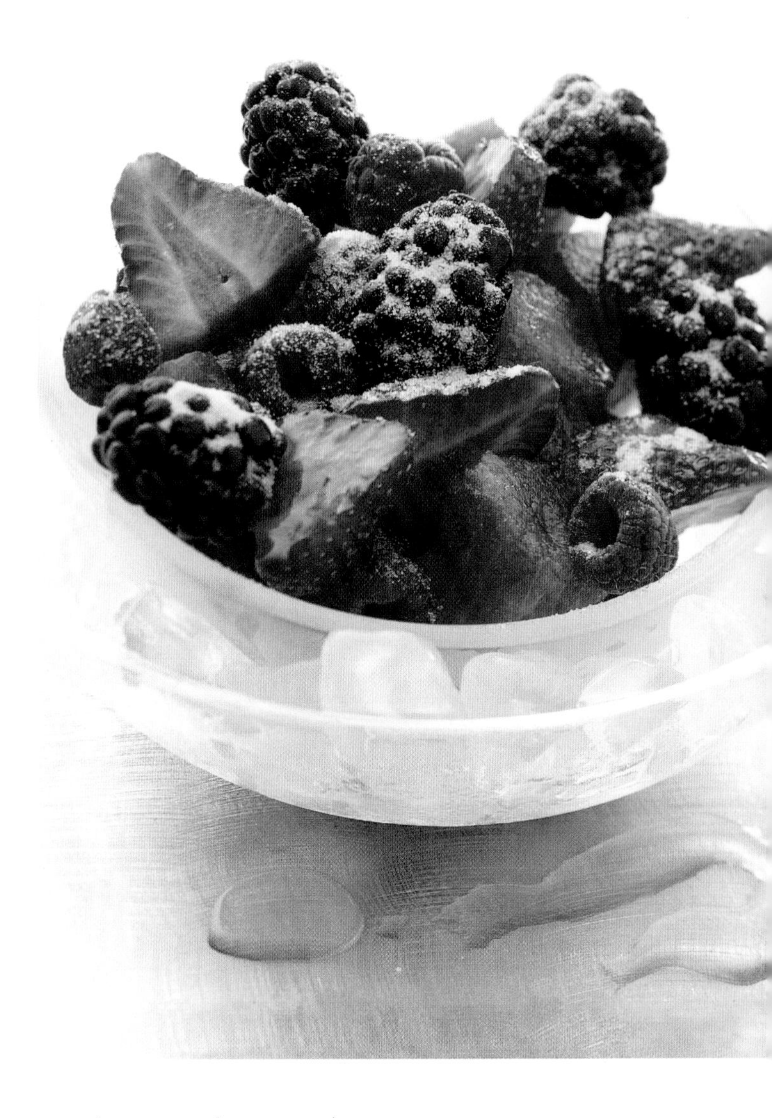

## watermelon and summer fruits *(right)*

1 small watermelon
Blackberries (frozen if out of season)*
Raspberries*
Strawberries*
Crushed ice
Caster sugar to taste
2 tbsp orange-blossom water (available in health shops and supermarkets)

* Use one quarter of the weight of the watermelon of each fruit.

Cut off the top of the watermelon and spoon out all the flesh. Remove the seeds and cut the flesh into rough cubes. Mix with the other fruit and a small amount of crushed ice. Use this fruit mixture to fill up the shell of the watermelon. Sprinkle on caster sugar and orange-blossom water. Alternatively, serve the fruit salad in individual bowls.

## banana and date salad

5 ripe bananas, peeled and sliced
250 g fresh dates, stoned and finely chopped
300 ml live yoghurt
To garnish: toasted chopped nuts (optional)

In glass bowls, arrange the bananas and dates in alternate layers and pour on the yoghurt. Refrigerate overnight. Sprinkled with the toasted chopped nuts if desired. Serve.

## lychee fruit salad

200 g lychees, peeled and stoned
200 g tangerines, peeled and separated into segments
6–8 kumquats, chopped
2 tbsp orange-blossom water
2 glasses crushed ice made with jasmine tea

Put the fruit in a bowl and pour over the orange-blossom water and crushed ice. Serve immediately.

## minted melon

2 tbsp granulated sugar
2 tbsp water
3 tbsp fresh mint leaves
Juice of ½ lemon
1 ripe honeydew melon, refrigerated
A few chunks of crystallized ginger or ginger preserved in syrup (optional)

In a small saucepan, over a low heat, completely dissolve the sugar in the water. Bring to the boil and add the mint and lemon juice. Cool. Slice the melon and place in glass bowls. Glaze the melon with the cold syrup. Add the ginger if desired. Serve.

## pumpkin in syrup

1 medium pumpkin
750 g sugar
½ litre water
To garnish: walnuts and toasted almonds, chopped

Cut the pumpkin into eight wedges, cut the flesh from the peel and remove the seeds and fibres. Dissolve the sugar completely in the water. Bring to the boil and add the pumpkin wedges. Simmer for 20 minutes or until tender: the bubbles should become bigger and slower. Allow to cool and serve the pumpkin and syrup sprinkled with the walnuts and toasted almonds.

# rhubarb and ginger tart

For the shortcrust pastry:
225 g plain flour
Pinch of salt
110 g butter
3 tbsp ice-cold water

For the filling:
500 g fresh rhubarb stalks, washed
100 g soft brown sugar
5-cm piece of ginger root, peeled and grated, or 1 tsp orange or lemon zest
1 tbsp lemon juice

To make the shortcrust pastry: blend the flour, salt and butter in a food processor until well combined. Mix in the water to bind. Chill for 30 minutes and then use the pastry to line a 25-cm tart tin. Cut the rhubarb into small chunks (about 1½ cm long). Stack the chunks tightly in the pastry case and sprinkle with the sugar, ginger, orange or lemon zest and lemon juice. Bake immediately in an oven preheated to 180°C/gas mark 4 for 35 minutes or until cooked. Serve with a little fresh cream or live yoghurt if desired.

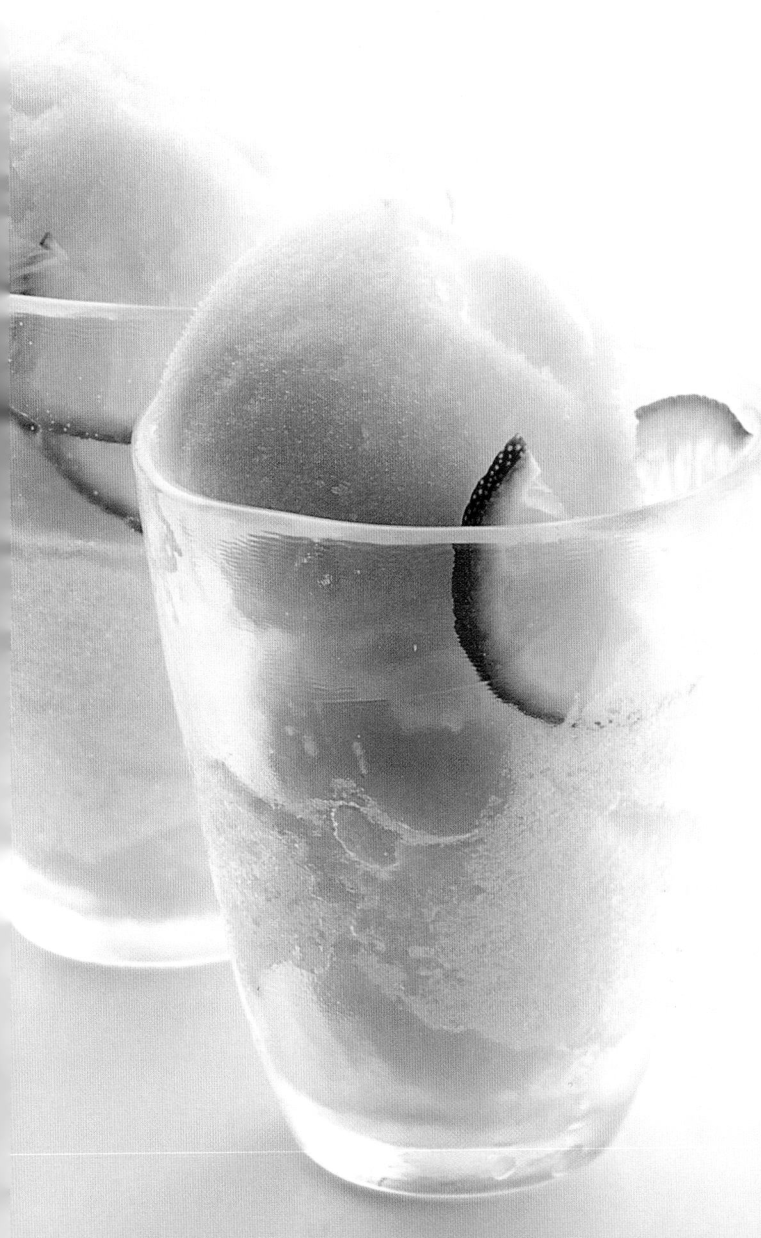

# fruit salad with lemon balm

100 g wild strawberries
100 g blackberries
100 g blueberries
100 g redcurrants
3 dessert apples, peeled, cored, sliced and sprinkled with lemon juice
100 g sugar
75 ml water
150 ml sparkling wine (optional)
2 tbsp lemon juice
10 lemon balm leaves, finely chopped

In a large bowl mix the fruit together. Over a low heat, dissolve the sugar in the water, wine (if using) and lemon juice. Bring to the boil and reduce to a syrup. When the syrup has cooled, pour it over the fruit and sprinkle the lemon balm leaves on top. Refrigerate for at least 2 hours before serving.

# red- and whitecurrants with raspberry coulis

250 g redcurrants
250 g whitecurrants
250 g raspberries
100 g sugar
To decorate: fresh mint leaves

Combine the red- and whitecurrants and arrange in individual glass bowls. Crush the raspberries with a fork or blend in a food processor. Transfer to a stainless steel, enamel or glass pan and cook over a medium heat for 2 minutes. Strain through a fine sieve into a clean pan and, over a low heat, dissolve the sugar in the juice. Pour, warm, over the red and whitecurrants. Decorate with the mint. Serve with fresh cream or live yoghurt if desired.

# fresh mint sorbet *(left)*

3 tbsp fresh mint leaves, washed and dried
200 g sugar
300 ml water
Juice of 2 lemons
1 egg white
To decorate: whole mint leaves or lime slices (optional)

In a large saucepan, over a low heat, dissolve the sugar completely in the water. Bring to the boil and reduce until syrupy. Meanwhile, chop the mint finely (setting some aside for the decoration if desired), add to the cooling syrup and allow to infuse for 1 hour. Strain, stir in the lemon juice and freeze until set. Break the frozen syrup into pieces and blend in a food processor. Whisk the egg white until stiff and fold in. Decorate with whole mint leaves or lime slices if desired and serve.

# pears with herbs

1 litre boiling water
1 handful lime flowers (linden)
2 tbsp dried mint
2 star anise
Zest of 1 orange
4 large pears
Sugar
Dried fruit such as apricots, sultanas or prunes (optional)
To garnish: toasted nuts (optional)

Pour the boiling water over the lime flowers, mint, star anise and orange zest, cover and infuse for 30 minutes. Strain the infusion and then pour it into a large steamer or pressure cooker. Steam the pears with the infusion until they are tender (in a pressure cooker this should take about 4–5 minutes). Remove the pears, reduce the infusion by half and add sugar to taste. Pour the infusion over the pears in a serving dish and allow to cool before serving. If desired, you can add some dried fruit such as apricots, sultanas or prunes to the infusion before you pour it over the pears. They will swell in the liquid and take up the fragrance of the herbs. Sprinkle the toasted nuts over the pears if desired. Serve.

# autumn fruit compote

1 kg dessert apples, peeled, cored and roughly chopped
1 kg pears, peeled, cored and roughly chopped
500 g black grapes, deseeded
1 lemon, juice and grated zest, or 1 tbsp grated fresh ginger
1 clove
½ tsp ground cinnamon
Pinch of nutmeg
150 ml water

In a heavy-based saucepan, place the apples, pears and grapes with the lemon juice or ginger, and add the remaining ingredients. Simmer for 25 minutes, or until all the fruit is cooked. Empty the fruit into a glass bowl and allow to cool. Serve with fresh cream or live yoghurt if desired.

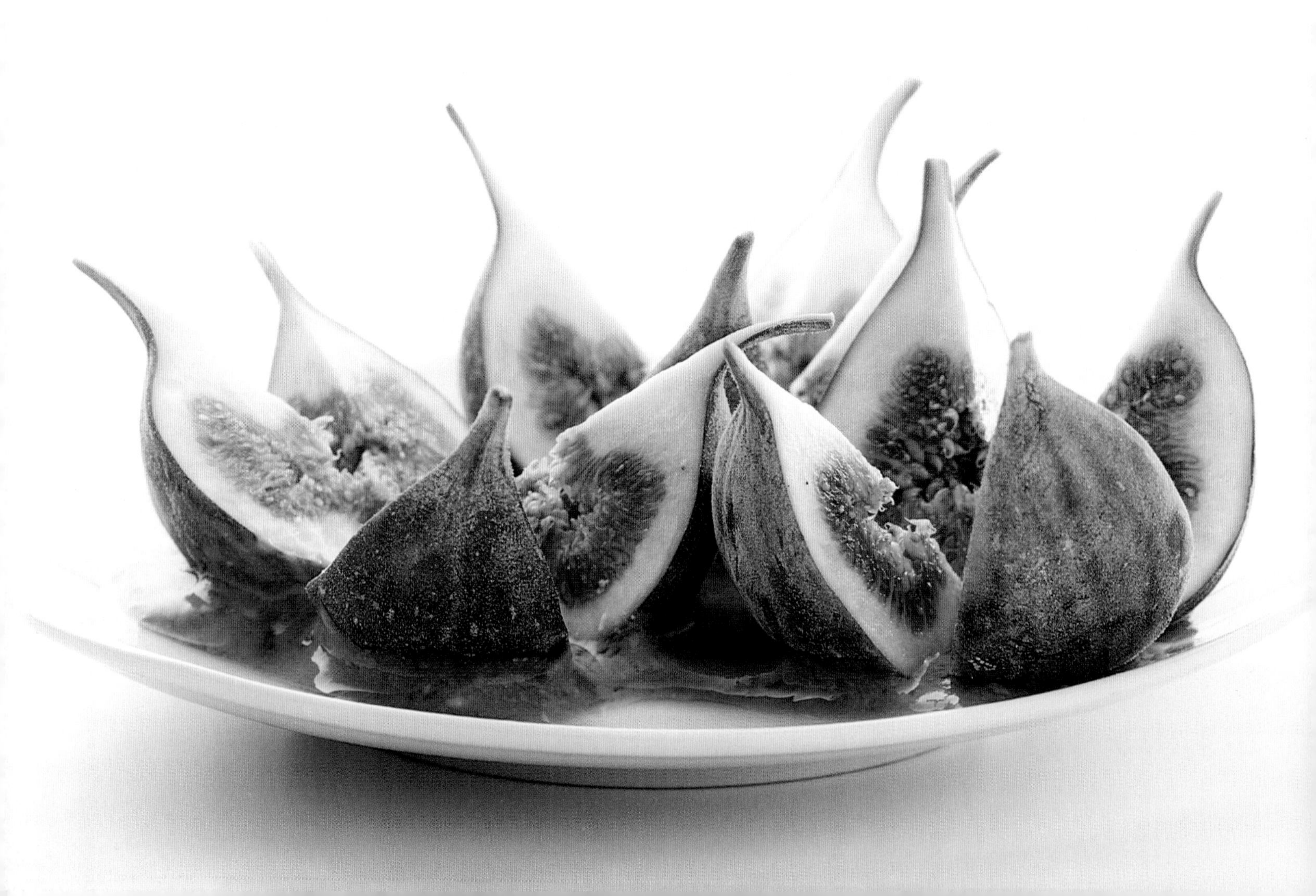

# baked papaya with ginger

3 papayas, halved and deseeded
60 g unsalted butter
5 chunks of preserved ginger, chopped
1 lime, juice and zest
1 tbsp of preserved ginger syrup
Brown sugar (optional)
honey (optional)

Place the papayas in a buttered ovenproof dish. Mash together or blend the butter and ginger with half the lime juice and zest. Pour the mixture into the halved papayas. Sprinkle with the remaining lime juice, followed by the ginger syrup (and sugar if desired). Bake in a preheated oven at 180ºC/gas mark 4 until tender, basting occasionally with the juices. Spoon a little honey over the top if desired. Serve.

# fresh figs with raspberry cheese *(left)*

12 figs
150 g raspberries
100 g cottage cheese
1 tbsp caster sugar
3 tbsp live yoghurt

Quarter the figs to within 1 cm of the base. In a food processor, blend the raspberries, then mix with the cottage cheese, sugar and yoghurt. Pour the mixture over the figs. Refrigerate for a few hours before serving.

# poached apricots with cardamom *(right)*

4 cardamom pods
600 ml water
100 g brown or white sugar
Zest of 1 lemon, cut into thin strips
12 apricots, stoned
Orange juice
To garnish: toasted nuts, chopped (optional)

Using a rolling pin, crush the cardamom pods and tie into a muslin bag. In a large saucepan, bring the water, sugar and lemon zest to the boil. Add the cardamom and simmer for a few minutes until the cardamom flavour is sufficiently strong (taste the syrup). Remove the muslin bag, add the apricots and poach for about 10 minutes over a low heat (the syrup should be barely simmering). Once the apricots are cooked, remove them and reduce the syrup by half by boiling rapidly. Add a little orange juice to taste and pour the syrup over the apricots. Sprinkle the toasted nuts over the apricots if desired. Serve chilled.

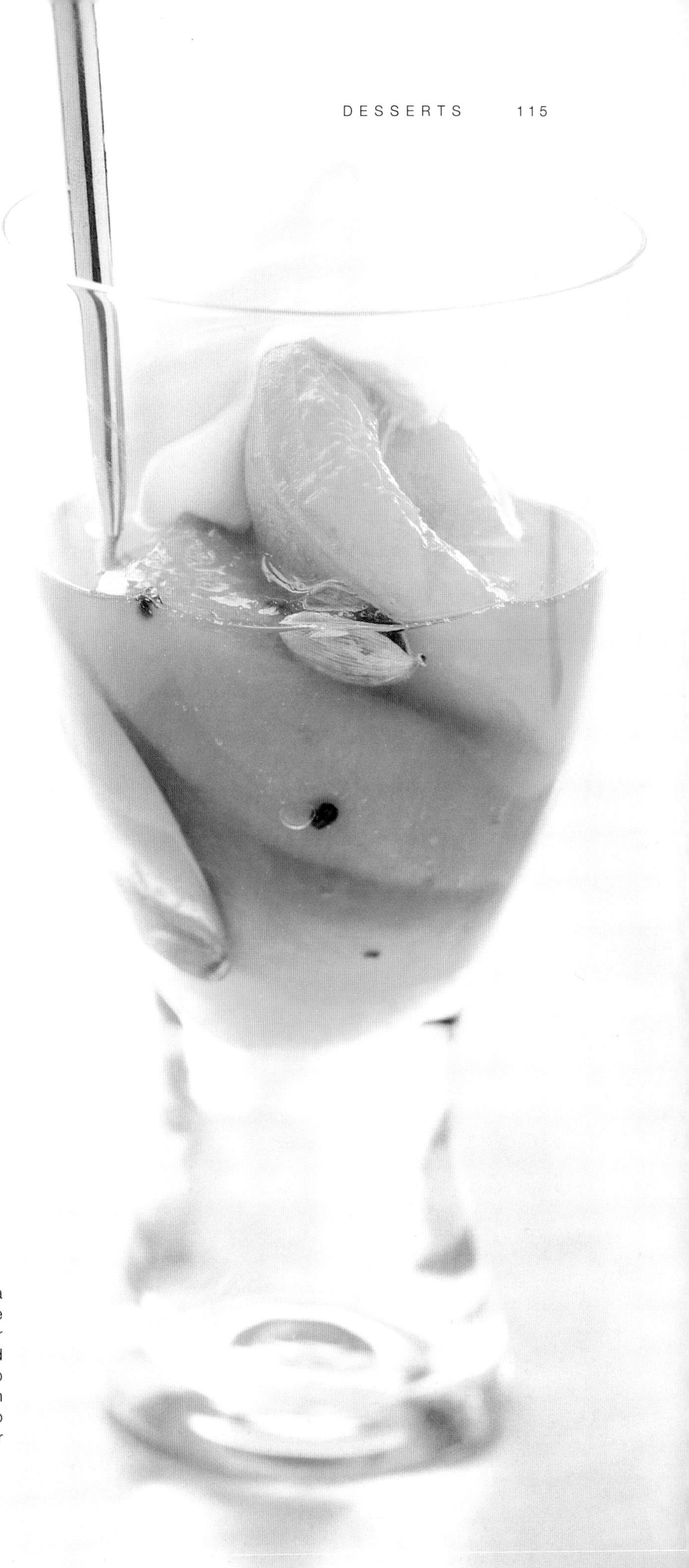

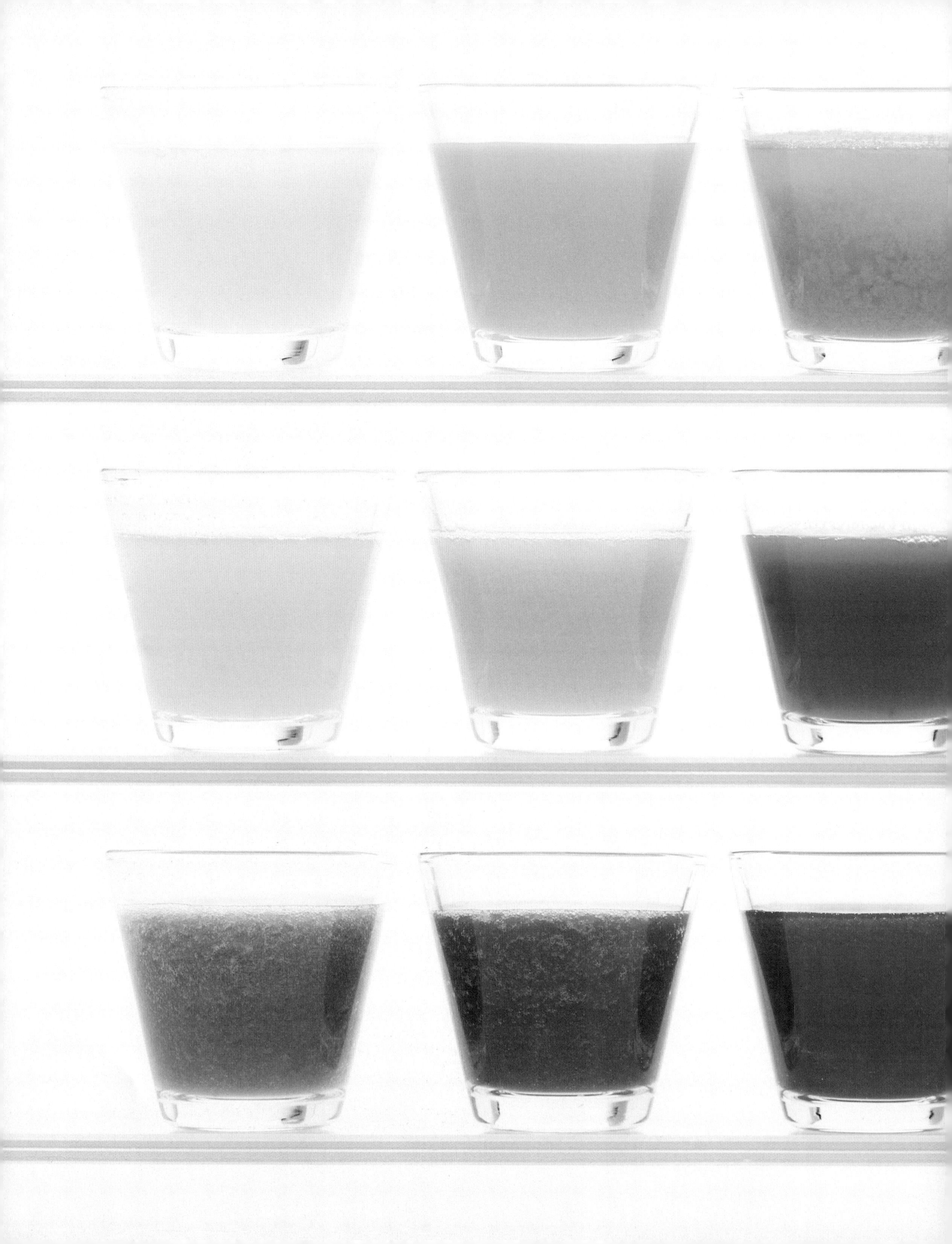

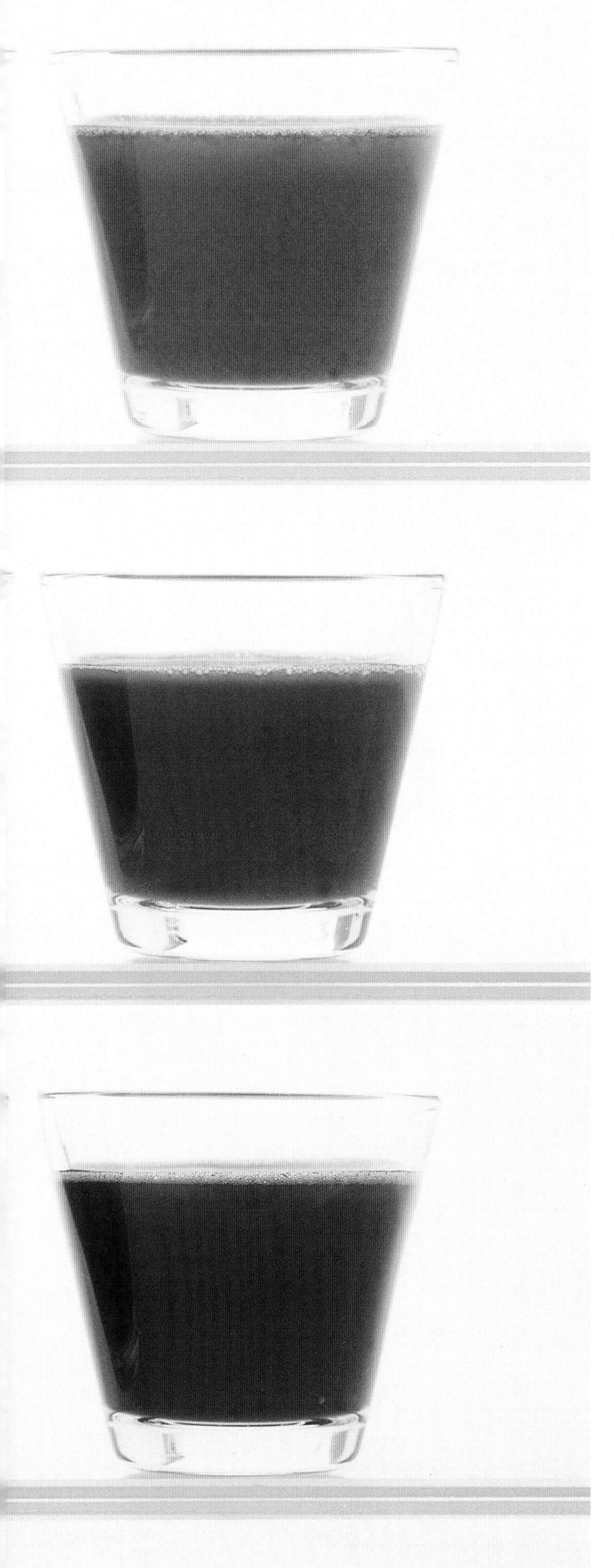

# juices

To maximize the nutritional value of juice, use the freshest possible ingredients and drink the juice as soon as you have made it (make a small quantity and drink it all at once rather than storing it). Where possible, harvest your own ingredients or use fresh, organic produce. Avoid using fruit and vegetables that are damaged or overripe and take care to wash ingredients thoroughly. If fruit is difficult to obtain, buy ready-made juice from a health-food shop – always choose brands that are organic and unsweetened.

The following juices are made using either a juicer or a blender. A juicer extracts the juice from fruit and vegetables, leaving behind the solid parts, such as the rind, peel, pith and pips – ideal for citrus fruit and apples. A blender simply liquidizes the whole fruit or vegetable – good for soft fruit such as strawberries and raspberries. If you do not have a juicer, you can add a little water to a recipe, blend the ingredients and then strain them through a sieve or a piece of muslin. Juices are best served cold, poured over crushed ice. Vegetable juices can be seasoned with salt and pepper.

Because is hard to predict how much juice individual fruits will yield, the amounts of fruit given in these recipes may need adjusting depending on water content (older, riper fruit yields more juice but may be less nutritious).

## FRUIT JUICES

### apple and raspberry juice

300 g dessert apples, peeled, cored and roughly chopped
100 g raspberries
2 tbsp rosewater or orange-blossom water
Ice cubes made from jasmine tea
Sugar to taste

Process the apples and raspberries in a blender. Add the rosewater or orange-blossom water, then pour the liquid over the jasmine tea ice cubes. Alternatively, crush the jasmine tea ice cubes in the blender with the fruit. Add sugar and serve.

### apricot, lime and mint juice

3 ripe apricots, stoned
3 tablespoons fresh lime juice
Honey to taste
1 tsp fresh mint, chopped

Blend the apricots and the lime juice. Sweeten with honey and pour into a glass half-filled with mint and crushed ice. Serve.

## cherry and raspberry juice

50 ml ready-made cherry juice
50 ml ready-made raspberry juice
Juice of ½ lemon

Mix the first 2 juices together, then add the lemon juice and serve over crushed ice.

## cherry and apple juice

3 dessert apples
50 ml ready-made cherry juice

Process the apples in a juicer, and then mix the apple juice with the cherry juice and serve.

## mango juice

2 medium-sized mangoes, peeled and stoned
2 tbsp orange-blossom water
A few ice cubes made from camomile tea

Blend the mango flesh with the orange-blossom water and the camomile ice cubes. Blend until the ice is well crushed, and serve.

## carrot, apple and ginger juice

6 carrots, cut into chunks
4 apples, peeled, cored and cut into chunks
1 tbsp root ginger, grated

Process the carrots, apples and ginger in a juicer. Serve over crushed ice.

## prune juice

1 tsp lemon juice
Maple syrup to taste
150 ml ready-made prune juice

Mix the lemon juice and maple syrup with the prune juice and serve.

## redcurrant, blackberry and blueberry juice

100 g redcurrants
100 g blackberries
100 g blueberries

Use frozen fruits if redcurrants, blackberries or blueberries are out of season. Blend the ingredients and serve.

## strawberry and raspberry juice

200 g strawberries
200 g raspberries
Lemon juice to taste
Water (optional)

Blend the strawberries and raspberries. Add the lemon juice and pour over crushed ice. Add a little water if necessary, and serve.

## pineapple shake

50 ml pineapple juice
100 ml soya milk
1 tsp coconut, grated
Sugar to taste

Process the pineapple, soya milk and coconut in a blender. Add the sugar and serve chilled.

# VEGETABLE JUICES

## celery and tomato juice

½ celery plant
2 tomatoes
1 cucumber

Trim the celery sticks and base. Juice all the ingredients and serve.

# cabbage, carrot and celery juice

This juice can be served hot or cold.

½ red or white cabbage
4 carrots, roughly chopped
5 sticks celery, roughly chopped
½ red onion (or 2 shallots)
Water
Salt and pepper to taste
1 tsp lemon juice

Blend the vegetables. Add a little water to thin the consistency and add the salt, pepper and lemon juice. Serve.

# green bean and garlic juice

230 g green beans
2 small lettuce hearts
2 tbsp water
2 cloves of garlic
Pinch of cayenne

Juice the vegetables with the water and garlic, mix with the cayenne and serve over crushed ice.

# black radish and carrot juice

100 g black radishes
50 g carrots

Process the ingredients in a juicer and serve.

# broccoli and green bean juice

A few stems and florets of broccoli
100 g green beans
2 tbsp lemon juice
2 tbsp water

Process the vegetables in a juicer, mix with the lemon juice and water and serve over crushed ice.

# celery and red onion juice

1 celery plant, leaves and outside sticks removed
2 red onions
Juice of ½ lemon

Trim the celery sticks and base. Juice the celery and onions and pour into a glass filled with the lemon juice and crushed ice. Serve.

# beetroot and celery juice

1 celery plant, leaves and outside sticks removed
2 medium-sized beetroots, cooked
Juice of ½ lemon or lime
1 tbsp olive oil

Trim the celery sticks and base. Process the celery and beetroots in a juicer and pour into a glass with the lemon or lime juice and olive oil. Serve.

# cucumber and lettuce heart juice

2 medium-sized cucumbers
1 lettuce heart

Process the ingredients in a juicer and serve.

# lettuce and basil juice

1 lettuce
1 radicchio
5 basil leaves
Juice of ½ lemon

Juice the lettuce, radicchio and basil, add the lemon juice and serve.

# pickles and preserves

When making preserves buy the best quality ingredients possible. Sterilize jars and bottles by pouring boiling water over them or leaving them in a hot oven for a few minutes. The main ingredient used in pickling is vinegar – this acts as a solvent, taking the aroma as well as the medicinally-active ingredients from the plants. Preserves should generally be consumed within three months.

## PICKLED VEGETABLES

### pickled turnips

Serve with main dishes, such as pork and potatoes.

1½ kg turnip, peeled and grated
30 g salt
40 juniper berries
30 black peppercorns

Place the ingredients in layers in a large glass or ceramic jar (do not use metal), then put a sterile cloth and a plate on the top layer. Place a weight on top of the plate and keep refrigerated. The turnips will start to ferment and will take 2–3 weeks to pickle. When pickled, rinse well in cold water and dry thoroughly. Serve raw in salad or cook and serve in the same way as sauerkraut (boiled and as an accompaniment for sausages or pork).

### pickled beetroot

1 kg baby beetroot, unpeeled
1 litre water
½ litre red wine vinegar
2 bay leaves
2 sprigs of thyme
12 black peppercorns
2 cloves of garlic
50 g salt
100 g granulated sugar
1 white onion, sliced

Wrap the beetroot in foil and bake in a preheated oven at 200ºC/gas mark 6 until tender. Meanwhile, bring the water, vinegar, herbs, peppercorns, garlic, salt and sugar to the boil and cook for 3 minutes. Leave to cool. Peel the beetroot and combine with the onion in hermetically-sealable pickling jars. Pour over the pickling vinegar and seal the jars tightly. Store for at least 2 weeks in a cool, dark place.

### pickled cauliflower *(right)*

Use in starters or salads.

1 medium cauliflower
20 g salt
White wine vinegar or cider vinegar (enough to cover the cauliflower)
1 tsp green peppercorns
1 tsp black peppercorns
1 tsp pink peppercorns
1–6 fresh green, red and yellow chillies according to taste (yellow chillies are optional, as they are not always available)

In a large saucepan, blanch the cauliflower in boiling, salted water for 5 minutes. Rinse under cold water, drain and pat dry with kitchen paper. Carefully cut away small florets from the main stalk and put them into a 1½ litre hermetically-sealable pickling jar. Using a stainless steel, glass or enamel saucepan, bring to the boil the white wine or cider vinegar, peppercorns and chillies and cook them for 30 seconds. Pour the vinegar mixture over the cauliflower florets in the pickling jar so that they are completely covered. Allow to cool and seal the jar tightly. Leave for 3 weeks in a cool, dark place.

## VINEGARS

### blackberry vinegar

Use in salad dressings or cooking.

300 g blackberries
1 tsp mustard powder in a small muslin bag
1 litre white wine vinegar

Wash the blackberries in cold water, trim away any stems and green parts, drain on kitchen paper, and place in a hermetically-sealable pickling jar with the mustard. Pour over the white wine vinegar and seal the jar tightly. Leave for 2 weeks in a cool, dark place. Strain and bottle the vinegar.

### raspberry vinegar

250 g raspberries
1 litre red wine vinegar

Put the raspberries in a hermetically-sealable pickling jar. Pour over the red wine vinegar and seal the jar tightly. Leave for 2 months in a cool, dark place. Strain and bottle the vinegar, pressing the fruit to extract the juice.

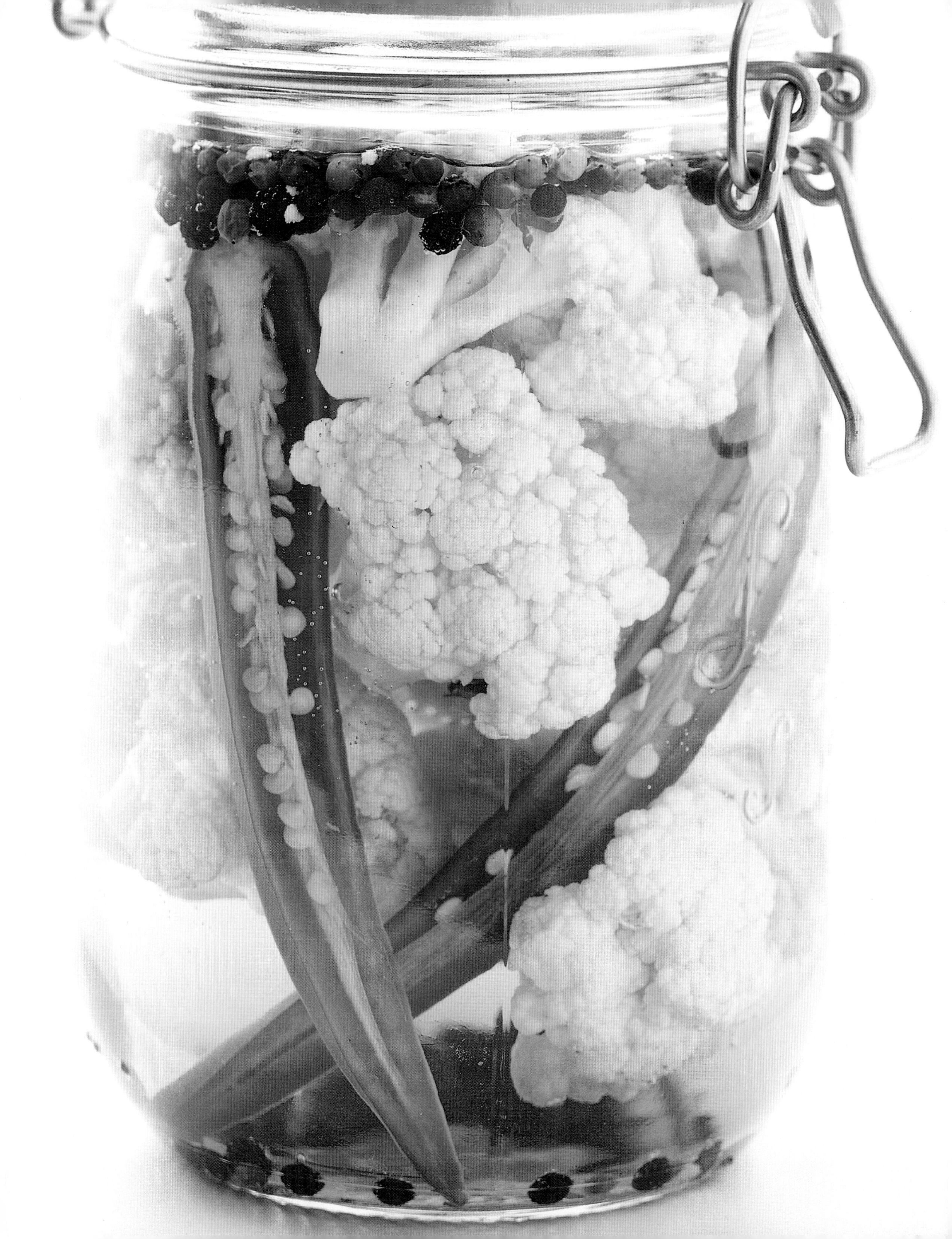

## borage leaves in vinegar

The leaves can be eaten on their own as a starter or added to salads or other dishes. The borage flowers give a blue colour to the vinegar.

110 g young borage leaves
A dash of white wine vinegar
Borage flowers (10% of the volume of borage leaves)
1 litre white wine vinegar (with 2 tbsp salt added)

Rinse the borage leaves in a bowl of cold water with a dash of vinegar added. Place the leaves in a single layer on a clean, dry cloth and leave them to wilt for 8 hours. Place them in a 1½ litre hermetically-sealable pickling jar and add the borage flowers. Pour over the salted white wine vinegar and seal the jar tightly. Leave for 1 month in a cool, dark place.

## tarragon vinegar

2 handfuls of fresh tarragon
10–12 very small pickling onions threaded onto toothpicks
A few borage flowers (optional)
1 litre white wine or cider vinegar

Put the tarragon into a hermetically-sealable pickling jar with the onions and the borage flowers (if using). Pour over the white wine or cider vinegar and seal the jar tightly. Leave for 2 weeks in a cool, dark place.

## shallot vinegar

1 litre white wine vinegar or cider vinegar
10 shallots
1 bay leaf
1 sprig of thyme
1 tsp black peppercorns

Pour the white wine or cider vinegar over the other ingredients in a hermetically-sealable pickling jar. Seal the jar tightly. Leave for 2 weeks in a cool, dark place. Strain and bottle.

## herb vinegar

1 litre red or white wine vinegar
1 sprig of marjoram
1 sprig of tarragon
1 sprig of thyme
1 clove or a few juniper berries
A few basil leaves
A few green and black peppercorns

Pour the vinegar over the other ingredients in a hermetically-sealable pickling jar. Seal the jar tightly. Leave for 1 month in a cool, dark place. Strain and bottle.

## amazingly aromatic vinegar

1 litre white wine or cider vinegar
2 handfuls of dill
2 handfuls of tarragon leaves and stems
1 handful of fresh basil leaves
1 handful of fresh thyme
1 handful of marjoram
10–12 small shallots threaded onto toothpicks
1 red chilli, whole (optional)

Pour the vinegar over the other ingredients in a hermetically-sealable pickling jar. Seal the jar tightly. Leave for 2–3 weeks in a cool, dark place. Strain and bottle, leaving the thyme in the vinegar.

## table mustard

2 tbsp celery leaves, chopped
2 tbsp chervil, chopped
2 tbsp chives, chopped
2 tbsp parsley, chopped
2 tbsp tarragon, chopped
2 tbsp thyme, chopped
1 clove of garlic
1 tsp salt
½ teaspoon black pepper
White wine vinegar (enough to cover the herbs)
Mustard powder
Olive oil

In a food processor, blend the herbs, garlic, salt and pepper. Transfer to a small, hermetically-sealable pickling jar and add white wine vinegar to cover. Seal the jar tightly. Leave for 1 week in a cool, dark place. Add mustard powder to make a thick paste and olive oil to create a smooth consistency. Mix well and store in a sealed container in the refrigerator.

# JAM

## physalis jam

1 kg physalis berries
Water
1 kg sugar

Remove the berries from their parchment skins, wash and cut them in half. Put them into a heavy-based saucepan, cover them with water and simmer for 30 minutes. Blend the berry mixture in a food processor, add the sugar and return to the heat for 30 minutes. Store in tightly-sealed jars.

# medicinal drinks, tinctures and syrups

Infusions, decoctions, wines, liqueurs, tinctures and syrups provide a valuable way of administering the active ingredients of various plants, herbs and spices. Each of the following recipes is accompanied by the recommended dosage, a brief explanation of its properties (some of the terms used are explained in the glossary; pages 276–78) and the ailments or body systems that it is good for. See Chapter 2 for more information about specific ailments and their remedies. Most of the recipes give amounts for dried herbs. If you wish to substitute fresh herbs, use two to three times the given amount. Dried herbs can be bought from health food shops and herbalists.

## INFUSIONS

Infusions can be prepared one day in advance, stored in the refrigerator and gently warmed when needed. They are relatively mild medicinal drinks and need to be taken frequently. Infusions made with lime flower, lemon balm and camomile are recommended for children.

### dandelion infusion

Dosage: 150 ml three times a day.
Properties: detoxifying, aids liver function.
Good for: bone and joint disorders, digestive system disorders, kidney and bladder disorders, eczema, high blood pressure.

1 tbsp dried dandelion root
1 tbsp dried dandelion leaves
1 litre boiling water

Pour the boiling water over the dandelion root and leaves, and cover. Leave to infuse for 10 minutes then strain.

### fennel infusion

Dosage: 150 ml three times a day. Alternatively, take a drop of fennel essential oil on a lump of sugar or in a teaspoon of honey.
Properties: anti-spasmodic, carminative, appetite and digestion stimulant.
Good for: digestive system disorders, women's health disorders, anaemia, candida, polymyalgia rheumatica, Raynaud's disease.

1 tbsp fennel seeds or root
150 ml boiling water

Pour the boiling water over the fennel seeds or root, and cover. Leave to infuse for 10 minutes then strain.

### raspberry-leaf infusion

Dosage: 150 ml of the warm infusion three times a day.
Properties: astringent.
Good for: fibrositis, period pain, polymyalgia rheumatica, pregnancy (especially the last few weeks).

1 tsp dried raspberry leaves
150 ml boiling water

Pour the boiling water over the raspberry leaves and cover. Leave to infuse for 5 minutes then strain.

### orange-zest infusion

Dosage: drink throughout the day instead of water.
Properties: stimulates the immune system.
Good for: blood and circulation disorders.

40 g orange zest
15 g bay leaves
1 litre boiling water

Pour the boiling water over the orange zest and bay leaves, and cover. Leave to infuse for 20 minutes then strain.

### marjoram infusion

Dosage: drink throughout the day instead of water. For ease of use, mix the herbs together and store them in a jar.
Properties: aids digestion, antiseptic, anti-spasmodic.
Good for: respiratory system disorders, immune system disorders, insomnia, thrush.

20 g dried marjoram
20 g dried mint
20 g dried thyme
½ litre boiling water
Honey to taste

Pour the boiling water over 15 g of the herb mixture and cover. Leave to infuse for a few minutes. Strain and add honey.

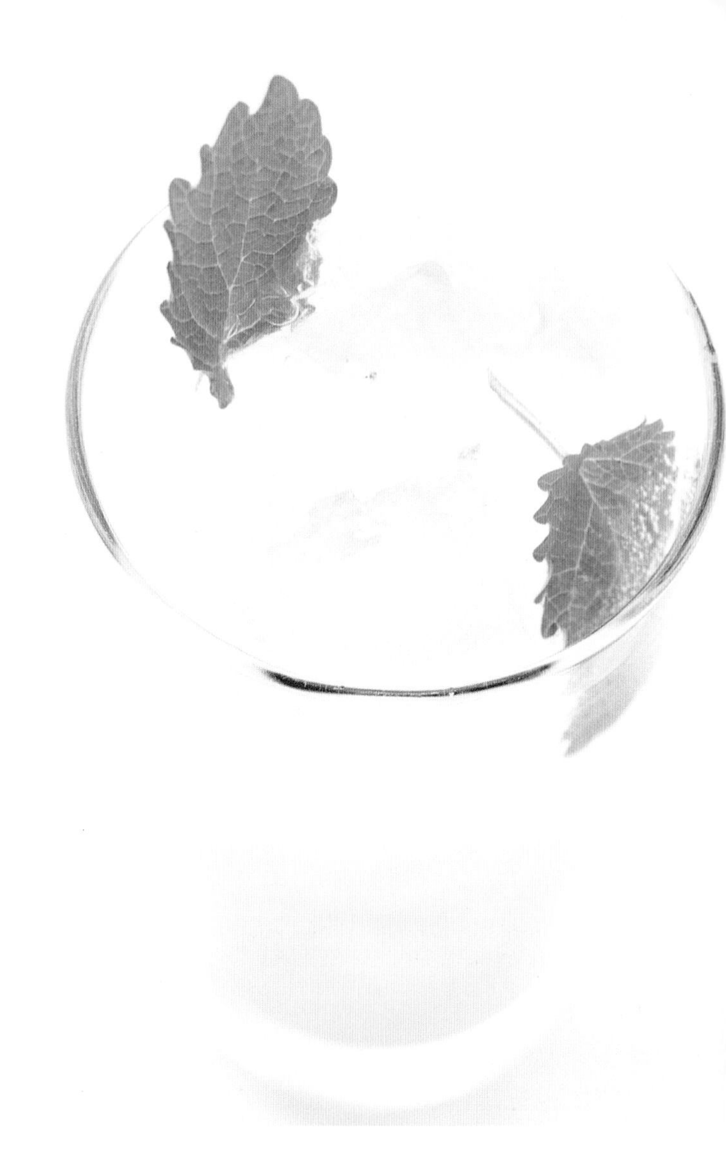

# lemon-balm and camomile infusion *(right)*

Dosage: 150 ml of the warm infusion two or three times a day. For ease of use, mix the herbs together and store them in a jar.
Properties: antispasmodic, sedative, detoxifying.
Good for: heart and circulation disorders, digestive system disorders, respiratory system disorders, nervous system disorders, women's health disorders, kidney stones, psoriasis, urticaria (hives).

100 g dried lemon balm leaves
30 g dried camomile flowers
20 g dried mint leaves
150 ml boiling water

Pour the boiling water over a tbsp of the herb mixture and cover. Leave to infuse for 5 minutes then strain.

# carrot-seed infusion

Dosage: 150 ml two or three times a day.
Properties: stimulates digestion, tonic, promotes bile flow, mild diuretic.
Good for: amenorrhoea.

5 g carrot seeds
300 ml boiling water

Pour the boiling water over the carrot seeds, and cover. Leave to infuse for 10 minutes then strain.

# pear and apple infusion

Dosage: drink throughout the day instead of water.
Properties: diuretic, anti-inflammatory, detoxifying.
Good for: bone and joint disorders, kidney and bladder stones.

50 g pear leaves
50 g dried apple peel
1 litre boiling water

Pour the boiling water over the pear leaves and apple peel and cover. Infuse for 20 minutes and strain.

# barley infusion

Dosage: drink throughout the day instead of water.
Properties: diuretic, calming, anti-inflammatory.
Good for: irritable bladder, prostatitis.

100 g barley grain
1 litre boiling water

Pour the boiling water over the barley and cover. Leave to infuse for 3 hours then strain.

# elder and camomile infusion

Dosage: 150 ml of the warm infusion three or four times a day. This infusion can be given to young children.
Properties: promotes sweating, detoxifying, sedative, anti-inflammatory.
Good for: digestive system, respiratory system, nervous system, immune system, endometriosis, premenstrual syndrome, psoriasis.

2 tbsp dried elderflowers
1 tbsp dried camomile flowers or 1 camomile teabag
250 ml boiling water
Sugar to taste

Pour the boiling water over the elderflowers and camomile flowers or camomile teabag and cover. Leave to infuse for 10 minutes. Strain and sweeten with sugar.

## sparkling lemon-balm infusion

Dosage: drink when desired. This recipe can be served as an aperitif for adults by replacing the sparkling water with sparkling wine.
Properties: refreshing, calming (excellent for children).
Good for: nervous system, women's health, angina, anxiety, cough, fear and nightmares in children, laryngitis, psoriasis, rhinitis, urticaria (hives).

For the infusion:
45 fresh lemon balm leaves
½ litre boiling water

For the drink:
½ litre sparkling mineral water (or wine if using)
Juice of 1 orange
Juice of 1 grapefruit
Sugar to taste
1 fresh lemon balm leaf
1 slice of lemon

Pour the boiling water over the lemon balm leaves and cover. Leave to infuse until cold and then strain. Mix the infusion with the sparkling mineral water, or wine if using, orange and grapefruit juice. Add the sugar and serve in a frosted glass with the lemon balm leaf and a slice of lemon.

## coriander-seed infusion

Dosage: 150 ml of the warm infusion two or three times a day.
Properties: anti-spasmodic, carminative, stimulates the digestive system.
Good for: digestive system, amenorrhoea, period pain.

1 tbsp coriander seeds
150 ml boiling water
Sugar to taste

Pour the boiling water over the coriander seeds and cover. Leave to infuse for 10 minutes. Strain and add the sugar.

## ginger infusion

Dosage: 150 ml of the warm infusion four times a day or when desired.
Properties: stimulates digestive system, anti-emetic.
Good for: heart and circulation, digestive system, respiratory system, nervous system, digestive problems and morning sickness during pregnancy.

2 tbsp fresh ginger root, grated
150 ml boiling water
Sugar to taste

Pour the boiling water over the ginger and cover. Allow to infuse for 5 minutes. Strain and sweeten with a little sugar.

# DECOCTIONS

As with infusions, decoctions can be prepared one day in advance, they are relatively mild and should be taken frequently. Decoctions involve boiling the tough or woody parts of plants, such as stems, roots, seeds and berries. Store decoctions in the refrigerator.

## carrot-leaf decoction

Usage: apply to the skin two or three times a day.
Properties: promotes healing and regeneration of damaged skin, anti-inflammatory, analgesic.
Good for: chilblains.

1 handful of fresh carrot leaves
150 ml water
Carrot juice (extracted using a juicer)

In a saucepan, boil the carrot leaves in the water for 5 minutes. Strain and mix with an equal quantity of fresh carrot juice.

## cherry-stem decoction

Dosage: 150 ml three or four times a day.
Properties: diuretic, detoxifying.
Good for: bone and joint disorders, measles, pleurisy, pneumonia.

30 g cherry stems
1 litre water

In a saucepan, boil the cherry stems in the water for 10 minutes and strain.

## corn-hair and fennel-seed decoction

Corn hair consists of black, hair-like threads that surround the corn beneath the outer leaves. It is available in specialist herb shops or from herbalists.

Dosage: 150 ml of the warm infusion three times a day.
Properties: detoxifying, diuretic, anti-inflammatory, stimulates the digestive system.
Good for: kidney and bladder disorders, women's health, chickenpox, prostatitis.

1 handful of dried corn hair
2 tsp fennel seeds
1 litre water

In a saucepan, bring the ingredients to the boil. Remove from heat, cover and leave to infuse for 20 minutes. Strain.

# lychee-seed decoction

Dosage: drink the warm decoction throughout the day.
Properties: analgesic, anti-spasmodic, astringent.
Good for: abdominal cramp and colic.

30 g lychee seeds
Zest of 1 lemon
1 tbsp fennel seeds
½ litre water

In a saucepan, boil the ingredients in the water for 20 minutes, then strain.

# physalis-berry decoction

Dosage: 150 ml four times a day.
Properties: diuretic, anti-inflammatory.
Good for: kidney and bladder disorders, prostatitis.

60 g physalis berries
1 litre water

In a saucepan, boil the berries in the water for 5 minutes. Allow to infuse for a further 10 minutes and strain.

# cherry-stem and apple decoction

Dosage: 150 ml three times a day.
Properties: detoxifying, anti-inflammatory, diuretic.
Good for: arthritis (rheumatoid), chickenpox, measles.

1 handful of cherry stems
1 litre water
2 or 3 apples, sliced

In a saucepan, boil the cherry stems in the water for 10 minutes. Strain and pour the decoction over the apple slices. Cover and leave to infuse for 20 minutes. Strain, pressing the apple slices to extract all the juice.

# lettuce-seed decoction

Dosage: 250 ml three times a day.
Properties: calming, sedative, anti-spasmodic.
Good for: respiratory disorders, anxiety, kidney stones.

1 tbsp lettuce seeds
250 ml water

In a saucepan, boil the lettuce seeds in the water for 10 minutes and then strain.

# dill-seed decoction

Dosage: 150 ml of the warm infusion two or three times a day.
Properties: anti-spasmodic, carminative, stimulates the digestive system.
Good for: digestive system disorders, amenorrhoea, period pain.

1 tbsp dill seeds
500 ml water
Sugar to taste

In a saucepan, boil the dill seeds in the water for 10 minutes. Strain and add the sugar.

# fennel-seed decoction

Dosage: 150 ml of the warm infusion once a day.

Properties: anti-spasmodic, carminative, stimulates the digestive system.
Good for: digestive system disorders, women's health disorders, anaemia, polymyalgia rheumatica, Raynaud's disease.

2 tsp fennel seeds
150 ml water
Sugar to taste

In a saucepan, boil the seeds in the water for 5 minutes. Strain and add the sugar.

# strawberry-leaf decoction

Dosage: drink throughout the day.
Properties: astringent, anti-inflammatory, detoxifying.
Good for: bone and joint, heart and circulation, respiratory system, kidney and bladder disorders, prostatitis.

1 handful of fresh strawberry leaves
1 handful of fresh strawberry roots
1 litre water

In a saucepan, bring the ingredients to the boil. Remove from the heat and allow to infuse for 10 minutes. Strain.

# cumin-seed decoction

Dosage: 150 ml of the warm infusion two or three times a day.
Properties: sedative, carminative, antiseptic.
Good for: digestive system, women's health.

1 tsp cumin seeds
150 ml water

In a saucepan, boil the cumin seeds in the water for 10 minutes. Strain.

## barley water

Dosage: drink throughout the day.
Properties: diuretic, calming, anti-inflammatory.
Good for: heart and circulation, digestive system, kidney and bladder.

30 g barley, germinated
1 litre water
Honey to taste

In a saucepan, bring the water and barley gently to the boil. Simmer until the barley is cooked. Strain and add the honey.

# WINES AND LIQUEURS

Only small amounts of the following drinks need to be taken for medicinal purposes. Wines should be stored in tightly corked bottles and kept for a few weeks. When preparing liqueurs, use the strongest alcohol available to help to extract the plants' active ingredients. Liqueurs can last for years. Store away from bright light. Wines and liqueurs should not be given to children.

## cinnamon wine *(right)*

Dosage: 50 ml when desired.
Properties: tonic, aphrodisiac, antiseptic, aids digestion.
Good for: Raynaud's disease.

50 g cinnamon bark
20 g vanilla pods
750 ml sweet red wine

Add the cinnamon and vanilla to the wine. Seal tightly and leave to macerate for 3 days. Strain through muslin and store in a tightly sealed bottle.

## blackcurrant wine

Dosage: 50 ml a day.
Properties: tonic, astringent, laxative, improves vitality and digestion.
Good for: anaemia, polymyalgia rheumatica, Raynaud's disease, ulcerative colitis.

200 g blackcurrants
750 ml dry white wine
150 g sugar
150 ml strong alcohol (such as vodka, eau de vie or grappa)

Crush the blackcurrants in a large bowl and pour over the dry white wine. Seal the bowl with clingfilm and refrigerate for a week. Press and strain the mixture through muslin. Add the sugar and over a low heat, bring to simmering point. Do not allow to boil. Cool and add the strong alcohol. Store in a tightly sealed bottle and leave to age for several months.

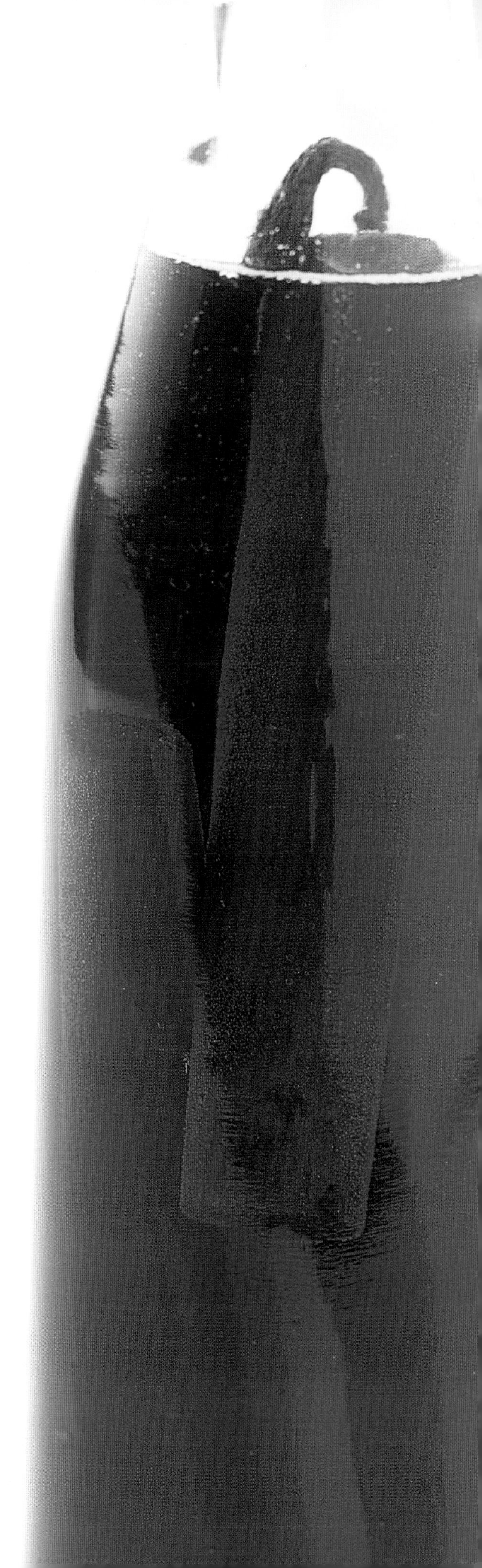

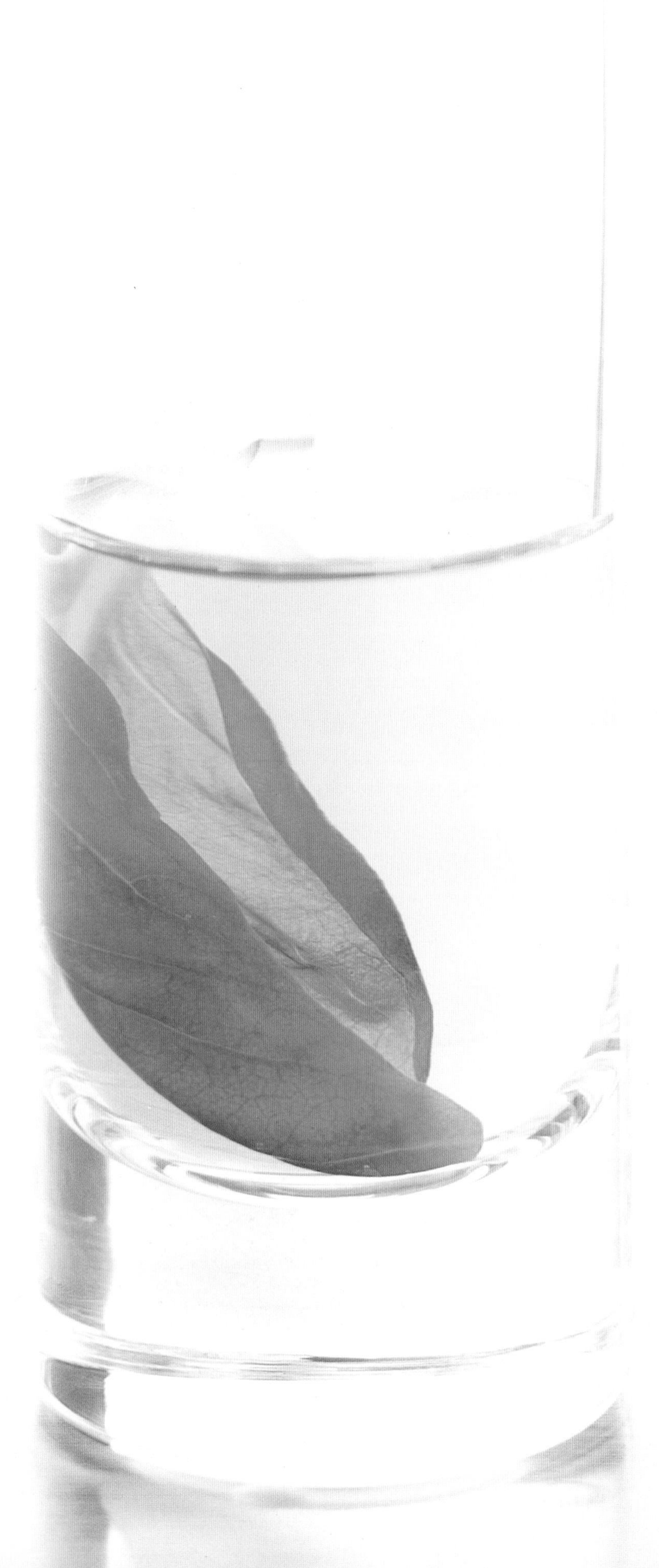

# artichoke-leaf wine

Dosage: 50 ml morning and evening before meals.
Properties: detoxifying, improves liver function, stimulates the flow of bile.
Good for: ankylosing spondylitis, arteriosclerosis, cholecystitis, gallstones, hyperlipidaemia.

50 g dried artichoke leaves, finely chopped
750 ml red wine

Add the artichoke leaves to the wine. Seal tightly and leave to macerate for 10 days. Strain through muslin and store in a tightly sealed bottle.

# cherry-leaf wine

Dosage: 50 ml a day (dilute to taste).
Properties: diuretic, detoxifying.
Good for: bone and joint disorders.

80 cherry leaves
5 tbsp sugar
750 ml red wine
150 ml kirsch

Add the cherry leaves and the sugar to the wine. Seal tightly and leave to macerate for 8 days. Remove the cherry leaves and add the kirsch.

# blueberry wine

Dosage: 50 ml a day.
Properties: tonic, aids digestion.

200 g fresh blueberries
100 g fresh raspberries or blackcurrants
700 ml dry white wine
150 g sugar
150 ml strong alcohol (such as vodka, eau de vie or grappa)

In a large bowl, crush the fruit. Cover with the white wine, seal the bowl and refrigerate for 1 week. Then press and strain the mixture, add the sugar to the liquid and, in a stainless steel pan, bring slowly to simmering point. Cool and add the alcohol. Age in a tightly sealed bottle for several months.

# juniper-berry wine

Dosage: 50 ml a day.
Properties: tonic, diuretic, analgesic, aids digestion.
Good for: kidney and bladder disorders, diabetes mellitus.

75 g fresh juniper berries, crushed
10 g lemon zest
750 ml white wine

Add the juniper berries and the lemon zest to the white wine. Seal tightly and leave to macerate in a cool, dark place for 1 week. Strain through muslin and store in a tightly sealed bottle.

# camomile and citrus wine

Dosage: 50 ml when desired.
Properties: sedative, bitter tonic, stimulates digestion.
Good for: digestive system disorders, anxiety, endometriosis, insomnia.

60 g camomile flowers
Zest of 1 unwaxed lemon
Zest of 1 unwaxed orange
1 tsp tea leaves (optional)
750 ml dry white wine
60 g sugar
150 ml strong alcohol (such as vodka or gin)

Mix all the ingredients together. Seal in an airtight container and leave to macerate in a cool, dark place for 1 week. Strain through muslin and store in a tightly sealed bottle.

# anisette

Dosage: 1 tablespoon (neat or diluted in 75 ml water) when desired.
Properties: anti-spasmodic, carminative.
Good for: digestive system disorders, women's health disorders, headaches and migraine.

25 g green anise seeds or star anise
15 g coriander seeds
½ g mace
1 g cinnamon bark
700 ml vodka
250 g sugar
100 ml water

Add the anise, coriander seeds, mace and cinnamon bark to the vodka. Seal tightly and leave to macerate in a cool, dark place for 1 month. In a saucepan over a low heat, dissolve the sugar in the water, then boil for 30 seconds. Allow to cool. Strain the vodka through muslin, pressing the seeds to extract as much liquid as possible. Mix with the cooled syrup, store in a tightly sealed bottle and keep in a cool, dark place for 2 weeks before using.

# camomile aperitif

Dosage: 50 ml in the evening.
Properties: sedative, bitter tonic, enhances digestion and sleep.
Good for: endometriosis.

60 g camomile flowers
750 ml white wine

Add the camomile flowers to the wine. Seal tightly and leave to macerate in a cool, dark place for 1 month. Strain through muslin and store in a tightly sealed bottle.

# lemon liqueur

Dosage: 25 ml when desired.
Properties: carminative, aids digestion, astringent, aperitive.
Good for: cholecystitis, gallstones.

Zest of 3 lemons, cut into thin strips
50 g almonds
1 small vanilla pod or cinnamon stick
700 ml strong vodka
250 g sugar
100 ml water
1 almond or clove

Add the lemon zest, almonds and vanilla pod or cinnamon stick to the vodka. Seal tightly and leave to macerate in a cool, dark place for 1 month. In a heavy-based pan, dissolve the sugar in the water and then boil for 30 seconds. Strain the infused alcohol and combine with the cooled syrup. Add an almond or clove and some of the original lemon zest to the mixture. Seal tightly and leave to mature for a few months.

# basil liqueur *(far left)*

Dosage: 25 ml when desired.
Properties: antiseptic, anti-spasmodic, stimulates appetite.
Good for: digestive system disorders, headaches and migraine.

80 fresh basil leaves
700 ml strong vodka
250 g sugar
100 ml water

Add the basil leaves to the vodka. Seal tightly and leave to macerate in a cool dark place for 1 month. In a heavy-based pan, dissolve the sugar over a low heat in just enough water to make it wet. When all the crystals have dissolved, boil for 30 seconds. Mix the cooled syrup with the vodka, seal tightly and leave for a further 3 weeks. To keep the green colour of the liqueur remove some of the basil leaves (they can be used to make basil ice cream in an ice-cream maker).

# quince liqueur

Dosage: 50 ml when desired.
Properties: astringent.
Good for: digestive system disorders.

1 kg quince, mashed
200 g sugar
2 cloves
Pinch of ground cinnamon
Vodka or brandy

Refrigerate the mashed quince for 48 hours, then press through muslin to extract the juice. Add the sugar, cloves and cinnamon and an equal volume of vodka or brandy. Seal tightly and leave to macerate for 2 months. Strain through muslin and store in a tightly sealed bottle. Leave to age for a further 2 or 3 months.

# TINCTURES

Tinctures are made with alcohol and provide a very concentrated way of taking the active ingredients of a plant. As with liqueurs, very strong alcohol should be used. Tinctures can have a lifespan of years. Store away from bright light.

## artichoke-leaf tincture

Dosage: 30 drops in 75 ml of water, morning and evening.
Properties: detoxifying, improves liver function, stimulates the flow of bile.
Good for: bone and joint disorders, cholecystitis, gallstones.

500 g dried artichoke leaves
750 ml strong alcohol (such as vodka, gin or brandy)

Add the artichoke leaves to the alcohol. Seal tightly and leave to macerate in a cool, dark place for 3 weeks. Strain through muslin and store in a tightly sealed bottle away from bright light.

## aniseed tincture

Dosage: 20 drops in 150 ml of water one to three times a day.
Or take 10 drops of tincture on a lump of sugar.
Properties: anti-spasmodic, carminative, stimulates the digestive system.
Good for: digestive system disorders, women's health disorders, headaches and migraine.

170 g aniseed (the seeds of the anise plant)
700 ml strong alcohol (such as vodka, eau de vie or gin)

Add the aniseed to the alcohol. Seal tightly and leave to macerate in a cool, dark place for 1 month. Strain through muslin and store in a tightly sealed bottle away from bright light.

## coriander-seed tincture

Dosage: 15 drops in 75 ml of water after a meal.
Properties: anti-spasmodic, carminative, aids digestion, aids lactation.
Good for: gastritis, amenorrhoea.

5 g coriander seeds
500 ml strong alcohol (such as vodka, gin or brandy)

Add the coriander seeds to the alcohol. Seal tightly and leave to macerate in a cool, dark place for 1 week. Strain through muslin and store in a tightly sealed bottle away from bright light.

# SYRUPS

The active ingredients of plants can be administered in the form of a syrup. Syrups should always be stored in a refrigerator and used within a few days (except crème de cassis, which will keep for several months).

The following test can help to determine the point during preparation at which a syrup should be removed from the heat: take a teaspoon of the syrup and drop it into a glass of cold water; if it breaks into droplets, it needs further boiling; if it forms a single droplet, it is ready.

## leek syrup

Dosage: 1 tablespoon three times a day.
Properties: soothing, expectorant, anti-inflammatory.
Good for: respiratory system disorders, fibrositis, polymyalgia rheumatica, sore throat, tonsillitis.

1 medium leek, chopped
1 litre water
150 g sugar

In a saucepan, simmer the leek in the water. When the water has reduced by approximately one-third, press the leek to squeeze out the juice. Remove the leek, add the sugar and boil for a few more minutes. Allow to cool and pour into a sterilized bottle. Seal tightly and refrigerate.

## peach syrup

Dosage: 3–4 tablespoons a day (2 tablespoons for children).
Properties: calming, laxative.
Good for: constipation in children.

20 g fresh peach flowers
150 ml boiling water
250 g honey

In a saucepan, pour the boiling water over the flowers, cover and leave to infuse for about 6 hours. Strain through muslin, add the honey, then bring to the boil, reduce the heat and simmer for a few minutes. Allow to cool and pour into a sterilized bottle. Seal tightly and refrigerate.

## black radish syrup

Dosage: 1 tablespoon three times a day.
Properties: soothing, anti-inflammatory, expectorant.
Good for: sore throat, tonsillitis, whooping cough.

1 black radish, peeled and sliced
Caster sugar

Place the radish slices in a dish, covering each layer with plenty of sugar. Cover with clingfilm and leave overnight. Press the radish slices to extract the syrup and strain into a sterilized bottle. Seal tightly and refrigerate.

# mint syrup

Dosage: 1 teaspoon in a glass of water. Mint syrup can be added to water or served with sorbet.
Properties: stimulates the digestive system, anti-spasmodic.
Good for: colitis, cough, endometriosis, food poisoning, rhinitis.

100 g fresh mint leaves
1 litre boiling water
1 kg sugar

Pour the water over the mint leaves. Seal tightly and leave to infuse for 24 hours. Strain. In a pan, bring the infusion and sugar to the boil and simmer for 3 minutes. Cool. Pour into a sterilized bottle. Seal tightly and refrigerate.

# blackberry syrup *(right)*

Dosage: 1 tablespoon in 150 ml of water two or three times a day.
Properties: astringent.
Good for: diarrhoea, dysentery.

1 kg blackberries
1 kg sugar
150 ml water

In a pan, bring the ingredients to the boil. Reduce the heat and simmer for 10 minutes. Cool. Pour into a sterilized bottle. Seal tightly and refrigerate.

# crème de cassis

Dosage: take as desired. This vitamin C-rich syrup can be diluted with water for children or added to dry white wine for adults.
Properties: tonic.
Good for: general well-being.

6 kg blackcurrants
6 kg sugar

Fill up 1-kg jars with equal amounts of blackcurrants and sugar in thin, alternating layers. Seal the jars and leave in a cool, dark place for 6 months. Strain and pour into sterilized bottles. Seal tightly and refrigerate.

# asparagus syrup

Dosage: 2 tablespoons morning and evening.
Properties: diuretic and sedative.
Good for: nervous system disorders, endometriosis, palpitations, premenstrual syndrome, psoriasis.

200 ml asparagus tips juice (extracted using a juicer)
400 g sugar

In a saucepan, boil the asparagus juice and sugar until a thick syrup forms. Allow to cool and pour into a sterilized bottle. Seal tightly and refrigerate.

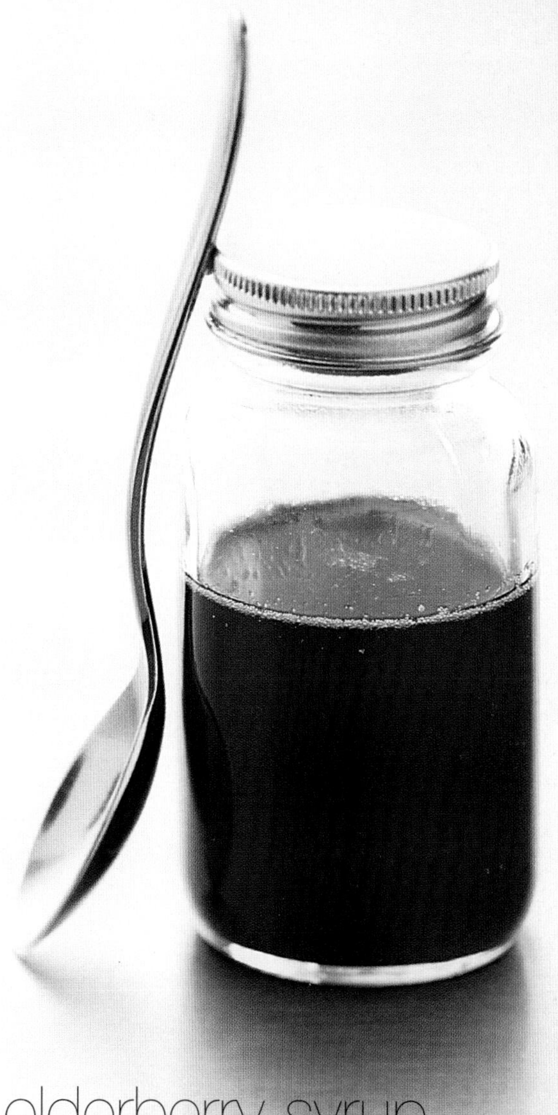

# elderberry syrup

Dosage: 1 tablespoon every morning.
Properties: gentle laxative.
Good for: colic, constipation, irritable bowel syndrome (recommended for elderly people).

1½ kg fresh elderberries, slightly unripe (red rather than black), with the stems cut off
150 ml water
350 g sugar
3 g cloves

In a saucepan, crush the berries and simmer them in the water for 30 minutes. Put the berry mixture in a piece of muslin and allow the juice to drip into a bowl overnight. In a non-reactive saucepan, bring the juice, sugar and cloves to the boil. Reduce the heat and simmer for 5 minutes. Allow to cool and pour into a sterilized bottle. Seal tightly and refrigerate.

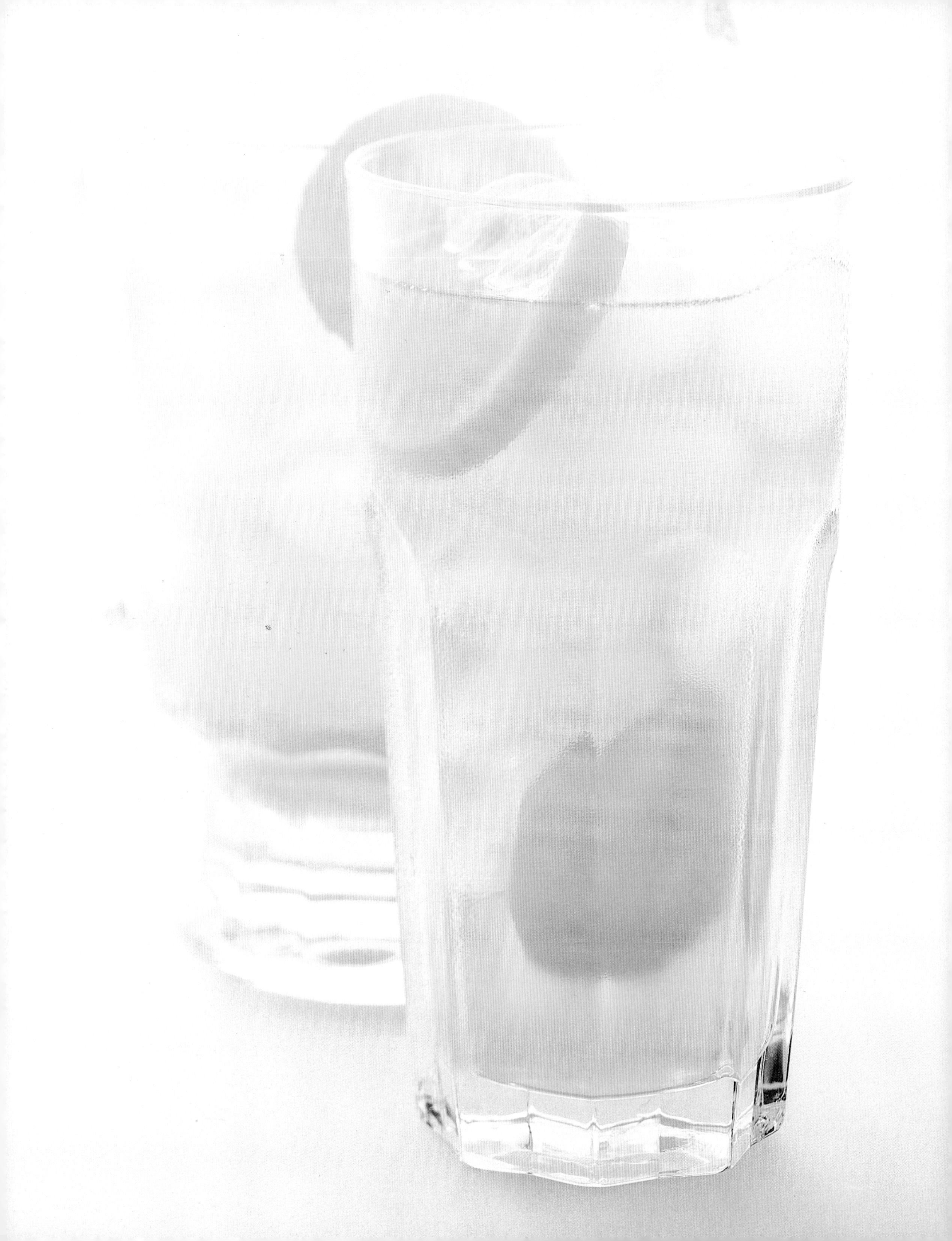

chapter four

# diet in practice

Sometimes the best way to fortify the body against illness is to simplify the diet to a few basic ingredients that are easy to digest and assimilate. This enables the body to rid itself of toxins and emerge stronger and more resilient. The detoxification programme on the following pages – a four-week prescription of healing foods, drinks and exercise – is the ideal way to accomplish this. It can be followed successfully by most adults regardless of their level of health and fitness. This chapter also presents the vitamins, minerals and other nutrients, such as antioxidants and essential fatty acids, that are needed for health, together with a selection of the foods in which they are found. There is also a short review of two basic elements of our everyday diet that have important health-giving properties but are often overlooked: culinary oils and bottled mineral waters.

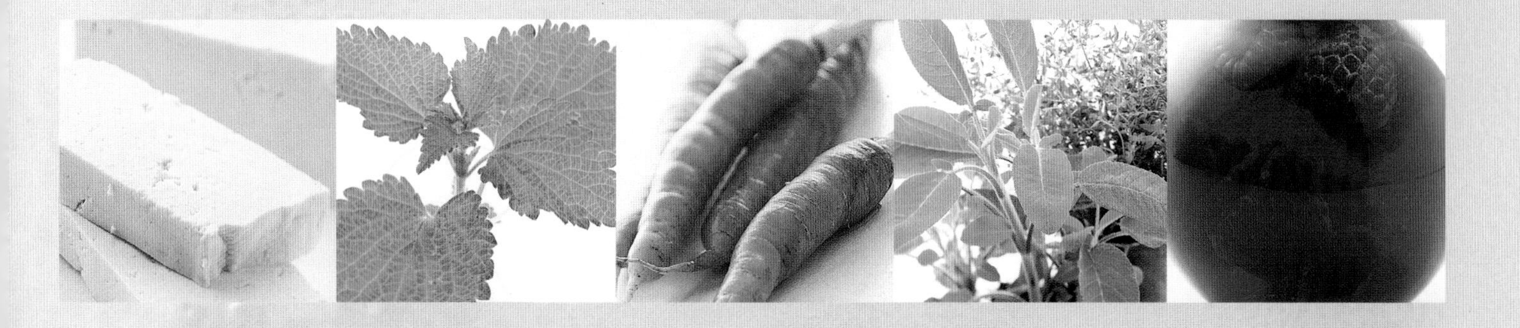

# the detox programme

During digestion, a certain amount of acids are produced – these are partly a result of normal digestive processes and partly a result of the incomplete degradation of animal proteins. The body gets rid of a small amount of these acids rapidly via the lungs but denser acids, such as uric, phosphoric and sulphuric acid, which are generated by the breakdown of animal protein, are eliminated slowly by the kidneys. If acid is not eliminated quickly enough, it creates toxicity.

A series of complex operations involving a variety of secretions – each acting under different pH – takes place in the digestive tract. The result of these operations is the breakdown of food into nutrients that can be used by the body. However, if the pH in one section of the gut is wrong, the digestive process is impaired and fats, sugars and proteins are only partially broken down. Food starts to putrefy in the gut and a pathogenic flora develops to the detriment of the beneficial flora. This also creates toxicity in the body.

According to the late Dr Kousmine, a nutrition and cancer specialist, acids that are not eliminated from the body during the day are stored in extra-cellular fluid (known as serous fluid) in the peritoneum. At night when the body is resting the acids are filtered and disposed of. Over a period of time, however, acids build up in the body's tissues causing an accumulation of toxins and a condition known as chronic acidosis. This can give rise to a variety of symptoms including fatigue, disturbed sleep, regurgitation, heartburn, lack of appetite or bulimia, diarrhoea or constipation, migraine, bad breath, cold perspiration, lowered resistance to infections, muscular pain, rheumatism, bronchitis and excessive mucus production resulting in chronic catarrh.

In the past 50 years, there has been an increase in heart disease, cancer and auto-immune or degenerative disorders such as rheumatoid arthritis. Rather than having mechanical, bacterial or viral causes, these illnesses are directly or indirectly linked to food processing and preserving methods and the excessive consumption of refined sugar, cereals, oils, meat, dairy and animal fat. The use of hormones, chemical fertilizers, antibiotics, insecticides and anti-fungal agents has also contributed to the build-up of toxins in the food chain.

A detoxification diet can facilitate the rapid and efficient elimination of toxins and improve both short- and long-term health. The plan described here combines diet and exercise with herbal medicine and nutritional supplements. Although it is suitable for the majority of adults, it should not be followed by children, elderly people or pregnant or breast-feeding women. If you are on long-term medication, such as hormone replacement therapy (HRT), or drugs for hypertension or thyroid problems, you should continue to take them throughout the programme (consult your doctor if you are in any doubt about whether it is safe for you to follow a detox plan). It is useful to be aware of some possible side-effects of detoxification. These vary depending on the stage of the programme but they tend to include mild headache, mood changes and energy fluctuations. If side effects do not abate after the first week, or you experience persistent or troublesome symptoms, consult your doctor.

Although the detox plan requires a few changes to your normal routine and some careful planning, it should be fairly easy to implement. Most people start to feel the benefits of detox about 10 days into the programme.

## week one

### WHAT TO DO

During the first week you should eliminate all dairy and wheat-based products from your diet, reduce your salt intake, avoid meat and animal fat, tea, coffee, white sugar, sweets, alcohol and tobacco. Remember that foods such as pasta, biscuits and bread all contain wheat; use rice, buckwheat or quinoa as a substitute. Soya milk is available from most supermarkets and can be used as a replacement for cow's milk. In addition, you should:

- Drink 1–2 litres of mineral water every day; choose water that has a low mineral content (page 144).
- If you experience an excessive amount of abdominal gas and bloating, take two capsules of activated charcoal three times a day after meals.

- Eat a handful of fresh or dried blueberries every day.
- Drink herbal teas made from fennel, ginger or camomile before and after your meals.
- Use plenty of herbs such as thyme, basil, rosemary, garlic and shallots in your cooking.

### HOW TO SUCCEED

- Revise your usual shopping list to include plenty of fresh fruit and vegetables, fish, rice, lentils, beans, millet, buckwheat flour, fresh herbs and herbal teas such as ginger, peppermint, camomile and fennel.
- Follow the recipes in this book and use a cookery book with an emphasis on healthy food (Provençal and Mediterranean cooking are recommended).
- Start the day with a protein-based breakfast (mushrooms are a good source of protein) and eat well at lunchtime. This will provide you with enough energy to get through the day. In contrast, your dinner should be very light.
- Resist the temptation to have the occasional sugary snack, cup of tea or coffee or alcoholic drink.

### POSSIBLE SIDE-EFFECTS

You may experience mild headaches, bursts of energy alternating with fatigue, muscle aches and pains, sudden hunger, irritability, cravings for sweet foods, intestinal gas, abdominal distension, and regurgitation. These are most common during the first 48 hours. Side-effects vary from one person to another and you certainly won't experience all of these.

### THE BENEFITS

Towards the end of week one, you may notice that your energy levels, appetite and quality of sleep are improving.

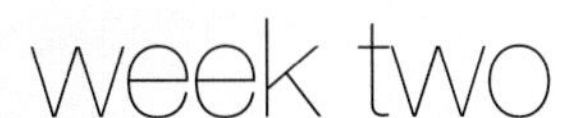

## week two

### WHAT TO DO

Follow exactly the same guidelines as for week one but increase the percentage of raw fruit and vegetables so that they make up 70 per cent of your daily food intake. In addition, avoid eating after seven o'clock in the evening.

- To accelerate the detoxification process, drink 150 ml dandelion infusion (page 123), three times a day. Or drink 50 ml artichoke leaf wine (page 128) at lunchtime and early evening.
- Take propolis tablets to help reduce bacterial activity in the gut. Follow the dosage instructions on the package.

### HOW TO SUCCEED

- Drink as much herbal tea as you like after seven o'clock in the evening.
- Try to go to bed earlier than usual – rest is an important aid to detoxification.
- Keep following the tips for success for week one.

### POSSIBLE SIDE-EFFECTS

Cravings for sweets and carbohydrates and feelings of hunger are common during week two. You may feel tired or cold immediately after you have had a meal and you may start to lose weight.

### THE BENEFITS

Towards the end of week two you will start to feel more energetic both physically and mentally. Your digestion, breathing and sleep patterns will be better and you may start to notice an improvement in chronic conditions, such as poor skin, eczema, rheumatism or arthritis.

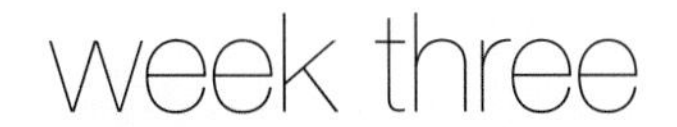

## week three

### WHAT TO DO

You should continue the programme of diet and rest that you followed in week two but, to accelerate detoxification, you should build in a programme of daily exercise. Do some low intensity exercise for 45 minutes twice daily. The best types of exercise are brisk walking, cycling or swimming.

You should also step up your intake of vitamins, minerals and trace elements by drinking a glass of fruit or vegetable juice twice every day. Recommended fruit juices are blackberry, blueberry, cherry or apricot. Good vegetable juice combinations include broccoli, green bean and lemon juice or carrot, cabbage and green or red pepper.

Before breakfast in the morning, drink the juice of half a lemon mixed with an equal amount of cold-pressed olive oil. This facilitates the emulsion and flow of bile into the digestive system. Other important dietary measures for week three are:

- Eat more of the following foods: rice, root vegetables such as carrot, celeriac, Jerusalem artichoke and turnip, germinated pulses, green vegetables, raw apple, fig and brazil nut.
- Eat fish at least twice a week.
- Drink 1–2 litres of mineral water every day; preferably with a medium to high mineral content (page 144).

### HOW TO SUCCEED

- Drink some water or herbal tea before you exercise, but avoid exercising on a full stomach.
- Eat a light snack after exercise, but nothing too heavy.
- Keep following the tips for success for weeks one and two.

### POSSIBLE SIDE-EFFECTS

Weight loss will continue as you burn calories during exercise. Exercise may also give rise to symptoms such as muscular aches (a recommended remedy for this is homeopathic arnica tablets of 30 or 200 potency; take when needed). However, if you experience a strong tightening or gripping pain in the centre of your chest after a few minutes of exercise, you must rest immediately and consult your doctor. Any sharp pains in weight-bearing joints or your lower back, should also be reported to your doctor.

### THE BENEFITS

You should continue to experience the benefits described in week 2. You will continue to feel more energetic, and your digestion, breathing and sleep patterns will improve further.

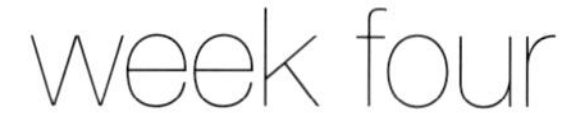


### WHAT TO DO

Continue to follow a wheat- and dairy-free diet but reduce your raw fruit and vegetable consumption to 50 per cent of your total food intake. Start to eat lightly after 7 o'clock in the evening. Continue your twice-daily exercise programme and keep taking the olive oil and lemon juice mixture before breakfast as in week 3. Drink fruit or vegetable juice twice a day and at least 1½ litres of a mineral water that has a medium-to-high mineral content.

### HOW TO SUCCEED

- Take a fish oil supplement every day for the next few weeks.
- Keep following the tips for success for weeks one to three.

### POSSIBLE SIDE-EFFECTS

At this stage of your programme, you should not experience any noticeable side-effects.

### THE BENEFITS

You should be feeling really fit and healthy by week four. Your energy levels should be consistently high, you should be sleeping well and any minor digestive problems should have completely disappeared. Chronic conditions such as eczema or rheumatism should be more manageable and may even have disappeared. Your immune system will be stronger and you will be more resistant to colds and influenza.

## your diet after detox

Once you have completed your four-week detoxification programme you can either follow the week-four guidelines for a further two weeks or you can return to a normal diet.

If you return to a normal diet, gradually reintroduce wheat products in the first week. If you experience any symptoms in response to them, eliminate wheat from your diet permanently. Dairy products should be reintroduced during the second week and any symptoms monitored. Again, if you have an adverse response, eliminate dairy products from your diet permanently.

Continue to practise as many aspects of the detox diet as you can and make sure that you apply the following principles to your long-term diet and lifestyle:

- Keep drinking plenty of water. Drink mineral water with a low mineral content (page 144), unless advised and supervised by a doctor or nutritionist.
- Eat meat and drink wine, coffee and tea in moderation.
- Keep up your exercise programme.
- Follow the detox programme annually and repeat the first two weeks of the plan twice a year: once in the autumn and once in the spring.

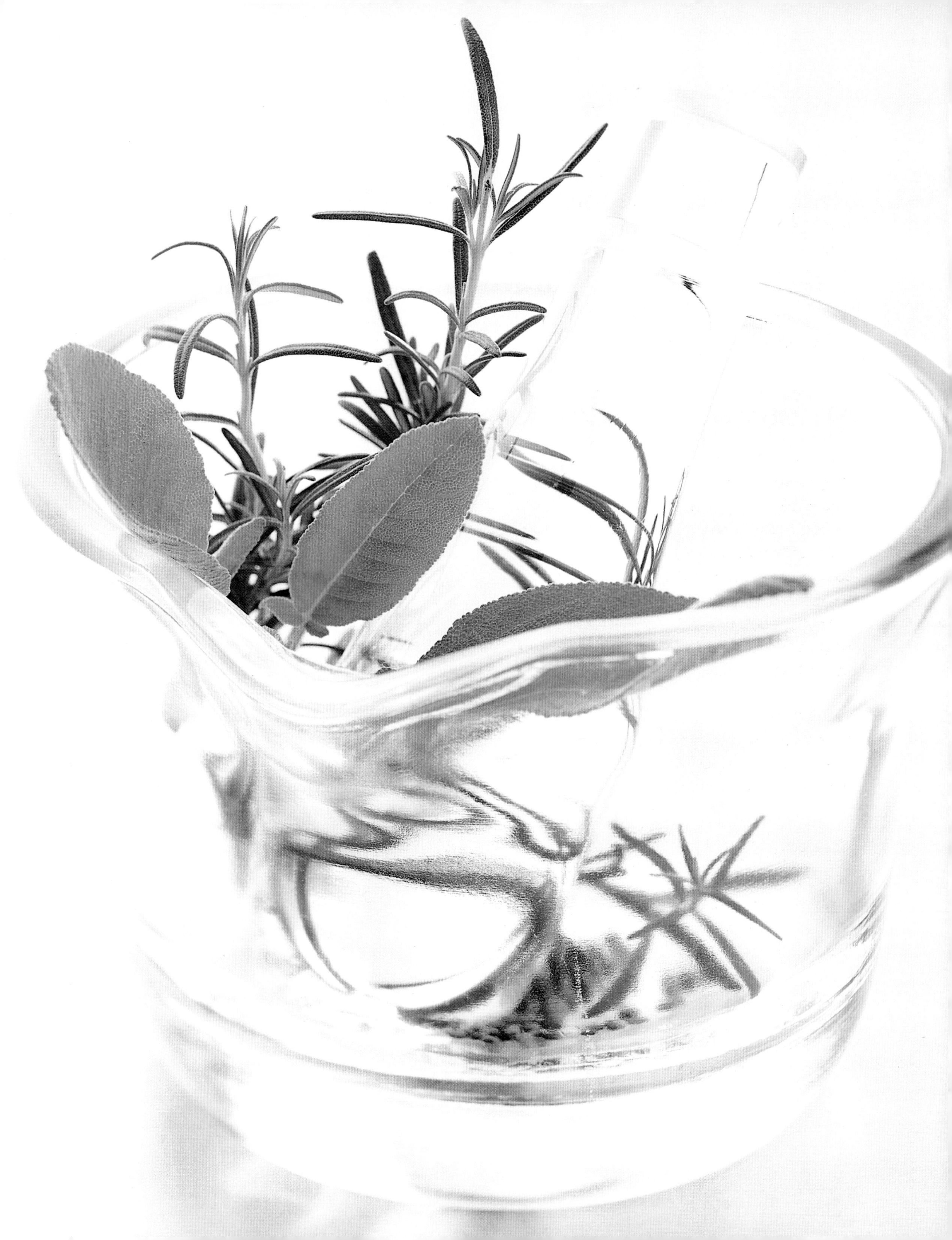

# directory of vitamins, minerals and other nutrients

THIS CHART LISTS VITAMINS, MINERALS AND OTHER NUTRIENTS THAT FORM AN IMPORTANT PART OF OUR DIET. THE BENEFITS OF EACH ARE GIVEN, AS WELL AS EXAMPLES OF FOODS THAT ARE PARTICULARLY GOOD SOURCES OF A NUTRIENT.

| VITAMIN | BENEFITS | SOURCES |
|---|---|---|
| **VITAMIN A** (Retinol) | Vitamin A is important for maintaining healthy skin. It also helps prevent frequent infections of the upper respiratory tract, such as colds and sore throats, and improves night vision. Retinol is found in animal products but vitamin A can also be produced from carotenes found in plant foods. | • carrot (pages 20–21)<br>• watercress (page 23)<br>• cabbage (pages 24–5)<br>• mango (page 36)<br>• melon (page 38) |
| **VITAMIN B1** (Thiamine) | Vitamin B1 increases concentration. It is easily destroyed by cooking or exposure to ultra-violet light. A low intake of vitamin B1 can cause depression and irritability. | • watercress (page 23)<br>• cabbage (pages 24–5)<br>• courgette (page 26) |
| **VITAMIN B2** (Riboflavin) | Vitamin B2 is essential for the metabolism of fats, sugars and proteins in the body. | • watercress (page 23)<br>• cabbage (pages 24–5)<br>• asparagus (page 29)<br>• milk (page 61) |
| **VITAMIN B3** (Niacin) | Vitamin B3 reinforces the skin's natural protection against exposure to the sun. Deficiency can cause fatigue, depression, poor concentration and dermatitis. | • cabbage (pages 24–5)<br>• courgette (page 26) |
| **VITAMIN B5** (Pantothenic acid) | Vitamin B5 is important for the health of the immune system and helps the body extract energy from food. | • watercress (page 23)<br>• cabbage (pages 24–5)<br>• celery (page 26)<br>• avocado (page 29)<br>• strawberry (page 39) |

| VITAMIN | BENEFITS | SOURCES |
|---|---|---|
| **VITAMIN B6** (Pyridoxine) | Vitamin B6 is necessary for healthy blood and for the metabolization of protein. | ● onion (page 18)<br>● watercress (page 23)<br>● cabbage (pages 24–5)<br>● banana (page 36) |
| **VITAMIN B12** | Vitamin B12 is needed for the health of the nerves and to make red blood cells. Low intake can cause fatigue and dry skin. | ● milk and cheese (page 61)<br>● egg (page 61) |
| **BIOTIN** | Biotin plays an important part in the metabolism of carbohydrate and fat. | ● cabbage (pages 24–5)<br>● cherry (page 39)<br>● grapefruit (page 43)<br>● milk (page 61)<br>● egg (page 61) |
| **FOLATE** (folic acid; part of the vitamin B complex) | Folate is crucial for making genetic material and red blood cells. Women should take 400 mcg of folate daily during pregnancy. | ● broccoli (page 22)<br>● cauliflower (page 22) |
| **VITAMIN C** | Vitamin C promotes tissue repair and wound-healing and is important for the general health of the immune system. It is an antioxidant and plays a major role in the absorption of iron and the formation of antibodies and collagen. | ● broccoli (page 22)<br>● cabbage (pages 24–5)<br>● pepper (page 26)<br>● lemon (pages 44–5) |
| **VITAMIN D** (Calciferol) | Vitamin D is essential for healthy bones and skin. Sunlight is our main source of this vitamin, although low levels are present in some foods. When the skin is in contact with sunlight it manufactures its own vitamin D. | ● lettuce (page 23)<br>● date (page 36)<br>● cottage cheese (page 61)<br>● egg (page 61) |
| **VITAMIN E** (Tocopherol) | A powerful antioxidant, vitamin E prevents the degeneration of nerves and muscles. It helps keep the skin healthy and helps to prevent cardiovascular disease. | ● wheat (page 33)<br>● peanut (page 47) |

| MINERAL | BENEFITS | SOURCES |
| --- | --- | --- |
| CALCIUM | A major constituent of bone and teeth, calcium is also vital to nerve transmission, blood clotting and muscle function. It regulates the heartbeat and helps maintain a proper acid-alkaline balance. A good calcium intake is also important for healthy skin. | ● seaweed (page 29)<br>● prune (page 38)<br>● almond (page 47)<br>● milk, cheese, butter, yoghurt (page 61) |
| COPPER | Copper is a trace element that is vital in forming connective tissue and for the growth of healthy bones. It helps the body absorb iron from food and is present in many enzymes, which protect against free radical damage. | ● fig (page 36) |
| FLUORIDE | This mineral protects against tooth decay. | ● asparagus (page 29) |
| IODINE | Iodine is required by the thyroid gland in order to produce the thyroid hormone, which regulates physical and mental development, including growth, reproduction and many other essential functions. | ● barley (page 33)<br>● banana (page 36)<br>● grape and raisin (page 38)<br>● shellfish (page 61)<br>● egg (page 61) |
| IRON | Essential for the production of haemoglobin, the pigment in red blood cells that transports oxygen to every cell, iron also boosts energy levels, prevents anaemia and increases the body's resistance to disease. | ● bean (page 30)<br>● lentil (page 30)<br>● prune (page 38)<br>● walnut (page 47)<br>● parsley (page 49) |
| MAGNESIUM | Magnesium is an important constituent of bones and teeth and is important for muscle contraction. It also calms the nervous system and regulates the heartbeat. It is required for normal calcium function. | ● hazelnut (page 47)<br>● almond (page 47)<br>● pine nut (page 47)<br>● walnut (page 47) |

| MINERAL | BENEFITS | SOURCES |
|---|---|---|
| PHOSPHORUS | Phosphorus regulates protein activity and is essential for the release of energy in the body's cells. It also helps to form and maintain healthy bones and teeth and is necessary for the absorption of many nutrients. | ● present in most foods |
| POTASSIUM | Potassium has a variety of functions: it regulates body fluids; it is essential for correct functioning of the cells and the transmission of nerve impulses; it keeps the heartbeat regular and maintains normal blood pressure. | ● cauliflower (page 22)<br>● cabbage (pages 24–5)<br>● celery (page 26)<br>● mushroom (page 30) |
| SELENIUM | An antioxidant that protects from heart disease, some cancers and premature ageing, selenium is required for normal growth and fertility, thyroid action, proper liver function and healthy skin and hair. | ● mushroom (page 30)<br>● buckwheat (page 31)<br>● walnut (page 47)<br>● shellfish (page 61)<br>● egg (page 61) |
| SILICA | Vital to the development of bones, silica also promotes healthy skin and connective tissues. | ● leek (page 19)<br>● green bean (page 22)<br>● nettle (page 22)<br>● chickpea (page 31)<br>● strawberry (page 39) |
| SODIUM | Sodium regulates the balance of body fluids and controls levels of electrolytes in blood plasma. It is essential for nerve and muscle function. Most people in the Western world consume far more sodium than they need. | ● seaweed (page 29)<br>● oat (page 33)<br>● grape and raisin (page 38) |
| SULPHUR | In its pure form sulphur works as an antifungal and antibacterial agent – it is used in creams for treating skin disorders such as acne. Sulphur also helps form proteins. It is present in every cell. | ● radish (page 19)<br>● cucumber (page 26)<br>● fennel (page 29)<br>● mango (page 36)<br>● horseradish (page 56) |
| ZINC | Zinc benefits the reproductive system, fertility and the skin. It also helps wounds to heal and regulates the sense of taste. Zinc is required for a healthy immune system and good night vision and is vital for normal growth. | ● red meat (page 61)<br>● shellfish (page 61)<br>● egg (page 61) |

| OTHER NUTRIENTS | BENEFITS | SOURCES |
|---|---|---|
| ALLIUM COMPOUNDS | Allium compounds aid the proper function of the cardiovascular and immune systems. | ● onion and shallot (page 18)<br>● leek (page 19)<br>● chive (page 50)<br>● garlic (pages 54–5) |
| ALPHA-LINOLEIC ACID | This is an essential fatty acid that is also known as omega-3 fatty acid. It has an anti-inflammatory effect that makes it good for rheumatoid arthritis, it helps to lower blood pressure and cholesterol, and reduce the likelihood of blood clots and heart attacks. It maintains cell membranes and transports fats around the body. | ● oily fish (pages 62–3) |
| ANTHOCYANOSIDES | These antioxidants inhibit a variety of dangerous bacteria including E. coli. | ● blueberry (pages 40–41) |
| BIOFLAVONOIDS | Bioflavonoids are antioxidants that facilitate the absorption of vitamin C. They strengthen the capillaries, which improves poor circulation and helps to prevent cardiovascular disease. | ● blueberry (pages 40–41)<br>● mandarin and tangerine (page 43)<br>● grapefruit (page 43) |
| CAPSAICIN | An antioxidant, capsaicin can act as a pain reliever and anti-inflammatory agent. It also helps to reduce blood cholesterol and the risk of blood clots, aids digestion and may kill harmful bacteria. Capsaicin may also prevent DNA damage. | ● chilli (page 52) |
| CAROTENOIDS (CAROTENE) | Carotenoids give the orange or yellow colour to vegetables such as carrots. They have antioxidant properties that help to prevent cellular damage caused by free-radical attack. They also reduce the risk of cancer and cardiovascular disease. | ● carrot (pages 20–21)<br>● spinach (page 23)<br>● pumpkin (page 30)<br>● mango (page 36) |

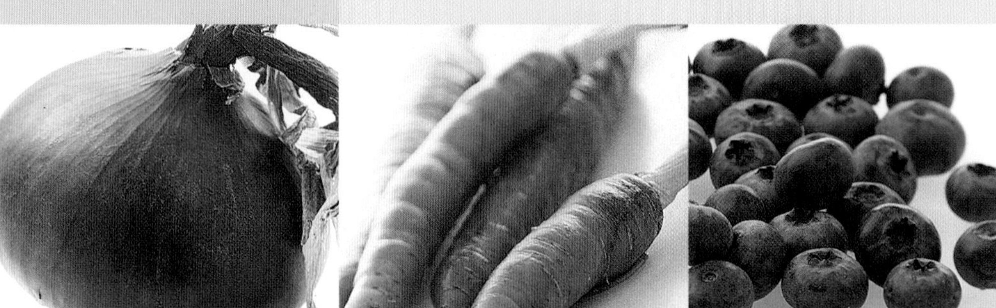

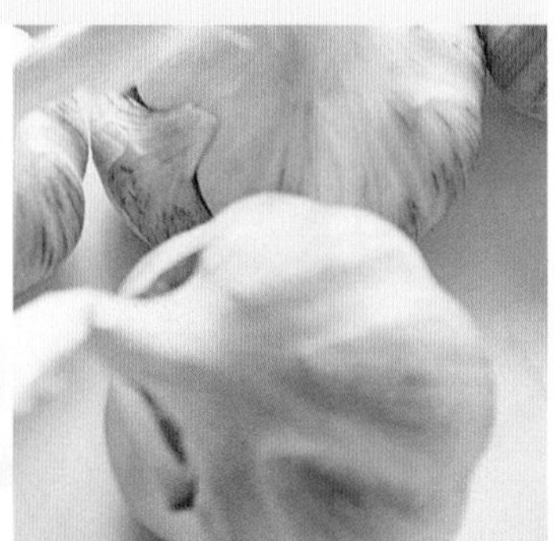

| OTHER NUTRIENTS | BENEFITS | SOURCES |
|---|---|---|
| CHLOROPHYLL | Chlorophyll is the substance that gives plants their characteristic green colour. It is thought to help keep blood healthy, promote wound healing and kill bacteria. It may provide some protection against cancer and certain forms of radiation. | • green bean (page 22)<br>• dandelion (page 22)<br>• lamb's lettuce (page 23)<br>• rocket (page 23)<br>• sorrel (page 51) |
| ELLAGIC ACID | A flavonoid found in fruits, ellagic acid appears directly to protect genes from attack by carcinogens. | • cherry (page 39) |
| GAMMA-LINOLEIC ACID | By helping to keep the blood thin, gamma-linoleic acid contributes to the prevention of blood clots and blockages. It also reduces inflammation and relieves pain and improves nervous- and immune-system function. | • borage oil (page 51) |
| LINOLEIC ACID | This essential fatty acid is also known as omega-6 fatty acid. It can help to lower blood cholesterol. | • olive (pages 34–5)<br>• sunflower seed (page 57)<br>• walnut (page 47) |
| MALIC ACID | Malic acid makes it possible for the body to convert sugars and fats into energy. | • apple (page 43) |
| OLEIC ACID | High levels of oleic acid can lower cholesterol levels. | • olive (pages 34–5) |
| PECTIN | Pectin lowers blood pressure and blood cholesterol, softens stools to help prevent bulges in the colon and haemorrhoids, and reduces the risk of colon cancer. | • orange (page 39)<br>• apple (page 43)<br>• pear (page 43)<br>• persimmon (page 43)<br>• quince (page 43) |
| PHYTOESTROGEN | May help to alleviate menopausal symptoms and lower the risk of breast cancer. Mimics the activity of oestrogen in the body. | • soya beans (page 31) |

# mineral water and culinary oils

## water

Water is essential to life in any form. It makes up approximately two-thirds of the human body and is constantly being lost in the form of sweat, water vapour, urine and faeces. We need to replace this by drinking 1–2 litres water every day.

Water varies greatly in content. The quality of the tap water in large urban areas is often poor. It may have been recycled three or four times and contain traces of hormones, nitrates and metals such as lead (lead pipes are still common in many old houses). Bottled mineral water is significantly richer than tap water in a range of minerals including calcium, magnesium, potassium, bicarbonate, chloride, sulphate, silica, fluoride, zinc, manganese, selenium and borate (check for these minerals on the label). Once opened, bottled water should be stored in the refrigerator and drunk quickly; it can rapidly become a breeding ground for bacteria. Some mineral waters are inappropriate for long-term daily use due to their high mineral content.

- Bottled waters with a low mineral content are excellent for every-day use and can be given to infants. They include Volvic and Evian.
- Bottled waters with a medium mineral content are beneficial when used every day for a limited amount of time. They include Vittel and Contrex. Mineral waters that are rich in calcium (San Pellegrino and Contrex) are recommended for the kidneys. Those rich in magnesium (Badoit and Hepar) are better for the liver.
- Bottled waters with a high mineral content, such as Vichy, have a stronger therapeutic action and should be drunk occasionally or as part of the detox programme (pages 134–37): they are diuretic, facilitate the elimination of toxins, strengthen teeth and bones and improve kidney and liver function. They are often recommended for rheumatism and arthritis, circulatory disorders, hypertension, kidney problems, low immunity and digestive and metabolic problems.

## culinary oils

When selecting culinary oils try to choose cold-pressed ones which are made by simple mechanical cleaning and crushing processes and retain their nutritional and therapeutic properties. Industrially-extracted oils have a longer shelf-life, but have lost most of their taste and therapeutic qualities. Industrial extraction is lengthy, complicated and involves chemical processing and heating the oil to high temperatures. Recent research suggests that the industrial manipulation of fatty acids may make these oils detrimental to our health. The most common culinary oils are:

- Olive oil: in my opinion, this is the most nutritional and therapeutic type of oil (page 34).
- Sunflower oil: this is rich in vitamin E, oleic and linoleic acid. It can be used for cooking and in salads. Sunflower and walnut oil are excellent in combination – the sunflower oil moderates the strong taste of walnut and increases the shelf-life; the walnut oil supplies alpha-linoleic acid.
- Corn oil: this is rich in polyunsaturated fat (see Corn, page 31).
- Walnut oil: a mineral-rich, strong-tasting oil favoured in south-west France. It is best diluted with sunflower or corn oil. A tablespoon can be added to vegetable juices to enhance their taste and therapeutic value.
- Hazelnut oil: this has a delicate taste, is very nutritious and is best used in salads. Both hazelnut and walnut oils are traditionally given to children to support their growth and to treat mild digestive problems and worms, including tapeworm.
- Peanut oil: this can stand very high temperatures which makes it good for frying. It is of little therapeutic or nutritional value. Organic peanut oil is difficult to find.
- Sesame oil: widely used in Asian countries, this oil is comparable to olive oil in its therapeutic and nutritional value.

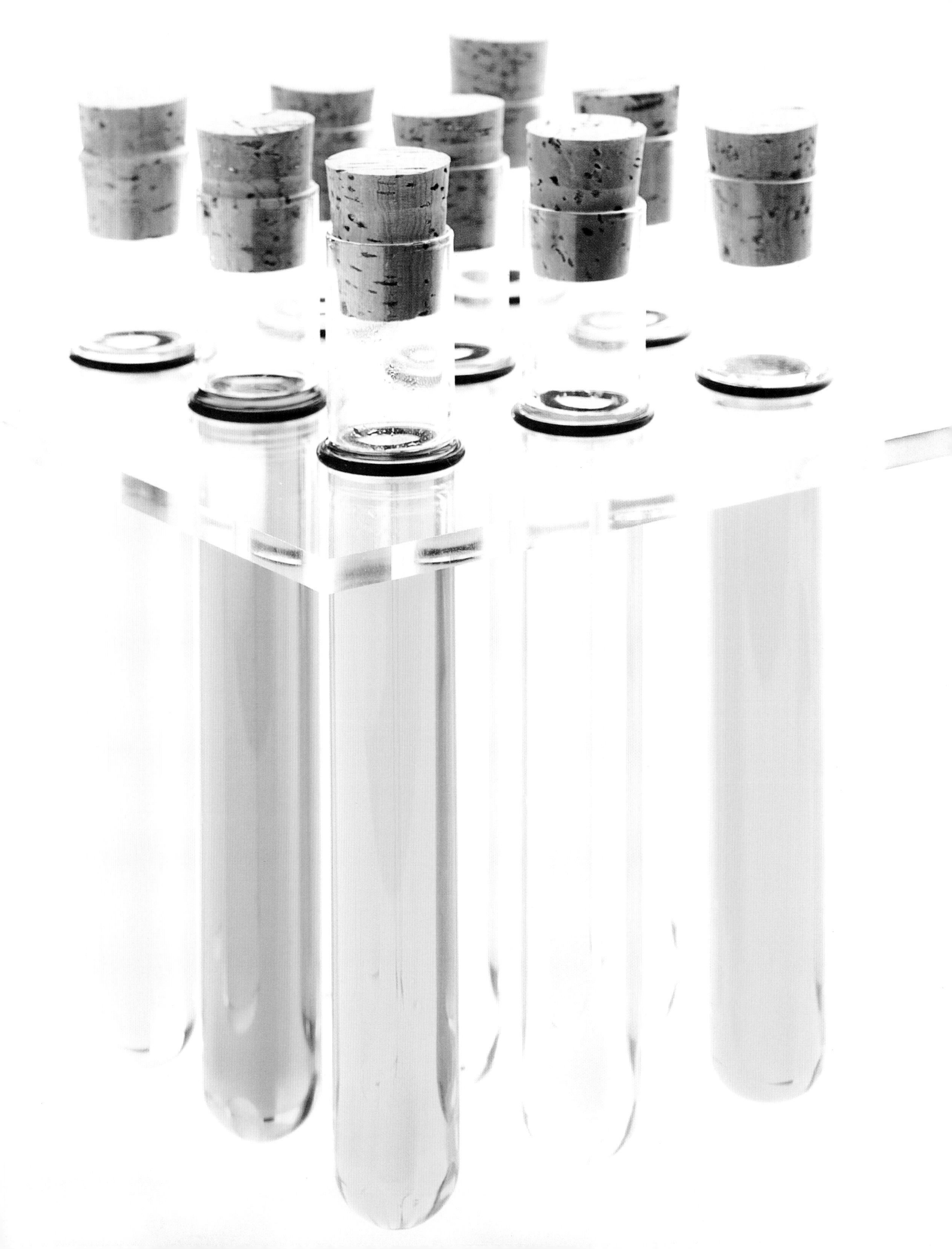

# part two: eat for immunity

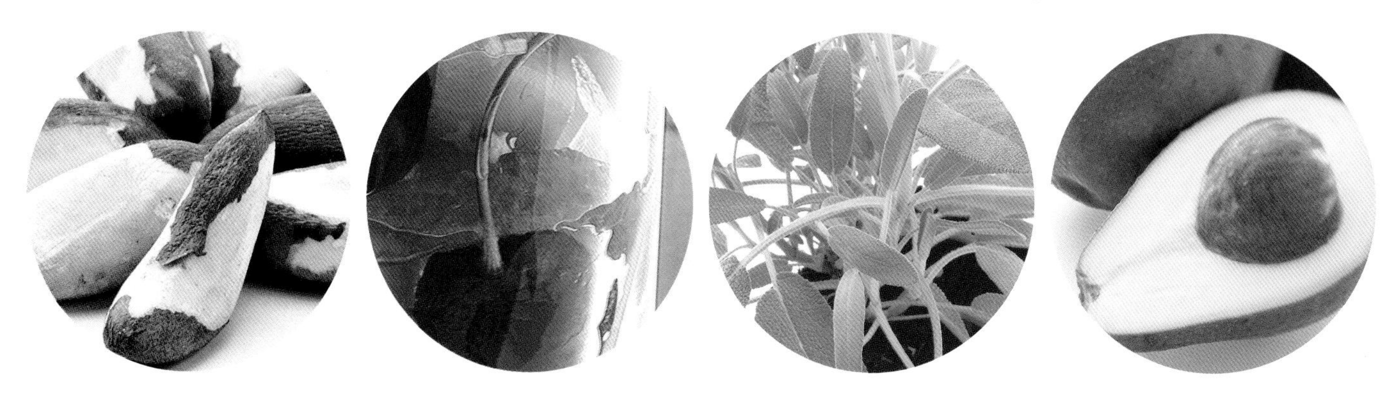

kirsten hartvig

# introduction

## using Part Two – Eat for Immunity

Eat for Immunity gives you a strategy to maximize your self-healing potential and develop a better understanding of health and disease. It is divided into four chapters:

- Chapter Five, A Guide to the Immune System, explains the components of the immune system and how they work together to maintain health and combat disease.
- Chapter Six, Superfoods for the Immune System, looks in detail at 150 foods that support the immune system.
- Chapter Seven, Coping with Common Ailments, highlights some common ailments, and explains how you can use the foods described in Chapter Six to prevent illness and promote health.
- Chapter Eight, Immune Foods in Practice, shows you how to incorporate immune-enhancing foods into your daily diet with 180 recipes and a range of diet plans.

You don't need to read Eat for Immunity from cover to cover before using it. Keep it in the kitchen and use it as a reference source of good food and better health.

When making the recipes in Chapter Eight, choose organic ingredients whenever possible, since chemical farming involves the use of many different substances that are harmful to immunity. Eating organic is also the best way of avoiding genetically engineered foods, the long-term health effects of which are unknown.

## food for life

Over the last 30 years, systematic scientific studies have confirmed that poor nutrition impairs the immune response, and that a diet based primarily on minimally processed and chemically unadulterated plant foods is the most effective way of enhancing immunity.

A recent global survey carried out by the World Cancer Research Fund together with the American Institute for Cancer Research concluded that plant-based diets protect against cancer. Hundreds of reliable studies show that fresh vegetables, fruits, nuts, grains and pulses are packed with immune-boosting phytochemicals.

Since the early 1960s, research has repeatedly confirmed that a diet high in natural fibre from vegetables, fruits and unrefined grains protects from a wide range of serious diseases.

Nutrition experts and scientists worldwide agree that high intakes of saturated fats from meat, dairy products and convenience foods are linked with coronary heart disease, and that the activity of the immune system is improved by decreased total fat intake.

Large numbers of fish caught for human consumption have been shown to contain toxic heavy metals, hydrocarbons and radioactive contaminants, and those reared in fish farms are commonly dosed with antibiotics and treated with dyes. Oily fish contain unsaturated fatty acids that may protect against coronary thrombosis, but increasing fish oil intake without reducing saturated fat intake is unlikely to have any significant effect on the development of coronary heart disease.

Taking fish oils in a concentrated form may cause excessive production of free radicals, which can interfere with immunity. Unlike fish oils, plant sources of polyunsaturated fatty acids are high in natural antioxidants, which combat the effects of free radicals.

Despite its reputation as a natural staple food, cow's milk may compromise immunity. Some people (particularly children) are allergic to milk protein and may develop eczema, hay fever or asthma as a result of consuming it, and people with catarrhal problems and allergies often experience substantial relief when they exclude milk products from their diet. Milk is also high in cholesterol and thus associated with an increased risk of heart problems.

Milk sugar (lactose) is digested in the stomach by an enzyme (lactase) that most humans stop producing at around the age of five, making it difficult to digest milk products efficiently. Contamination of milk products with hormones, antibiotics and other agricultural chemical residues may also produce unpredictable and unexpected adverse reactions.

Based on this overwhelming evidence, Eat for Immunity follows a plant-based approach to improving immunity that is relevant to every style of eating – carnivore, piscivorous, vegetarian and vegan. It is designed to help you tailor your personal food choices to the benefit of your immune system, increasing your intake of health-enhancing foods and cutting down on those that increase immune system workload.

## dos and dont's

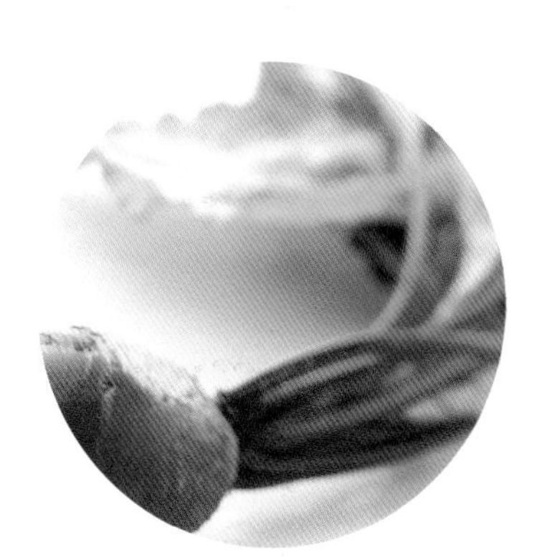

Eat for Immunity can be used by nearly everyone, although people suffering from serious acute illness and young people under the age of eighteen are advised to follow the diet recommendations under the guidance of a suitably qualified medical practitioner. During pregnancy and while breast-feeding, stringent diet regimes are not recommended, but eating a varied diet rich in fresh fruits, nuts, seeds, grains and vegetables is beneficial for both mother and baby.

The health suggestions in this book are intended to complement and enhance other treatments, not to replace them. Increasing your intake of some foods can change your body's reaction to medication (for example, cholesterol-lowering drugs), so if you are currently under medical treatment consult your practitioner before making any major dietary changes. If you are being treated for diabetes, you should follow your normal dietary guidelines and discuss the implications of change with your medical adviser.

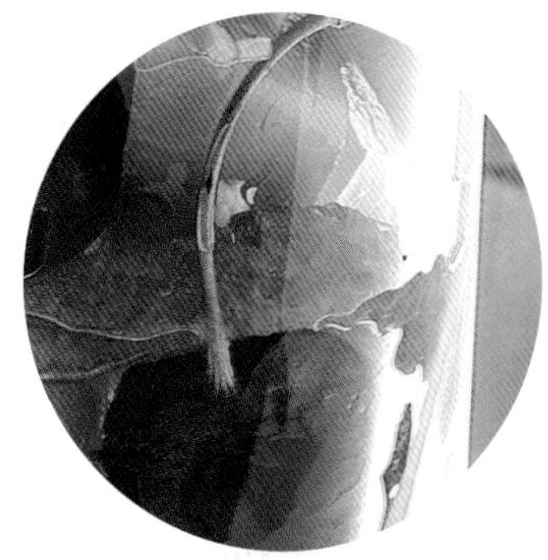

## side effects

The diet plans in Eat for Immunity are extremely unlikely to produce any unpleasant adverse reactions, but you may notice that withdrawing from caffeinated tea and coffee, and abstaining from alcohol and smoking makes you feel more edgy, headachey, lethargic and short-tempered for a few days. An increase in fruit and vegetable intake may also make your bowels more loose, and the extra fibre may cause wind. Such symptoms soon pass and are not a cause for concern.

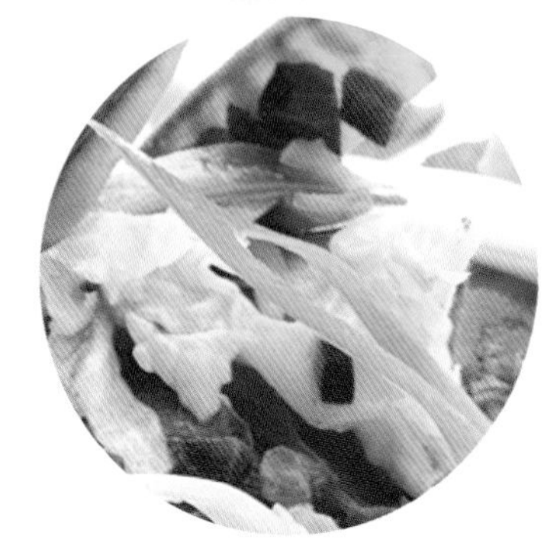

As always, if you have any particular concerns or worries, or if you have any doubt about the suitability of the advice contained in this book in relation to your current situation, you should seek advice form your doctor (or, if he or she should feel unable to offer advice, from a registered naturopath or other suitably qualified medical practitioner).

Happy – and healthy – eating!

**Kirsten Hartvig**

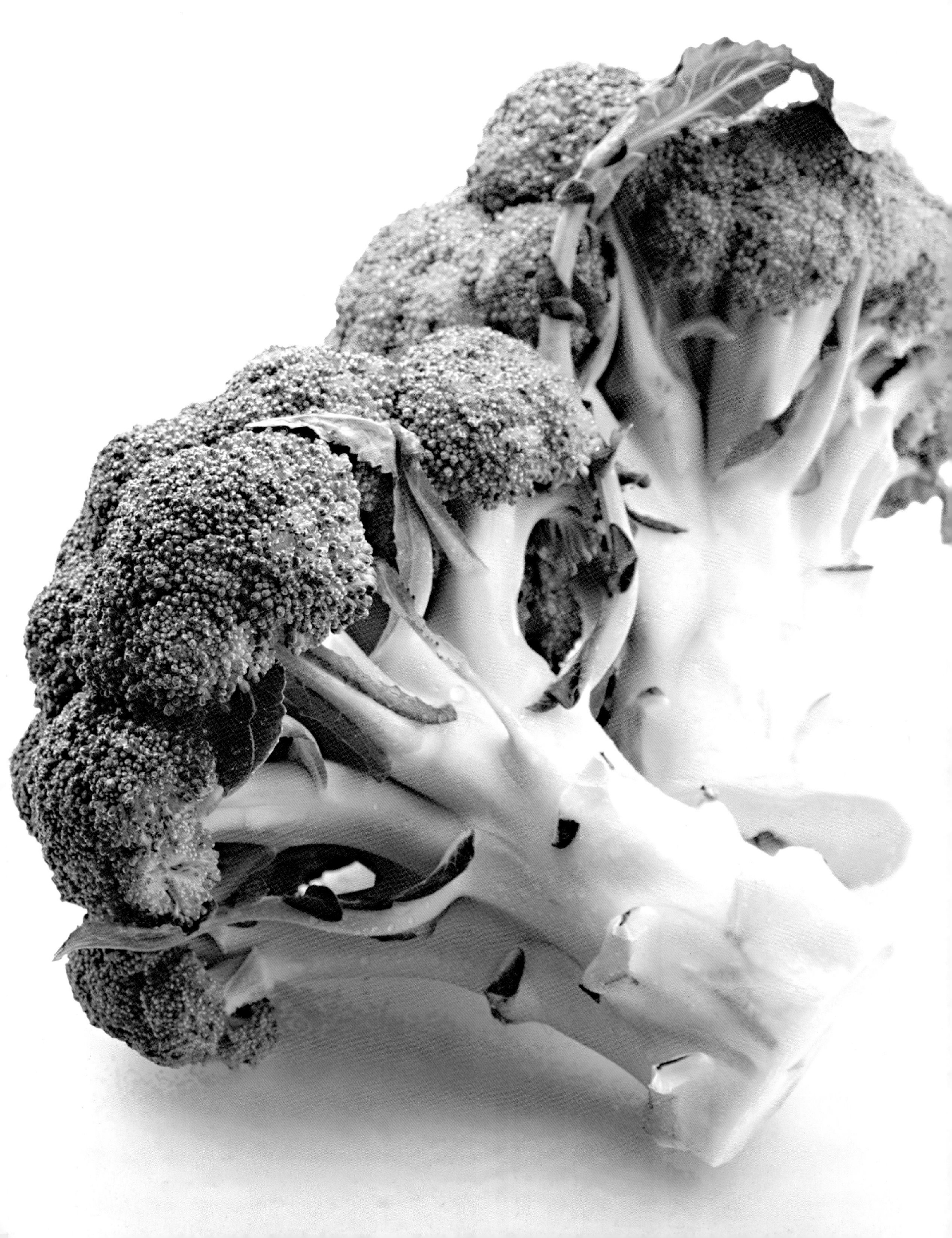

chapter five

# a guide to the immune system

A fully functioning immune system is one of the most vital aspects of a healthy body, helping to prevent and combat disease. However, for many people, the immune system does not function as effectively as it should. In some cases, the immune response fails to offer protection from disease, such as infection or cancer. In other cases, the immune system actively turns against its host, triggering a range of autoimmune and other disorders, such as rheumatoid arthritis or allergies, that are increasingly prevalent in the modern world. Chapter Five explains how the immune system works, why it sometimes breaks down, and what you can do to strengthen it and keep it in tip-top condition.

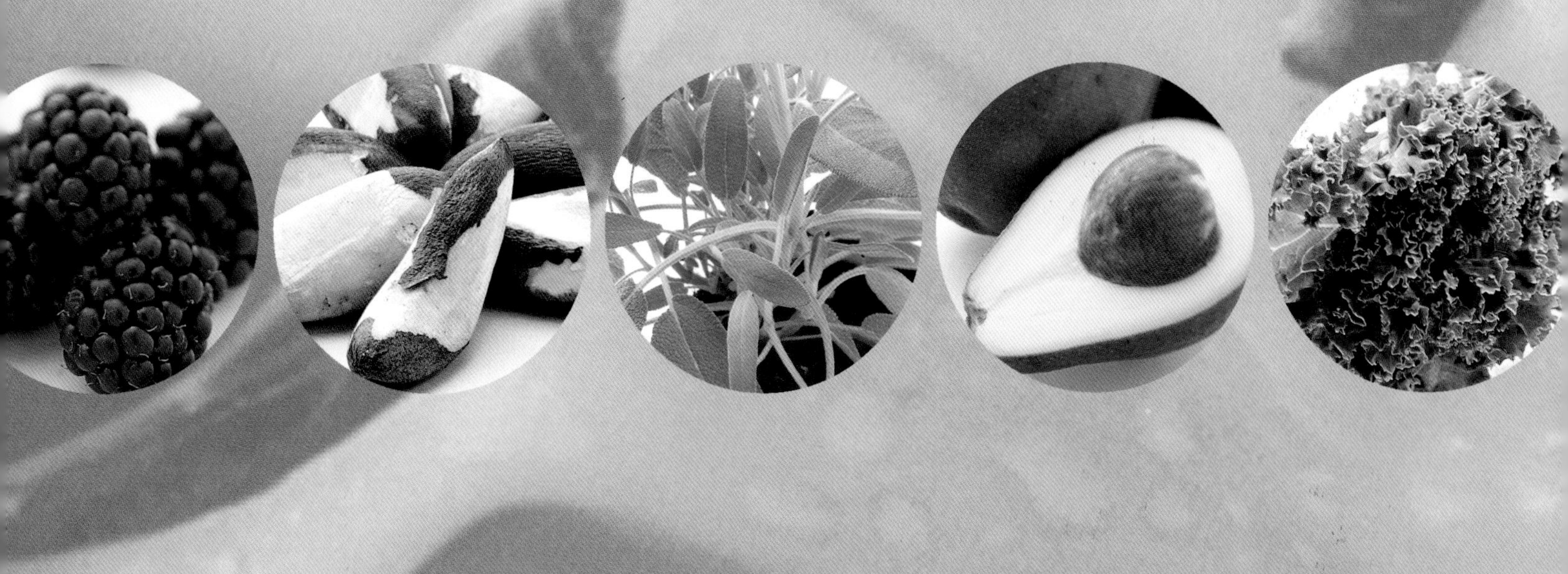

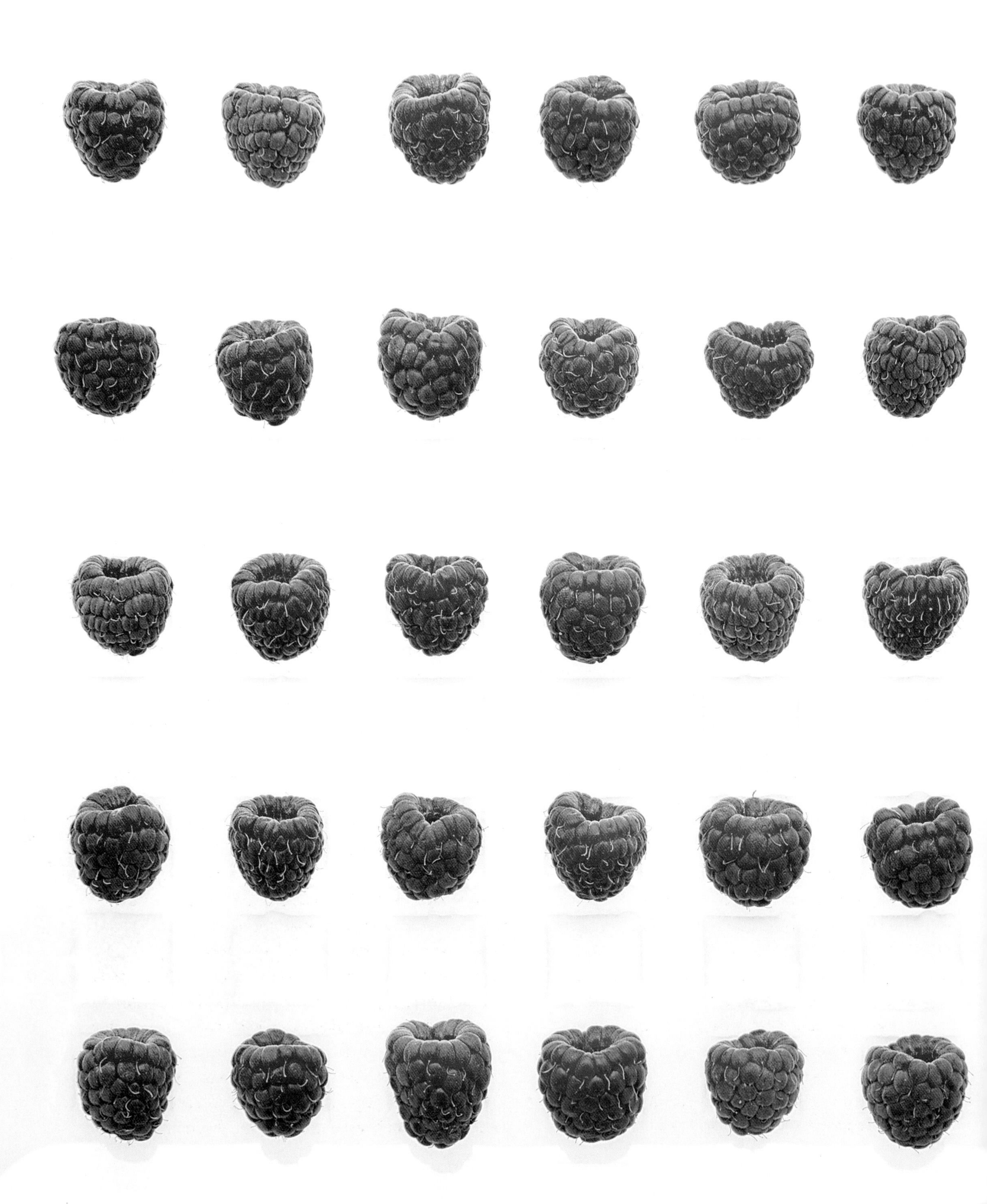

# NATURAL DEFENCE

When it comes to maintaining good health, the immune system is the body's most precious asset. By helping the body to resist infection and avoid cancer, it offers protection against many of the world's most widespread and deadliest diseases. Yet, despite modern scientific understanding and major advances in medical treatments, infection is still the commonest cause of illness and death worldwide. And cancer of the lung, stomach, breast, cervix, bowel and prostate continue to be scourges of the world – responsible for over two and a half million deaths worldwide per year.

What is going wrong? Why hasn't our detailed knowledge of the immune system enabled us to enhance our body's defence mechanisms in a sustainable way? In the process of developing ever more powerful means of attacking and destroying micro-organisms and cancer cells, have we lost sight of the need to strengthen our innate protective systems and nurture our inner environment?

In the early 1950s, with antibiotic therapy, general vaccination programmes, radical cancer surgery, radiotherapy and chemotherapy moving into the medical front line, it seemed clear to most people that scientific know-how was going to provide more effective solutions to disease than old-fashioned naturopathic methods designed to encourage the self-healing processes. Now, 50 years on, we are faced with the spectre of malaria and tuberculosis on the rise once again, new strains of drug-resistant superbugs outwitting our most powerful technologies, vaccinations that may harm as well as protect, a rising incidence of cancer and the engulfing tide of collapsed immunity that is AIDS.

History suggests that, when things go wrong, human beings have a tendency to continue doing what doesn't work – only doing it harder. Despite valuable short-term tactical advances in the management of infectious disease and cancer, we are signally failing in our strategic goal of improving world health in a sustainable manner. This is because we have attempted to usurp the power of the natural world, attacking it with crude weapons and losing ourselves in a maze of technical detail, instead of working with nature and doing everything we can to enhance our natural powers of healing and self-defence.

Just as the pioneers of microbiology – Didier Béchamp, Claude Bernard and Louis Pasteur – explained that micro-organisms should be thought of as agents of disease and not as causes, we need to understand that our detailed, valuable and hard-won knowledge of the process of immunity is not the same as an understanding of its purpose. We have superimposed a dualistic, male-oriented, warlike model on to the remarkable scientific observations we have made, and are assuming that life is a battle between ourselves and the micro-organisms and cancer cells; that we inhabit a dog-eat-dog, kill-or-be-killed biological universe.

The effect has been to focus our attention on external factors, while neglecting an inward-looking, broader approach to healing that attempts to observe the interaction between the physical, mental, emotional and spiritual aspects of self, and to understand how these affect health and our susceptibility to disease. As a result, we have developed a range of medical weapons that are becoming increasingly hazardous to use.

As a society, we seem to find it easier to spend our money on weapons and drugs rather than on good food, basic sanitation and clean water for those most at risk of disease. Therefore, we do not even keep faith with the knowledge that we do possess – that immunity is profoundly compromised by malnutrition; that poverty creates the perfect environment for the spread of infectious disease; that the typical Western diet and lifestyle lead to cardiovascular problems and cancer; that fear and stress create an internal bodily environment that is prone to disease and degeneration.

This section is written in the knowledge that good health involves paying attention to body, mind and spirit, that the immune response is the fundamental physical process of healing, and that health and healing are encouraged and enhanced by good food. On the following pages, we take a look at the history, mechanisms, language and science of immunity, and explain how it operates both in health and disease, and how it can be influenced by diet and lifestyle. You are welcome to use it as a reference as you explore other parts of the book, and as an aid to a better understanding of how the body heals and protects itself.

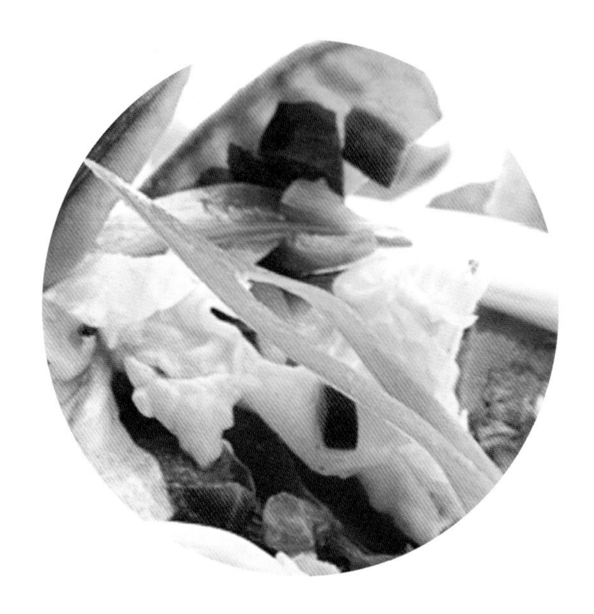

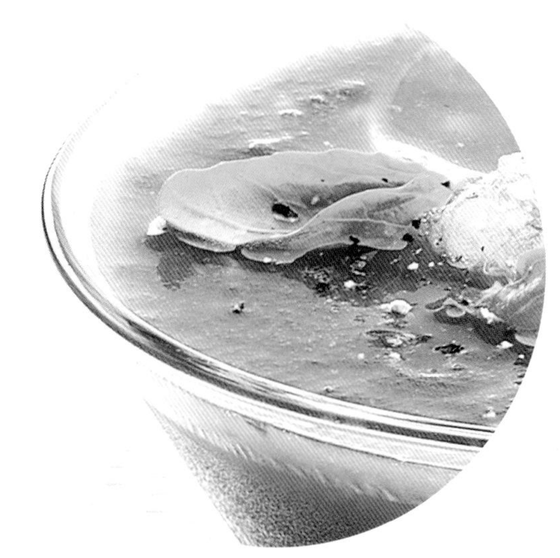

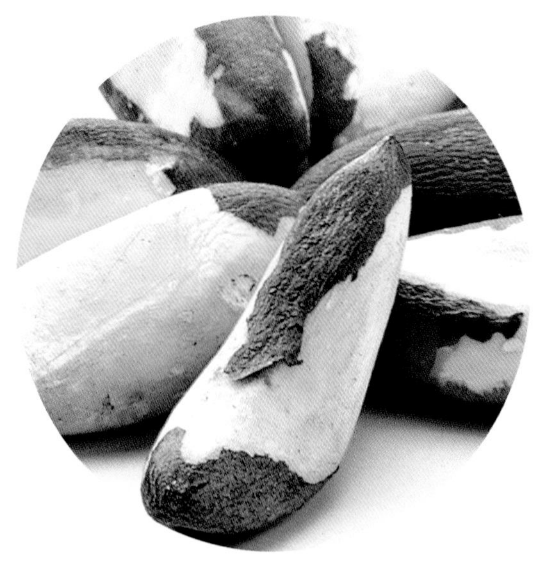

# WHAT IS IMMUNITY?

At the beginning of the 18th century, Mary Pierrepont, an English noblewoman living in Constantinople, became interested in the local method for preventing smallpox, which involved taking scrapings from smallpox crusts and scratching them into the skin. This was an early form of vaccination. Although successful in some cases, the risk of actually developing smallpox from this procedure was very high, and her attempts to introduce inoculation into Britain were largely unsuccessful. However, with smallpox ravaging the 18th-century world (approximately 50 million people died from the disease in Europe between 1700 and 1800), the search for an effective preventive strategy continued.

Some years later, Edward Jenner, an English country doctor from the county of Gloucestershire, noticed that dairymaids who caught cowpox (a relatively minor condition causing spots on the hands) had a strong capacity to resist smallpox. In 1796, he inoculated a young boy with material taken from cowpox spots and then, in an experiment that caused much controversy at the time, inoculated the same boy several times with actual smallpox, without causing any ill effects! Not surprisingly, this dramatic demonstration led to large numbers of people visiting Jenner's country home seeking vaccination, and the success of his smallpox-prevention treatment paved the way for the development of the worldwide vaccination programmes we see today.

However, at the time, Jenner's work did little to stimulate new thinking on the nature and causes of infectious disease. Since Roman times, doctors had been trying to discover the reason for the epidemics that decimated the population periodically, but the "germ" theory central to our current understanding of infection did not gain wide acceptance until the mid-19th century. It was then that an Italian, Agostino Bassi, proved that a disease of silkworms was caused by micro-organisms. Although not directly related to human health, his research formed the basis for later discoveries by the "giants" of microbiology – Pasteur, Robert Koch, Joseph Lister and Paul Ehrlich – that revolutionized biomedicine.

Modern-day research into infectious disease follows two parallel tracks – the first investigating the form, nature and lifestyle of pathogenic (or disease-causing) micro-organisms and the chemicals that can be used to destroy them; the second looking into the nature of the body's inherent capacity to resist infection, and how this in-born immunity can be stimulated.

While this research has produced much valuable information and given us important new treatments, the commonly-held belief that germs are malign micro-foes, constantly out to get us – and that the best way of dealing with them is to zap them with increasing doses of powerful antibiotics – is, in fact, a misunderstanding of what the pioneers of microbiology and immunology were saying.

Pasteur, together with the other early holistic medical thinkers – Béchamp, Bernard and Max von Pettenkofer – emphasized that microbes are only a part of the story, best thought of as agents of disease rather than the causes, their effects largely dependent on the nature of the bodily "terrain" they encounter. In other words, he understood that the state of the body's natural defence systems was paramount to the maintenance of good health.

# what the immune system does

The immune system is the body's first line of defence against invasion by micro-organisms and "foreign" materials, and the basis for vaccination and the differences between blood groups. It also protects against the development of cancer by destroying mutant (abnormal) cells. However, immune reactions are not always helpful. If the immune system overreacts to the presence of harmless substances, it produces allergic conditions such as hay fever and asthma. When it is weakened and fails to protect us from infection, the body suffers from immunodeficiency states such as AIDS. When it starts to attack its own body cells as if they were "foreign," the immune system causes autoimmune diseases such as rheumatoid arthritis and systemic lupus erythematosus (SLE).

Thus, the immune system can help or harm the body, depending on the nature and strength of its reactions. There is no fundamental difference between the mechanisms underlying "protective" immunity and those that cause disorders such as allergy and autoimmunity. The part that the immune system plays in health and disease can be divided into two helpful effects – active and passive immunity – and two harmful effects – overactivity and underactivity:

- Active immunity involves the body's own defensive cells and chemicals, which act against bacteria, viruses, fungi, parasites, tumours and foreign blood groups. Some forms of vaccination stimulate active immunity in the body.
- Passive immunity includes the antibodies acquired by a foetus from its mother, and also refers to vaccination with pre-formed antibodies taken from people or animals.
- Overactivity includes allergy and hypersensitivity to external substances, autoimmunity and adverse blood transfusion reactions (rhesus incompatibility).
- Underactivity includes inherited immunodeficiency and acquired immunodeficiency (for example, associated with HIV infection, drugs, radiation, or environmental toxins).

# components of the immune system

The immune system is an elaborate, interactive system of cells, chemicals and tissues distributed throughout the body. When any of these components come into contact with any cells or substance to which they are programmed to respond (such as bacteria, viruses and pollen grains), a series of reactions is triggered that results in the "foreign invader" being destroyed or rendered harmless.

Any cell or chemical substance that triggers a reaction by the immune system is known as an antigen. The reaction may be innate or adaptive (see page 158) and a property of adaptive immunity is that it is specific to the antigen that stimulated it. The cells and antibodies involved in an adaptive immune reaction to a particular antigen won't respond to any other antigen unless it is very similar indeed to the original.

Among the most important components of the immune system are the lymphocytes, or white blood cells, chemicals such as cytokines, antibodies and the complement system and tissues such as the lymph nodes ("glands"). These form the "sharp end" of the immune system. They are the tools that the body uses to dismantle, destroy and eliminate harmful antigens such as bacteria, viruses and tumour cells. The way in which these various components interact determines how efficiently the immune system will function.

# cells

The principal cells of the immune system are T cells, B cells, antigen-presenting cells (APCs), neutrophils and mast cells. All have clearly defined roles in the immune system.

- T cells are a type of white cell, or lymphocyte, found in the blood, bone marrow and lymph nodes. They stimulate B cells (see below) to produce antibodies and can also act directly to destroy antigens (such as viruses) that invade the body's own cells, by secreting chemicals called cytokines. T cells are divided into three groups, according to function – T helper cells, cytotoxic T cells and T suppressor cells.
- B cells are another group of white cells, also found in the blood, bone marrow and lymphoid tissues. When stimulated by T cells and cytokines, they turn into plasma cells and secrete antibodies, which enhance the body's response to a disease. Antibodies produced by any group of plasma cells react against only one specific antigen. After infection, some B cells remain in the circulation as "memory" cells, capable of recognizing the disease should it strike again. This function is described in more detail on page 161.
- Antigen-presenting cells are a group of cells found in the skin and throughout the lymphoid tissues. These process antigens in a way that ensures the T cells recognize the presence of foreign cells and other substances as efficiently as possible, and do not confuse them with naturally occurring cellular material. Macrophages – a type of APC whose name means "big eaters" – are the waste-disposal units of the immune system, eating up all types of foreign matter and the debris that results from immune activity.
- Neutrophils are the commonest form of white blood cells. Like macrophages, they are capable of engulfing bacteria and foreign matter.
- Mast cells are found throughout the body. When activated by antibodies during an immune reaction, they release chemicals (such as histamine) that trigger inflammation.

# chemicals

Antibodies are also known as immunoglobulins (Ig). They are proteins secreted by plasma cells that activate enzymes and stimulate various blood and tissue cells to destroy bacteria and other pathogens. There are five types of antibody:

- IgG is the most abundant immunoglobulin, found in the blood and throughout the body tissues. It activates the complement system (see opposite), and stimulates neutrophils and macrophages to destroy antigens.
- IgM is also found in the bloodstream. It, too, activates the complement system and is particularly important in the fight against bacteria.
- IgA is found in tears, saliva and the secretions from mucous membranes (such as the lining of the intestines and the respiratory and reproductive tracts) and so is one of the first lines of defence against invading micro-organisms. It helps resist gastro-intestinal infections and maintains a healthy gut flora. Like IgG and IgM, it also activates complement enzymes (see below).
- IgE is found in the body tissues and can trigger allergic reactions, such as hay fever, by stimulating mast cells to release histamine.
- IgD is present in the body in very low concentrations. Its role in the immune response is unclear.

Surface membrane molecules (also known as CD molecules) are antibody-like molecules found on the outer surface of T cells. They enhance the ability of T cells to trigger immune responses and help them to recognize the difference between antigens and our own body cells. The number of T cells in the blood carrying CD surface molecules is important in the diagnosis of some diseases. A low level of CD4-carrying T cells is characteristic of AIDS.

Cytokines are a group of chemicals secreted by T cells and other white cells (including macrophages, mast cells and neutrophils). They stimulate the immune response and improve its efficiency. Four are particularly important:

- Interleukin 1 is secreted by blood cells in response to injury and tissue damage.
- Interleukin 2 is secreted by T cells in response to the presence of antigens. It increases the rate of production of B cells and other T cells.
- Tumour necrosis factor alpha (TNF) is secreted by lymphocytes, macrophages and neutrophils. As the term "tumour necrosis" (tumour death) suggests, TNF attacks and destroys tumour cells. It also plays a role in activating the immune response to disease and is responsible for a

number of symptoms of illness (including fever, weight loss and feeling generally unwell).

- Interferon gamma is produced by activated T cells (and other white blood cells) after they have been exposed to an antigen. It encourages macrophage activity and has a strong anti-viral action. It also works with TNF to destroy tumour cells and, like TNF, is responsible for some of the general symptoms of acute illness.

Complement is a group of enzyme proteins, made in the liver and found in the blood. When an immune reaction is triggered, antibodies start attaching themselves to antigens and this triggers a chain reaction by the complement enzymes that amplifies the immune response and produces the classic symptoms of inflammation – swelling, redness and pain.

- Human leucocyte antigen (HLA) markers were discovered in the latter half of the 20th century by scientists researching the phenomenon of transplant rejection. The scientists found a cluster of genes on chromosome six of human DNA that they called the major histocompatibility complex. As well as containing the instructions for making some of the complement proteins, these "histocompatibility genes" are responsible for the presence of so-called HLA "markers" on the surface of body cells. These markers identify cells as belonging uniquely to that body. They provide the means by which the immune system can distinguish between its "own" body cells and "foreign" cells (such as bacteria).

A T cell will respond to the presence of an antigen only when it comes across that antigen stuck to an HLA marker on the surface of an antigen-presenting cell. The fact that HLA markers are genetically determined explains some of the variation in immune response shown by different individuals.

## tissues

While many immune reactions happen in the bloodstream, there are other "lymphoid" tissues equally important to immunity – namely lymph nodes, mucosa-associated lymphoid tissue (MALT), the spleen, the bone marrow and the thymus.

- Lymph nodes are collections of lymphoid cells found throughout the body, including the neck, the armpits and the groin. They are joined by a network of lymph-carrying vessels (the lymphatics), and are the main sites of storage, activation and production of the lymphocytes. They are also places where macrophages swallow up and process foreign antigenic particles. Lymph is a pale

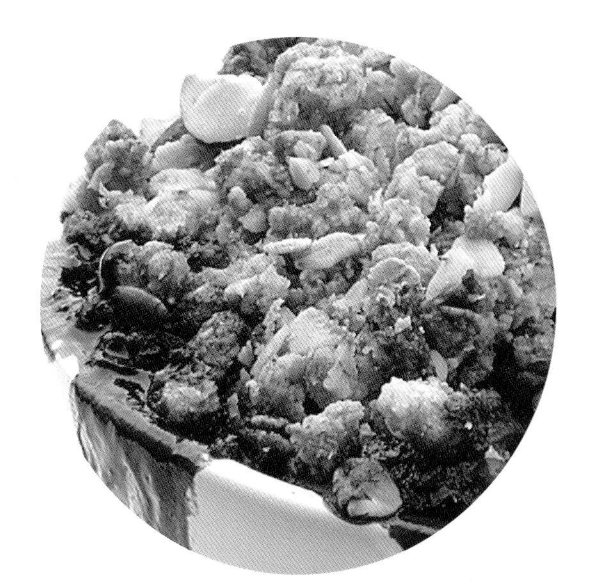

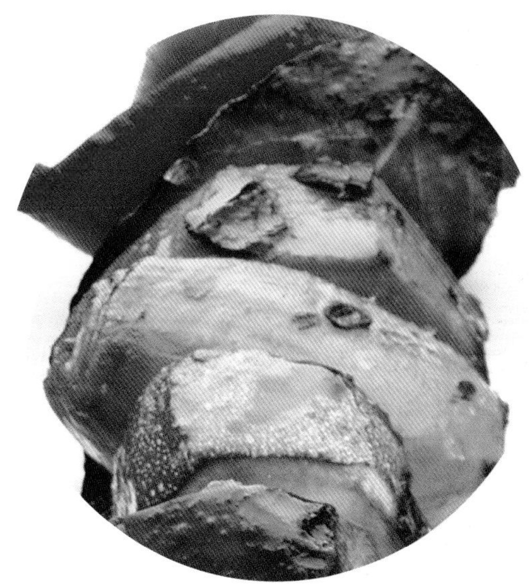

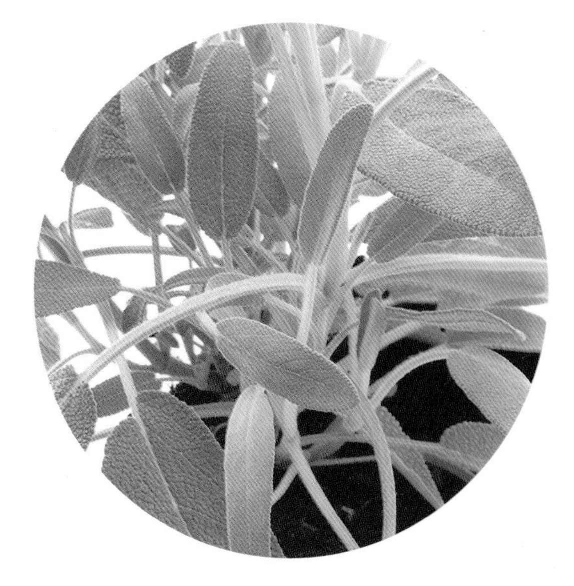

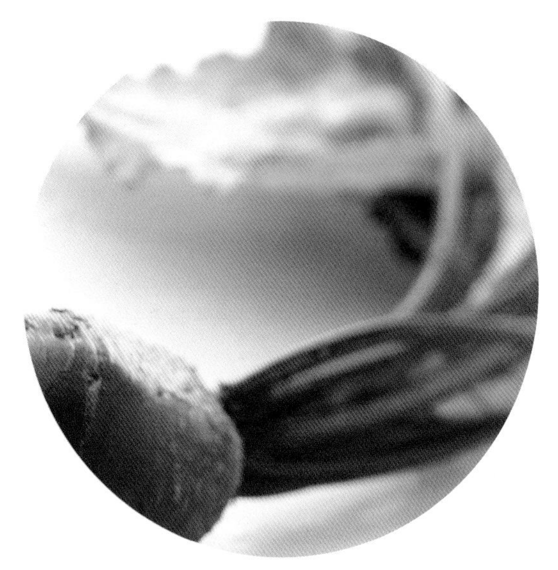

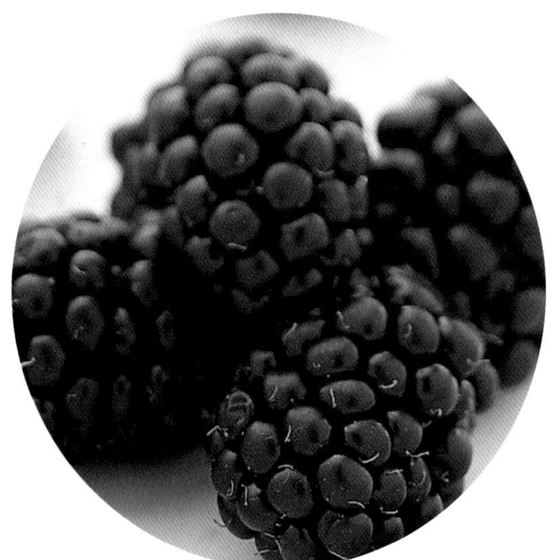

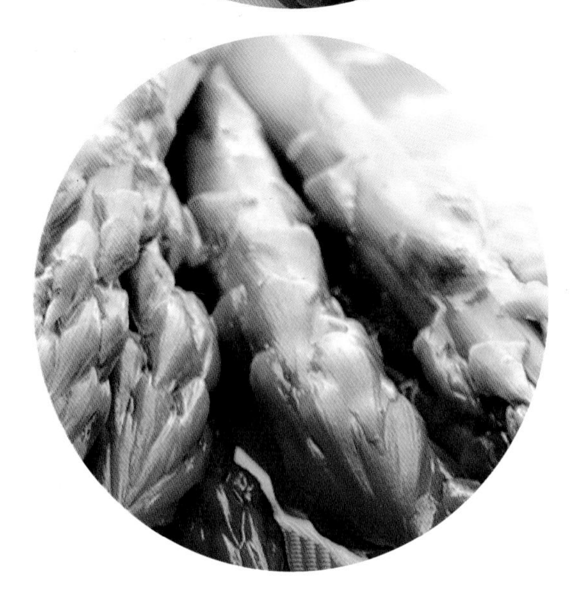

straw-coloured fluid, similar to blood plasma, from which it is produced, but more watery and containing only lymphocytes plus some protein, fats and salts. It circulates throughout the body, via the lymphatics, and acts as a transport and communications medium for immune cells.

- MALT is a diffuse collection of patches of lymphoid tissue found in many parts of the body, including the lining of the gastro-intestinal tract, the appendix, the tonsils, the breasts and the lungs. It contains clusters of B cells, T cells and mast cells.
- The spleen, like other lymphoid tissues, contains B cells, T cells and macrophages. In the developing foetus, the spleen also produces red blood cells.
- The bone marrow is the main production site for red and white blood cells and is a constantly renewing reservoir of small, "primitive" immune system cells. Immature B cells leave the bone marrow to take up residence in the other lymphoid tissues. Immature T cells leave the bone marrow at an even earlier stage of development and migrate to the thymus (hence the name "T" cell) where they are taught to recognize the difference between "self" (the body's own cells) and "other" (foreign cells and other material) before moving on to other lymphoid tissues. The thymus was named by the second-century physician Galen, who thought it looked like a bunch of thyme flowers. It is situated in the upper part of the chest and is crucial to the proper development of T cells and thus to the function of the immune system as a whole.

## how the immune system works

We all have an innate, genetically determined ability to produce an immediate, non-specific immune response to disease-causing antigens that enter the body. Cells in the lymphoid tissues (including macrophages and primitive lymphocytes) are genetically pre-programmed to secrete cytokines when foreign antigens enter the body. These cytokines stimulate B cells to change into plasma cells and secrete antibodies against the invader, and also stimulate T cells to turn into "killer" cytotoxic T cells that are capable of destroying pathogens directly. However, there is such a wide variety of potentially pathogenic organisms in the world that we have also evolved a powerful system of adaptive immunity that enables us to mount a massive, specific defence against individual pathogens, and also protects us against future exposure to those same pathogens. This adaptive immune response is triggered by an interaction between antigen-presenting cells and T helper cells, which leads to the production of antibodies, cytokines and cytotoxic T cells specifically directed against the particular strain of invading pathogen that is posing a threat.

The first time the immune system is exposed to a new antigen, the adaptive response takes about 10 days to reach full intensity, during which time the balance between resisting and succumbing to the disease can be very fine. Assuming we recover, the next time the immune system meets the same pathogen, the defensive response is powerful and immediate, giving us resistance to the disease.

## recognition and defence

Innate or adaptive, our immune response is always a two-stage process. First, we have to recognize that a foreign, potentially harmful antigen has entered (or is trying to enter) the body. Second, we have to do something to defend ourselves from the invasion. In the process of recognition, we have to be sure as far as possible that we are not mistaking the surface characteristics of our own cells (or other harmless substances) for those of pathogens.

In the defence process, we have to be able to adapt and respond efficiently to a huge variety of potentially harmful antigens, yet without letting the intensity of the immune response cause damage to the body. And we have to do it fast enough to ensure that the invaders don't get the upper hand. Then we have to be able to remember past battles, in order to respond more quickly and effectively if faced with the same challenge in the future.

In summary, for antigen recognition we have primitive T cells, T helper cells, antigen-presenting cells, "virgin" killer T cells and B cells. For defence, we have T helper cells, cytotoxic "killer" T cells, macrophages, antibody-producing plasma cells, mast cells, neutrophils, macrophages and the complement system, all kicked into action by cytokines.
As well as these specific responses, the body also has a number of non-specific protective mechanisms that amplify the effects of immunity, and which are triggered by immune activity. These non-specific responses can be grouped together under the general term "inflammation".

## inflammation

This is one of the oldest recognized features of disease, first described by the Roman medical writer Celsus. It is the body's initial response to tissue or cell damage (internal or external), and the symptoms of heat, redness, swelling and pain it causes are well known. Much orthodox medical treatment of illness is directed toward the suppression of inflammation, and in many cases (especially in chronic inflammatory conditions such as arthritis) this is both rational and humane.

However, the bad press that inflammation usually receives is misleading because, for most people, it is the process of inflammation that actually allows the immune system to do its work quickly and efficiently. To the naturopathic physician, inflammation is not an unwelcome event but the primary sign that the body is starting to heal itself. Naturopathic treatment seeks to keep the patient comfortable while allowing natural healing mechanisms to do their work unsuppressed.

The inflammatory process follows a set course. First, a cell or tissue is injured, or attacked by pathogens. As a result, chemicals are released from damaged cells or immune cells that cause blood vessels in the damaged area to widen, bringing more blood to the damaged area and slowing down the rate of blood flow. In addition, the blood vessels around the area become "leaky", allowing the free flow of immune cells and fluid into the tissues.

White cells in the blood line up along the blood vessel walls and pass into the damaged area. These cells come into contact with micro-organisms and foreign particles, triggering an immune reaction. Swelling caused by the fluid immobilizes and localizes the damage, and the other components of the immune system – including antibodies, cytotoxic T cells and complement – then come into play and neutralize the antigens. The debris is swallowed up by macrophages and neutrophils.

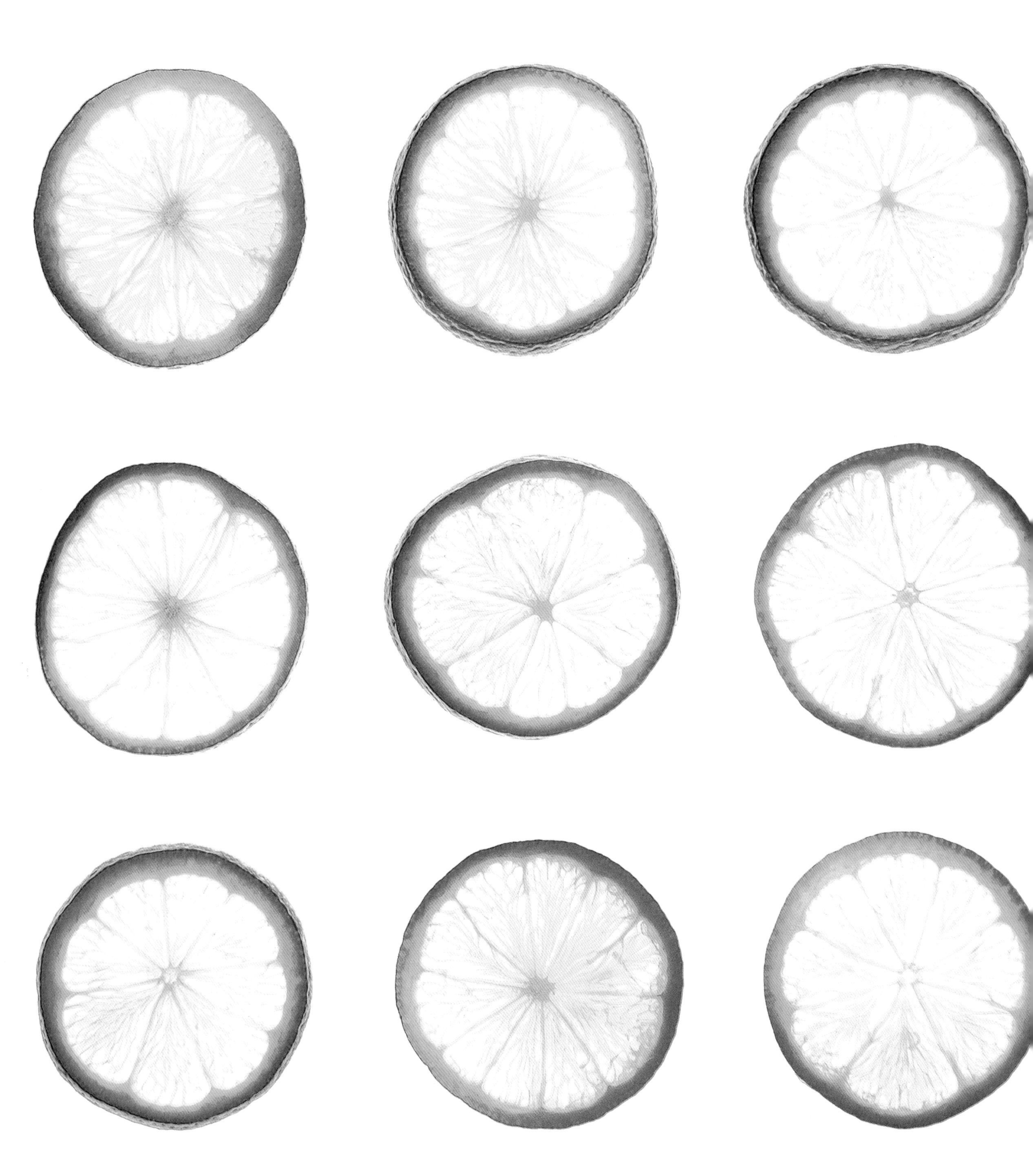

# control of immune reactions

With all this cellular and chemical firepower at its disposal, the immune system needs to include certain safeguards to ensure that its reactions do not get out of hand and start attacking healthy body cells. One simple control mechanism built into the system is that, because the intensity of the immune response depends on the amount of antigen present, as soon as immunity starts destroying antigen, the strength of the response fades naturally. This means that the immune response is inherently self-limiting.

As a further safeguard, some of the cytokines damp down the immune response, and there is also a sub-group of T cells, called T suppressor cells, that act to keep immune system activity in check. (In cases of deficient T-cell function, such as immunodeficiency states and malnutrition, this suppression function is lost, leading to an increase in allergic and autoimmune reactions; see pages 164–65.)

# immune memory, tolerance and vaccination

The capacity for immunological memory is one of the most important features of the immune system. When B cells are activated by the presence of antigens, many of them turn into plasma cells that produce antibodies, but a proportion remain as B cells and form a "memory population" capable of multiplying rapidly and mounting a swift immune response if the body is exposed to the same antigen at a later date.

This response to the antigen may be so effective that the symptoms of disease are much milder than on the first occasion – or there may be no symptoms at all (in which case, the person is said to be immune to that disease). However, each antigen is recognized by its unique chemical characteristics and immunological memory relates only to those antigens that have been encountered before. An individual who is immune to one kind of pathogen does not have immunity to other pathogenic organisms. The capacity for immunological memory underlies the concept of vaccination in its two forms – "active" and "passive". In active vaccination, immunity is induced artificially by exposing the body to small amounts of dead or inactivated micro-organisms, usually by injection. The protective response generated in the body by this form of vaccination can last for many years. However, for some diseases, it is not possible to produce a safe, active vaccine, but some measure of short-term protection can be given by passive vaccination – which involves injecting "ready-made" antibodies against the disease, usually derived from animals.

The debate over the safety and effectiveness of vaccination continues to smoulder, with protagonists pointing to successes in the control of epidemic diseases such as smallpox, diphtheria, polio and tuberculosis, and opponents claiming that it can cause brain damage and autism and pointing to the increased incidence of allergy and autoimmune disease that has coincided with the widespread use of vaccination.

Whatever view you hold over the risks and benefits of vaccination, it is important to remember that vaccines necessarily contain antigens that have been altered from their original state, and that our understanding of the body's reactions to such antigens is far from complete.

Another extremely important property of the immune system is that, in general, it can distinguish between cells from its "own" body and "foreign" cells and antigens. As already explained, this is owing to the presence of "markers" on our body cells that signal "self" to the immune system.

In the developing foetus, these surface markers are "learned" by the immune system because the only cells passing through the unborn baby's lymphoid tissues are its own. In fact, if a newborn baby (whose immune system has not yet fully matured) is exposed to antigenic material there is a good chance that it will develop tolerance to the antigen rather than mount an immune response against it. (The same is true in some elderly people whose immune systems become progressively less efficient.) This means that it is ineffective to vaccinate very young babies, because their capacity to develop tolerance to antigens at this stage in life might leave them unprotected, despite the vaccination.

# IMMUNITY AND DISEASE

For many years, it was thought that the symptoms and signs of infectious disease were caused by pathogens, and that the immune system was purely a protective shield, destroying microbes and eliminating dangerous toxins from the body. While the second part of this idea is still held to be true, it is now known that many of the unpleasant, painful and damaging effects of infection are a direct result of the immune response itself, and that the protection we enjoy from the immune system carries a cost.

When it comes to infectious disease, most of us are happy to pay the price of short-term discomfort as long as we receive the longer-term benefit of recovering from the illness. If, on the other hand, the immune system begins to react to substances in the environment that would ordinarily pose no threat to health – or worse, starts attacking our own body tissues for no apparent reason – we get justifiably concerned. Before looking in detail at allergy and autoimmunity, it is helpful to look at the ways in which the immune system causes illness, and at what it is that makes us susceptible to immune-based diseases.

The following are important conditions caused by immune system activity:

- Heart – carditis in rheumatic fever, cardiomyopathy and post-heart attack syndromes
- Lungs – alveolitis and asthma
- Gastro-intestinal and liver – coeliac disease, ulcerative colitis and some forms of hepatitis
- Skin – contact dermatitis, pemphigus, pemphigoid and dermatitis herpetiformis
- Endocrine – Addison's disease, thyroiditis and type I, insulin-dependent (early onset) diabetes mellitus
- Ear, nose and throat – hay fever, otitis media ("glue ear")
- Eyes – uveitis, allergic conjunctivitis and keratoconjunctivitis sicca
- Children – atopic eczema, milk allergy, food allergies, juvenile chronic arthritis and Henoch-Schönlein purpura
- Blood – pernicious anaemia, autoimmune haemolytic anaemia, thrombocytopenia and blood transfusion reactions
- Reproductive – rhesus disease of newborn and infertility
- Kidneys – glomerulonephritis
- Joints – rheumatoid arthritis, SLE and dermatomyositis
- Nerves – multiple sclerosis, myasthenia gravis, polyneuritis, polymyositis, post-vaccination/post-infection encephalitis
- Infections – immune activity is responsible for a variety of syndromes associated with tuberculosis, malaria, Chagas' disease and leprosy
- General – anaphylaxis, graft rejection, serum sickness.

## immune-based disease

Anaphylactic (reaginic) immune reactions are caused by the release of histamine and other chemicals from mast cells, resulting in inflammation, oedema and contraction of smooth muscle. Anaphylaxis evolved to protect us against parasites and to provide an immediate response to foreign antigens, but it is also responsible for allergic asthma, hay fever, atopic eczema and food allergies. In its most severe form, acute anaphylaxis, reaction to an antigen causes a rapid onset of nausea, wheezing, itching, low blood pressure, abdominal pain, urticaria (nettle rash) and loss of consciousness. Untreated, acute anaphylaxis can be fatal.

Cell-reactive immune reactions involve antibodies sticking to the surface of body cells and triggering various inflammatory responses. Originally designed to destroy invading micro-organisms, these reactions are also responsible for blood transfusion incompatibility, rhesus disease of the newborn, acute graft rejection and a variety of autoimmune conditions including haemolytic anaemia, thyrotoxicosis, pemphigoid and myasthenia gravis.

Immune complex reactions are caused by antibodies binding with soluble antigens (such as bacterial toxins) in the blood or body fluids. The resulting "immune complexes" are then deposited in the tissues, clogging small blood vessels and triggering inflammation. Intended as a way of ridding the body of toxins, these reactions are a common cause of immune-related disorders including rashes, vasculitis, alveolitis, serum sickness, glomerulonephritis, rheumatoid arthritis and systemic lupus erythematosus.

Cell-mediated reactions (or delayed hypersensitivity reactions) involve T cells and macrophages and offer protection against parasitic infection. They are also responsible for the clinical features of tuberculosis, leprosy, pernicious anaemia, "contact" dermatitis, type I, insulin-dependent (early onset) diabetes mellitus, graft rejection and "sensitization" to common substances (such as household chemicals and latex).

## susceptibility to immune disease

One of the big unanswered questions in modern immunology is: "Why are some people more prone to immune-based diseases than others?" Research into this subject is ongoing but scientists have uncovered important clues that might point to possible answers. The first involves an immune phenomenon called "atopy". At least 5 per cent of the population have an inherited tendency to produce high levels of IgE, which reacts with common substances, such as pollen and food additives, to cause atopic allergic reactions – such as itching and sneezing. A popular but unproven theory suggests that children develop atopy because they are raised in oversanitized environments and eat "non-natural" diets (such as formula infant milks and convenience foods). The theory is that, because modern children are exposed to few disease microbes but are repeatedly in contact with artificial substances, such as industrial chemicals, the immune system directs too much of its attention toward harmless environmental antigens and hence lacks an adequate response to disease organisms. The allergic child, constantly suffering upper respiratory-tract infections, is an example of this mechanism at work.

There is some evidence that an inherited lack of some of the components of the complement system is responsible for the tendency to develop some immune disorders. Research has also shown that an individual's inherited HLA type has a bearing on the development of a wide range of immunologically based diseases, including ankylosing spondylitis, coeliac disease, Graves' disease, SLE, rheumatoid arthritis and pernicious anaemia.

Research in West Africa has shown an association between HLA type and the capacity to resist malaria. Although useful in the diagnosis of some conditions, the reason for these associations is not yet clear.

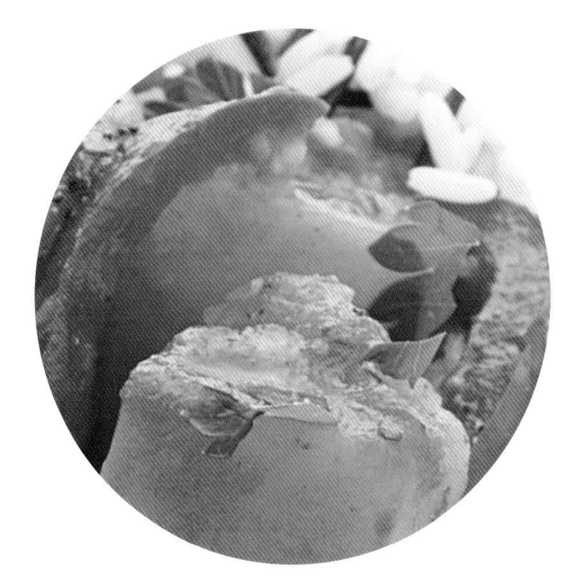

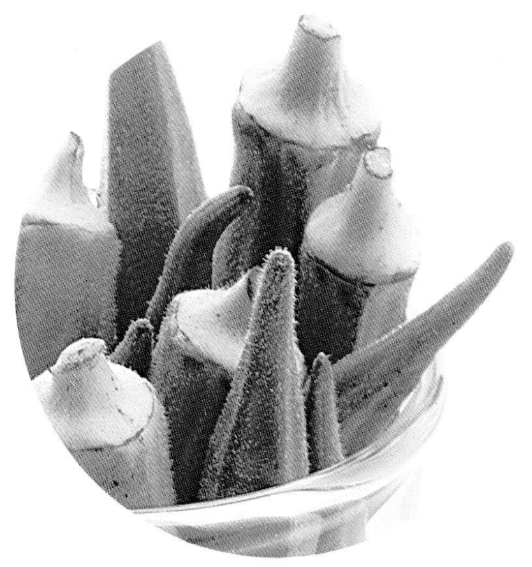

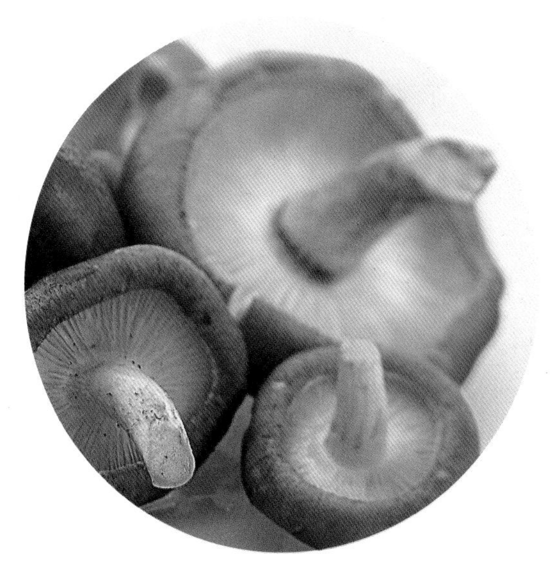

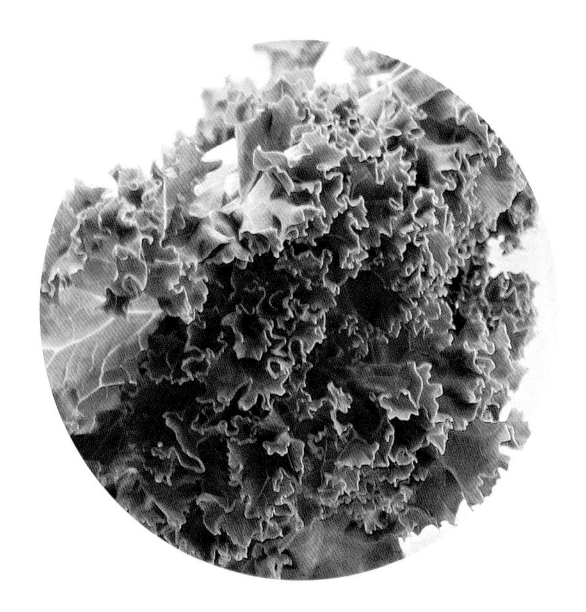

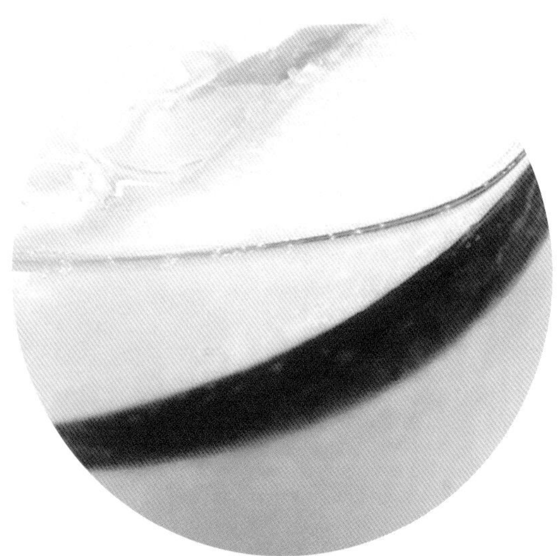

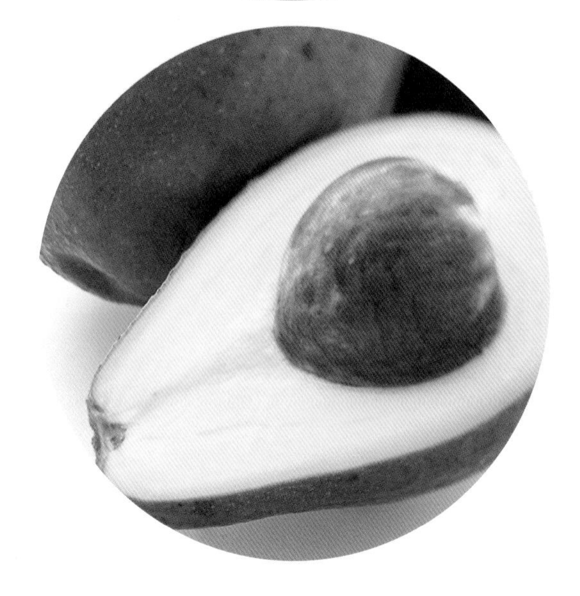

# allergy, autoimmunity and immunodeficiency

Allergy (an unpleasant reaction to non-microbial, "harmless" environmental antigens) and autoimmunity (an immune response against one's own body tissues) are now major causes of illness, particularly in the Western world. Between them they are responsible for much of the daily workload of family doctors, and also generate a huge market for pharmaceutical products that control or suppress the immune response.

## allergy

As we saw on page 162, allergic reactions fall into two categories: anaphylactic (or reaginic), rapid allergic responses caused by histamine released from mast cells; and cell-mediated, a slower response to environmental antigens involving T cells and macrophages. A significant proportion of the population have an inherited atopic tendency to anaphylactic allergic reactions of the skin, lungs, eyes, nose and digestive tract causing conditions such as eczema, hay fever, conjunctivitis, asthma and food allergy.

Coeliac disease (an allergy to wheat gluten, which causes malabsorption), dermatitis herpetiformis (a blistering skin disease also caused by gluten) and allergic alveolitis (for example, farmer's lung, a potentially serious allergic lung inflammation usually caused by occupational exposure to moulds) are other important conditions caused by allergy to environmental antigens. Allergic asthma is most often caused by tiny particles of antigenic material. Allergic rhinitis or hay fever is triggered by larger particles. The commonest environmental antigens are plant pollens, house dust mites, insect stings, pet dander (fur and feathers), fungal moulds, food proteins, vaccines, drugs, household/industrial chemicals, latex and heavy metals (especially chromium, cobalt and nickel).

However, not all adverse reactions to environmental substances are caused by allergies. The term "allergy" is sometimes wrongly attached to any unpleasant reaction to a food or drug. Favism is a haemolytic anaemia caused by an inherited lack of the enzyme glucose-6-phosphatase dehydrogenase, which is vital for the health of red blood cells. When a sufferer eats broad beans, inhales broad bean pollen or takes certain drugs, including sulphonamide antibiotics and certain anti-malarial drugs, red blood cells are rapidly destroyed causing fever, abdominal pain and, in severe cases, coma and even death. The sensitivity of some asthma sufferers to drugs such as aspirin is more often a chemical, rather than an immunological, problem.

Orthodox treatment of allergy is a two-stage process. First, it involves reducing exposure to the allergen responsible (where possible) and, second, the use of drugs. Common drugs used for allergies include:

- Nasal sprays and inhalers (such as antihistamines and sodium cromoglycate) to inhibit the release of histamine from mast cells.
- Bronchodilators to reduce muscle spasm in the lungs and open the airways.
- Corticosteroid drugs ("steroids"), which counteract inflammation.

# autoimmunity

In normal circumstances, the immune system is able to distinguish clearly between "self" and "non-self". During their "education" in the thymus, developing T cells that may react to the body's own tissues are destroyed, and any self-reacting cells that do survive are suppressed by other cells in the immune system. However, for reasons not yet clearly understood, these safety mechanisms sometimes break down, resulting in an autoimmune disease.

Autoimmune diseases are usually chronic and cause slow, progressive damage to organs and tissues. These conditions cover a spectrum ranging from "organ specific" disorders, in which only one "target" organ is damaged, to "multi-system" diseases involving a variety of body systems and producing complex patterns of symptoms and signs.

Organ-specific autoimmune diseases include:

- Thyroid – Hashimoto's thyroiditis and Graves' disease
- Adrenal gland – Addison's disease
- Pancreas – Type I (early onset) diabetes mellitus
- Nerves and muscles – multiple sclerosis and myasthenia gravis
- Skin – pemphigus, pemphigoid and vitiligo
- Kidney – Goodpasture's syndrome
- Liver – primary biliary cirrhosis
- Stomach – pernicious anaemia
- Hair – alopecia
- Ovaries – premature ovarian failure
- Reproductive organs – endometriosis.

Autoimmune disease is growing increasingly common, so the search for a cause is generating an enormous research effort. This research has uncovered important clues suggesting possible trigger mechanisms for autoimmune reactions. It seems, for example, that certain infections (particularly viruses), vaccinations and environmental factors can cause subtle changes in lymphocyte function that lead to a breakdown in self-recognition by the immune system.

Some microbes even stimulate B cells to produce "auto-antibodies" directly, by mimicking the actions of T helper cells, and it is possible that other micro-organisms contain proteins that closely resemble those of human tissues. If the immune system makes antibodies to such micro-organisms, it will unwittingly produce antibodies that damage the body's own cells as well.

Many of those suffering from autoimmune diseases have an inherited immunological instability that affects their ability to control immune responses. In particular they may lack T suppressor cells, which normally keep stray "auto-reactive" T helper cells under control.

# immunodeficiency

In order to cope with the huge diversity of potentially harmful micro-organisms (and other antigens) that we are exposed to in life, the immune system has evolved into a highly complex system of many inter-related components. Although this gives a wide repertoire of immune responses, it also means that damage or deficiency in any part of the system makes us susceptible to illness.

Immunodeficiency is now an increasingly common cause of disease worldwide. The basic feature of immunodeficiency is the tendency to suffer more frequent and more serious infection than normal, often from micro-organisms not usually considered dangerous.

Immunodeficiency can be divided into two categories: primary – a genetic defect involving the lack of a vital immune system component; and secondary – the direct result of another disease process, or the consequence of exposure to drugs, chemicals or ionizing radiation. Primary immunodeficiency is usually diagnosed early in life (most often in a child suffering frequent ear, nose, throat and chest infections), and in some cases (such as in severe combined immunodeficiency – SCID) it may lead to early death. When primary immunodeficiency is owing to a lack of B cells (such as X-linked hypogammaglobulinaemia – Bruton's disease), lifelong injections of immunoglobulin are necessary to maintain health. Deficiency of complement enzymes can also be managed with drugs and enzyme injections.

Secondary immunodeficiency is more common than the primary type and has a wide variety of possible causes. The commonest are leukaemia, Hodgkin's lymphoma, myeloma, burns, severe kidney disease, Down's syndrome, chronic inflammation, chronic infection (such as malaria and leprosy), congenital rubella (German measles), surgery/radiation of lymphoid tissues, drug therapy (especially corticosteroids and anti-cancer drugs) and poverty.

Of these, poverty is probably the most common cause of immunodeficiency worldwide. Protein-energy malnutrition causes decreased cellular immunity, atrophy of lymph nodes, a reduction of T cells, and an overall decrease in the capacity of the immune system to deal with infection.

# HIV and AIDS

Of all the possible causes of immunodeficiency, in the last 20 years the most important has undoubtedly been acquired immune deficiency syndrome (AIDS). This is a slow, progressive deterioration of immune function and to date has been responsible for more than 15 million deaths worldwide, with the brunt of the disease borne by the populations of sub-Saharan Africa, south and south-eastern Asia and South America. AIDS is now probably responsible for more deaths per year than malaria and is a major factor in the re-emergence of tuberculosis as a world health problem.

As in other immunodeficiency states, the central problem faced by the AIDS sufferer is susceptibility to severe infections by viruses, bacteria, fungi and parasites. The other important feature of full-blown AIDS is the development of tumours such as lymphoma (cancer of lymphoid tissue) and Kaposi's sarcoma (a type of skin tumour). When HIV is active, the number of CD4 T cells in the blood (see page 156) falls progressively.

The commonest AIDS-related infections are Herpes simplex, Herpes zoster, cytomegalovirus (CMV), tuberculosis, salmonella, toxoplasma, cryptosporidium, giardia, pneumocystis, cryptococcus, histoplasma, candida and strongyloides.

There has been extensive worldwide debate over the cause of AIDS, but the current consensus is that infection with either the HIV1 or HIV2 virus is at the root of the problem. HIV viruses belong to a family of retroviruses thought to have originated in primates. HIV2 infection is most common in West Africa.

How HIV causes immunodeficiency is not well understood, but it is known that the HIV virus has the ability to stick on to CD4 molecules on the surface of T helper cells, which seriously interferes with T-cell function. HIV infection also damages the thymus (where T cells develop), and affects antigen-presenting cells such as macrophages, altering their pattern of cytokine release.

The fact that the HIV virus is able to fuse with T cells and commandeer their internal workings – and that it is capable of assuming a wide range of antigenic forms during the course of the disease – enables it to evade the body's protective immune response, and makes the development of effective treatments very difficult.

Combination anti-viral drug therapy with reverse transcriptase inhibitors helps raise the CD4 lymphocyte count, and antibacterial and antifungal drugs are also used to treat infections. Health education programmes about the need for safer sex, safe blood transfusion procedures and reducing shared-needle use by intravenous drug users are the mainstays of prevention, and much research is being devoted to the development of a safe and effective vaccine.

Given the close link between nutrition and immunity, it is not surprising that diet and the treatment of HIV infection are also intimately related. It has been shown that good nutrition greatly improves the outcome of drug therapy and chances of long-term survival. Maximizing the quality of the diet can also play a major role in improving the quality of life of AIDS sufferers (see pages 232–33).

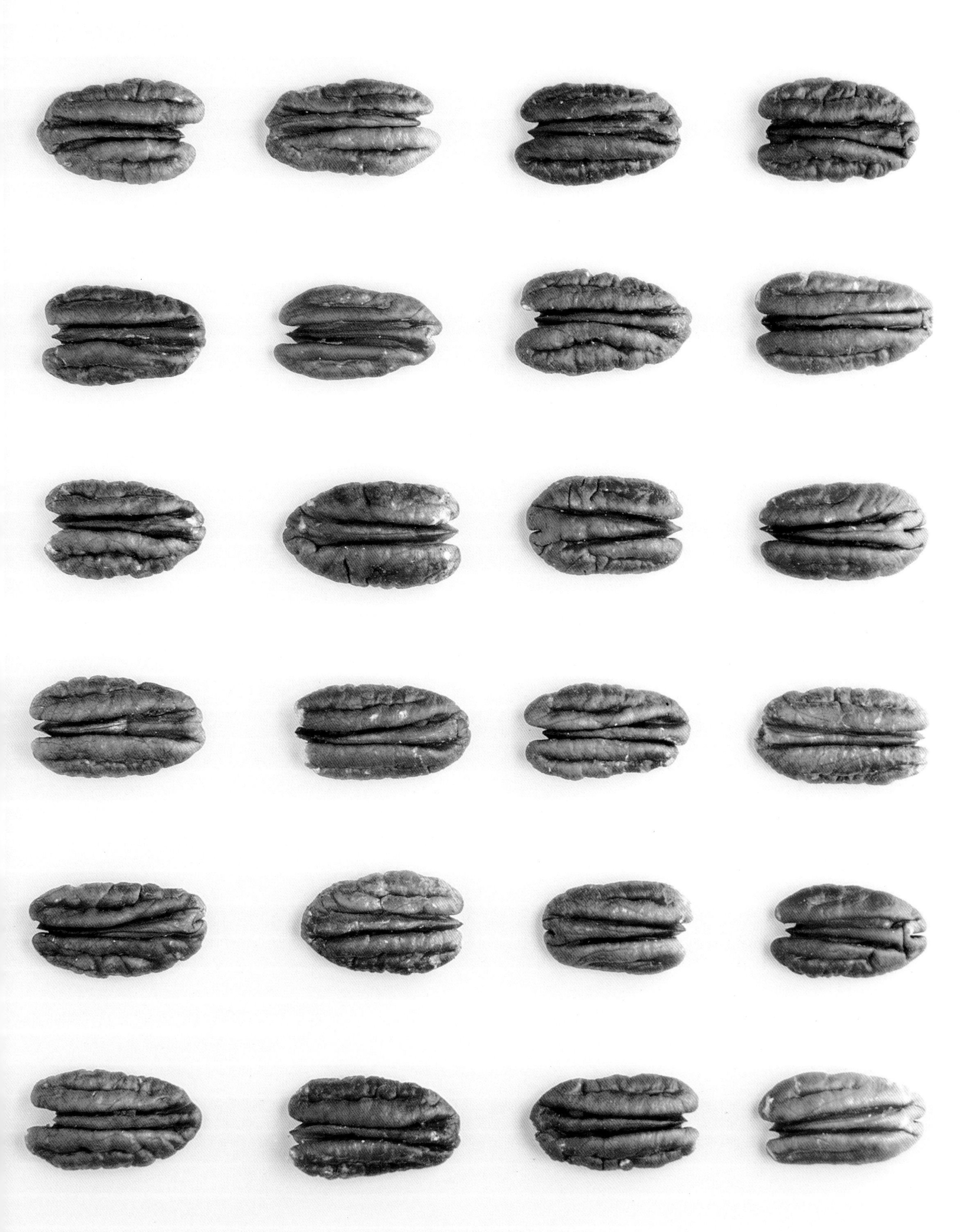

# IMMUNITY AND FOOD

Like the lungs, the gastro-intestinal tract is a major "meeting place" in which the body comes into contact with the outside world. All food and drink has to pass through it before being absorbed and used for nutrition, and its lining is rich in lymphoid tissue called Peyer's patches.

The challenge for the immune system is that it has to be tolerant of the wide variety of "foreign" food proteins that we consume habitually, while at the same time being able to recognize and destroy potentially harmful micro-organisms that might contaminate our food and water.

It manages this by suppressing the production of any IgG and IgM antibodies that might react against food protein molecules, and by increasing the amount of IgA antibody in gut secretions. IgA has the ability to bind directly to pathogenic micro-organisms and to neutralize them without activating the complement system or causing inflammation.

However, when the immune system is combating an infection elsewhere in the body, gastro-intestinal lymphoid tissue can get caught up in the action and start attacking harmless food antigens. This, in turn, causes inflammation and damage to the lining of the gastro-intestinal tract. Severe malnutrition can also damage the lining of the intestines and disturb the pattern of immune responses.

## allergy or intolerance?

Sometimes – and especially in those with a family tendency to atopic conditions such as eczema, asthma and hay fever – the immune system reacts against certain foods. In addition to triggering general allergic symptoms, this causes inflammation of the intestinal lining and increased contraction of intestinal muscle, leading to wind, abdominal discomfort, diarrhoea and poor absorption of nutrients. Deficiencies of vitamins, minerals and other nutrients can, in turn, affect the immune system. For example:

- Essential fatty acid deficiency causes atrophy of lymphoid tissues and decreased ability to produce antibodies.
- Vitamin A and E deficiency affects the immune defences of skin and mucous membranes, decreases T-cell activity and antibody production, and so increases infection risk.
- Vitamin B6, folate and pantothenate deficiency decreases T and B cell activity.
- Iron deficiency (or excess iron) increases infection risk.
- Zinc deficiency causes atrophy of lymphoid tissue, decreases B and T cell responses and inhibits development of the immune system in the foetus.

There is a tendency these days to label all unpleasant reactions to food as "food allergy", but for accurate diagnosis and effective treatment, it is necessary to classify such reactions under their correct headings: food intolerance; food allergy and psychological intolerance.

Food intolerance is a general term covering all negative reactions to foodstuffs, including those caused by inherited enzyme deficiencies, interactions with drugs and medicines and chemical irritations (for example, by chilli pepper).

Food allergy means that a particular food is triggering a specific immune response. True food allergy is more common in children, and can express itself in a variety of ways including eczema, asthma, urticaria (nettle rash), mood disturbance, severe anaphylactic reactions, epilepsy, poor growth, diarrhoea, vomiting and gastro-intestinal bleeding. (The association between childhood hyperactivity and food allergy is not clearly established.)

Food allergy in adults tends to cause urticaria, asthma, migraine, or "irritable bowel syndrome"-type symptoms such as nausea, bloating, abdominal pain and alternating constipation and diarrhoea. There is also some evidence implicating food allergy in arthritis and depression. Accurate diagnosis of food allergy is time-consuming and usually involves elimination diets followed by "challenges" with the suspect food(s). Patch and scratch tests, cytotoxic blood testing, hair analysis, applied kinesiology, vega testing and iridology are also used, with varying degrees of success.

Psychological intolerance means reacting to a food which, although causing unpleasant symptoms when eaten in a recognizable form, causes no reaction when it is disguised or made unrecognizable by mixing with other foods. Generally speaking, orthodox medical practitioners tend to over-diagnose psychological intolerance, whereas complementary therapists tend to under-diagnose it.

# cow's milk allergy

Despite its status as a staple food in the West, cow's milk is a common cause of food allergy in children and is responsible for a variety of symptoms – including eczema, asthma, diarrhoea, vomiting and malabsorption of nutrients, causing slow growth.

The allergen responsible is beta-lactoglobulin, a protein that forms part of milk whey, and most children (and many adults) have antibodies to milk protein in their blood. Babies can become sensitized to milk protein via breast milk if the mother's diet contains cow's milk and milk products. Although the majority of children have developed "tolerance" to cow's milk by about one year old, the lining of the intestine continues to show abnormalities. Excluding cow's milk from the diet resolves the problem.

Allergy to cow's milk is not the same as lactose intolerance, another common cause of gastro-intestinal upset in children. Babies and young children produce the enzyme lactase, which can digest lactose, a sugar found in breast milk. Production of this enzyme drops sharply after weaning and in most races (except Western Caucasians) is practically non-existent in adults. If an individual with lactase "deficiency" drinks cow's milk, the lactose will not be digested and so will pass into the colon, causing diarrhoea, wind and abdominal discomfort. Lactose intolerance is a common cause of "unexplained" abdominal pain in children and is also common after bouts of gastroenteritis.

# coeliac disease

Coeliac disease is another immune-related gastro-intestinal condition, in which eating wheat gluten causes inflammation and damage to the lining of the small intestine. This leads to severe malabsorption of important nutrients resulting in multiple health problems including diarrhoea, weight loss, flatulence, oedema, anaemia, muscle wasting, bone problems and disturbance of heart rhythm. The exact nature of the immune reaction that causes coeliac disease is unclear, but it is known that people with the condition have an inherited genetic susceptibility, and that the components of gluten that cause the problem are called gliandins. Although potentially serious, coeliac disease can be managed by eating a gluten-free diet. This means avoiding wheat, barley, rye and, usually, oats for life. However, rice, maize and soya products are safe and not everyone with the disorder is sensitive to oats.

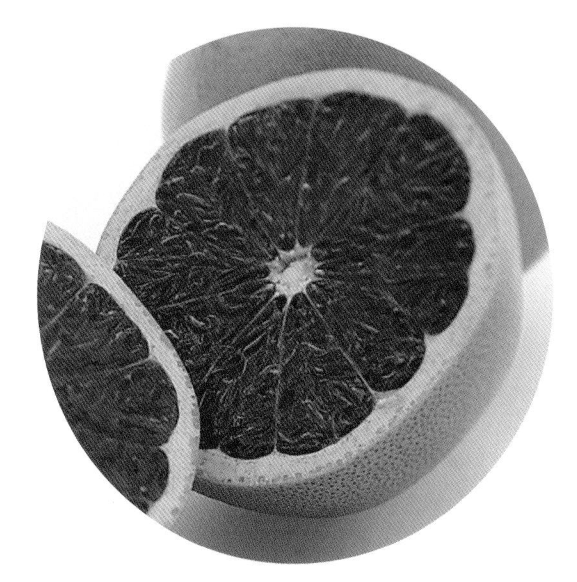

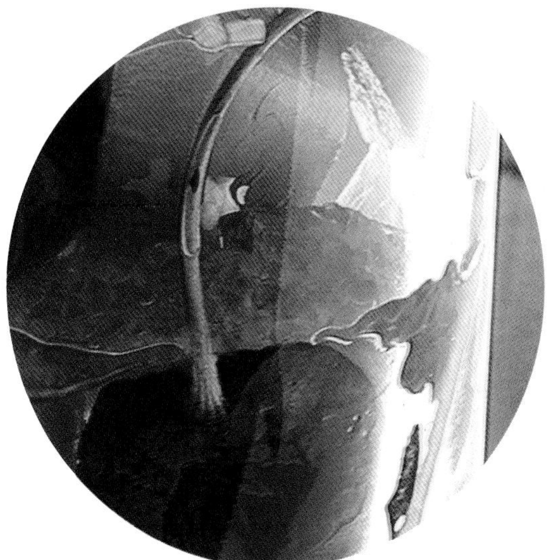

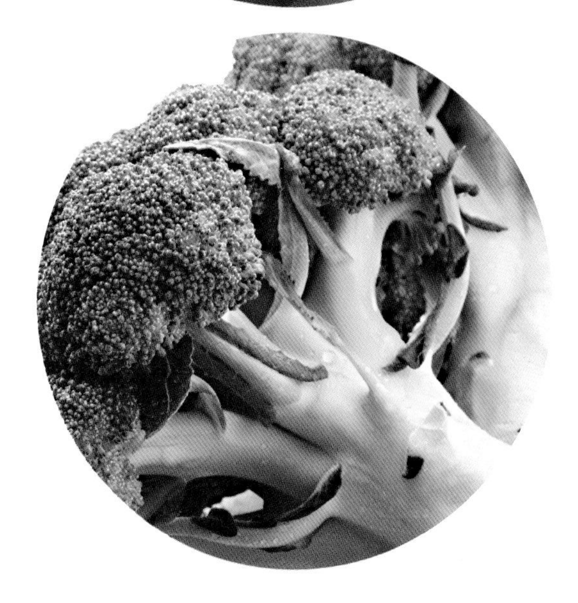

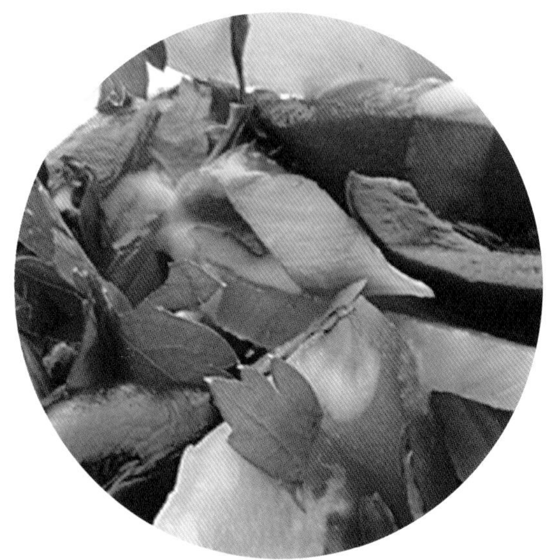

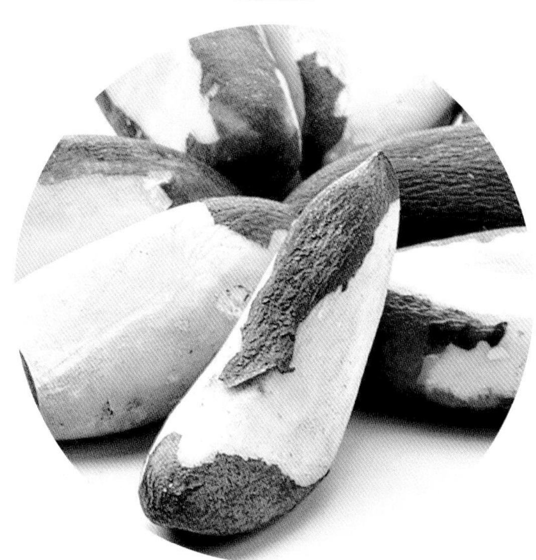

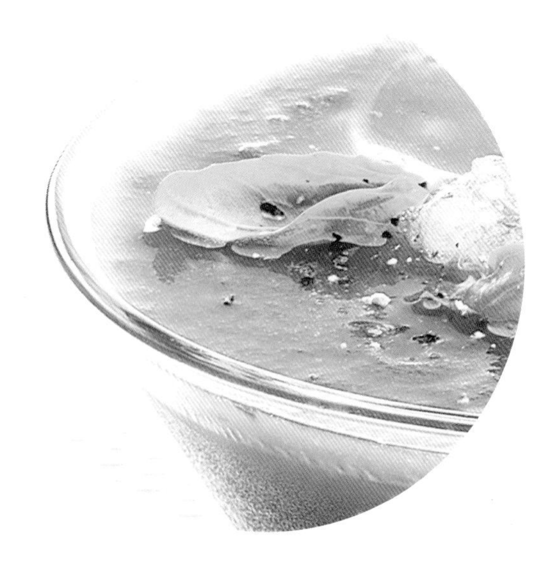

# IMPROVING IMMUNITY

Immunity that harms and immunity that heals are both caused by the same basic mechanisms, so knowing which nutritional and lifestyle factors influence immunity gives us a powerful way of enhancing personal health and of coping with many common ailments that have immune disturbance at their root. A healthy immune system is the basis of well-being, so making it more efficient, and avoiding anything that might compromise or weaken it, are the fundamental steps to life-long health.

Later sections of this book look in detail at how you can select the right foods to optimize immune function, but clinical experience and modern research also show that other factors have powerful effects on immunity, particularly stress, environmental pollution, alcohol, cigarettes and recreational drugs, medical interventions, obesity, lack of exercise and age factors.

## managing stress

Chronic stress causes the adrenal glands to secrete higher levels of corticosteroids, which depress immune function. In acute stress reactions, high adrenaline levels also decrease T-helper-cell activity, increase T-suppressor-cell activity and lead to degeneration of lymphoid tissues. Changes in mood alter the amount of IgA present in secretions from mucous membranes, and depression interferes with T and B cell function. Therefore, chronic stress is a major risk factor for illness, particularly cancer and heart disease, and making the lifestyle changes necessary to reduce its impact on our lives is a vitally important preventive health strategy. Stress-management techniques such as yoga, deep breathing, meditation and autosuggestion can also have a significant effect on immune function and reduce our susceptibility to disease.

## avoiding pollution

Environmental pollutants are broadly divided into three categories:

- Radiation – from microwave appliances, television and radio transmitters, mobile phones, television and computer screens, high-tension overhead electricity cables and nuclear installations and reprocessing plants.
- Chemicals – including garden and agricultural pesticides and herbicides, aerosols, industrial emissions, engine exhaust fumes,

smoke, paints, fungicides and household products such as air fresheners, detergents and furniture polish.

- Biological – such as house dust and dust mites, pet dander and moulds.

All of these can compromize immunity and should be avoided where possible. Minimizing the use of household chemicals, buying organic produce, using dust-covers on mattresses, exchanging carpets for wood or tiled flooring, avoiding smoking and smokers, ensuring good ventilation in the house, limiting the amount of time spent in front of television screens and computer monitors and regular household maintenance to avoid damp and mould formation are all achievable ways of improving immune-system health.

## avoiding alcohol, cigarettes and drugs

In many parts of the world, alcohol is one of the most important controllable risk factors for serious illness. It depresses the immune response and is clearly associated with heart disease, hypertension, stroke, gastritis, pancreatitis, peptic ulcers, serious liver damage and deterioration of mental function. As with hard-drug use, it is a major cause of poor nutrition, which further damages immune competence. Tobacco smoke contains high concentrations of dangerous chemicals including benzene, carbon monoxide and cadmium (a powerful immuno-suppressant also found in fungicides, fertilizers and rubber tyres). Cannabis inhibits both T cell and macrophage activity. Put simply, drinking, smoking and recreational drug use are not compatible with a healthy immune system.

## taking treatment – with caution!

Medicinal remedies used to control the symptoms of allergic reactions – antihistamines, bronchodilators, decongestants, sodium cromoglycate, corticosteroids – are designed to dampen immune system activity, but many other drugs – including anti-inflammatories, blood thinners, oral contraceptives, hormone replacement therapy (HRT), antibiotics and anti-cancer drugs – can cause unintentional suppression of normal immune responses. Diagnostic and therapeutic X-rays and other ionizing radiations also carry a risk of immune-system damage. Informed and appropriate use of medical drugs, plus avoidance of unnecessary high-energy imaging procedures, should form part of any strategy for immune health.

## controlling weight

Obesity is a global epidemic, which is clearly related to the high incidence of coronary heart disease worldwide, and strongly implicated as a risk factor for cancer, especially of the breast, uterus, cervix and ovary in women, the prostate in men, and the colon and rectum in both sexes. As immunity plays a major role in protecting against cancer, and as it is proven that obese people are more likely to die earlier than the non-obese, maintaining a healthy body weight is a common-sense way of encouraging long-term immune health, as well as improving general well-being.

## taking exercise

Research confirms that regular moderate exercise enhances immune function and protects against cancer, heart disease and osteoporosis, as well as being an effective way to relieve stress. Three or more 30-minute exercise sessions a week, such as brisk walking, jogging, cycling or swimming, are ideal for optimizing immunity, but beware of overexertion – it suppresses T-cell function and other immune responses.

## for young and old

At both extremes of age, the immune system is less efficient, so paying special attention to the above factors is particularly important for children and the elderly. As far as children are concerned, breast-feeding, avoiding cow's milk, allowing minor illnesses to take their course without suppressing the symptoms with drugs, and eliminating unnecessary exposure to environmental antigens, are the basics of healthy immune-system development.

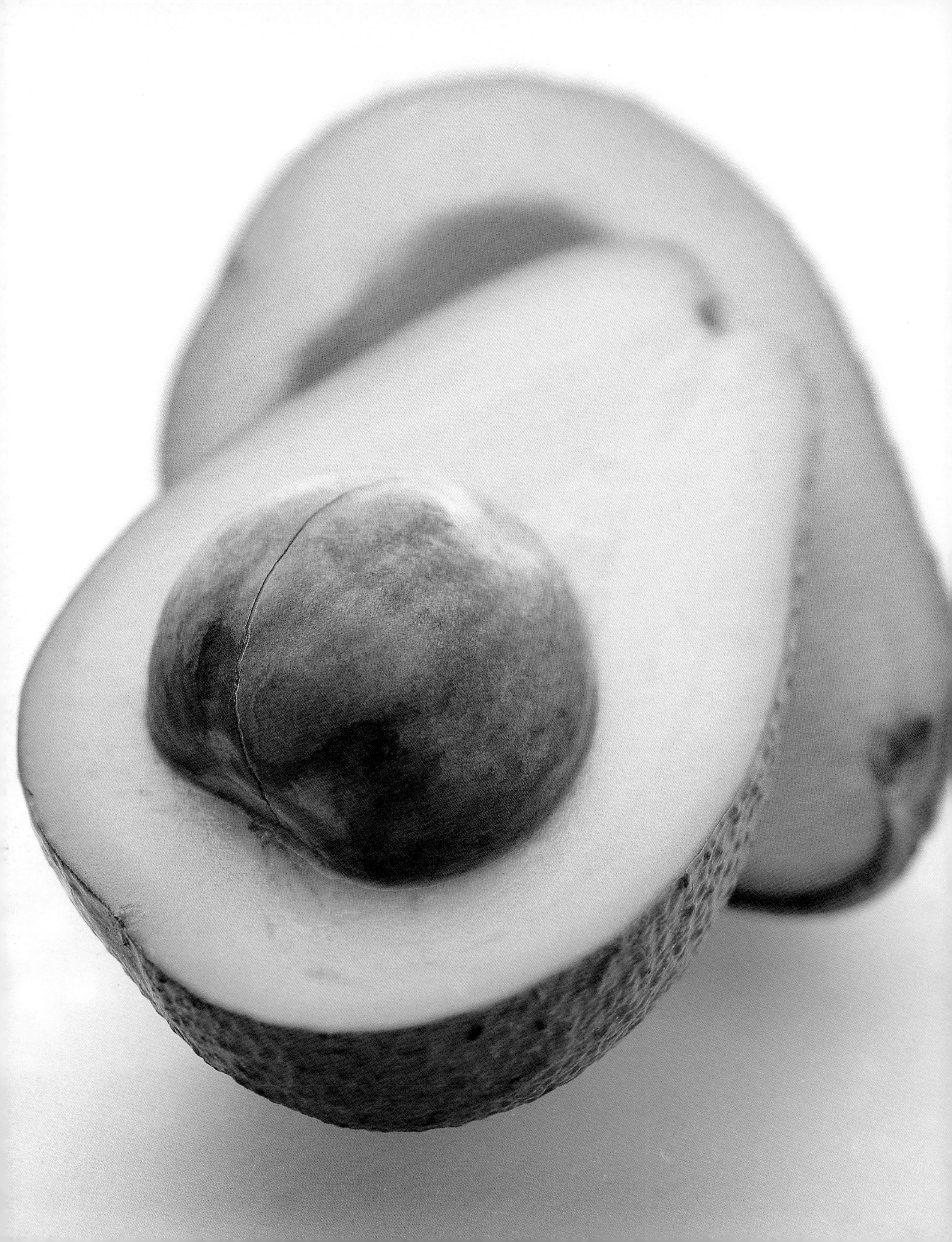

chapter six

# superfoods for the immune system

The medicinal value of food for warding off illness has been acknowledged for thousands of years. More recently, scientific research has discovered hundreds of beneficial nutrients in the foods we eat. By applying our knowledge of these nutrients and of how they work to our diet, we can eat foods that boost our immune system and so help protect ourselves against a host of ailments. Chapter Six presents profiles of 150 foods packed with disease-fighting nutrients, including nine "star foods", such as beetroot and shiitake mushrooms, that are particularly effective in boosting the body's natural defences. All recipes serve four people unless otherwise stated.

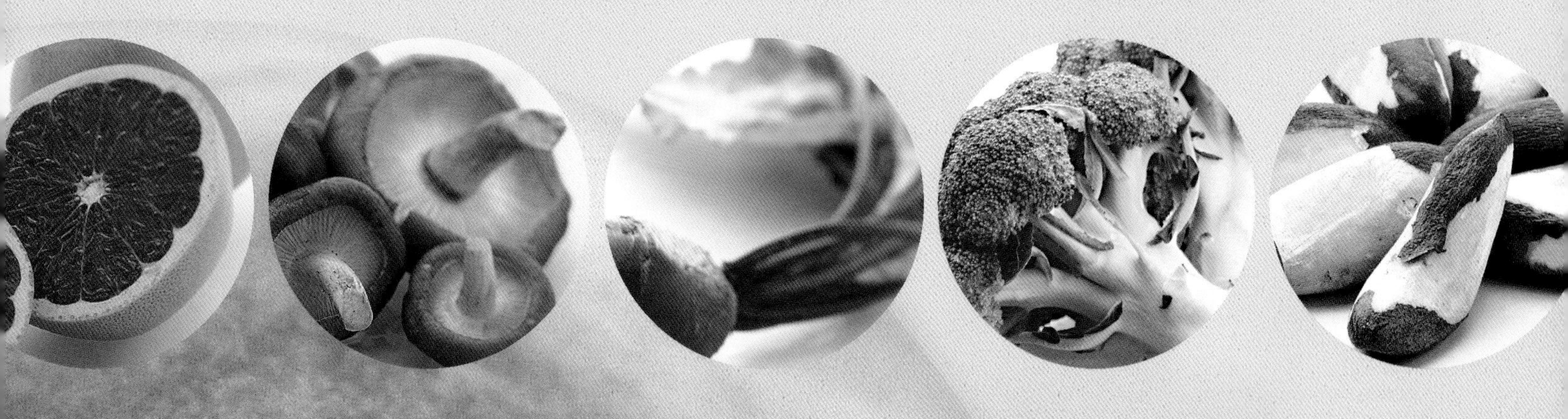

# fruits and vegetables

## ROOTS AND BULBS

### CARROT

★ VITAMINS A, K, FOLATE; CALCIUM, MANGANESE, PHOSPHORUS; CHROMIUM, IRON, ZINC; CAROTENOIDS; FIBRE

✓ ANTI-CANCER, ANTIOXIDANT, GOOD FOR SKIN AND EYES

! HIGH CARROT INTAKE CAUSES ORANGE/YELLOW SKIN COLOURING; THIS EFFECT IS HARMLESS AND GOES ONCE INTAKE IS REDUCED

Carrots (*Daucus carota*) support the immune system, aid wound healing and promote healthy skin. They can also be useful in treating chronic viral infections, such as herpes simplex. Carrots help prevent the formation of cancer cells and can protect against heart disease and arthritis. They play a role in regulating blood-sugar levels and thus may help protect against diabetes.

**RECIPES** *healing soup (page 244), carrot 'n' beetroot salad (page 259), carrot and lemon with garlic (page 264)*

### ONION

★ VITAMINS B1, B6; SULPHUR COMPOUNDS

✓ ANTI-ASTHMATIC, ANTIBACTERIAL, ANTI-CANCER, ANTISEPTIC, DIURETIC, LOWERS BLOOD PRESSURE, LOWERS CHOLESTEROL

! MAY CAUSE INDIGESTION IN THOSE WITH GASTRO-INTESTINAL DISORDERS

Onion (*Allium cepa*) is a natural antibacterial that also helps the body's metabolism by lowering blood cholesterol, blood fat and blood sugar. Onions decrease the formation of blood clots, too. They inhibit the activity of *Helicobacter pylori* (the bacterium thought to be responsible for gastritis and stomach ulcers), and may protect against stomach cancer by decreasing the conversion of nitrates to nitrites in the stomach. Onion syrup (prepared like garlic oxymel – page 269) is a useful remedy for colds and coughs.

**RECIPES** *samosa parcels (page 248), tofumasalata (page 248), french onion tart (page 255)*

### POTATO

★ VITAMINS C, B1, FOLATE; POTASSIUM; IRON; SOLANIDINE ALKALOIDS; FIBRE, COMPLEX CARBOHYDRATES, PROTEIN

✓ ANTIOXIDANT, ENERGY-BOOSTING, NUTRITIONAL VALUE

! GREEN AND DAMAGED POTATOES HAVE AN INCREASED ALKALOID CONTENT THAT MAKES THEM TASTE BITTER, AND WHICH CAN BE TOXIC IN LARGE AMOUNTS

Potatoes (*Solanum tuberosum*) boost energy and strengthen immunity. They lower blood-fat levels, improve tissue oxygenation, promote a healthy nervous system and improve wound healing. They help the body absorb and use other nutrients and alleviate digestive and malabsorption disorders. For most benefit, eat in their skins. Hot potato water and raw potato juice are traditional remedies for arthritis and gout.

**RECIPES** *welsh leek and potato soup (page 246), shepherdess' pie (page 256), hasselbach potatoes (page 258)*

### SWEET POTATO

★ VITAMINS A, B1, B3, FOLATE; CAROTENOIDS (IN YELLOW VARIETY); COMPLEX CARBOHYDRATES, FIBRE, SUGARS

✓ ANTIOXIDANT, ANTIVIRAL (YELLOW VARIETY), ENERGY-BOOSTING

There are two varieties of sweet potato (*Ipomoea batatas*) – yellow and white. The yellow variety contains high levels of vitamin A and carotenoids, which enhance the immune response and help the body deal with viral infections and cancer. Therefore sweet potato is useful in the treatment of ailments such as cancer and AIDS, in which the immune response is compromised. Both kinds boost resistance to infection and help maintain optimum energy levels. They nourish the nervous system, help maintain healthy muscles, and keep skin and mucous membranes in good condition.

**RECIPES** *nettle and sweet potato mash (page 185), vegetable kebabs (page 247), sweet potato curry (page 256)*

### YAM

★ VITAMINS A, B1; CAROTENOIDS (IN YELLOW YAM); COMPLEX CARBOHYDRATES, FIBRE, PROTEIN

✓ ANTIOXIDANT, ANTIVIRAL (YELLOW YAM), ENERGY-BOOSTING

There is a yellow and a white variety of yam (*Dioscorea spp.*). The yellow kind aids immunity and inhibits cancer growth. Both kinds help maintain healthy heart, nerves, muscles and metabolism.

**RECIPES** *use as sweet potato (above)*

# VEGETABLE FRUITS

## BUTTERNUT SQUASH

★ VITAMINS A, E; MAGNESIUM; CAROTENOIDS

✓ ANTI-CANCER, ANTIOXIDANT

Butternut squash (*Cucurbita sp.*) helps protect against cancer, heart disease and mental dysfunction. It aids normal blood cell function and encourages healthy skin, muscles and nerves.

**RECIPES** *butternut squash with red pepper and tomato* *(page 253)*

## OKRA (GUMBO, LADIES' FINGERS)

★ FOLATE; CALCIUM, MAGNESIUM, PHOSPHORUS, POTASSIUM; IRON; FIBRE

✓ ANTIDEPRESSANT, IMMUNO-STIMULANT

Okra (*Abelmoschus esculentus*) helps protect against colon cancer and other disorders related to low fibre intake, such as diverticulitis. It strengthens the immune system by supporting lymphatic tissue and white blood cells, aids the development and maintenance of a healthy nervous system and reduces the risk of heart disease.

**RECIPES** *okra in sweet and sour tamarind sauce* *(page 256)*

## PUMPKIN

★ VITAMIN A; CAROTENOIDS

✓ ANTIOXIDANT, ANTI-CANCER

Like butternut squash, pumpkin (*Cucurbita maxima*) helps prevent the formation of cancer cells and promotes healthy skin.

**RECIPES** *pumpkin soup* *(page 245)*

## RED PEPPER

★ VITAMINS A, C, B6; CAROTENOIDS; FIBRE

✓ ANTI-ALLERGIC, ANTIOXIDANT, ANTI-CANCER, SUPPORTS NERVES

! ONE OF SOLINACEAE FAMILY OF VEGETABLE FRUITS – MAY CAUSE ADVERSE REACTIONS IN THOSE WITH FOOD ALLERGIES OR ARTHRITIS

Red pepper (*Capsicum sp.*) boosts immunity and helps protect against cancer. It also helps maintain normal blood-fat levels and aids production of haemoglobin by the red blood cells. It encourages a healthy nervous system and may protect against asthma, migraine and depression.

**RECIPES** *grilled red peppers (page 247), vegetable kebabs (page 247), paella (page 252), catalan salad (page 260)*

## TOMATO

★ VITAMINS A, C, B3; LYCOPENE; FIBRE

✓ ANTI-CANCER, ANTIOXIDANT, ANTIVIRAL

! ONE OF SOLINACEAE FAMILY OF VEGETABLE FRUITS – MAY CAUSE ADVERSE REACTIONS IN THOSE WITH FOOD ALLERGIES OR ARTHRITIS

Tomatoes (*Lycopersicon sp.*) are packed with antioxidants, including vitamins A and C and lycopene. They improve the immune response while also helping to maintain energy levels. This combination makes tomatoes a useful addition to the diet of those suffering from energy-compromising conditions such as cancer and AIDS. They boost resistance to infectious disease, encouraging wound healing and keeping the skin and mucous membranes in good condition.

**RECIPES** *baked tomatoes on toast (page 242), beans and tomatoes on toast (page 242), cool tomato soup (page 244), tomato and cucumber canapés (page 250), tomato ketchup (page 251), tomato salsa (page 258), tomato cocktail (page 267)*

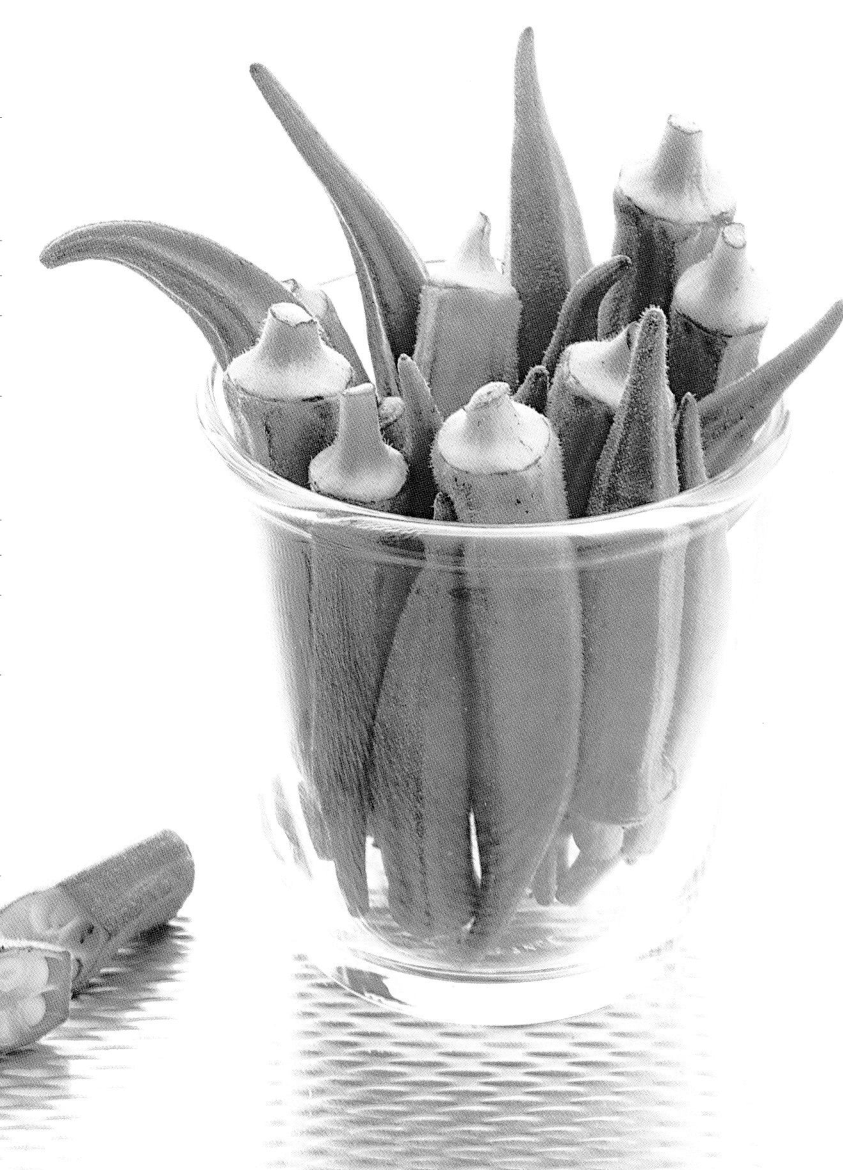

# beetroot

**BEETROOT HAS BEEN USED AS A FOOD AND A MEDICINE SINCE EARLY TIMES. ITS UNIQUE MIXTURE OF MINERALS AND PHYTOCHEMICALS RESISTS INFECTION, BOOSTS CELLULAR INTAKE OF OXYGEN AND TREATS DISORDERS OF THE BLOOD, LIVER AND IMMUNE SYSTEM.**

## The origin of beetroot

A native of southern Europe, beetroot (*Beta vulgaris rubra*) is now cultivated worldwide. It is derived from the sea beet, which grows wild around the Mediterranean. Beetroot has an unmistakable sweet flavour that is strongest when the food is eaten raw. Its leaves taste like spinach and, as with spinach, can be cooked, or eaten raw in salads. Modern Western medicine makes little use of the healing power of beetroot, but the vegetable is held in high regard by practitioners of natural medicine all over the world.

Beetroot was prized in ancient Greece, where people would offer it up to the god Apollo. Legend has it that Aphrodite ate beetroot to retain her beauty. In the old English medical tradition, beetroot was regarded as an important remedy for blood ailments. Herbalists and naturopaths of today still use beetroot as an effective treatment for disorders of the blood and the immune system and often refer to it as "the vitality plant".

## Immune-boosting properties

Beetroot stimulates the immune system by improving cell respiration and tissue oxygenation. It does this by encouraging the production of new red blood cells (a process called erythropoiesis). The enhanced cell respiration helps keep the heart, muscles and nerves in good condition. There is evidence that eating beetroot causes cancer cells to revert to normal or die, by altering their rate of cell respiration. This may not cure the disease, but may help to boost the length and quality of life of sufferers. Beetroot also helps stabilize the body's pH (acid–alkaline balance). This is important for immunity because bacteria thrive when the body's pH is disturbed. Beetroot can be used to treat cancers (particularly leukaemia), skin problems, chronic infections, inflammatory bowel disease, liver disease and in the prevention and treatment of heart disease and rheumatoid arthritis. It also aids fat metabolism and liver function.

## Using beetroot

Beetroot has no harmful side effects and is well tolerated by most people. It needs to be eaten over a relatively long period of time to improve general health and vitality in all cases of chronic illness. The average dose is two medium-size beetroots per day. Beetroot is just as effective cooked as it is eaten raw or juiced. Try this recipe for a blood-purifying drink: juice equal amounts of beetroot, carrot, celery, tomato and a lemon. Drink 1 to 2 wineglassfuls per day for three weeks.

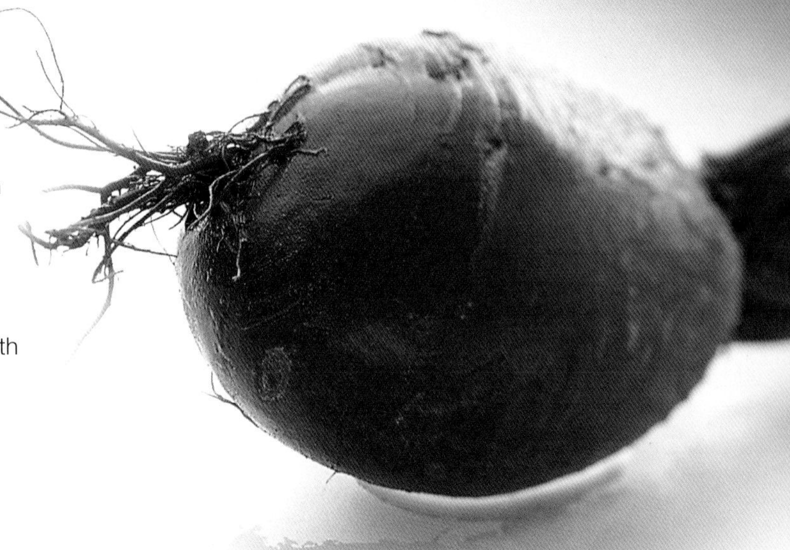

**IMMUNE-BOOSTING PROFILE**

★ FOLATE; CALCIUM, MANGANESE, POTASSIUM; IRON; BETANIN, MALONIC ACID, PHYTOSTEROL, SAPONIN; FIBRE, PROTEIN, SUGARS

✓ ANTI-CANCER, ANTI-INFLAMMATORY, ANTIOXIDANT, DETOXIFYING, IMMUNO-STIMULANT, BOOSTS CELL OXYGENATION, REJUVENATING

! BETANIN, THE PIGMENT IN BEETROOT, MAY COLOUR FAECES AND URINE RED; THIS IS HARMLESS AND THE EFFECT DISAPPEARS ONCE YOU STOP EATING THE VEGETABLE

! THE LEAVES CONTAIN OXALIC ACID AND SHOULD BE AVOIDED BY PEOPLE SUFFERING FROM KIDNEY STONES OR ARTHRITIS

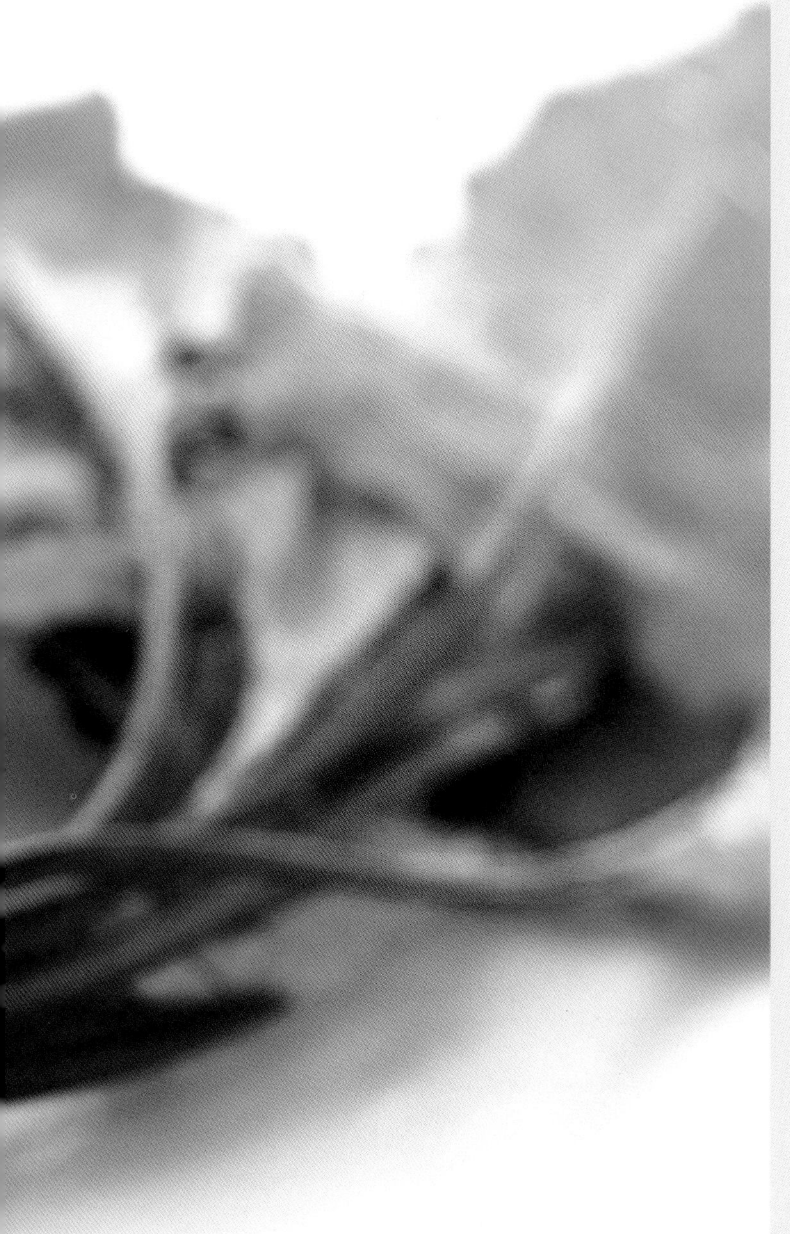

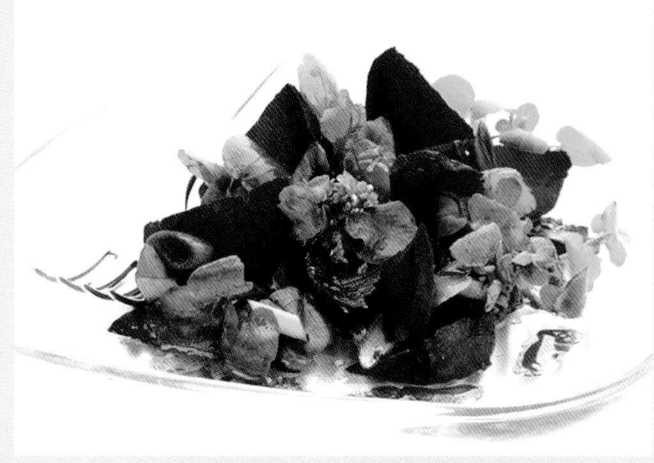

## baked beetroot salad *(above)*

2 beetroots, washed but not peeled
1 spring onion, finely chopped
1 bunch of watercress, finely chopped
2 tbsp safflower oil
1 tbsp balsamic vinegar

Dry the beetroots gently and rub in a little oil. Bake at 180°C/gas mark 4 for about one hour. Cool under running water, peel and chop into sticks. Place in a salad bowl and mix with the other ingredients.

## beetroot and horseradish salad

200 ml plain soya yoghurt
1 or 2 tbsp fresh horseradish, grated
Salt to taste
3 medium beetroots, grated
4 tbsp fresh mint, finely chopped

Mix the yoghurt, horseradish and salt. Gently fold the beetroot into the dressing and garnish with mint.

## scandinavian beetroot burgers

350 g white rice, well cooked
125 g firm tofu, grated
2 medium beetroots, grated
2 tbsp breadcrumbs
1 tbsp balsamic vinegar
1 tbsp olive oil
1 tbsp marjoram
Salt and pepper to taste
Flour for dipping
Oil for frying

Mix the rice, tofu, beetroot, breadcrumbs, vinegar, oil and marjoram in a bowl. Season and shape into flat cakes. Dip in flour and fry at high temperature for 2 minutes on each side. Turn down the heat and continue frying for about 5 minutes on each side. Serve in burger buns, with salad, slices of tomato, cucumber, raw onion, mustard and tomato ketchup (*see page 251*).

# LEAVES AND FLOWERS

## AMARANTH LEAVES (LOVE LIES BLEEDING)

★ VITAMINS A, C, B2, FOLATE; CALCIUM, MAGNESIUM, MANGANESE, PHOSPHORUS, POTASSIUM; IRON; FIBRE, PROTEIN

✓ ANTI-ALLERGIC, ANTI-CANCER, ANTIOXIDANT, ENERGY-BOOSTING

! AMARANTH HAS A HIGH PROTEIN CONTENT, WHICH MAY MAKE IT HARDER FOR CHILDREN TO DIGEST LARGE AMOUNTS

The leaves of amaranth (*Amaranthus candatus*) are high in protein and other important nutrients. This makes amaranth a useful support to the immune system and a good source of energy. Amaranth leaves aid liver function and wound healing, help regulate blood-fat levels and are good for the digestion. They may also help protect against heart disease, cancer and rheumatoid arthritis. The leaves can be used like other greens in salads, or steamed or creamed like spinach. Amaranth tisane is taken to treat bronchitis and irritable bowel syndrome.

***RECIPES*** *amaranth and tofu puffs (page 252)*

## ASPARAGUS

★ VITAMINS B3, FOLATE; POTASSIUM; ZINC; RUTIN, SAPSONIN, TANNIN; FIBRE, PROTEIN

✓ ANTISPASMODIC, DIURETIC, GENTLY LAXATIVE, SOOTHING TO THE URINARY TRACT, WOUND HEALING

Asparagus (*Asparagus officinalis*) is a gentle diuretic that is used to stimulate urine flow and hence alleviate water retention. As a general tonic, it helps keep the skin and mucous membranes in good condition and maintains the health of blood-vessel walls. It may have a role in regulating blood cholesterol levels and inhibiting the growth of cancer cells.

***RECIPES*** *scrambled tofu (page 242), asparagus with ravigote (page 246), asparagus asian-style (page 253), catalan salad (page 260), pasta salad (page 260)*

## BELGIAN ENDIVE

★ VITAMINS A, B1, FOLATE; PHOSPHORUS; BITTER PRINCIPLE; FIBRE

✓ ANTI-ALLERGIC, ANTI-CANCER, ANTIOXIDANT, ANTI-STRESS

Belgian endive (*Cichorium intybus*) has a delicate, slightly bitter taste that is popular in France. It stimulates the liver and digestion, supports the immune system and helps to regulate and maintain energy levels. Endive is also good for the health of the skin and mucous membranes.

***RECIPES*** *grapefruit salad (page 189), grilled endive and brazil nut salad (page 197)*

## BROCCOLI (GREEN- AND PURPLE-SPROUTING)

★ VITAMINS A, C, E, B3, B5, FOLATE; CALCIUM, PHOSPHORUS, POTASSIUM; IRON, ZINC; GLUCOSINOLATES

✓ ANTI-CANCER, ANTIOXIDANT, ANTI-STRESS, ENERGY-BOOSTING

SEE GLOSSARY FOR INFORMATION ON GLUCOSINOLATES

Broccoli (*Brassica oleracea var.*) is a useful aid to detox and boosts energy and strength. It protects the health of the heart, skin, nerves and muscle tissue and helps prevent heart disease, cancer and immune disorders.

***RECIPES*** *sweet potato curry (page 256)*

## BRUSSELS SPROUT

★ VITAMINS C, B2, B5, B6, FOLATE; POTASSIUM; GLUCOSINOLATES; FIBRE, PROTEIN, SUGARS

✓ ANTI-ALLERGIC, ANTIOXIDANT, ANTI-STRESS

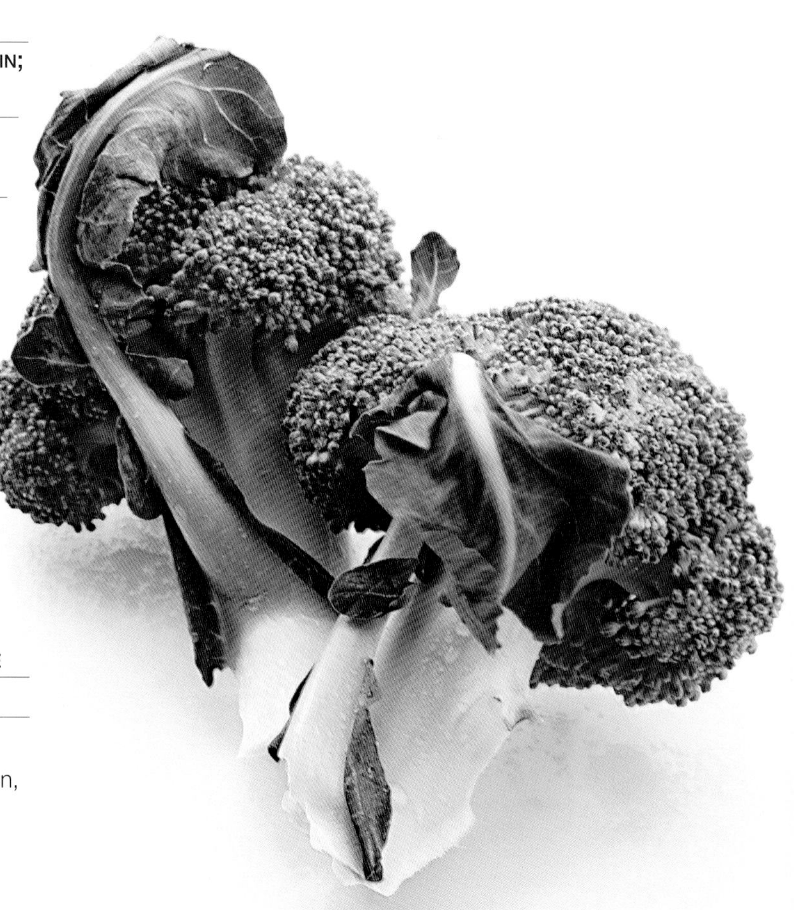

SEE GLOSSARY FOR INFORMATION ON GLUCOSINOLATES

Brussels sprouts (*Brassica oleracea gemmifera*) strengthen the immune system and help maintain the health of the skin, nerves and mucous membranes. They also help maintain normal energy and blood-fat levels and may protect against asthma, migraine, depression and cancer.

**RECIPES** *serve steamed or grilled as a side dish*

### BUTTERHEAD LETTUCE

★ VITAMINS A, C, B3, FOLATE; CALCIUM, POTASSIUM; ZINC

✓ ANTI-CANCER, ANTIOXIDANT

Butterhead lettuce (*Lactuca sativa sp.*) improves oxygen transport in the blood and aids liver function and wound healing. It also helps to regulate blood-fat levels and maintain the strength of the heart, nerves and muscles.

**RECIPES** *provençal mesclun salad (page 259)*

### CAULIFLOWER

★ VITAMINS C, B3, B5, B6; PHOSPHORUS, POTASSIUM; ZINC; GLUCOSINOLATES; FIBRE, PROTEIN

✓ ANTI-ALLERGIC, ANTI-CANCER, ANTIOXIDANT, ANTI-STRESS

SEE GLOSSARY FOR INFORMATION ON GLUCOSINOLATES

Cauliflower (*Brassica oleracea botrytis*) encourages antibody and haemoglobin production and protects against allergy, asthma, migraine and depression. It improves the health of the skin and mucous membranes, helps maintain energy levels and regulates blood-fat concentration.

**RECIPES** *creamy cauliflower soup (page 245), green lentil salad (page 260)*

### FLORENCE FENNEL

★ VITAMIN B3, FOLATE; POTASSIUM; ZINC; VOLATILE OILS, BITTER PRINCIPLES; FIBRE

✓ ANTI-INFLAMMATORY, CARMINATIVE, DIURETIC, CIRCULATORY STIMULANT

Fennel (*Foeniculum vulgare dulce*) is an important remedy for digestive upsets. It also helps regulate blood-fat levels and maintains the health of the heart, muscles, skin, mucous membranes and nerves.

**RECIPES** *black-eye bean and wild marjoram soup (page 245), florence fennel salad (page 260), green party (page 264)*

### GLOBE ARTICHOKE

★ VITAMINS B3, B5, BIOTIN, FOLATE; ZINC; BITTER PRINCIPLE; PROTEIN

✓ ANTI-ALLERGIC, ANTI-STRESS

Globe artichoke (*Cynara scolymus*) stimulates the appetite and enhances liver function. It is a good source of energy, which improves the health of the skin, hair, bone marrow, mucous membranes and nervous system and helps regulate blood-fat levels.

**RECIPES** *artichoke hearts, broad beans and shiitake (page 252), paella (page 252), artichoke salad (page 259)*

### MUSTARD CRESS

★ VITAMINS A, C, B3, FOLATE; CALCIUM; IRON, ZINC; GLUCOSINOLATES, SULPHUR, VOLATILE OIL; FIBRE

✓ ANTI-ALLERGIC, ANTIBACTERIAL, ANTI-CANCER, ANTIOXIDANT, STIMULANT

! LARGE QUANTITIES OF MUSTARD CRESS CAN CAUSE DIGESTIVE UPSET BECAUSE OF THE SULPHUR AND MUSTARD OIL CONTENT

SEE GLOSSARY FOR INFORMATION ON GLUCOSINOLATES

Mustard cress (*Brassica hirta*) improves iron absorption, oxygen transport and wound healing, and helps balance blood-fat levels. It is also good for the heart, liver, nerves, skin and muscles.

**RECIPES** *provençal mesclun salad (page 259)*

### NASTURTIUM

★ VITAMIN C; GLUCOSINOLATES, VOLATILE OIL

✓ ANTIBACTERIAL, ANTIMICROBIAL, ANTIOXIDANT, ANTIVIRAL

SEE GLOSSARY FOR INFORMATION ON GLUCOSINOLATES

Nasturtium (*Tropaeolum majus*) leaves and flowers are powerful natural antibiotics and are particularly useful in relieving respiratory-tract infections such as bronchitis, influenza and colds.

**RECIPES** *green leafy salad (page 181), toasted tempeh with herb salad (page 248), tropical sunshine salad (page 261)*

### RADICCHIO

★ VITAMINS B2, B3; POTASSIUM; ANTHOCYANIN, BITTER PRINCIPLES; FIBRE

✓ ANTI-CANCER, ANTIOXIDANT

Eating radicchio (*Cichorium var.*) helps the body maximize energy release from food and prevents cholesterol buildup and the formation of blood clots.

**RECIPES** *orange mango salad (page 260)*

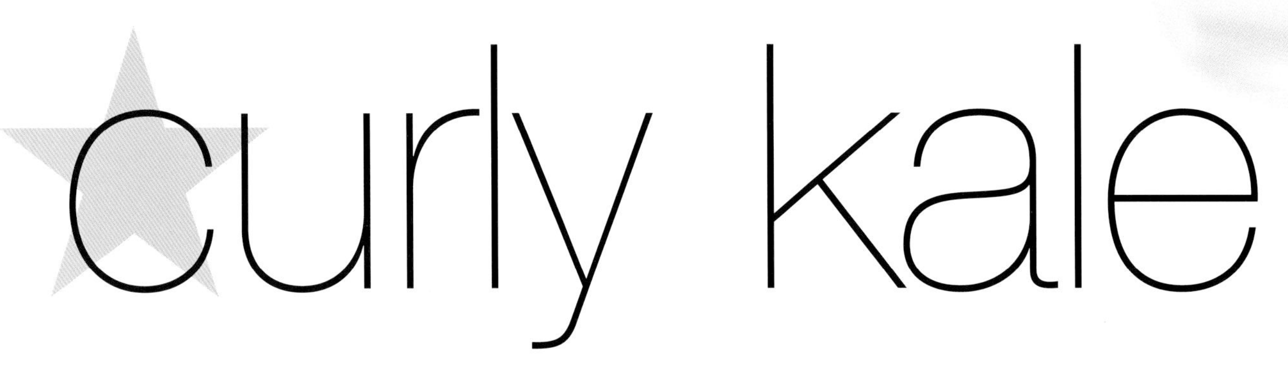


**CURLY KALE IS A MEMBER OF THE BRASSICA FAMILY, WHICH INCLUDES CABBAGE, BROCCOLI AND BRUSSELS SPROUTS. IT IS PACKED WITH VITAMINS, MINERALS AND PHYTOCHEMICALS THAT GUARD AGAINST BACTERIAL AND VIRAL INFECTION, HEART DISEASE AND CANCER.**

## The origin of curly kale

Curly kale (*Brassica oleracea acephala*) is also known as "Borecole", from the Dutch word "Boerenkool" meaning "peasants' cabbage." It is derived from the wild cabbage (*Brassica oleracea*), which is a native of southwestern Europe and the Mediterranean region and grows on seaside cliffs. Opinions differ over when the wild cabbage was first cultivated (estimates range from a few hundred to thousands of years ago!) but it has been developed into a number of edible varieties.

Other members of the cabbage family form "heads" but curly kale retains its ancestral shape – leaves set loosely on a stem. The leaves are blue-green and, as the name implies, curly and crimped. Although kale and the other edible brassicas originated in temperate zones, they are now cultivated all over the world.

A characteristic of the brassicas is that they hold a lot of water in their leaves, making them fleshy and succulent foods. Like other members of the family, curly kale is a biennial – it grows for two years, storing a large amount of nutrients in its leaves. We can benefit from this nourishment only if the leaves are harvested during its first year. In its second (final) year, the plant will use the stored nutrients to produce flowers and seed.

## Immune-boosting properties

Curly kale is a valuable winter vegetable, highly nutritious and rich in vitamins, minerals and protective phytochemicals. It is one of the tastiest of the cabbage family and easily overwinters to provide important nutrients when little else is growing in temperate regions. Its phytochemicals facilitate oxygen transport to the tissues, support the immune system, aid liver function, and play a part in controlling blood-fat levels, and helping the body to release and utilize the energy contained in food. Curly kale thus promotes the health of the heart, nerves and muscles and protects against high blood pressure, vascular disease and rheumatoid arthritis.

Curly kale is good for the skin, encourages wound healing and the maintenance of healthy cell membranes, and may protect against oestrogen-linked cancers such as those of the breast and ovaries. It helps regulate protein and fat metabolism and, because of its vitamin K content, encourages normal blood clotting. It also improves iron absorption from food and facilitates the production of haemoglobin and red blood cells. It may offer protection against asthma, migraine and depression, and aid the nervous system.

## Packed with protection

Curly kale contains three important groups of protective phytochemicals: glucosinolates, bioflavonoids and sterols (phenylpropanoids). Glucosinolates include indoles, dithiolthiones, sulphoraphane and isothiocyanates. Indoles, in particular, protect against various carcinogens. They also help reduce the activity of oestrogen in the body and therefore have a dual role in protecting against oestrogen-related cancers.

Bioflavonoids stimulate the immune system. They chelate (combine with) metals and make blood platelets less sticky, thus protecting against abnormal blood clotting and preventing heart disease.

Sterols influence the absorption of cholesterol from food and its metabolism in the body. They also affect the production of steroid hormones.

## IMMUNE-BOOSTING PROFILE

★ VITAMINS A, C, E, K, B2, B3, B6, FOLATE; CALCIUM, MAGNESIUM, PHOSPHORUS, POTASSIUM, MANGANESE; IRON, ZINC; BIOFLAVONOIDS, GLUCOSINOLATES, KAEMPFEROL, STEROLS; FIBRE, PROTEIN

✓ ANTI-ALLERGIC, ANTI-CANCER, ANTIOXIDANT, DETOXIFYING, IMMUNO-STIMULANT

SEE GLOSSARY FOR INFORMATION ON GLUCOSINOLATES

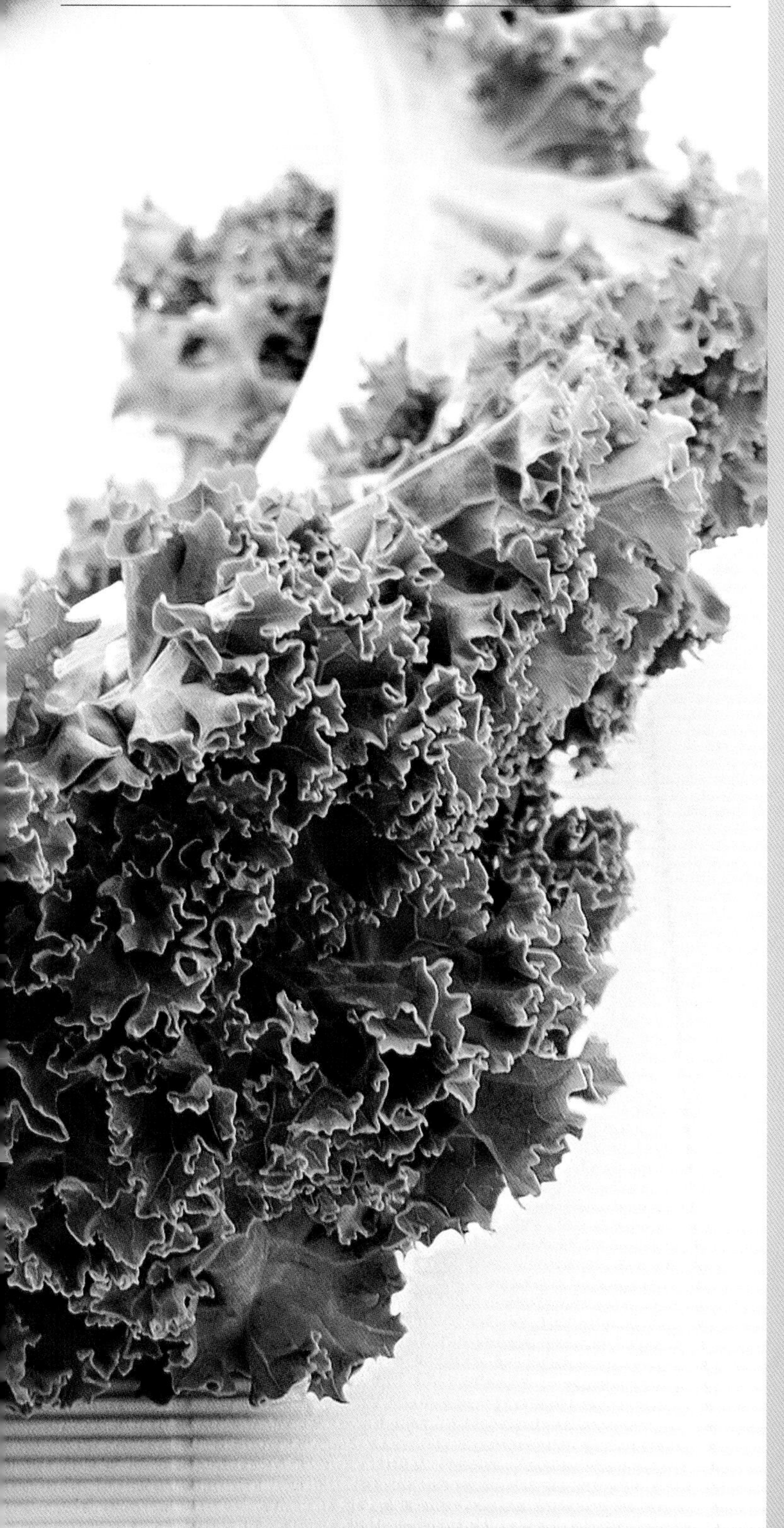

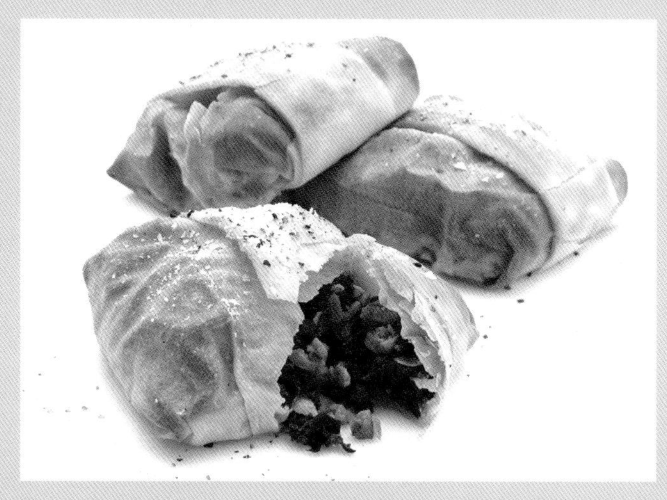

## curly kale parcels *(above)*

2 tbsp olive oil
450 g curly kale, chopped
250 g tempeh, cut into small cubes
1 tbsp soy sauce
2 garlic cloves, finely chopped
1 onion, finely chopped
1 tsp turmeric
1 tsp cumin
Pinch of cayenne
Salt and pepper to taste
1 packet filo pastry

Stir-fry the curly kale in the oil for 2 minutes. Add the next 8 ingredients one by one, stirring in between. Add a little water and simmer gently for 5 minutes (until the kale is soft). Open out sheets of filo pastry (as many as you have filling for), brush with oil and place a generous portion of filling in the middle of each one. Fold each sheet into a parcel. Brush each parcel with oil and bake at 220°C/gas mark 7, until golden.

## curly kale, tomato & broad beans

3 tbsp olive oil
1 red onion, chopped
900 g fresh broad beans, shelled
500 g lb curly kale, chopped
500 g tomatoes, in wedges
4 garlic cloves, finely chopped
Salt and pepper to taste
2 tbsp lemon juice
2 spring onions, chopped

Heat the oil gently in a deep saucepan. Sauté the onion for 2 minutes, add the beans and cook for 5 minutes. Add the curly kale and the tomatoes and stir-fry for 2 minutes, then add the garlic and salt and pepper. Add enough water to cover, bring to the boil and simmer for 30 minutes (or until all the liquid is reduced). Add lemon juice, adjust seasoning, garnish with spring onions and serve with couscous.

## green leafy salad

1 handful of fresh curly kale, finely chopped
1 handful of iceberg lettuce, shredded
1 handful of lamb's lettuce
1 small handful of parsley sprigs, finely chopped
1 small handful of fresh mint, finely chopped
1 small handful of nasturtium flowers and marigold (calendula) petals (optional)
Lemon tahini dressing (see page 251)

Mix the green leaves in a bowl. Decorate with the flowers. Pour the dressing over and mix gently. Serve with bread or cooked bulgur.

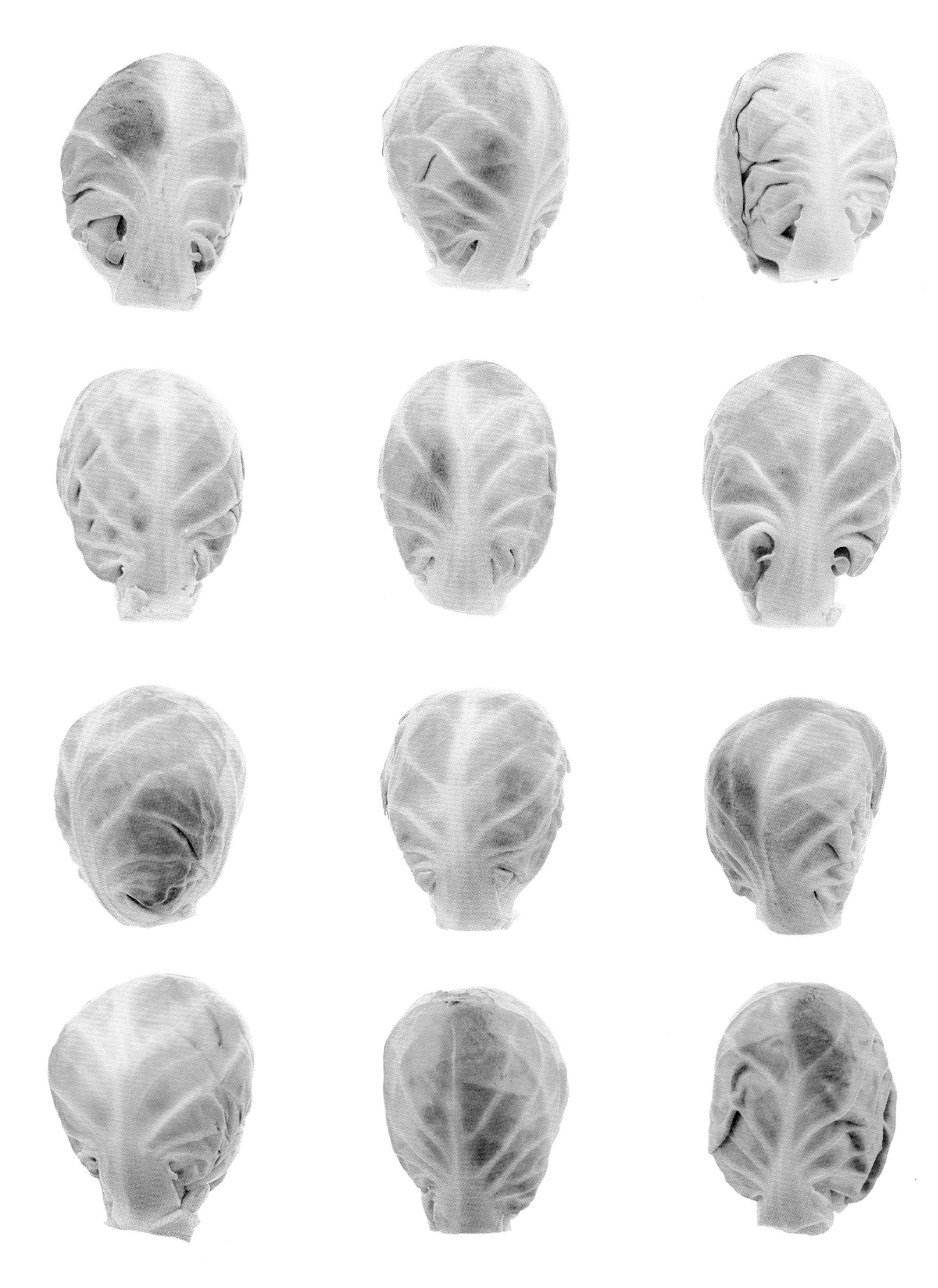

## ROCKET

★ VITAMINS A, C; BITTER PRINCIPLE, VOLATILE OIL; FIBRE

✓ ANTI-CANCER, ANTISCORBUTIC, ANTIOXIDANT

Rocket (*Eruca sativa*) keeps the skin in good condition, and improves immunity and wound healing as well as helping the body to maintain healthy blood-fat levels.

**RECIPES** *shiitake salad (page 215), rocket salad (page 259), sweetcorn and sun-dried tomato salad (page 260), green party (page 264), vegetable cocktail (page 267)*

## SAVOY CABBAGE

★ VITAMINS A, C, B3, FOLATE; CALCIUM, POTASSIUM; IRON; GLUCOSINOLATES; FIBRE, PROTEIN

✓ ANTI-CANCER, ANTIOXIDANT, ENERGY-BOOSTING

SEE GLOSSARY FOR INFORMATION ON GLUCOSINOLATES

Savoy cabbage (*Brassica oleracea capitata*) aids the liver's detoxifying capabilities and improves oxygen transport in the blood and tissues. It is a good source of vitamin B3, which boosts energy and strength, and helps keep the heart, muscles, skin, mucous membranes and nerves healthy.

**RECIPES** *garlic and savoy cabbage (page 209)*

## SPINACH

★ VITAMINS A, E, B2, B3, FOLATE; CALCIUM, MAGNESIUM, MANGANESE, POTASSIUM; ZINC; CAROTENOIDS, OXALIC ACID; FIBRE, PROTEIN

✓ ANTI-CANCER, ANTIOXIDANT, ANTIVIRAL, IMMUNO-STIMULANT

! FOODS CONTAINING OXALIC ACID ARE BEST AVOIDED IF YOU SUFFER FROM KIDNEY OR BLADDER STONES, OR RHEUMATOID ARTHRITIS

Spinach (*Spinacia oleracea*) originated in Iran and spread east via China, Korea and Japan. It reached Spain with the Arabs in the 11th century and was being used throughout Europe by the 18th century. It stimulates the immune response and helps protect against heart disease and some cancers, particularly of the lung, breast and cervix, as well as keeping the skin, mucous membranes, blood, muscles and nerves in good condition. It is a good source of energy, aids normal liver function and regulates blood-fat levels.

**RECIPES** *spinach bouillabaisse (page 255), sweet potato curry (page 256), tomato cocktail (page 267)*

## SPRING GREENS

★ VITAMINS A, C, B2, B3, B5, FOLATE; CALCIUM, PHOSPHORUS, POTASSIUM; IRON, ZINC; GLUCOSINOLATES; PROTEIN, FIBRE

✓ ANTI-ALLERGIC, ANTI-CANCER, ANTIOXIDANT, ANTI-STRESS, DETOXIFYING, ENERGY-BOOSTING, WOUND HEALING

SEE GLOSSARY FOR INFORMATION ON GLUCOSINOLATES

Spring greens (*Brassica oleracea var.*) evolved from wild cabbage, which is a native of southwestern Europe and the Mediterranean region. They support the liver's detoxifying action and enhance the action of the immune system as a whole. Spring greens help protect against cancer and help maintain the health of the heart, skin, mucous membranes and nerves, and maintain energy levels.

**RECIPES** *spring greens and macadamia nuts (page 258)*

## SWISS CHARD

★ VITAMINS A, C, FOLATE; POTASSIUM; IRON

✓ ANTI-CANCER, ANTIOXIDANT

Also known as "seakale-beet", Swiss chard (*Beta vulgaris cycla*) is closely related to beetroot and spinach beet. It increases natural resistance by supporting oxygen transport via the blood to nerves, muscles and liver, and helps in the regulation of blood-fat levels.

**RECIPES** *swiss chard and juniper berries (page 259)*

## WATERCRESS

★ VITAMINS A, C, E, B3, B6; CALCIUM, MANGANESE; IRON; GLUCOSINOLATES, VOLATILE OIL; PROTEIN, FIBRE

✓ ANTI-CANCER, ANTIOXIDANT, ANTISCORBUTIC, EXPECTORANT, PURGATIVE

! EXCESSIVE INTAKE OF WATERCRESS MAY CAUSE KIDNEY PROBLEMS AND SHOULD BE AVOIDED IN THOSE WITH KIDNEY DISEASE

SEE GLOSSARY FOR INFORMATION ON GLUCOSINOLATES

Traditionally used in spring cures to stimulate metabolism and aid detoxification, watercress (*Nasturtium officinale*) was once considered a specific cure for tuberculosis. Nowadays, the principal medicinal use of watercress is in the relief of arthritic conditions and congestion problems affecting the upper respiratory tract. Watercress stimulates the immune and lymphatic systems.

**RECIPES** *baked beetroot salad (page 177), grapefruit salad (page 189), avocado, watercress and cumin salad (page 193), green lentil salad (page 260), chinese salad (page 260)*

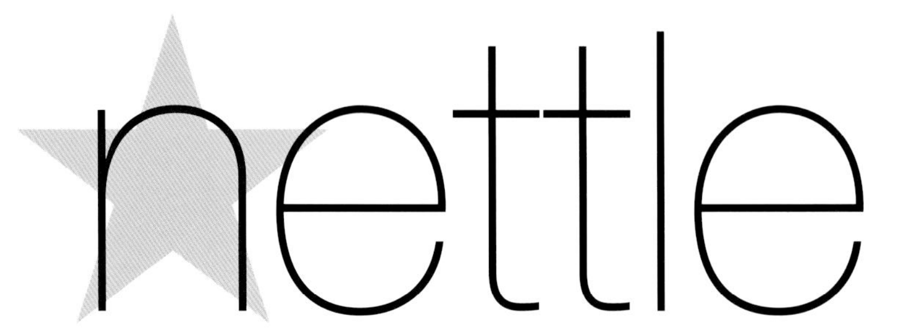

# nettle

**THE NETTLE MAY BE JUST A HUMBLE WEED, BUT IT IS PACKED WITH NUTRIENTS THAT STRENGTHEN THE IMMUNE SYSTEM AND FORTIFY THE BODY AGAINST DISEASE. THIS VERSATILE PLANT CAN ALSO ENRICH AND PURIFY THE BLOOD TO HELP ALLEVIATE CIRCULATORY DISORDERS.**

## The origin of nettle

The nettle (*Urtica dioica*) is one of the world's commonest weeds. It quickly colonizes any piece of reasonably fertile and well-watered land, and is found in fields, gardens, woodland and wasteground throughout the world's temperate zones. Being a "greedy" plant, the nettle stores up large quantities of vital nutrients that promote health and restock depleted tissues and body systems. This makes nettle a fortifying remedy that strengthens the whole body.

## Immune-boosting properties

In immunodeficiency states, chronic degenerative diseases, and cancer, nettle has a unique ability to revitalize and replenish, helping the body to cope better in difficult circumstances, and providing many of the building blocks necessary for health and healing. As a gentle but efficient diuretic, nettle can be very effective in the management of disorders of the heart and circulation, helping to rid the body of excess fluid while toning up blood-vessel walls. It has a beneficial effect on the kidneys, enhancing their ability to excrete uric acid and so relieving gout (which is caused by excess uric acid in the tissues and joints). The nettle's ability to cleanse the body of accumulated waste also promotes the healing of chronic skin problems such as eczema. Being rich in iron, nettle is a useful treatment for anaemia.

## Using nettle

Nettle tea has been used for centuries as a blood purifier and "spring tonic", and is an excellent aid during convalescence from illness. As both a circulatory stimulant and a diuretic, it is a powerful aid to detox and thus helpful in the management of arthritis, urinary-tract disorders and skin problems such as psoriasis. Cold nettle tea is a useful external remedy for the relief of burns and minor wounds. The green tips of the plant can be used fresh or dried. For drying, it is best to pick the young shoots on a fine morning, after the sun has dried the dew. The young tips can be harvested almost all year round to provide a nutritious, healing and tasty addition to any diet. Pick and wash the nettle tops. Boil them in a little water for about 10 minutes, then remove them with a slotted spoon (preserve the liquid for use as a stock or a medicine). Chop finely and use with other vegetables in soups, stews and pasta sauces. As a side dish, precooked nettles are delicious stir-fried with leeks, garlic, salt and pepper. They can also be used as a substitute for spinach (although they need a little more cooking water). Cooked nettles have a full-bodied flavour. Try nettle lasagne, using cooked nettles and lentils for the filling instead of meat.

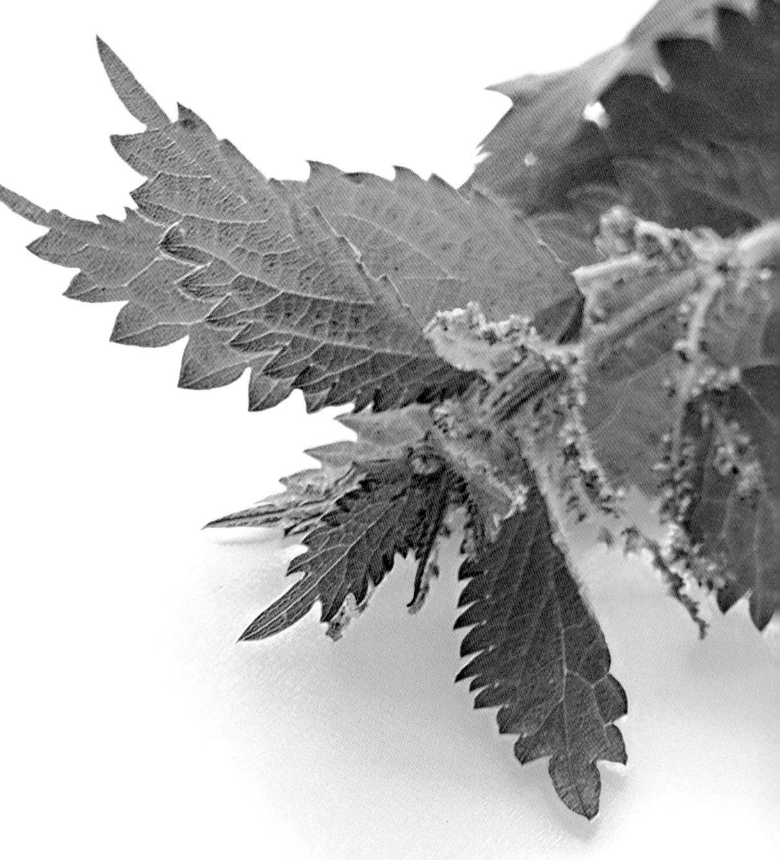

## IMMUNE-BOOSTING PROFILE

★ VITAMINS A, C, K, B1, B2, B3, B5; CALCIUM, MAGNESIUM, PHOSPHATE, PHOSPHORUS, POTASSIUM; BORON, BROMINE, COPPER, IRON, SELENIUM, SILICA, ZINC; ACETYLCHOLINE, CHLOROPHYLL, FORMIC ACID, LYCOPENE, GLUCOQUINONE, HISTAMINE, SEROTONIN, TANNIN; FIBRE, OMEGA-3, -6 AND OLEIC FATTY ACIDS

✓ ANTI-CANCER, ANTI-INFLAMMATORY, ANTIOXIDANT, ASTRINGENT, CIRCULATORY STIMULANT, DETOXIFYING, DIURETIC, LOWERS BLOOD SUGAR, TONIC

! USE GLOVES WHEN HANDLING THE FRESH PLANT; NETTLE SHOULD NOT BE EATEN UNCOOKED

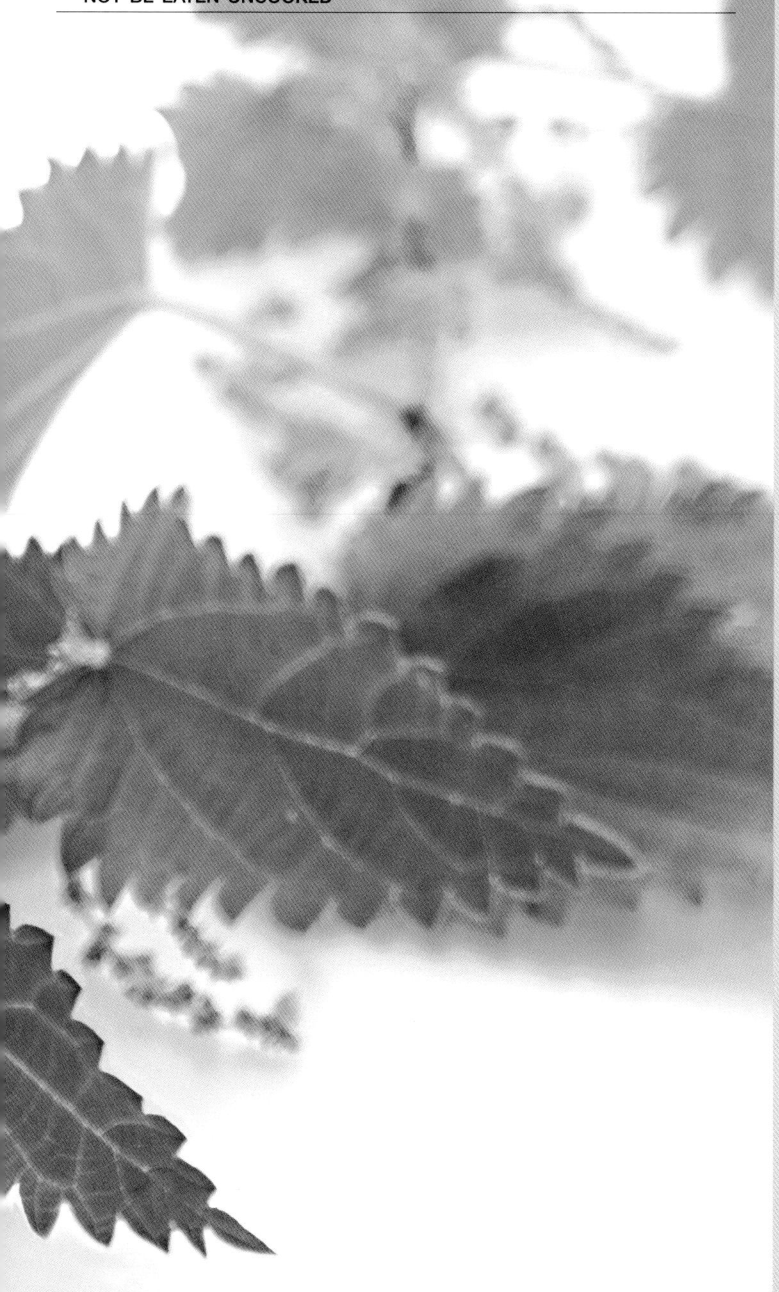

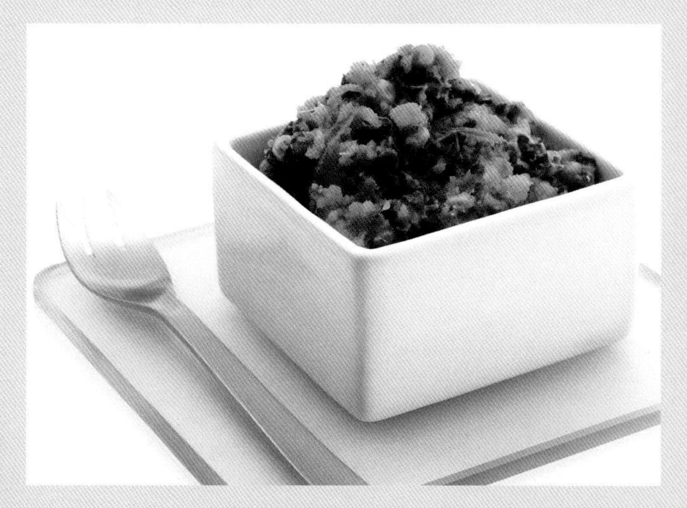

## nettle and sweet potato mash *(above)*

500 g sweet potatoes, peeled and chopped
250 g fresh nettle tips
3 tbsp olive oil
1 red onion, sliced
200 g green peas
Sea salt and freshly ground black pepper, to taste

Pick and wash the nettles (wearing gloves). Boil the sweet potatoes in lightly salted water until soft. Mash and set aside. Boil the nettles in a little water until soft. Remove from water and chop. Heat the oil in a pan or wok and stir-fry the onion until soft. Add the peas, then the nettles and the sweet potato. Mix well, season, and serve hot.

## spiced nettle soup

250 g fresh nettle tips
2 tbsp olive oil
½ tsp cayenne
1 tsp turmeric
1 bay leaf
1 garlic clove, chopped
1 leek, chopped
2 potatoes, chopped into cubes
1 carrot, chopped
1 parsley root or parsnip, chopped
2 tbsp flour
1½ litres diluted basic vegetable stock (*see page 244*)
Sea salt and freshly ground black pepper, to taste

Pick and wash the nettles (wearing gloves). Steam in a little water until soft, then chop finely. Heat the oil gently in a big saucepan. Add the spices, stir for ½ minute, then add the vegetables. Stir-fry for a few minutes, but don't let them brown. Sprinkle with the flour at low heat, mix well and add the stock. Bring to the boil and simmer for 10–15 minutes, then add the nettles (together with their cooking water). Heat through and simmer for another 5 minutes. Season and serve.

## nettle and lime tisane

2 fresh nettle tips or 1 tsp dried nettle
1 cup boiling water
1 thick slice of lime

Wearing gloves, place the nettle in a tea filter in a large cup or mug. Add the boiling water and the lime. Leave to infuse, covered with a lid, for 5 minutes.

# SWEET FRUITS

## APPLE

★ VITAMIN C; POTASSIUM; MALIC ACID, TANNIN, VOLATILE OIL; FIBRE, PECTIN, SUGARS

✓ DETOXIFYING, LOWERS CHOLESTEROL

Apples (*Malus domestica*) stimulate the secretion of digestive juices and aid protein digestion. They contain pectin, which binds with cholesterol and bile acids, enhancing their excretion from the body. The pectin makes apples a remedy for simple diarrhoea. Apples protect the body against the effects of some environmental toxins.

**RECIPES** *yoghurt with fruit (page 243), baked apples (page 262), beetroot and apple (page 264), guava and apple (page 266)*

## APRICOT (FRESH AND DRIED)

★ VITAMINS A, B2, B3, B5; CALCIUM, MAGNESIUM, POTASSIUM; COPPER, IRON, ZINC; FIBRE, SUGARS

✓ ANTIOXIDANT, DETOXIFYING, IMMUNO-STIMULANT

! BRIGHT-ORANGE DRIED APRICOTS HAVE BEEN TREATED WITH SULPHUR AND SHOULD BE AVOIDED

Apricots (*Prunus armeniaca*) promote detoxification and waste elimination. They also contribute to efficient antibody production. Apricots help stabilize blood-sugar levels, keep muscles, nerves, enzymes and hormones working properly, facilitate the release of energy from food and tissue stores, and enhance the transport of oxygen in the blood.

**RECIPES** *muesli (page 243), fruity pancakes (page 243), apricot and ginger (page 264), nirvana (page 267), soft tutti fruity (page 267)*

## BANANA

★ VITAMINS C, B3, B5, B6, BIOTIN; MAGNESIUM, MANGANESE, POTASSIUM; FIBRE, SUGARS

✓ ANTI-STRESS, ENERGY-BOOSTING, DIGESTIVE STIMULANT

Bananas (*Musa cavendishii*) help prevent high blood pressure, heart disease, cancer and rheumatoid arthritis. They enhance the metabolism of protein, carbohydrate and fats, stabilize blood-sugar levels, and promote healthy skin, hair, nerves and bone marrow. Easy to digest, they are useful in the management of gastro-intestinal disorders.

**RECIPES** *baked apples (page 262), blackberry cream (page 264), caribbean smoothie (page 264), creamy mango (page 264)*

## CANTALOUPE MELON

★ VITAMINS A, C, B3; CAROTENOIDS; SUGARS

✓ ANTIOXIDANT

With its high level of carotenoids, cantaloupe melon (*Cucumis melo cantalupensis*) may inhibit the growth of cancer cells, and also help maintain vitality. It aids wound healing, and helps maintain the health of all body tissues, including the skin. It also enhances release of energy from other foods.

**RECIPES:** *ruby red melon salad (page 242), mint and melon soup (page 245), melon and orange (page 266)*

## GRAPE

★ VITAMINS B3, B6, BIOTIN; MAGNESIUM, PHOSPHORUS; COPPER, IRON, SELENIUM, ZINC; ANTHOCYANIN, TARTARIC ACID; SUGARS

✓ ANTI-INFLAMMATORY, ANTIOXIDANT, DETOXIFYING

Fresh grapes (*Vitis vinifera*) and dried grapes (sultanas, raisins and currants), are "biological response modifiers" – inhibiting the action of allergens, viruses and carcinogens. They also act as free-radical scavengers, making them ideal detoxifiers, particularly of the skin, liver, kidneys and bowels. (See traditional grape fast – page 273.)

**RECIPES** *fresh fruit salad (page 242), porridge with dried fruit and quinoa (page 242), grape and raisin smoothie (page 267)*

## GUAVA

★ VITAMINS A, C, B3; FIBRE, SUGARS

✓ ANTIOXIDANT, DETOXIFYING, IMMUNO-STIMULANT

Guava (*Psidium guajava*) is an excellent natural antioxidant, combining vitamins A and C, which mop up free radicals before they can do the body harm. It has a major role to play in serious immunodeficiency disorders, heart disease and cancer, as well as reducing the severity of autoimmune diseases.

**RECIPES** *fruity pancakes (page 243), guava and apple (page 266)*

## KIWI (CHINESE GOOSEBERRY)

★ VITAMINS A, C, B3; FIBRE, SUGARS

✓ ANTIOXIDANT

An advantage of kiwi fruit (*Actinidia chinensis*) is that it keeps well for a long time after harvesting with little loss of its nutritional value – even after 6 months' storage, 90 per cent of the vitamin C is still intact. Kiwi fruits encourage the health and repair of all body tissues and promote the release of the energy from other foods.

**RECIPES** *fresh fruit salad (page 242), tropical fruit salad (page 263)*

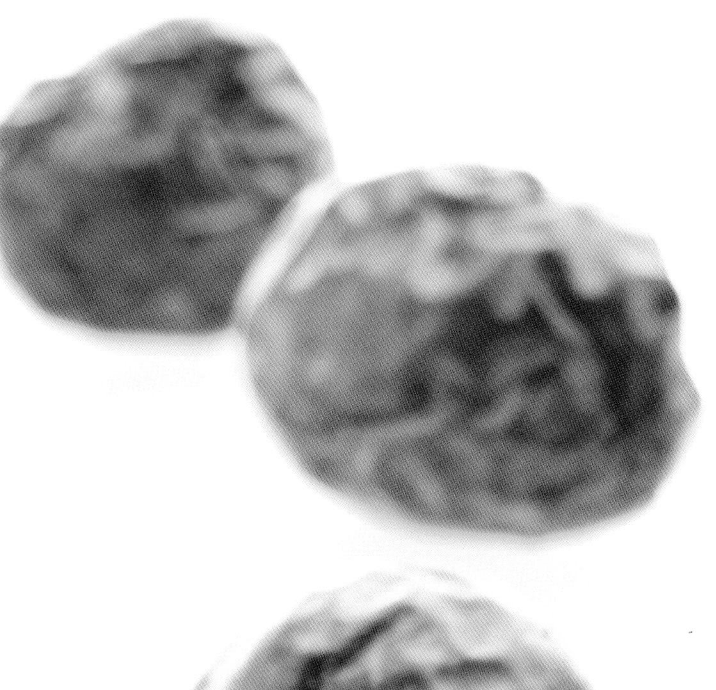

## MANGO

★ VITAMINS A, C, E, B3; CITRIC ACID, PAPAIN; FIBRE, SUGARS

✓ ANTI-ALLERGIC, ANTIBACTERIAL, ANTI-CANCER, ANTIOXIDANT, DETOXIFYING, ENERGY-BOOSTING, IMMUNO-STIMULANT

! IN RARE CASES, MAY CAUSE DERMATITIS

Mango (*Mangifera indica*) stimulates the immune system and helps protect mucous membranes from pathogens. Mango contains papain, a protein-digesting enzyme that may help anyone suffering gluten intolerance or wheat allergy.

**RECIPES** *creamy mango (page 264), mango and lime (page 266)*

## PAPAYA (PAW-PAW)

★ VITAMINS A, C; CAROTENOIDS, PAPAIN; FIBRE, SUGARS

✓ ANTI-ALLERGIC, ANTIBACTERIAL, ANTIOXIDANT, DETOXIFYING

Papaya (*Carica papaya*) can help prevent skin disorders, gastro-intestinal ulcers, pancreatic disorders, cancer and other conditions related to dysfunctional immunity. The papain in papaya promotes the breakdown of protein and can play an important role in alleviating digestive disorders and detoxifying the body.

**RECIPES** *fresh fruit salad (page 242), papaya power (page 267)*

## PASSION-FRUIT

★ VITAMINS A, C, B2, B3; MAGNESIUM, PHOSPHORUS; IRON, ZINC; CITRIC ACID; FIBRE, SUGARS

✓ ANTI-ALLERGY, ANTI-CANCER, ANTIOXIDANT

Passion-fruit (*Passiflora edulis*) helps ensure healthy nerves, skin and mucous membranes, boosts energy levels, relieves muscle cramps and alleviates insomnia and depression.

**RECIPES** *passion-fruit sorbet (page 262), height of passion (page 266), passion and lime (page 267)*

## PINEAPPLE

★ CALCIUM, MAGNESIUM, MANGANESE, PHOSPHORUS, POTASSIUM; COPPER, IRON, ZINC; BROMELAIN, CITRIC ACID; FIBRE, SUGARS

✓ ANTI-CANCER, ANTI-INFLAMMATORY

Pineapple (*Ananas comosus*) modifies the body's inflammatory response, speeds up tissue repair and alleviates fluid retention. It aids digestion, helps prevent blood clots and atherosclerosis, relieves angina and lowers blood pressure.

**RECIPES** *piña colada (page 267), pink pineapple (page 267)*

# grapefruit

**GRAPEFRUIT IS A POWERFUL DETOXIFIER, HELPING TO RID THE BODY OF HARMFUL MICROBES AND STRENGTHENING THE IMMUNE SYSTEM AGAINST FURTHER ATTACK. IT MAY ALSO AID TISSUE REPAIR AND HELP RESIST THE GROWTH OF TUMOURS.**

## The origin of grapefruit

Grapefruit (*Citrus paradisi*) is thought to have originated in Jamaica, possibly as a mutation of the pomelo (*Citrus maxima*), or as a hybrid between the pomelo and the sweet orange (*Citrus sinensis*). By 1750 it had become popular throughout the West Indies, and its fame then spread rapidly to the American mainland and the rest of the world. Depending on the variety, grapefruits are lemon-yellow or orange-yellow when ripe, with a juicy, fragrant, light yellow, pink or ruby-red pulp, and a distinct sweet-sharp acid flavour. When buying grapefruits, choose ones that feel heavy for their size, with firm, shiny skin. Avoid very soft or dull-coloured fruits. The nutritional content varies with type and colour. Fruits with ruby-red and pink pulp contain more vitamin A than yellow ones.

## Immune-boosting properties

Grapefruit is a natural detoxifier, acting on the digestive system and liver. Its detoxifying action, combined with a strong growth-inhibiting effect on bacteria, fungi, parasites and viruses, means that grapefruit can be beneficial in immunodeficiency states, as well as for colds and flu. Grapefruit contains a wealth of protective phytochemicals that enhance immunity and wound healing, and may inhibit tumour growth. Although citrus fruits in general are best avoided by those suffering from autoimmune disorders, there is evidence that grapefruit improves some inflammatory conditions.

Grapefruit is an effective pick-me-up when stress takes its toll on energy levels. It also aids healing by strengthening bones, blood vessels and other tissues. The soluble fibre in grapefruit helps lower blood cholesterol (and other blood fats) by binding with excess cholesterol and bile acids and promoting their excretion from the body. This makes it useful in the prevention and treatment of heart and artery disease and gallstones. By aiding digestion and waste elimination, grapefruit relieves constipation. The fruit also inhibits the formation of calcium oxalate kidney stones by reducing the amount of calcium salts in the urine.

Grapefruit boosts fat metabolism, which explains its popularity as a "fat burning" aid in weight-loss diets. An average serving of grapefruit is less than 100 calories and yet its high fibre content helps satisfy hunger. Its bitter principles aid the digestion of other foods, thus enabling dieters to gain maximum nutritional value from their meals, while keeping their appetite under control.

Citricidal – grapefruit seed extract – is a natural, broad-spectrum antimicrobial agent active against streptococci, staphylococci, salmonella, mycobacteria and other pathogens. Grapefruit oil is a powerful astringent and antiseptic that can be used to cleanse oily skin and as a gentle treatment for acne and other minor skin conditions.

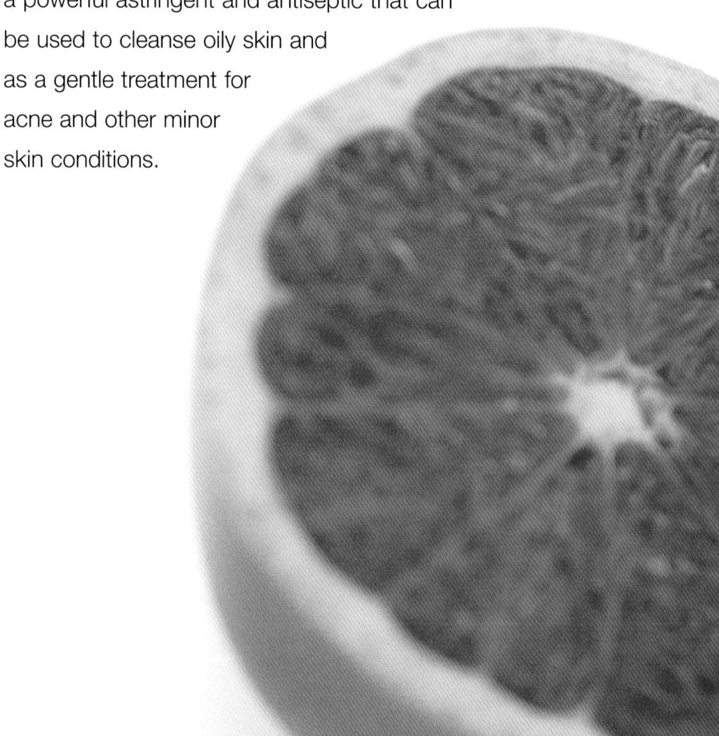

## IMMUNE-BOOSTING PROFILE

★ VITAMINS A, C, FOLATE; POTASSIUM; BITTER PRINCIPLE, BIOFLAVONOIDS, CITRIC AND PHENOLIC ACIDS, LYCOPENE; FIBRE, PECTIN, SUGARS

✓ ANTI-ALLERGIC, ANTI-CANCER, ANTIMICROBIAL, ANTIOXIDANT, LOWERS BLOOD PRESSURE, LOWERS CHOLESTEROL LEVELS, DETOXIFYING, DIGESTIVE STIMULANT, IMMUNO-STIMULANT

! GRAPEFRUIT JUICE MAY INTERACT WITH SOME PRESCRIBED DRUGS SO CHECK WITH YOUR MEDICAL PRACTITIONER IF YOU ARE TAKING ANY MEDICINES

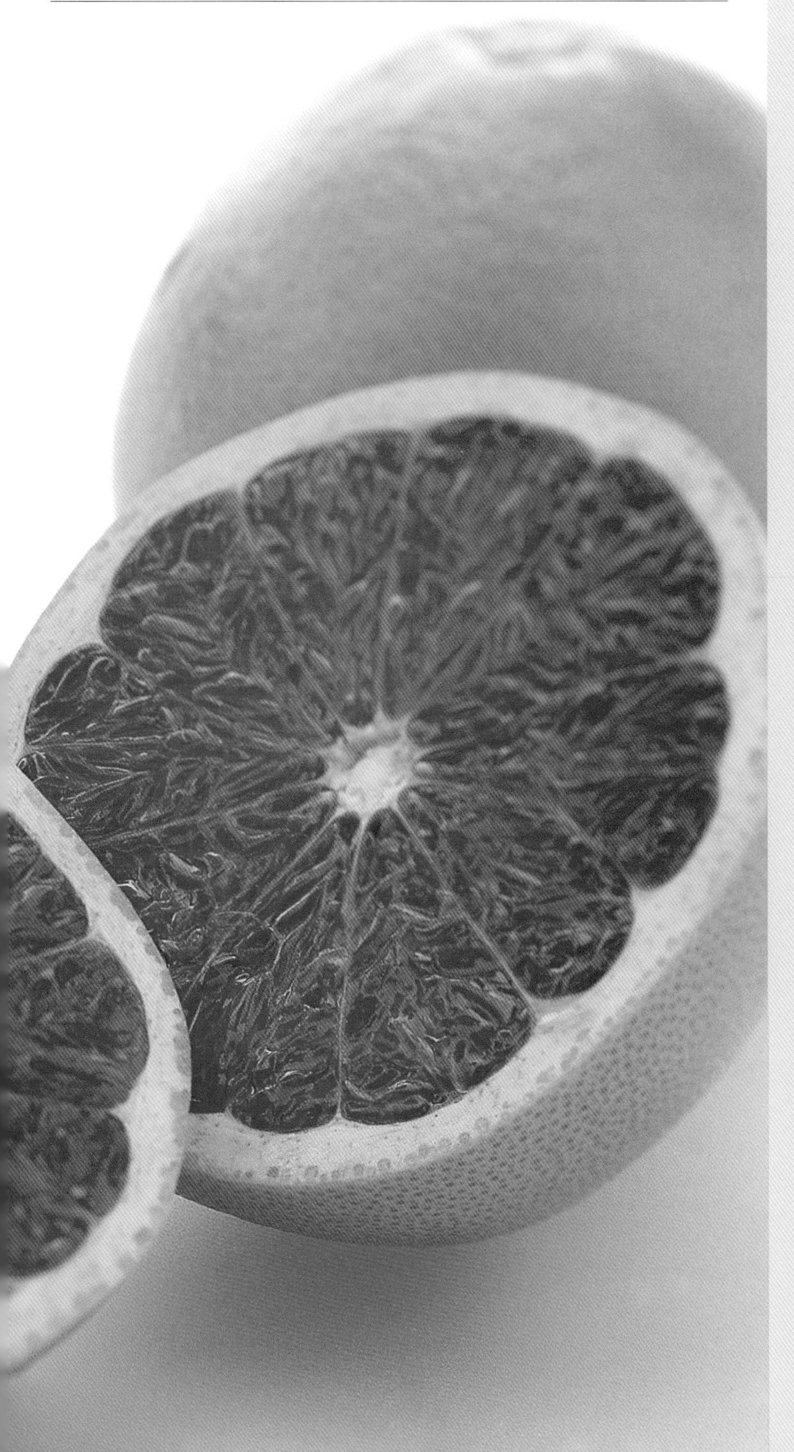

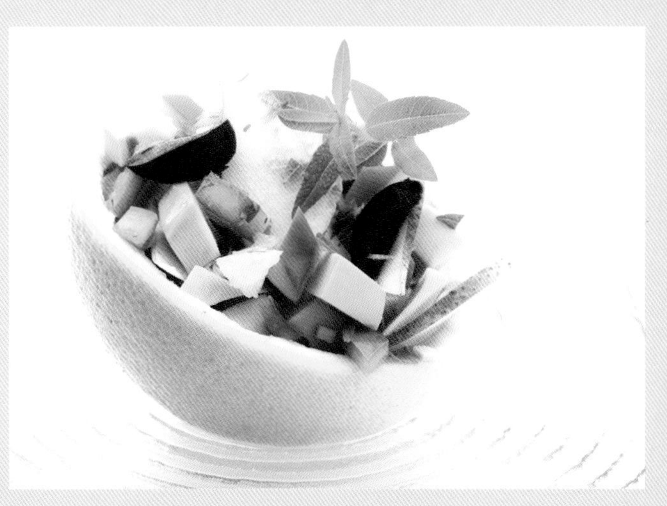

## stuffed grapefruit *(above)*

2 grapefruits, halved, flesh removed and chopped
1 avocado, stoned and peeled, in cubes
2½-cm cube of fresh ginger root, finely chopped
1 pear, core removed, in cubes
1 small green pepper, deseeded, finely chopped
To garnish: 2 black olives,stoned, 2 tbsp fresh lemon balm, finely chopped

Mix the grapefruit flesh with the avocado, ginger, pear and green pepper. Divide the filling between the two half shells. Garnish with olives and lemon balm.

## grapefruit and peppermint fizz

1 bunch of fresh peppermint
500 ml boiling water
2 tbsp maple syrup
2 ruby-red grapefruits
1 lime

Put the mint in a teapot or bowl, pour the boiling water over and then leave to infuse for 5 minutes. Add the maple syrup and leave to cool. Squeeze the grapefruit and the lime and divide the juice between four tall glasses. Add the peppermint infusion when cool. Serve with ice.

## grapefruit salad

1 grapefruit, peeled and cut into segments
1 avocado, peeled, stoned and sliced
1 endive, thinly sliced
2 stalks of celery, thinly sliced
100 g bean sprouts
1 bunch of watercress
Lime dressing (*see page 251*)

Combine all the ingredients in a salad bowl. Add some lime dressing, garnish with watercress and serve immediately.

# CITRUS FRUITS

## LEMON

★ VITAMIN C, FOLATE; CALCIUM, POTASSIUM; CITRIC ACID; FIBRE

✓ ANTI-ALLERGIC, ANTIBACTERIAL; ANTIOXIDANT

Lemons (*Citrus limon*) contain high levels of vitamin C, which boosts the body's resistance to infection, as well as enhancing iron absorption, aiding efficient wound healing and strengthening cell membranes. Lemons also lower blood-fat levels and help maintain the health of the heart, nerves and muscle tissue.

**RECIPES** *guacamole (page 250), lemon tahini dressing (page 251), carrot and lemon with garlic (page 264), cold buster (page 268)*

## LIME

★ VITAMIN C, FOLATE; CALCIUM, POTASSIUM; CITRIC ACID, FIBRE

✓ ANTI-ALLERGIC, ANTIBACTERIAL, ANTIOXIDANT

Like lemon, lime (*Citrus aurantifolia*) improves the health of all body tissues and enhances iron absorption. It may speed up wound healing and increase the efficiency of the immune system. It therefore has a role in the prevention and treatment of cancer.

**RECIPES** *nettle and lime tisane (page 185), tempeh kebabs (page 203), lime dressing (page 251), mango and lime (page 266), piña colada (page 267), passion and lime (page 267)*

## ORANGE

★ VITAMINS C, B3, B5, FOLATE; POTASSIUM; BETA-SITOSTEROL; FIBRE, SUGARS

✓ ANTIOXIDANT, ANTI-STRESS, LOWERS CHOLESTEROL

! ORANGES CAN TRIGGER MIGRAINE ATTACKS IN SOME CASES

! IT MAY BE BEST TO AVOID ORANGES IN YOUR DIET IF YOU SUFFER FROM RHEUMATOID ARTHRITIS

The high vitamin C content in oranges (*Citrus sinensis*) helps to maintain healthy blood cells and increases resistance to infections. Oranges also lower blood cholesterol, improve iron absorption and wound healing, and may help protect against cancer. Eating oranges helps to maintain optimum energy levels, keeps skin and mucous membranes in good condition, aids antibody production and protects against high blood pressure and allergy.

**RECIPES** *oriental salad with tempeh (page 203), orange mango salad (page 260), melon and orange (page 266), pink pineapple (page 267), sunrise (page 267)*

# BERRIES

## BILBERRY (BLAEBERRY, WHORTLEBERRY, WINBERRY)

★ VITAMIN C; ANTHOCYANIN; FIBRE, SUGARS

✓ ANTIBACTERIAL, ANTI-INFLAMMATORY, ANTIOXIDANT, ANTISEPTIC, TONIC

Bilberries (*Vaccinium myrtillus*) are helpful in the treatment of rheumatoid arthritis. They inhibit free radicals, strengthen blood capillaries, tone up the cardiovascular system and help prevent abnormal blood clots. Bilberries can be used for gastro-intestinal disorders and throat infections, and are effective as a tisane (1 tablespoon per cup).

**RECIPES** *use in place of blackberries, raspberries or cranberries*

## BLACKBERRY

★ VITAMINS C, E, B3, FOLATE; MANGANESE; IRON; CITRIC ACID; FIBRE

✓ ANTIOXIDANT, TONIC

Blackberries (*Rubus ulmifolius or R. alleghanensis*) improve iron absorption, increase energy release from food and enhance oxygen transport to the tissues. They aid liver function, speed up protein and fat metabolism, help regulate blood-fat levels and encourage wound healing. They may also offer a degree of protection against heart disease and some cancers.

**RECIPES** *yoghurt with fruit (page 243), blackberry crumble (page 263), blackberry cream (page 264)*

## SWEET CHERRY

★ POTASSIUM; ANTHOCYANIN, MALIC ACID; FIBRE, SUGARS

✓ ANTI-INFLAMMATORY, ANTIOXIDANT, DETOXIFYING, REJUVENATING

TISANES MADE FROM CHERRY STALKS ARE A TRADITIONAL REMEDY FOR CYSTITIS

Cherries (*Prunus avium*) boost energy and are beneficial to the heart, muscles and nerves. Eating cherries can lower uric acid levels in the blood and so is a traditional way of avoiding gout. They reduce platelet "stickiness" and help prevent blood clots, and can help relieve the symptoms of rheumatoid and osteoarthritis.

**RECIPES** *ruby red melon salad (page 242)*

## CRANBERRY

★ VITAMIN C; IRON; ANTHOCYANIN, BENZOIC, CITRIC AND QUINIC ACIDS; FIBRE

✓ ANTI-CANCER, ANTIOXIDANT

The juice of cranberries (*Vaccinium vitis-idaea*) prevents harmful bacteria from sticking to the bladder wall and so has long been used to relieve urinary-tract infections. Cranberry juice has powerful antioxidant effects that improve cardiovascular health and help prevent cancer. It may also reduce kidney stones.

***RECIPES*** *cranberry spritzer (page 264)*

## ELDERBERRY

★ VITAMINS A, C, B2, B3, B6, BIOTIN; IRON; ANTHOCYANIN, TANNIN; SUGARS

✓ ANTI-ALLERGIC, ANTI-CANCER, ANTIOXIDANT, ASTRINGENT, DIURETIC, ENCOURAGES SWEATING, LAXATIVE

Elderberries (*Sambucus nigra*) are an effective remedy for disorders of the upper respiratory tract, such as catarrh, colds and flu, and can be used to relieve all types of inflammation, including rheumatic complaints. They improve iron absorption from food and aid haemoglobin production, benefit blood-fat levels and fat metabolism, aid liver function and boost energy.

***RECIPES*** *elderberry cordial (page 268)*

## HAWTHORN

★ VITAMIN C; ANTHOCYANIN, GLYCOSIDES, SAPONINS, TANNIN

✓ ANTI-INFLAMMATORY, ANTIOXIDANT, LOWERS BLOOD PRESSURE, TONIC

Hawthorn berries (*Crataegus monogyna*) benefit the whole cardiovascular system. They are gentle in action and can help support the heart in heart failure, as well as being used to treat hypertension, arteriosclerosis and angina. They reduce the "stickiness" of blood platelets and so may help prevent thrombosis (abnormal blood-clot formation). They may also inhibit the growth of some cancers, especially of the lung, skin and oesophagus.

***RECIPES*** *circulation booster (page 268)*

## MULBERRY

★ VITAMINS C, B3, BIOTIN, FOLATE; MANGANESE, POTASSIUM; IRON; ANTHOCYANIN, CITRIC ACID; FIBRE, SUGARS

✓ ANTIOXIDANT

! UNRIPE MULBERRIES CAN BE TOXIC AND SHOULD NOT BE EATEN

Mulberries (*Morus nigra*) boost energy and strength, support nerve, heart, liver, muscle and bone marrow function, and help to keep cell membranes healthy. They enhance iron absorption, reduce blood-fat levels, improve oxygen transport to the tissues and aid protein and fat metabolism. They may also protect against heart disease, cancer and rheumatoid arthritis.

***RECIPES*** *use in place of blackberries in recipes*

## RASPBERRY

★ VITAMINS C, B3, BIOTIN, FOLATE; MANGANESE; IRON; CITRIC ACID; FIBRE, SUGARS

✓ ANTIOXIDANT, DETOXIFYING, LAXATIVE, TONIC

💡 RASPBERRY LEAVES ARE ALSO USED MEDICINALLY TO HELP ENSURE HEALTHY PREGNANCY AND BIRTH

Raspberries (*Rubus idaeus*) activate the body's natural self-cleansing ability and improve the health of the skin, hair, sweat glands, nerves, liver, bone marrow and mucous membranes. They enhance wound healing and their powerful antioxidant properties mean they also help protect against heart disease, cancer and rheumatoid arthritis. Raspberries boost the body's energy levels, and also encourage efficient protein and fat metabolism.

***RECIPES*** *fruity pancakes (page 243), raspberry gateau (page 262), raspberry sorbet (page 263)*

## ROSEHIP

★ VITAMIN C; CAROTENOIDS, TANNIN; PECTIN

✓ ANTI-ALLERGIC, ANTIOXIDANT, HEALING, MILD LAXATIVE

Rosehips (*Rosa canina*) are extremely rich in vitamin C and therefore improve immunity to infections – especially the common cold. They boost energy levels, help maintain healthy mucous membranes, enhance wound healing and help prevent heart disease and the formation of cancer cells.

***RECIPES*** *pick-me-up (page 270), rosehip syrup (page 270), tea for ear infections (page 271)*

## STRAWBERRY

★ VITAMINS C, B3, B5; CITRIC ACID; FIBRE, SUGARS

✓ ANTIOXIDANT, ASTRINGENT, DIURETIC, LAXATIVE

Strawberries (*Fragaria* x *ananassa*) can be used to treat fever and to relieve the symptoms of rheumatoid arthritis. Good for the health of the skin and mucous membranes, strawberries improve wound healing, encourage iron absorption and reduce blood-fat levels. They may reduce the tendency to develop high blood pressure and allergic reactions. They can also help the body cope with stress.

***RECIPES*** *fruity pancakes (page 243)*

# avocado

**AVOCADO IS PACKED WITH ENERGY AND IMMUNE-BOOSTING PHYTOCHEMICALS THAT CAN HELP GUARD AGAINST CERTAIN CANCERS AND PREVENT FUNGAL DISEASES. THIS TASTY FRUIT ALSO STABILIZES BLOOD FATS AND HELPS MAINTAIN HEALTHY BLOOD PRESSURE.**

## The origin of avocado

The avocado pear is thought to have originated in Central America, where it was an important component of the diet of the native Aztec people. It was discovered by the Spanish conquistadors in the 16th century, but was little-known to the rest of the world until the early 20th century. Avocados are now popular all over the world and are grown commercially in many tropical and subtropical regions, mainly in Australia, Brazil, USA, Israel, Mediterranean Europe, South Africa and southeast Asia.

Avocados are usually thought of as a savoury food, even though, botanically speaking, they are fruits. The avocado grows on an evergreen tree (*Persea americana*) with small green-yellow flowers. The tree starts producing fruit when it is three years old. A mature tree can display one million flowers on its branches, of which only 100 to 400 will set fruit. Healthy avocado trees can continue to produce fruit for hundreds of years.

Avocados are normally picked before they are fully ripened. On average, an avocado takes about a week to ripen at room temperature. The process can be accelerated by placing the unripe avocado in a paper bag along with an apple. The flesh of the fruit is yellow/green and discolours easily when exposed to the air. You can prevent this by rubbing lemon juice on to the exposed surface of the flesh.

## Immune-boosting properties

The avocado is a highly nutritious food that houses several important nutrients and phytochemicals. It contains glutathione, a powerful antioxidant phytochemical that mops up free radicals – the destructive molecules known to trigger the development of cancer and heart disease. In particular, glutathione has been shown to reduce the risk of cancer of the mouth and throat. Recent research has discovered a new group of phytochemicals in the avocado that have strong antifungal properties. They work by inhibiting the germination of fungal spores and so make avocado useful in the treatment of internal and external yeast infections.

The particular combination of nutrients and micro-nutrients found in the avocado offers other beneficial effects. It stimulates the immune system, enhances antibody production and acts as a mild vasodilator, relaxing the muscles surrounding blood vessels and thus reducing blood pressure. The avocado can help protect the skin by slowing down the effects of ageing, and maintaining hair, mucous membranes, sweat glands, nerves, muscles and bone marrow in good condition. New research suggests that avocados can enhance male fertility by improving sperm health.

## Energy-rich

Avocados differ markedly from other vegetable fruits in being extremely high in calories – about 90 per cent is fat. Some 80 per cent of this fat is oleic acid. There are many health benefits associated with eating a diet high in monounsaturated fat such as this. In particular, such fats reduce levels of LDL cholesterol in the blood and have a beneficial effect on the composition of blood fats in general. Monounsaturated fat also helps to stabilize blood-sugar levels. Most of the rest of the fat found in avocados is polyunsaturated. As the fruit ripens, the small amount of saturated fat it contains steadily turns into polyunsaturated fat. Avocados also contain phytochemicals called beta-sitosterols, which reduce the absorption of cholesterol from food (these chemicals are widely used in the manufacture of blood-cholesterol-lowering drugs).

### IMMUNE-BOOSTING PROFILE

★ VITAMINS E, K, B1, B2, B3, B5, BIOTIN, FOLATE; POTASSIUM; ZINC; BETA-SITOSTEROLS, CAROTENOIDS, GLUTATHIONE; FIBRE, UNSATURATED FATTY ACIDS (INCLUDING OLEIC)

✓ ANTI-CANCER, ANTIFUNGAL, ANTIOXIDANT

! PEOPLE WHO ARE ALLERGIC TO NATURAL RUBBER (LATEX) HAVE A ONE IN TWO CHANCE OF BEING ALLERGIC TO AVOCADO

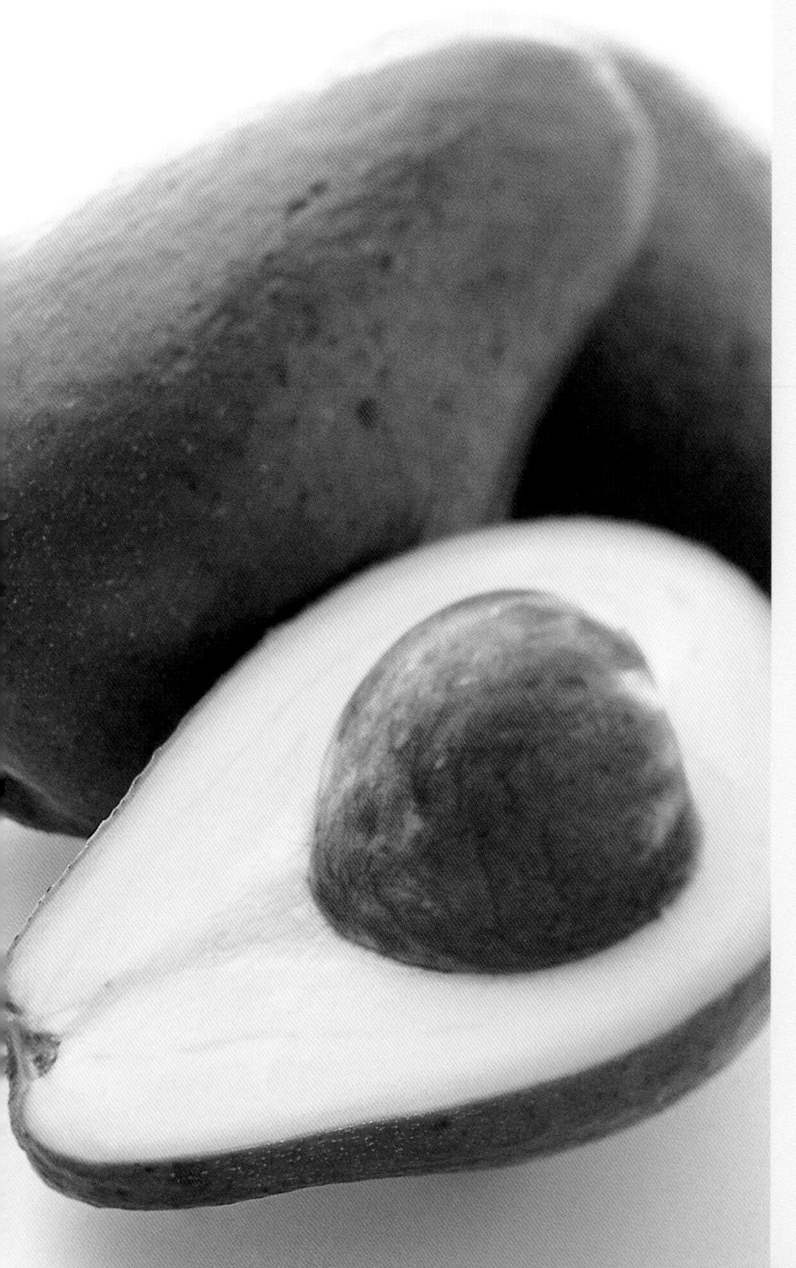

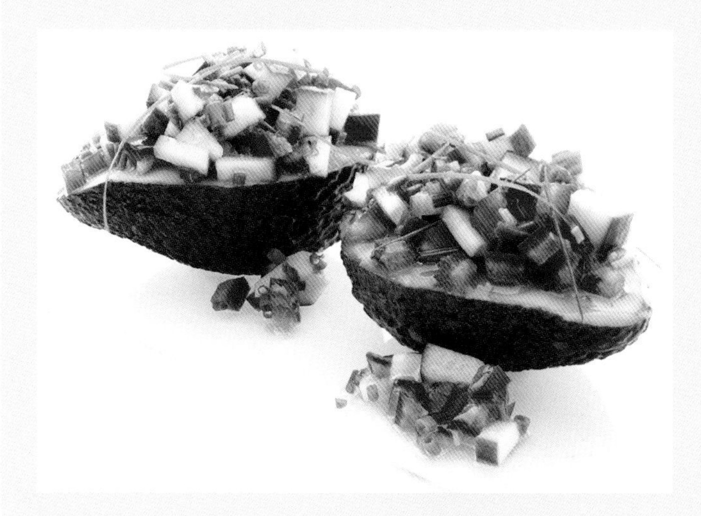

## filled avocados *(above)*

2 avocados, halved, stone removed
2 ripe tomatoes, finely chopped
½ cucumber, finely chopped
1 bunch of chives, finely chopped
4 tbsp sunflower oil
1 tbsp tarragon vinegar (or wine vinegar)
1 garlic clove, crushed
½ tsp soy sauce
½ tsp tabasco

Place the avocado halves on separate plates. Gently mix the tomato, cucumber and chives, and divide on top of the avocado halves. Beat the dressing ingredients together and drizzle over the avocados. Serve with French bread.

## avocado smoothie

Per serving:
1 avocado, peeled and chopped
1 pear, peeled, deseeded and chopped
½ grapefruit, squeezed
1 tsp fresh ginger root, finely chopped
100 ml soya milk
4 tbsp plain soya yogurt

Blend all the ingredients. Serve immediately in a glass.

## avocado, watercress and cumin salad

To garnish: 2 tsp cumin seeds
1 bunch of watercress, chopped
3 large ripe avocados, thinly sliced
Lemon tahini dressing (see page 251)

Roast the cumin seeds in a dry frying pan. Remove and crush. Place the watercress on a large plate. Arrange the avocado on top. Sprinkle with dressing and garnish with the roasted cumin.

# nuts and seeds

## ALMOND

★ VITAMINS E, B2, B5, BIOTIN, FOLATE; CALCIUM, MAGNESIUM, MANGANESE, PHOSPHORUS, POTASSIUM; BORON, COPPER, IRON, SELENIUM, ZINC; STEROLS; FIBRE, PROTEIN, UNSATURATED FAT

✓ ANTIOXIDANT, LOWERS CHOLESTEROL, NUTRIENT-RICH

! BEWARE BITTER-TASTING ALMONDS – THEY CAN BE TOXIC

Almonds (*Prunus dulcis*) help maintain healthy blood-fat levels, strengthen the cardiovascular system and reduce the risk of coronary heart disease. They also enhance antibody production, strengthen cell membranes and help protect against cancer.

**RECIPES** *muesli (page 243), toasted nuts and seeds (page 248)*

## CASHEW

★ VITAMINS B1, B2, B3, B5, B6, BIOTIN, FOLATE; MAGNESIUM, MANGANESE, PHOSPHORUS, POTASSIUM; BORON, COPPER, IODINE, IRON, SELENIUM, ZINC; FIBRE, PROTEIN, UNSATURATED FAT

✓ ANTIOXIDANT, LOWERS CHOLESTEROL

Cashews (*Anacardium occidentale*) help to maintain healthy blood-fat levels, aid haemoglobin production and fat metabolism, enhance the body's ability to cope with stress, and help keep skin, hair, glands, nerves, mucous membranes, blood cells and bone marrow in good condition.

**RECIPES** *toasted nuts and seeds (page 248), paella (page 252)*

## LINSEED (FLAXSEED)

★ GLYCOSIDES; MUCILAGE, OMEGA-3 AND -6 FATTY ACIDS, PROTEIN

✓ ANTI-COUGH, LOWERS CHOLESTEROL, IMMUNO-STIMULANT, LAXATIVE

Linseeds (*Linum usitatissimum*) can help treat coughs, bronchitis, chronic constipation and psoriasis. They also help maintain healthy blood-fat levels and may be protective against cardiovascular disease and cancer.

**RECIPES** *muesli (page 243)*

## HAZELNUT

★ VITAMINS E, B1, B2, B3, B5, B6, BIOTIN, FOLATE; CALCIUM, MAGNESIUM, MANGANESE, PHOSPHORUS, POTASSIUM; BORON, COPPER, IRON, ZINC; FIBRE, PROTEIN, UNSATURATED FAT

✓ ANTIOXIDANT, LOWERS CHOLESTEROL

! SOME PEOPLE ARE ALLERGIC TO HAZELNUTS

Hazelnuts (*Corylus avellana*) help regulate blood fats and aid cell renewal and repair. They help protect cells against free-radical damage and benefit skin, hair, nails, glands, nerves, bone marrow and mucous membranes.

**RECIPES** *toasted nuts and seeds (page 248)*

## MACADAMIA NUT (QUEENSLAND NUT)

★ VITAMINS B1, B3, B5, B6, BIOTIN; MAGNESIUM, MANGANESE, PHOSPHORUS; COPPER, IRON, SELENIUM, ZINC; FIBRE, PROTEIN, UNSATURATED FAT

✓ ANTIOXIDANT, LOWERS CHOLESTEROL

Research shows that the unsaturated fat in macadamia nuts (*Macadamia ternifolia*) has a favourable effect on blood cholesterol.

**RECIPES** *spring greens and macadamia nuts (page 258)*

## MELON SEED

★ VITAMINS B2, B3, FOLATE; CALCIUM, MAGNESIUM, MANGANESE, POTASSIUM; COPPER, IRON, ZINC; PROTEIN, UNSATURATED FAT

✓ ANTIOXIDANT, LOWERS CHOLESTEROL

Melon (*Cucumis melo*) seeds support the immune and cardiovascular systems, help regulate healthy blood-fat levels, and provide the nutrients necessary to aid wound healing and help maintain healthy skin, nails and nerves.

**RECIPES** *toasted nuts and seeds (page 248)*

## PECAN NUT

★ VITAMINS E, B1, B2, B3, B5, FOLATE; CALCIUM, MAGNESIUM, MANGANESE, PHOSPHORUS, POTASSIUM; COPPER, SELENIUM, ZINC; FIBRE, PROTEIN, UNSATURATED FAT (MAINLY OLEIC ACID)

✓ ANTIOXIDANT, LOWERS CHOLESTEROL

! SOME PEOPLE ARE ALLERGIC TO PECAN NUTS

Pecan nuts (*Carya illinoensis*) are high in monounsaturated fat and health-protective vitamins and minerals, helping to prevent cancer and heart disease. Eating pecans regularly also lowers blood cholesterol and improves blood lipid balance, emphasizing the importance to health of the type of fat contained in the diet.

**RECIPES** *muesli (page 243)*

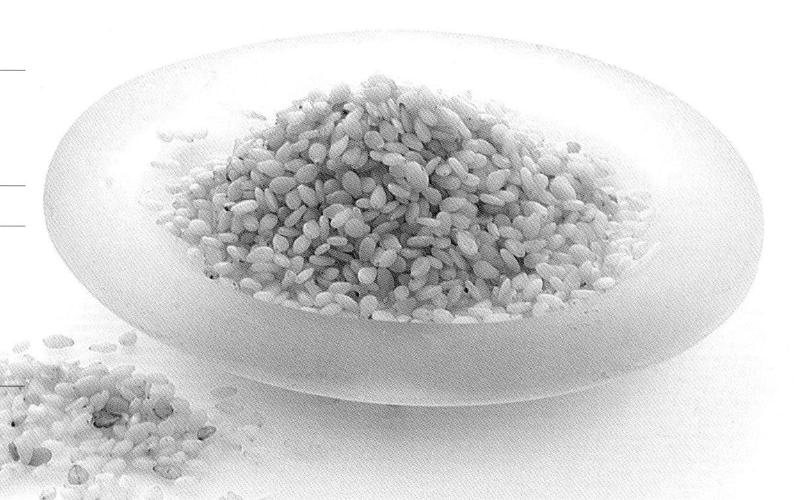

## PISTACHIO

★ VITAMINS E, B1, B2, B3, FOLATE; CALCIUM, MAGNESIUM, PHOSPHORUS, POTASSIUM; COPPER, IRON, SELENIUM, ZINC; FIBRE, PROTEIN, UNSATURATED FAT

✓ ANTIOXIDANT, LOWERS CHOLESTEROL

Pistachio (*Pistacia vera*) nuts protect against heart disease and some cancers, aid liver function and metabolism, boost energy, and improve the health and function of blood cells, muscles, nerves, mucous membranes and skin.

**RECIPES** *muesli (page 243), toasted nuts and seeds (page 248)*

## PINE NUT

★ VITAMINS E, B1, B2, B3; MAGNESIUM, MANGANESE, POTASSIUM; COPPER, IRON, ZINC; FIBRE, PROTEIN, UNSATURATED FAT

Pine (*Pinus spp.*) nuts protect against heart disease and some cancers. They aid liver function and metabolism, boost energy, and benefit the blood, muscles, nerves, mucous membranes and skin.

**RECIPES** *pasta, pesto and shiitake (page 215)*

## PUMPKIN SEED

★ VITAMINS B1, B2, B3; MAGNESIUM, PHOSPHORUS, POTASSIUM; COPPER, IRON, SELENIUM, ZINC; FIBRE, OMEGA-3 FATTY ACIDS, PROTEIN, UNSATURATED FAT

✓ ANTI-INFLAMMATORY, ANTIOXIDANT, DETOXIFYING, IMMUNO-STIMULANT

Pumpkin (*Cucurbita maxima*) seeds are highly nutritious, and a valuable aid in the prevention and treatment of cardiovascular, autoimmune and immunodeficiency disorders. They can also benefit the prostate gland.

**RECIPES** *carrot 'n' beetroot salad (page 259)*

## SESAME SEED/TAHINI

★ VITAMINS E, B1, B2, B3; CALCIUM, MAGNESIUM, MANGANESE, PHOSPHORUS, POTASSIUM; COPPER, IRON, ZINC; COMPLEX CARBOHYDRATES, FIBRE, OMEGA-6 FATTY ACIDS, PROTEIN, UNSATURATED FAT

✓ ANTIOXIDANT, LOWERS CHOLESTEROL, NUTRIENT-RICH

Sesame (*Sesamum indicum*) seeds are an excellent natural food supplement, aiding tissue repair and renewal and helping the body cope with stress. Tahini is a paste made from ground sesame and adds interest and nutritional value to many different dishes.

**RECIPES** *oriental salad with tempeh (page 203), lemon tahini dressing (page 251), green lentil salad (page 260)*

## SUNFLOWER SEED

★ VITAMINS E, B1, B2, B3; CALCIUM, MAGNESIUM, MANGANESE, PHOSPHORUS, POTASSIUM; COPPER, IRON, SELENIUM, ZINC; COMPLEX CARBOHYDRATES, FIBRE, OMEGA-6 FATTY ACIDS, PROTEIN, UNSATURATED FAT

✓ ANTIOXIDANT, NUTRIENT-RICH

Sunflower (*Helianthus annuus*) seeds improve skin health, help regulate blood-fat levels and aid tissue repair. They may also be beneficial in treating eczema.

**RECIPES** *muesli (page 243), toasted nuts and seeds (page 248)*

## SWEET CHESTNUT (SPANISH CHESTNUT)

★ VITAMINS B3, B5, B6; MAGNESIUM, MANGANESE, PHOSPHORUS, POTASSIUM; COPPER, ZINC; COMPLEX CARBOHYDRATES, FIBRE, SUGARS, PROTEIN

✓ ENERGY-BOOSTING, IMMUNO-STIMULANT, NUTRIENT-RICH

Sweet chestnuts (*Castanea sativa*) are versatile and nutritious. Their energy is released slowly and steadily in the body, helping to stabilize blood-sugar levels and boosting energy and strength.

**RECIPES** *sweet chestnuts and kumquats (page 257)*

## WALNUT

★ VITAMINS E, B1, B2, B3, B5, B6, BIOTIN, FOLATE; CALCIUM, MAGNESIUM, MANGANESE, PHOSPHORUS, POTASSIUM; COPPER, IRON, SELENIUM, ZINC; FIBRE, OMEGA-3 FATTY ACIDS, PROTEIN

✓ ANTIOXIDANT, ANTI-INFLAMMATORY, LOWERS CHOLESTEROL

Walnuts (*Juglans sp.*) reduce the risk of heart disease and cancer, benefit blood cells, muscles and nervous system, aid brain function, boost energy and strength, and help us cope with stress.

**RECIPES** *rocket salad (page 259), florence fennel salad (page 260)*

# brazil nut

**THIS DELICIOUS SOUTH AMERICAN KERNEL IS ONE OF THE RICHEST NATURAL SOURCES OF SELENIUM AND VITAMIN E – TWO POWERFUL ANTIOXIDANTS WITH ANTI-AGEING PROPERTIES THAT CAN HELP GUARD AGAINST MANY DISORDERS INCLUDING HEART DISEASE AND CANCER.**

## The origin of the Brazil nut

The Brazil nut, also called the para nut, cream nut and castanea, is the edible seed of a giant tree (*Bertholletia excelsa*) that grows in the Amazon rainforest. It is an important source of nutrition – and income – to the local population. Most Brazil nuts are collected from wild trees. They grow in clusters of 8 to 24 nuts enclosed in a woody, fibrous fruit capsule that looks like a cross between a coconut and a cooking pot with a lid. The nut is enclosed in a hard, dark-brown, wedge-shaped shell. From January to June, the capsules ripen and fall to the ground, where they are collected. The kernels are taken out, sun-dried and washed before being sold and exported, mainly to North America and Europe. (After the nuts have been removed, the dried capsules are used as animal traps, a practice that has given them the name "monkey-pots".)

## Immune-boosting properties

The Brazil nut is extremely nutritious with high levels of protein, unsaturated fat, selenium, zinc and other minerals, plus substantial quantities of vitamins E and B-complex. It is the combination of vitamin E with selenium that gives the Brazil nut its special immune-enhancing properties. These two important antioxidants work synergistically, each improving the performance of the other to boost immune-system function. Antioxidants prevent cell damage by mopping up free radicals and thus preventing the "oxidative" chain reactions that can damage DNA. Some oxidation is normal and vital for health (the immune system actually uses oxidative reactions to destroy micro-organisms), but if the level of oxidation outstrips the body's own defensive capabilities, the resulting excess of free radicals can cause cellular damage.

Accumulated damage by free radicals is known to be an important factor in ageing and disease, and the role of antioxidants in the prevention and treatment of illness is well recognized. Antioxidants play a preventive role in many conditions including asthma, heart disease, immunodeficiency disorders and cancer.

Selenium enhances immunity by activating an enzyme in the body called glutathione peroxidase, which inhibits the formation of free radicals and suppresses tumour growth. Infection depletes the body's selenium levels. This, in turn, suppresses the immune system because a low level of selenium affects the normal antibody response to infection and cell damage. Thus even a moderate increase in selenium intake is beneficial to the body's self-defence mechanisms, and can help to reduce the risk of cancer, heart disease and fungal infections such as candidiasis. However, it is possible to get too much of a good thing. Taking excess selenium as a food supplement can result in selenium toxicity, which causes hair loss,

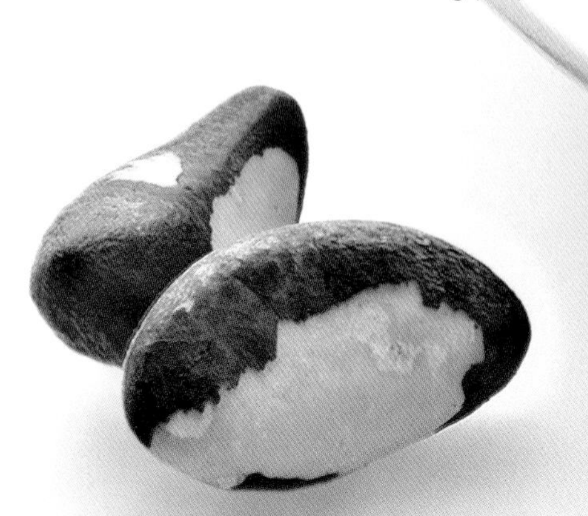

dizziness, fatigue and skin problems. Fortunately, the Brazil nut–selenium "package" provides a natural safety limit because Brazil nuts satisfy hunger long before selenium intake reaches toxic limits. Selenium is found in many other foods of plant origin – the amount depending on the plant's ability to absorb it from the soil. Unfortunately, in many parts of the world, modern agricultural practices have depleted the soil of selenium, providing yet another good reason for preserving the Amazon rainforest – Brazil nuts.

### IMMUNE-BOOSTING PROFILE

★ VITAMINS E, B1, B3, B5, B6, BIOTIN; CALCIUM, MAGNESIUM, MANGANESE, PHOSPHORUS, POTASSIUM; COPPER, IODINE, IRON, SELENIUM, ZINC; FIBRE, OMEGA-6 AND OLEIC FATTY ACIDS, PROTEIN

✓ ANTI-CANCER, ANTIOXIDANT, IMMUNO-STIMULANT

! SOME PEOPLE ARE ALLERGIC TO BRAZIL NUTS

! GENETICALLY MODIFIED SOYA BEANS MAY CONTAIN GENES FROM BRAZIL NUTS, AND SO MAY TRIGGER AN ALLERGIC REACTION

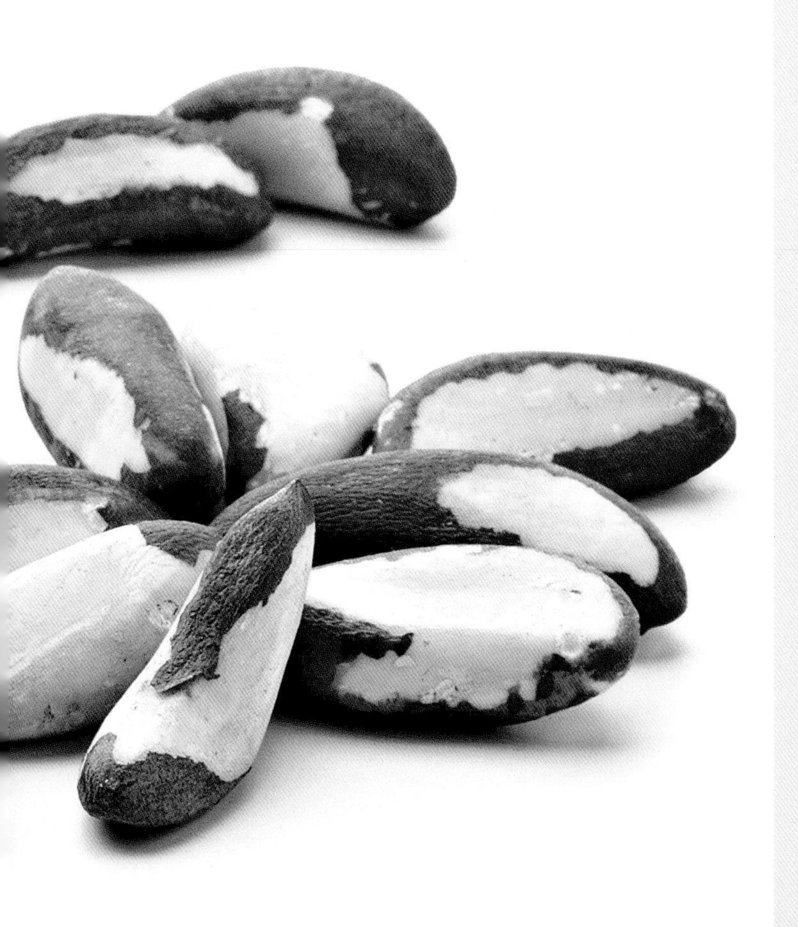

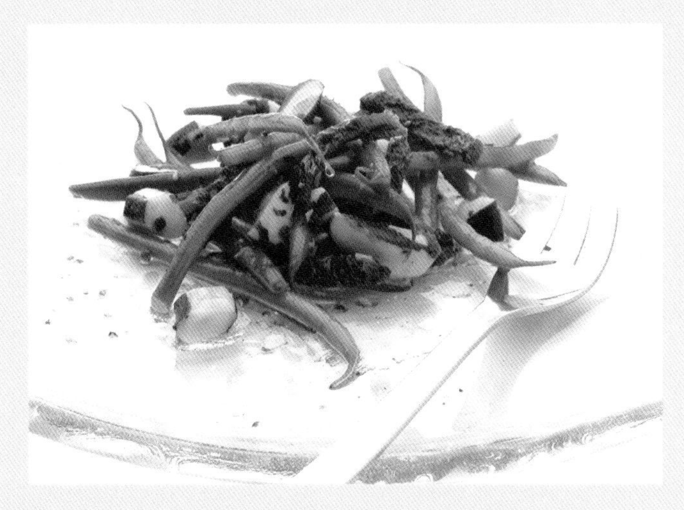

## brazil nuts and sun-dried tomatoes with beans *(above)*

500 g French beans, topped and tailed
200 g Brazil nuts, chopped
100 g sun-dried tomatoes, sliced
1 tbsp olive oil
Salt and pepper to taste

Steam the beans till tender. Place the rest of the ingredients in a bowl, add the beans while still hot, mix well and serve.

## grilled endive and brazil nut salad

4 endives, halved lengthways
3 tbsp olive oil
50 g Brazil nuts
Salt and pepper to taste

Brush the endives with olive oil, then grill a few minutes on each side until they begin to char and soften. Brush with more oil as you turn them, if necessary. Place on a serving dish, scatter with Brazil nuts and season with salt and pepper. Serve with vinaigrette.

## spicy brazil nut pâté

50 g Brazil nuts, chopped
Soy sauce
500 g mushrooms, chopped
200 g tofu, crumbled
3 tbsp olive oil
2 garlic cloves, chopped
1 tsp thyme
1 tsp garam masala
Pinch of cayenne
Salt and pepper to taste
To garnish: 2 tsp fresh parsley

Roast the Brazil nuts in a dry frying pan, add a little soy sauce, stir and remove from the pan. Sauté the mushrooms and the tofu in the oil with the garlic, thyme and the spices until soft. Blend all the ingredients to a coarse pâté, season with salt and pepper. Place in a serving dish, garnish with parsley and serve.

# grains

## BULGUR WHEAT

★ VITAMINS B1, B2, B3; MAGNESIUM, PHOSPHORUS; COPPER, IRON; COMPLEX CARBOHYDRATES, PROTEIN

✓ EASILY DIGESTIBLE, ENERGY-BOOSTING

! AVOID IF ALLERGIC OR SENSITIVE TO GLUTEN IN WHEAT

Bulgur is the cracked kernels of boiled and dried durum wheat (*Triticum durum*). Fine grains are used for salads and need very little cooking – cover with boiling water and leave for a few minutes to expand and soften. Larger grains are cooked like rice (but need less cooking time and water).

**RECIPES** *bulgur wheat salad (page 259)*

## MUESLI (SWISS STYLE, NO ADDED SUGAR)

★ VITAMINS E, B1, B2, B3, B5, B6, BIOTIN, FOLATE; CALCIUM, MAGNESIUM, PHOSPHORUS, POTASSIUM; IRON, ZINC; COMPLEX CARBOHYDRATES, FIBRE, PROTEIN, SUGARS

✓ ANTI-CANCER, ANTIOXIDANT, ANTI-STRESS, LOWERS CHOLESTEROL

Muesli contains a potent mixture of highly nutritious, vitality-enhancing ingredients.

**RECIPES** *muesli (page 243)*

## OATS

★ VITAMINS E, B1, B2, B3, B5; MAGNESIUM, MANGANESE, PHOSPHORUS, POTASSIUM; IRON, SELENIUM, ZINC; COMPLEX CARBOHYDRATES, FIBRE, PROTEIN

✓ ANTI-CANCER, ANTI-STRESS, LOWERS CHOLESTEROL, ENERGY-BOOSTING

Oats (*Avena sativa*) are high in protein, iron and soluble fibre. They lower blood cholesterol, ease stress and soothe tired nerves.

**RECIPES** *porridge with dried fruit and quinoa (page 242), muesli (page 243), blackberry crumble (page 263), pick-me-up (page 270)*

## PASTA (MADE FROM DURUM WHEAT)

★ VITAMINS B1, B3; MAGNESIUM, MANGANESE, PHOSPHORUS, POTASSIUM; IRON, ZINC; COMPLEX CARBOHYDRATES, FIBRE, PROTEIN

✓ ENERGY-BOOSTING

! AVOID IF ALLERGIC OR SENSITIVE TO GLUTEN IN WHEAT

Durum wheat (*Triticum durum*) is high in protein. When ground to flour and mixed with water, it is ideal for rolling into pasta shapes.

**RECIPES** *pasta, pesto and shiitake (page 215)*

## QUINOA

★ VITAMINS E, B2, B3; CALCIUM, MAGNESIUM, PHOSPHORUS, POTASSIUM; COPPER, IRON, ZINC; SAPONINS; COMPLEX CARBOHYDRATES, FIBRE, PROTEIN, SUGARS, UNSATURATED FAT

✓ ANTI-CANCER, ANTIOXIDANT, LOWERS CHOLESTEROL, ENERGY-BOOSTING

💡 CONTAINS NO GLUTEN

Quinoa (*Chenopodium quinoa*) is arguably the most nutritious of all grains. It is rich in protein and minerals and can be used to add nutritional value to breakfast cereals, biscuits and casseroles.

**RECIPES** *porridge with dried fruit and quinoa (page 242)*

## RICE

★ VITAMINS B1, B3, FOLATE; MAGNESIUM, MANGANESE, PHOSPHORUS; COPPER, IRON, ZINC; COMPLEX CARBOHYDRATES, FIBRE, PROTEIN

✓ ENERGY-BOOSTING, LOWERS CHOLESTEROL

💡 CONTAINS NO GLUTEN

Brown rice (*Oryza sativa*) is a rich source of energy, fibre, protein and B vitamins. It helps protect the cardiovascular system, nerves, digestion, muscles, mucous membranes, skin, hair, glands and bone marrow. Rice milk is a good alternative to cow's milk – ideal for those with irritable bowel syndrome and other gastro-intestinal disorders.

**RECIPES** *rice: paella (page 252), khichuri – rice with lentils (page 257); rice milk: muesli (page 243), heart chai (page 269)*

## SWEETCORN (CORN, MAIZE)

★ VITAMINS B3, B5, FOLATE; MAGNESIUM, PHOSPHORUS; ZINC; COMPLEX CARBOHYDRATES, FIBRE, OMEGA-6 FATTY ACIDS, PROTEIN

✓ ANTI-STRESS, AIDS DIGESTION

💡 CORN SILK (FINE THREAD ON FRESH CORN COBS) CAN BE USED IN

A TISANE TO SOOTHE IRRITATIONS OF THE BLADDER AND URETHRA

Sweetcorn (*Zea mays*) aids wound healing, strengthens the immune system by boosting antibody production, and keeps the skin and mucous membranes in good condition. It helps the body cope with stress, stabilizes blood sugar and maintains a healthy level of blood fats.

**RECIPES** *tempeh kebabs (page 203), pasta, pesto and shiitake (page 215), sweet potato curry (page 256)*

## WHEAT BRAN

★ VITAMINS B2, B3, B5, B6; CALCIUM, MAGNESIUM, MANGANESE, PHOSPHORUS, POTASSIUM; COPPER, IRON, ZINC; FIBRE, COMPLEX CARBOHYDRATES

✓ ANTIOXIDANT, DETOXIFYING, LAXATIVE

! THE PHYTATES IN BRAN INHIBIT ABSORPTION OF NUTRIENTS INCLUDING IRON, CALCIUM AND ZINC; HOWEVER, AS BRAN ALSO CONTAINS LARGE AMOUNTS OF THESE MINERALS, THE NET EFFECT OF EATING IT IN MODERATE AMOUNTS IS STILL HIGHLY BENEFICIAL

! ALWAYS DRINK PLENTY OF FLUIDS WHEN EATING BRAN TO AVOID INTESTINAL BLOCKAGE

Wheat bran, the outer layer of wheat (*Triticum sp.*) grain, is the richest source of insoluble fibre. It absorbs large amounts of water and increases in bulk, aiding the passage of waste through the bowel and relieving constipation. This helps prevent diseases such as diverticulitis and bowel cancer. Bran also helps regulate blood-fat and blood-sugar levels.

**RECIPES** *muesli (page 243)*

## WHEATGERM

★ VITAMINS E, B1, B2, B3, B5, B6, BIOTIN, FOLATE; MAGNESIUM, MANGANESE, PHOSPHORUS, POTASSIUM; COPPER, IRON, SELENIUM, ZINC; COMPLEX CARBOHYDRATES, FIBRE, PROTEIN, SUGARS, POLYUNSATURATED FAT

✓ ANTIOXIDANT, ANTI-STRESS

! AVOID IF ALLERGIC OR SENSITIVE TO GLUTEN IN WHEAT

Wheatgerm is the inner (embryo) layer of wheat (*Triticum sp.*) grain. It is a delicious natural source of zinc, vitamin E, folate, biotin and other B-complex vitamins. It helps the body maintain energy levels, enhances fat metabolism, and helps protect against heart disease, immunodeficiency disorders and some cancers.

**RECIPES** *muesli (page 243), try sprinkling on salads and desserts*

## WHEATGRASS

★ VITAMINS A, E; ZINC; CHLOROPHYLL; ESSENTIAL FATTY ACIDS, FIBRE, PROTEIN

✓ ANTIOXIDANT, DETOXIFYING

Wheatgrass (*Triticum sp.*) comes from young, newly sprouted wheat kernels. It is a highly concentrated source of immune-enhancing nutrients and is a powerful liver detoxifier. It stimulates haemoglobin production, lowers cholesterol and helps regulate blood-fat levels.

**RECIPES** *grow your own to eat in sandwiches or salads, or, buy wheatgrass juice, or add wheatgrass powder to other juices*

## WILD RICE

★ VITAMIN B1, B2, B3; PROTEIN; UNSATURATED FAT

✓ ENERGY-BOOSTING, LOWERS CHOLESTEROL

💡 WILD RICE IS UNRELATED TO COMMON RICE BUT AS NUTRITIOUS

Wild rice (*Zizania aquatica*) aids metabolism, improves the release of energy from food and helps the body to maintain optimum energy levels. It enhances the health of nerves, muscles, skin and mucous membranes, and helps prevent cardiovascular disease.

**RECIPES** *provençal-style kidney beans (page 255), sweet chestnuts and kumquats (page 257), wild rice salad (page 261)*

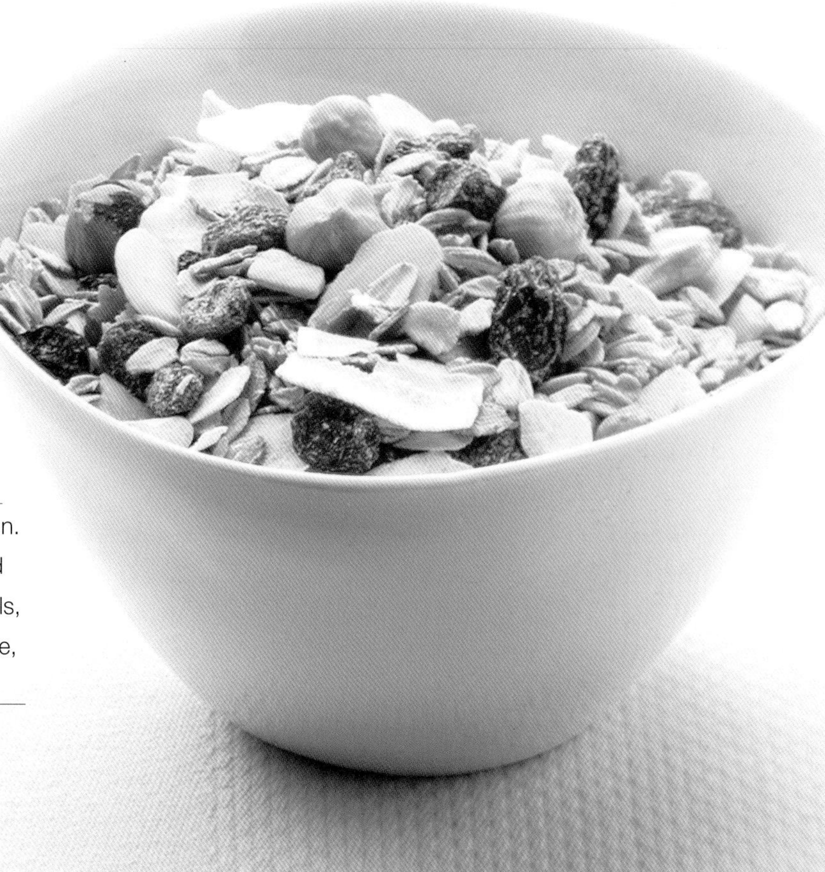

# pulses

## ADUKI BEAN (ADZUKI BEAN, AZUKI BEAN)

★ VITAMINS B1, B2, B3; CALCIUM, MAGNESIUM, MANGANESE, PHOSPHORUS, POTASSIUM; COPPER, IRON, ZINC; COMPLEX CARBOHYDRATES, FIBRE, PROTEIN

✓ HEALING, ENERGY-BOOSTING

Aduki beans (*Phaseolus angularis*) are small red beans with a sweet, nutty flavour. Their nutrients help release energy from food and keep skin and mucous membranes in good condition.

**RECIPES** *add to stews, casseroles and salads*

## BLACK-EYE BEAN (BLACK-EYE PEA, COWPEA)

★ VITAMINS B1, B2, B3, BIOTIN, FOLATE; CALCIUM, MAGNESIUM, MANGANESE, PHOSPHORUS, POTASSIUM; COPPER, IRON, SELENIUM, ZINC; COMPLEX CARBOHYDRATES, FIBRE, PROTEIN

✓ AIDS DIGESTION, LOWERS CHOLESTEROL, IMMUNO-STIMULANT

Black-eye beans (*Vigna sinensis*) are savoury and are used like haricot beans and butterbeans. Rich in micro-nutrients and energy, they enhance the body's ability to make amino acids and DNA.

**RECIPES** *beans and tomatoes on toast (page 242), black-eye bean and wild marjoram soup (page 245)*

## BROAD BEAN

★ VITAMINS C, B3, B5, BIOTIN, FOLATE; POTASSIUM, PHOSPHORUS; IRON, ZINC; COMPLEX CARBOHYDRATES, FIBRE, PROTEIN

✓ ANTI-STRESS, LOWERS CHOLESTEROL, DETOXIFYING

The high level of vitamin B5 and folate (the plant form of folic acid) in broad beans (*Vicia faba*) makes them a useful support for the body's defence against stress.

**RECIPES** *artichoke hearts, broad beans and shiitake (page 252)*

## BUTTERBEAN

★ VITAMINS B3, B5, FOLATE; POTASSIUM, PHOSPHORUS, MAGNESIUM, MANGANESE; IRON, ZINC; COMPLEX CARBOHYDRATES, FIBRE, PROTEIN

✓ ANTI-STRESS, LOWERS CHOLESTEROL

Butterbeans (*Phaseolus vulgaris sp.*) help the body to release energy from food and promote normal function of the immune and nervous systems. They also help maintain healthy skin, glands, hair and bone marrow.

**RECIPES** *italian butterbean soup (page 245)*

## CHICKPEA (GARBANZO BEAN)

★ VITAMINS E, B2, B3, B5, FOLATE; CALCIUM, MAGNESIUM, MANGANESE, PHOSPHORUS, POTASSIUM; ZINC; COMPLEX CARBOHYDRATES, FIBRE, PROTEIN

✓ ANTI-CANCER, ANTIOXIDANT, ANTI-STRESS, LOWERS CHOLESTEROL

One of the most nutritious and delicious of the pulses, chickpeas (*Cicer arietinum*) aid the absorption of nutrients and protect the cells from free radical damage. They support the function of nerves, muscles, enzymes and hormones and may help protect the body against heart disease and cancer.

**RECIPES** *spicy moroccan soup (page 246), hummus with crudités and warm pitta bread (page 246), winter hot pot (page 256)*

## HARICOT BEAN/GREEN BEAN

★ VITAMINS A, B3, FOLATE; IRON; FIBRE

✓ ANTI-CANCER, ANTIOXIDANT, LOWERS CHOLESTEROL

Haricot beans and green beans (*Phaseolus vulgaris sp.*) help keep cells well oxygenated and in good condition, particularly those of the skin and mucous membranes. They also enhance energy levels, support the nervous system and aid liver function.

**RECIPES** *beans and tomatoes on toast (page 242); okra in sweet and sour tamarind sauce (page 256), salad niçoise (page 259)*

## LENTIL

★ VITAMINS B3, B5, B6, FOLATE; CALCIUM, MAGNESIUM, MANGANESE, PHOSPHORUS, POTASSIUM; COPPER, IRON, SELENIUM, ZINC; COMPLEX CARBOHYDRATES, FIBRE, PROTEIN

✓ ANTIOXIDANT, ENERGY-BOOSTING, LOWERS CHOLESTEROL

Lentils (*Lens culinaris*) are an excellent source of antioxidants and so can help protect against heart disease and cancer. They improve the function of red blood cells and the integrity of cell membranes, and also help regulate blood-fat levels.

**RECIPES** *spicy moroccan soup (page 246), casserole de puy (page 252), shepherdess' pie (page 256), winter hot pot (page 256), khichuri – rice with lentils (page 257), green lentil salad (page 260)*

## MANGETOUT PEA

★ VITAMINS A, B1, B2, B3, B5, BIOTIN; CALCIUM; IRON; FIBRE, PROTEIN

✓ ANTI-CANCER, ANTIOXIDANT

Mangetout peas (*Pisum sativum sp.*) are good for the skin, hair, glands, nerves and muscles. They aid metabolism, liver function and antibody production, and help maintain energy levels.

**RECIPES** *chinese salad (page 260)*

## MUNG BEAN SPROUT

★ VITAMINS B3, B5, FOLATE; PHOSPHORUS; IRON; FIBRE, PROTEIN

✓ ANTI-STRESS, LOWERS CHOLESTEROL

Mung bean sprouts (*Phaseolus aureus*) help the body maintain optimum energy levels during stressful situations. They also aid antibody production and enhance liver function.

**RECIPES** *grapefruit salad (page 189), oriental salad with tempeh (page 203), asparagus asian-style (page 253), carrot 'n' beetroot salad (page 259), chinese salad (page 260)*

## PINTO BEAN

★ VITAMINS B1, B2, B3, B5, B6, FOLATE; CALCIUM, MAGNESIUM, MANGANESE, PHOSPHORUS, POTASSIUM; COPPER, IRON, SELENIUM, ZINC; COMPLEX CARBOHYDRATES, FIBRE, PROTEIN

✓ ANTIOXIDANT, ENERGY-BOOSTING, LOWERS CHOLESTEROL

Pinto beans (*Phaseolus vulgaris sp.*) help keep the skin, mucous membranes and muscles (including the heart) in good condition, maintain optimum energy levels, and aid the nervous system, helping to ease stress.

**RECIPES** *spicy moroccan soup (page 246)*

## SOYA BEAN

★ VITAMINS E, B1, B3, B6, BIOTIN, FOLATE; CALCIUM, MAGNESIUM, MANGANESE, PHOSPHORUS, POTASSIUM; COPPER, IRON, SELENIUM, ZINC; ISOFLAVONES, PROTEASE INHIBITORS, SAPONINS; COMPLEX CARBOHYDRATES, FIBRE, PROTEIN, UNSATURATED FAT

✓ ANTI-CANCER, ANTIOXIDANT, ENERGY-BOOSTING, LOWERS CHOLESTEROL, NUTRIENT-RICH

! SOME PEOPLE ARE ALLERGIC TO SOYA

! MUCH OF THE WORLD'S SOYA CROP HAS BEEN GENETICALLY MODIFIED: BUY ORGANIC

! SOME GENETICALLY MODIFIED SOYA BEANS CONTAIN GENES FROM BRAZIL NUTS AND SO MAY TRIGGER AN ALLERGIC REACTION

Soya beans (*Glycine max*) are a versatile and extremely nutritious food that can be eaten sprouted or cooked, and as tempeh, tofu, soya milk, flour, yoghurt, soy sauce or miso. They contain numerous phytochemicals beneficial to human health, some of which halt the growth of hormone-sensitive tumour cells. In particular, soya bean products are believed to reduce the risk of prostate and breast cancer, and can help both prevent and treat cardiovascular disease. Soya milk, which is made from soya beans, is a nutritious alternative to dairy milk.

**RECIPES** *see tofu (below) and tempeh (page 202)*

## SOYA YOGHURT

★ AS FOR SOYA BEAN, PLUS LACTOBACILLI

✓ ANTI-CANCER, ANTIOXIDANT, IMMUNO-STIMULANT, LOWERS CHOLESTEROL

! AS FOR SOYA BEAN

Live yoghurt contains lactobacilli, beneficial bacteria that help prevent the colonization of the gut by harmful micro-organisms. Live yoghurt is especially helpful after antibiotic treatment (which kills off beneficial bacteria in the digestive tract). It also helps in the treatment of urinary-tract infections, gastroenteritis, infection by *helicobacter pylori* (the bacterium that causes stomach ulcers), inflammatory bowel disease and colon cancer.

**RECIPES** *avocado smoothie (page 193), yoghurt with fruit (page 243), potato salad (page 260), raspberry gateau (page 262), blackberry cream (page 264), passion and lime (page 267)*

## TOFU (BEANCURD)

★ VITAMIN B3, FOLATE; CALCIUM, MAGNESIUM, MANGANESE, PHOSPHORUS; COPPER, IRON, ZINC; ISOFLAVONES, PROTEASE INHIBITORS, SAPONINS; PROTEIN, UNSATURATED FAT

✓ ANTI-CANCER, LOWERS CHOLESTEROL, CALCIUM-RICH

! AS FOR SOYA BEAN

Tofu is an extremely versatile food that is made from soya beans (*Glycine max*) in a process similar to cheese-making. It is high in protein, free from saturated fat, easy to digest and, like all soya products, has many health benefits. Soft tofu has a delicate texture and is generally mixed with other ingredients before being used in recipes. Firm tofu can be cut, sliced, chopped or crumbled and added to a wide variety of dishes. Both soft and firm types have a neutral taste and absorb flavours readily when marinated or cooked with herbs and spices. See also tempeh (page 202).

**RECIPES** *scrambled tofu (page 242), tofumasalata (page 248), tofu balls (page 250), amaranth and tofu puffs (page 252), spicy tofu burgers (page 257)*

# tempeh

**TEMPEH IS A VERSATILE AND NUTRITIOUS PRODUCT MADE FROM SOYA BEANS. PACKED WITH PHYTOCHEMICALS, IT IS ONE OF THE BRIGHTEST STAR FOODS FOR BOOSTING IMMUNITY AND PREVENTING CANCER, HEART DISEASE AND HORMONE-RELATED PROBLEMS.**

## The origin of tempeh

Tempeh is a form of beancurd, originally produced in Indonesia but now popular all over the world. It is a near-perfect source of protein. Unlike animal meat, it contains no saturated fats and it is also one of the few vegetable products to contain vitamin B12.

Tempeh is made by mixing dehulled, split and precooked soya beans (*Glycine max*) with a yeast culture in a process similar to cheese-making. The beans are packed tightly into perforated containers (traditionally banana leaves, but nowadays usually plastic bags) and moulded into flat cakes or sausages. These are set to incubate, in ovens or in the sun, at a temperature of 15–38°C/gas mark 1 until the process of fermentation transforms the mixture into a tight lump. The finished product is delicious, with a nutty taste resembling chicken or fish. Tempeh can be sliced and fried, or cut into cubes and added to stews and other dishes. The fermentation process initiates the partial breakdown of the beans, which makes tempeh easier to digest than other cooked beans, with less tendency to cause flatulence.

## Immune-boosting properties

Tempeh is packed with health-enhancing carbohydrates, fibre and protein and also contains a wealth of minerals, B vitamins, phytoestrogens (isoflavonoids), protease inhibitors and saponins that have anti-microbial and anti-cancer properties. Phytoestrogens are active against viruses and are known to inhibit the growth of cancers and halt the spread of malignant cells into surrounding tissues, reducing the risk of breast and prostate cancers in particular. They also appear to be protective against many other hormone-related health problems, such as fibrocystic breast disease, osteoporosis, endometriosis and uterine fibroids.

Protease inhibitors are believed to prevent cancer-causing agents from entering cells and so help to keep cellular DNA intact. They have also been found to inhibit the growth of some cancers and to stop the spread of tumour cells. Saponins support the immune system, reduce the growth rate of some cancer cells and help control blood cholesterol. Tempeh protein improves the efficiency of cell-mediated immunity.

## Heart protector

Heart disease is much less common in regions where soya bean protein is eaten in preference to animal protein. Like other soya products, tempeh helps lower blood cholesterol. It contains a protein that inhibits intestinal absorption of dietary cholesterol and helps remove cholesterol from the blood, thereby reducing the risk of cardiovascular disorders. Tempeh also contains antioxidants and genistein, which may help prevent cardiovascular disorders such as atherosclerosis. The nutrients in tempeh boost energy levels and make the body better able to cope with stress by supporting both the nervous and immune systems. They also keep hair, glands, blood cells, bone, bone marrow, skin and mucous membranes in good condition, and act as building blocks for proteins, carbohydrates and fats. The nutrients in tempeh aid in the production of haemoglobin (the chemical that transports oxygen in the blood), as well as supporting liver function and fat metabolism, and may also protect against high blood pressure, allergy, asthma, migraine, depression and prostate disorders.

### IMMUNE-BOOSTING PROFILE

★ VITAMINS B2, B3, B5, B6, B12, BIOTIN; CALCIUM, MAGNESIUM, MANGANESE, PHOSPHORUS, POTASSIUM; COPPER, IRON, ZINC; ISOFLAVONES, GENISTEIN, PROTEASE INHIBITORS, SAPONINS; COMPLEX CARBOHYDRATES, FIBRE, PROTEIN

✓ ANTI-CANCER, ANTI-STRESS, ANTI-VIRAL, LOWERS CHOLESTEROL, ENERGY-BOOSTING, IMMUNO-STIMULANT

! SOME PEOPLE ARE ALLERGIC TO SOYA PRODUCTS

! MUCH OF THE WORLD'S SOYA BEAN CROP HAS BEEN GENETICALLY MODIFIED: BUY ORGANIC

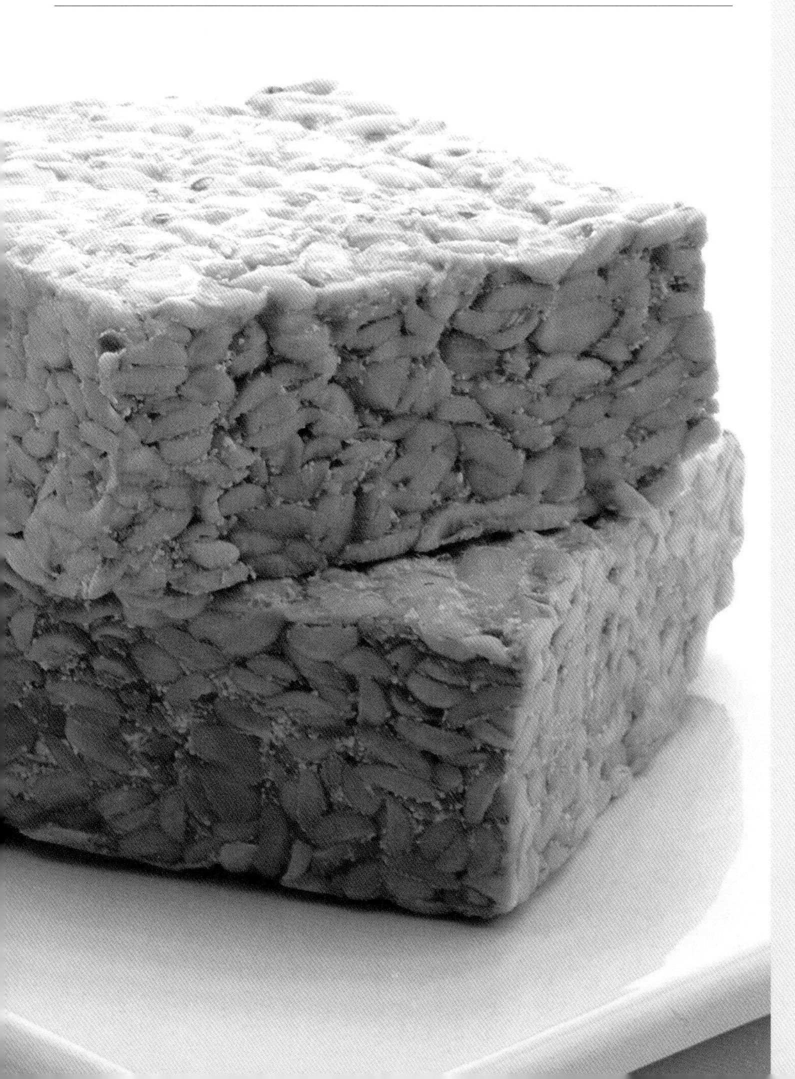

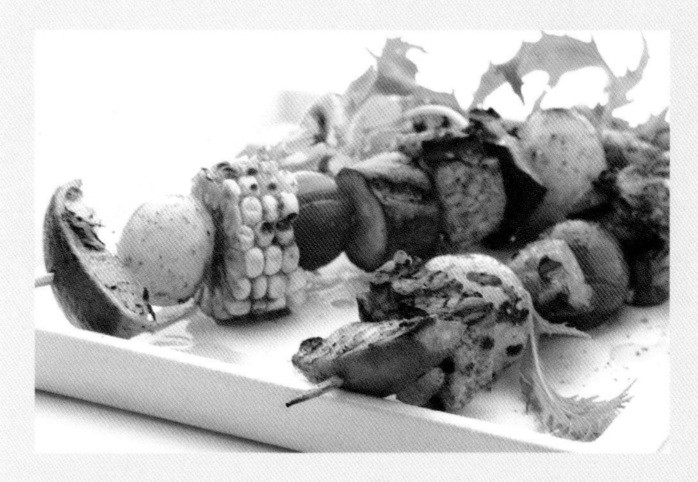

## oriental salad with tempeh *(above)*

2½-cm piece of fresh ginger root, finely chopped
1 garlic clove, finely chopped
10-cm stalk of lemon grass, finely chopped
4 tbsp lemon juice
1 tbsp balsamic vinegar
1 tbsp maple syrup
100 ml orange juice
4 tbsp soy sauce
8 tempeh rashers, cut into chunks
1 tbsp sesame oil
1 bunch of spring onions, thinly sliced
8 baby corn cobs, steamed
100 g bean sprouts
6 leaves of chinese cabbage, shredded
Salt and pepper
2 tbsp gomassio (sesame salt)

Mix the ginger, garlic, lemon grass, lemon juice, vinegar, maple syrup, orange juice and soy sauce in a bowl. Add the tempeh and leave to marinate for 1 hour. Remove the tempeh (leaving the marinade in the bowl) and fry it in the oil. Sprinkle with salt. Mix the spring onions, baby corn cobs, bean sprouts and chinese cabbage in a salad bowl, mix in the marinade, add the tempeh, season, and sprinkle with gomassio.

## tempeh kebabs

200 g tempeh, cubed
1 courgette, thickly sliced
1 lime, in wedges
8 garlic cloves
2 corn cobs, cut into chunks
16 cherry tomatoes
1 aubergine, diced
450 g small new potatoes, cooked

For the marinade:

2 tbsp lemon juice
2 tbsp sherry
2 tbsp olive oil
1 tbsp soy sauce
2 garlic cloves, crushed
4 tbsp tomato ketchup (see page 251)

Place the kebab ingredients in a bowl. Add the marinade ingredients and mix well. Leave covered for a couple of hours, stirring occasionally. Divide the mixed ingredients between 8 barbecue skewers. Brush with the leftover marinade and place on a hot barbecue for about 10 minutes, turning from time to time.

# herbs and spices

## HERBS

### BORAGE (BEEPLANT, TALEWORT)

★ VITAMINS A, C, B3; CALCIUM, MAGNESIUM, PHOSPHORUS, POTASSIUM; ZINC; MUCILAGE, SAPONINS, TANNIN, VOLATILE OIL; FIBRE

✓ ANTI-INFLAMMATORY, ANTIOXIDANT, DIAPHORETIC, EXPECTORANT

The leaves of borage (*Borago officinalis*) can be used to treat inflammation, fevers and coughs, and help the body recover from the effects of stress. They taste like cucumber and are delicious chopped finely and added to salads.

***RECIPES*** *cough mixture (page 268), immuni-tea (page 269), stress relief (page 270), tea for fever (page 271), tea for glands (page 271)*

### CATMINT (CATNIP, CATNEP)

★ CALCIUM, MAGNESIUM, PHOSPHORUS, POTASSIUM; ZINC; BITTER PRINCIPLE, TANNIN, VOLATILE OILS

✓ ANTISPASMODIC, ASTRINGENT, CIRCULATORY AND DIGESTIVE STIMULANT, DIAPHORETIC, FEBRIFUGE

Catmint (*Nepeta cataria*) leaves and flowering tops are particularly useful in treating childhood fevers and respiratory-tract infections, and help settle stomach upsets and diarrhoea.

***RECIPES*** *sleepy time (page 270), tea for fever (page 271)*

### CHAMOMILE (CAMOMILE – WILD, GERMAN, ANNUAL)

★ COUMARINS, MUCILAGE, RUTIN, SALICYLIC ACID, TANNIN, VALERIANIC ACID, VOLATILE OIL

✓ ANTI-ALLERGIC, ANTI-INFLAMMATORY, ANTISEPTIC, ANTISPASMODIC, SEDATIVE

Chamomile (*Matricaria recutita*) flowers relieve restlessness and tension, and are useful for headache, anxiety and sleeplessness. They also help relieve digestive upsets, and are particularly suitable for children.

***RECIPES*** *calming tea (page 268), chamomile tonic (page 268), hay fever relief (page 269), sleepy time (page 270), tea for fever (page 271)*

### CLEAVERS (CLIVERS, GOOSEGRASS)

★ BIOFLAVONOIDS, CITRIC ACID, COUMARINS, GLYCOSIDES, TANNIN

✓ ANTI-CANCER, ANTI-INFLAMMATORY, DETOXIFYING

Cleavers (*Galium aparine*) is a tonic for the lymphatic system, useful for treating swollen glands, eczema, psoriasis, joint problems, oedema, ulcers, tumours, infections of the urinary tract, and urinary stones.

***RECIPES*** *immuni-tea (page 269), tea for ear infections (page 271), tea for glands (page 271), tea for the skin (page 271)*

### ECHINACEA

★ ECHINACEIN, GLYCOSIDE (ECHINACOSIDE), RESIN, VOLATILE OIL

✓ ANTI-ALLERGIC, ANTI-CANCER, ANTI-INFLAMMATORY, ANTI-MICROBIAL, ANTISEPTIC, IMMUNO-STIMULANT

Echinacea (*Echinacea angustifolia*) enhances the body's natural resistance to infection, and is one of the most important natural remedies against colds and flu and other infectious diseases (including HIV) and cancer.

***RECIPES*** *hay fever relief (page 269), immuni-tea (page 269), tea for fungal infections (page 271), tea for glands (page 271)*

### ELDERFLOWER (BLACK, EUROPEAN)

★ CHOLINE; BIOFLAVONOIDS (INCLUDING RUTIN AND KAEMPFEROL), CYANOGLYCOSIDE; MUCILAGE, OMEGA-3 AND -6 FATTY ACIDS, PECTIN, TANNIN, VOLATILE OIL

✓ ANTI-CATARRHAL, ANTI-INFLAMMATORY, CIRCULATORY AND IMMUNE STIMULANT, DIAPHORETIC, EXPECTORANT

Elderflower (*Sambucus nigra*) enhances natural resistance to disease and promotes perspiration – excellent for colds, flu and high temperature, as well as allergic symptoms and catarrh.

***RECIPES*** *cold buster (page 268), elderflower spritzer (page 268), hay fever relief (page 269), lung-cleansing tea mix (page 270), tea for ear infections (page 271)*

### FEVERFEW (MIDSUMMER DAISY)

★ BITTERS, VOLATILE OIL

✓ ANTI-INFLAMMATORY, DIGESTIVE STIMULANT, PAINKILLING, VASODILATOR

! CHEWING FRESH FEVERFEW LEAVES MAY CAUSE MOUTH ULCERS

! STIMULATES UTERUS AND SO BEST AVOIDED DURING PREGNANCY

The leaves of fresh feverfew (*Tanacetum parthenium/ Chrysanthemum parthenium*) are used to relieve headache. They offer an effective way of preventing migraine, and can help relieve the pain of rheumatoid arthritis.

***RECIPES*** *tea for headache (page 271)*

## LAVENDER

★ TANNIN, VOLATILE OIL

✓ ANTIDEPRESSANT, ANTISPASMODIC, RELAXING, SEDATIVE

Lavender (*Lavandula angustifolia*) is an effective treatment for headaches, and for nervous exhaustion, depression and skin irritations. Soothing and relaxing, it promotes healing by bringing body and mind into balance.

***RECIPES*** *calming tea (page 268), pick-me-up (page 270), sleepy time (page 270), stress relief (page 270)*

## LEMON BALM

★ BITTERS, ROSMARINIC ACID, TANNIN, VOLATILE OIL

✓ ANTI-DEPRESSANT, ANTI-VIRAL, LOWERS BLOOD PRESSURE, MILD SEDATIVE, RELAXANT

Lemon balm (*Melissa officinalis*) is a sweet-tasting herb that can help prevent and treat cold sores, and is thought to reduce the growth rate of tumours. It has a calming effect on the nerves and the digestion, and is useful in the management of heart problems.

***RECIPES*** *calming tea (page 268), immuni-tea (page 269), pick-me-up (page 270), stress relief (page 270)*

## MARIGOLD (CALENDULA)

★ VITAMIN C; BITTERS, CAROTENOIDS, LUTEIN, LYCOPENE, QUERCETIN, MUCILAGE, RESIN, RUTIN, SALICYLIC ACID, SAPONINS, VANILLIC ACID

✓ ANTI-MICROBIAL, ANTI-INFLAMMATORY, ANTIOXIDANT, WOUND HEALING

Marigold or calendula (*Calendula officinalis*) flowers are a natural antibacterial, antifungal and antiviral treatment for mouth and skin infections, inflammation and ulcers (both internal and external). Marigold helps relieve gall-bladder disorders, and may have a role in the management of cancer.

***RECIPES*** *green leafy salad (page 181), tea for ear infections (page 271), tea for fungal infections (page 271), tea for glands (page 271), tea for the skin (page 271)*

## PEPPERMINT

★ VITAMINS A, C, E, B2, B3, FOLATE; CALCIUM, MAGNESIUM, POTASSIUM, PHOSPHORUS; IRON; BITTERS, PECTIN, RUTIN, TANNIN, VOLATILE OILS (INCLUDING MENTHOL)

✓ ANTI-CANCER, ANTIMICROBIAL, ANTIOXIDANT, ANTISEPTIC, ANTISPASMODIC, CARMINATIVE, COOLING, DIGESTIVE STIMULANT

Peppermint (*Mentha* x *piperita*) is an effective treatment for colds and coughs, helping to clear airways and make breathing easier. It also stimulates the secretion of digestive juices and helps to relieve symptoms of indigestion, ulcerative colitis and Crohn's disease.

***RECIPES*** *grapefruit and peppermint fizz (page 189), mint and melon soup (page 245), nectarine surprise (page 263), green tea with mint (page 269), lung-cleansing tea mix (page 270)*

## ROSEMARY

★ VITAMIN A; CALCIUM, MAGNESIUM; IRON, ZINC; BIOFLAVONOIDS, BITTERS, SAPONINS, VOLATILE OILS (INCLUDING CAMPHOR)

✓ ANTI-MICROBIAL, ANTIOXIDANT, ANTISPASMODIC, ASTRINGENT, CARMINATIVE, CIRCULATORY AND DIGESTIVE STIMULANT, TONIC

Rosemary (*Rosmarinus officinalis*) stimulates the circulation and the nervous system. It is a traditional tonic for the heart, and it has a calming effect on the digestion. It is also an effective treatment for tension headaches.

***RECIPES*** *scrambled tofu (page 242), pick-me-up (page 270), tea for aches and pains (page 271), tea for headache (page 271)*

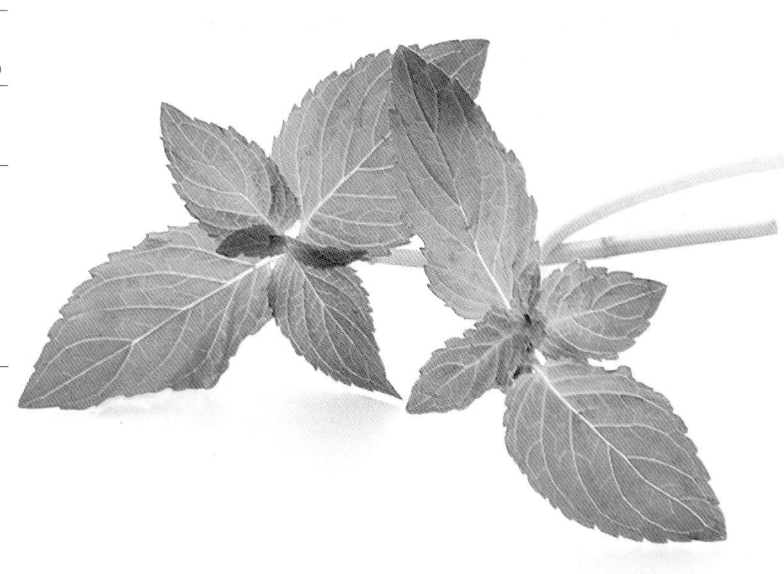

### SAGE (RED, GARDEN)

★ VITAMIN A; CALCIUM, MAGNESIUM, MANGANESE, POTASSIUM; ZINC; BIOFLAVONOIDS, GLYCOSIDES, PHYTOESTROGENS, SAPONINS, TANNIN, VOLATILE OIL

✓ ANTI-MICROBIAL, ANTIOXIDANT, DIGESTIVE, DRYING, PERIPHERAL VASODILATOR

! AVOID DURING PREGNANCY

Sage (*Salvia officinalis*) is an antiseptic herb that improves the health of mucous membranes. It can also reduce perspiration.

**RECIPES** *mushrooms with sage and thyme stuffing (page 256), sage mix for sore throats (page 270)*

### ST JOHN'S WORT (HYPERICUM)

★ VITAMIN C; BIOFLAVONOIDS, CAROTENOIDS, GLYCOSIDES, PECTIN, RESIN, TANNIN

✓ ANTIDEPRESSANT, ANTISEPTIC, ASTRINGENT, ANTI-INFLAMMATORY, ANTIOXIDANT, EXPECTORANT, HEALING, PAINKILLING

! MAY INHIBIT THE EFFECT OF PRESCRIPTION DRUGS: IF RECEIVING MEDICATION, SEEK YOUR DOCTOR'S ADVICE BEFORE TAKING

St John's wort (*Hypericum perforatum*) is helpful in the management of post-viral disorders. It is an effective remedy for mild depression and can also be used as a mild painkiller.

**RECIPES** *calming tea (page 268), tea for aches and pains (page 271), tea for joints (page 271)*

### THYME (COMMON, GARDEN)

★ VITAMIN A; CALCIUM, MAGNESIUM, MANGANESE; ZINC; BITTERS, BIOFLAVONOIDS, RESIN, VOLATILE OIL (INCLUDING THYMOL AND CAMPHOR); OMEGA-3 AND -6 FATTY ACIDS

✓ ANTIMICROBIAL, ANTIOXIDANT, ANTISEPTIC, ANTISPASMODIC, ASTRINGENT, CARMINATIVE, EXPECTORANT

Thyme (*Thymus vulgaris*) contains the volatile oil thymol, a powerful antiseptic and one of the most effective of all herbal antibiotics. It is useful in the treatment of respiratory-tract infections, such as bronchitis, laryngitis and whooping cough, and helps relieve the symptoms of asthma. Thyme is also beneficial in the treatment of gastro-intestinal disorders including colic and diarrhoea.

**RECIPES** *beans and tomatoes on toast (page 242), italian butterbean soup (page 245), marinated olives (page 248), mushrooms with sage and thyme stuffing (page 256), catalan salad (page 260), cough mixture (page 268), eucalyptus mix (page 269)*

### VIOLET (BLUE, SWEET)

★ ALKALOID, METHYL SALICYLATE, RUTIN, SAPONINS, VOLATILE OIL

✓ ANTI-CANCER, ANTI-INFLAMMATORY, EXPECTORANT

Violet (*Viola odorata*) leaves and flowers have a role in the management of malignant tumours and may help inhibit the spread of cancer. They are also useful in the treatment of chronic bronchitis, chronic nasal catarrh, skin problems and arthritis.

**RECIPES** *yoghurt with fruit (page 243), cough mixture (page 268), lung-cleansing tea mix (page 270), tea for the skin (page 271)*

### WILD MARJORAM (EUROPEAN OREGANO)

★ VITAMIN A; CALCIUM, MAGNESIUM, MANGANESE, PHOSPHORUS, POTASSIUM; COPPER, IRON, ZINC; BIOFLAVONOIDS, BITTERS, PHYTOSTEROLS, TANNINS, VOLATILE OILS; OMEGA-3, -6 AND OLEIC FATTY ACIDS

✓ ANTIMICROBIAL, ANTIOXIDANT, DIAPHORETIC, EXPECTORANT, STIMULANT, WARMING

Wild marjoram (*Origanum vulgare*) is an excellent warming remedy for coughs (including whooping cough), colds and influenza. It can also be used to relieve headache and indigestion.

**RECIPES** *black-eye bean and wild marjoram soup (page 245), cold buster (page 268), cough mixture (page 268), tea for headache (page 271), scandinavian beetroot burgers (page 177)*

### YARROW (MILFOIL)

★ BIOFLAVONOIDS, BITTERS, RESIN, SALICYLATES, TANNIN, VOLATILE OILS (INCLUDING CINEOL, AZULENE AND CAMPHOR)

✓ ANTI-INFLAMMATORY, ANTISEPTIC, ASTRINGENT, BLOOD PRESSURE LOWERING, DIAPHORETIC, DIGESTIVE TONIC, PERIPHERAL VASODILATOR

! EXCESS YARROW INTAKE CAN CAUSE HEADACHE

Yarrow (*Achillea millefolium*) has a long tradition as a remedy for colds and flu but in fact this versatile herb has a multitude of beneficial effects on health. As an anti-inflammatory and diaphoretic it helps to relieve catarrh, bronchitis, cystitis and gastro-intestinal inflammation, and enables the body to deal more effectively with infections. As a cardiovascular restorative, it improves peripheral circulation and lowers blood pressure. As an external remedy, it has a longstanding reputation for stopping bleeding and healing wounds.

**RECIPES** *cold buster (page 268), circulation booster (page 268), cystitis relief (page 268), tea for ear infections (page 271)*

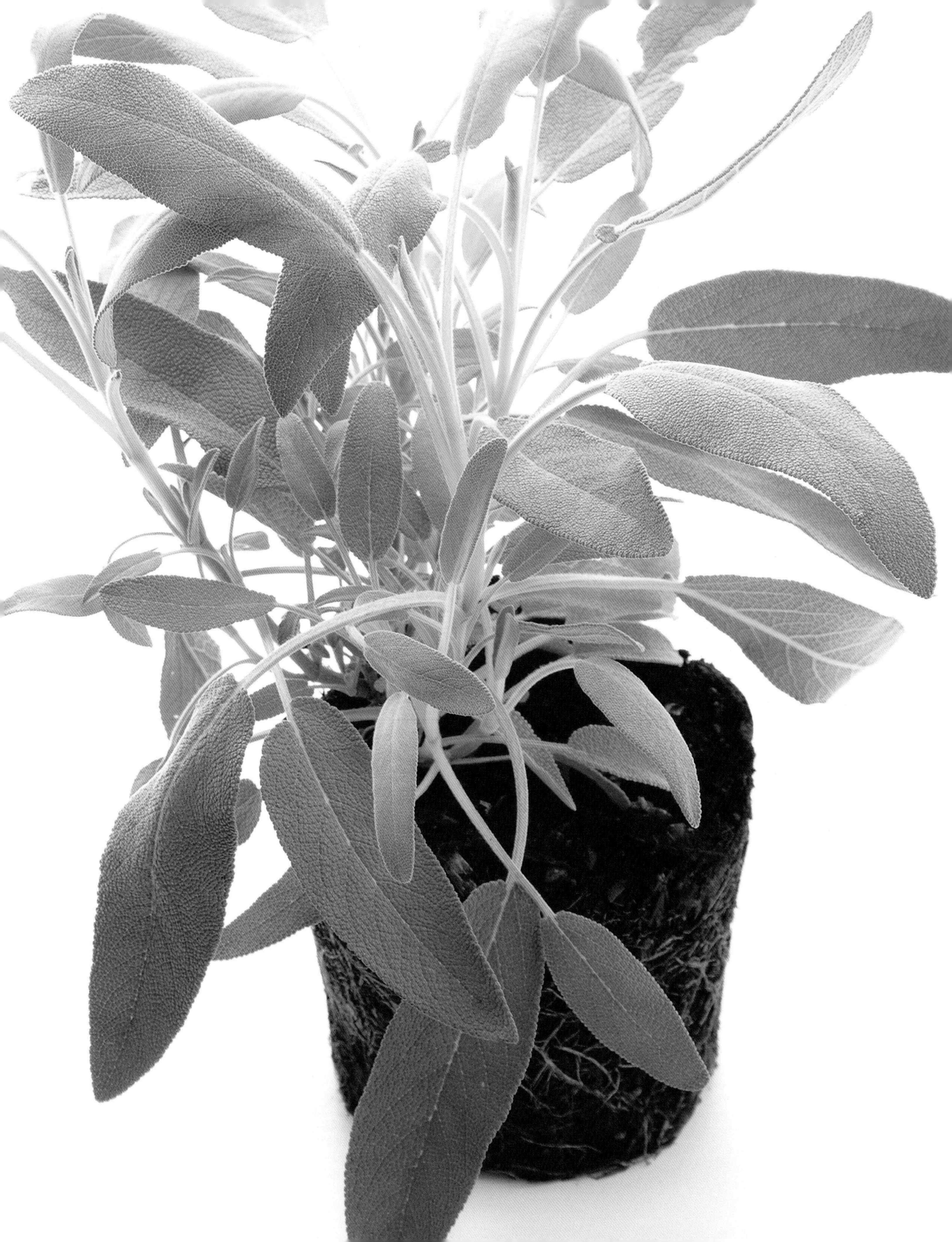

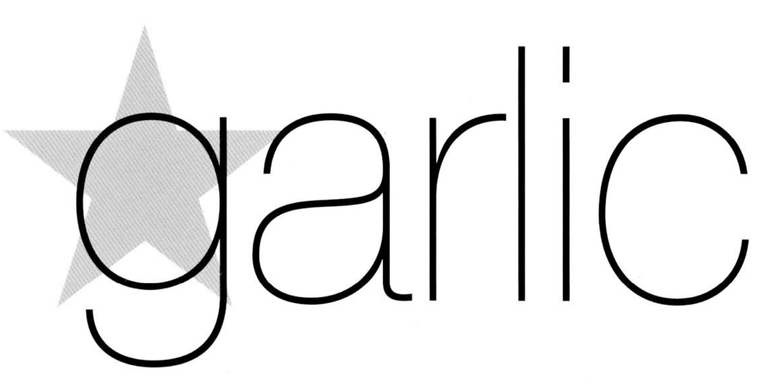

# garlic

**THIS AROMATIC HERB DOESN'T JUST KEEP VAMPIRES AT BAY! GARLIC PROTECTS AGAINST A WIDE RANGE OF BACTERIAL, FUNGAL AND VIRAL INFECTIONS. IT ALSO STRENGTHENS THE HEART AND BLOOD VESSELS AND HELPS PREVENT CANCER.**

## The origin of garlic

Garlic (*Allium sativum*) is a plant so ancient that no one is really sure of its origins. It is thought to have evolved from the wild garlic (*Allium longicuspis*) of central Asia, and is known to have been cultivated in Egypt and Mesopotamia before 2000BCE. According to Pliny, it had a semi-divine status in the ancient world and was called upon in the swearing of oaths. Now one of the world's most popular herbs, it is cultivated and used worldwide as both a food and medicine.

## Immune-boosting properties

Garlic grows best where warm and dry summers prevail, and is itself a warming and drying herb. It is also one of the most effective natural anti-microbials, stimulating the production of white blood cells and acting against a wide range of bacteria, fungi, parasites and viruses. Even with the development of modern antibiotics and a more sophisticated understanding of microbiology, garlic is still regarded by many health practitioners as first-line treatment for infectious disease. Garlic fights various gastro-intestinal infections and infestations such as dysentery, typhoid, threadworm and tapeworm. It contains a volatile oil that is mostly excreted through the lungs, making it an excellent remedy for respiratory disorders such as bronchitis, catarrh, influenza and whooping cough. This oil is also active against tuberculosis and plays a role in the management of asthma. Garlic combats fungal infections such as yeast infections, athlete's foot and ringworm, and is a standard ingredient in anti-candida diets, encouraging the growth of beneficial bacteria and inhibiting pathogens. It may also reduce the virulence of the HIV virus.

One of the most popular modern uses for garlic is in dealing with cardiovascular disease. It acts on the circulatory system to reduce the level of blood fat and cholesterol, and decreases the tendency of the blood to clot.

Over time, garlic will also lower blood pressure significantly, and it prevents the formation of atheroma (fat deposits on artery walls). Recent studies have also shown that garlic reduces the arteriosclerotic changes (hardening of the arteries) that appear with age. These changes are accelerated by smoking and eating a typical Western diet high in saturated fats and sugar.

Allicin is one of the active ingredients responsible for garlic's ability to suppress the formation of cancer cells and enhance the immune system's ability to slow the spread of malignant tumours. This corresponds with epidemiological findings that cancer is less common in areas with high garlic consumption.

Even the idea that garlic keeps vampires away may be based on fact, not fiction. In Central Asia, a rare variety of the disease porphyria

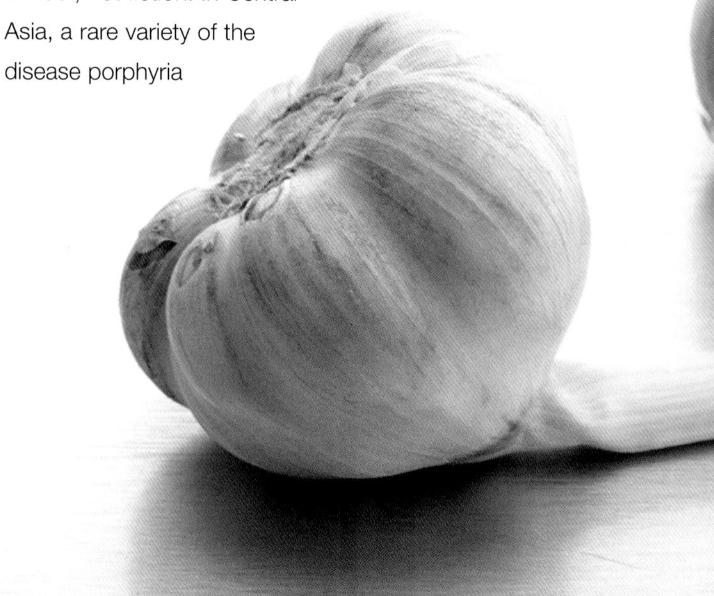

was once relatively common. Symptoms included extreme paleness and a complete intolerance to sunlight. Relief from some of these might have been found in garlic's medicinal properties.

## IMMUNE-BOOSTING PROFILE

- ★ VITAMIN B6; MAGNESIUM, PHOSPHORUS, POTASSIUM; IRON, ZINC; BIOFLAVONOIDS, GLUCOKININ, MUCILAGE, PHYTOHORMONES, VOLATILE OILS (INCLUDING ALLICIN)
- ✓ ANTIBACTERIAL, ANTICOAGULANT, ANTI-CATARRHAL, ANTIOXIDANT, ANTISEPTIC, DETOXIFYING, EXPECTORANT, LOWERS BLOOD PRESSURE AND CHOLESTEROL
- ! THE SULPHUR COMPOUNDS IN GARLIC CAN IRRITATE ULCERS
- ! HIGH DOSES OF GARLIC CAN EXAGGERATE THE EFFECTS OF ANTICOAGULANT AND BLOOD-PRESSURE-LOWERING DRUGS
- EAT WITH PARSLEY TO AVOID GARLIC ON THE BREATH

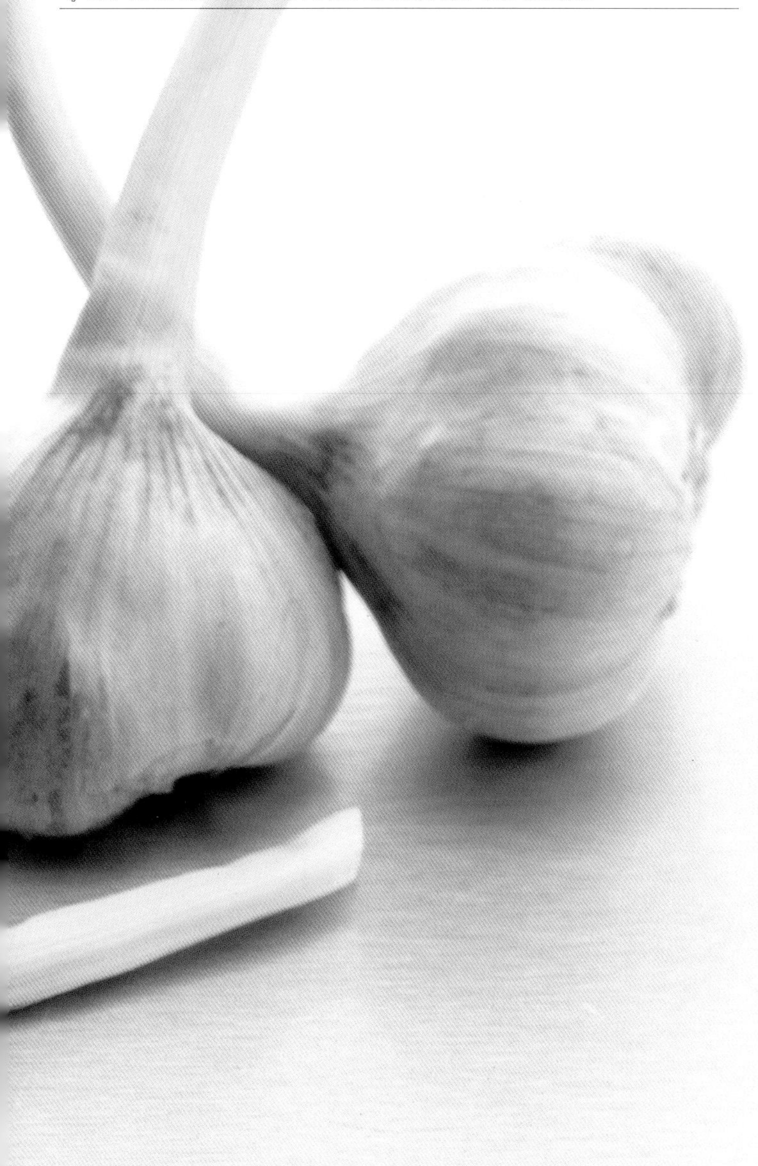

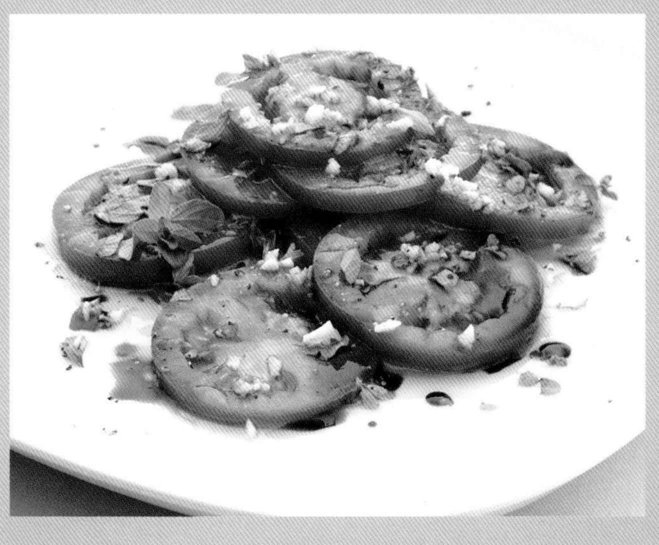

## tomato, wild marjoram and garlic salad *(above)*

1 kg ripe tomatoes, sliced
4 tbsp fresh wild marjoram, chopped
2 garlic cloves, finely chopped
6 tbsp olive oil
2 tbsp balsamic vinegar
Salt and pepper to taste

Arrange the tomatoes on a large plate and sprinkle with marjoram, garlic, oil, vinegar, and salt and pepper. Serve.

## garlic and savoy cabbage

3 tbsp olive oil
1 tsp curry powder
1 tbsp black mustard seeds
1 medium savoy cabbage, finely shredded
3 garlic cloves, finely chopped
2 tbsp desiccated coconut
1 tbsp maple syrup
2 tbsp lemon juice
Salt and pepper to taste

Heat the oil in a large frying pan or wok. Add the spices and stir-fry until the mustard seeds begin to pop. Add the cabbage and the garlic and stir-fry until the cabbage begins to wilt. Add the coconut and stir-fry for 1 minute more, then add the maple syrup and lemon juice. Mix well and season with salt and pepper. Serve hot.

## rich garlic dressing

4 tbsp balsamic vinegar
1 tbsp maple syrup
1 tbsp Dijon mustard
2 garlic cloves, crushed
Salt and pepper to taste
150 ml olive oil

Whisk or hand-blend the vinegar, maple syrup, mustard, garlic, and salt and pepper with a little oil. Add the oil very slowly, a little at a time until the dressing starts to emulsify. Then add more oil, still a little at a time, until the taste is right. Adjust seasoning if necessary and serve.

# SPICES

## BLACK CUMIN

★ VITAMINS A, B1, B2, B3; CALCIUM, MAGNESIUM, MANGANESE, PHOSPHORUS, POTASSIUM; COPPER, IRON, ZINC; OMEGA-3 AND -6 FATTY ACIDS

✓ ANTI-ALLERGIC, ANTI-INFLAMMATORY, ANTIMICROBIAL, ANTIOXIDANT

Black cumin (*Nigella sativa*) has been used for centuries in Asia and the Middle East as a treatment for allergy, eczema and upper respiratory-tract disorders such as asthma and bronchitis. It may also help in the prevention of immunodeficiency disorders.

**RECIPES** *beans and tomatoes on toast (page 242), spicy moroccan soup (page 246), baba ganoush (page 248), garlic oxymel (page 269), heart chai (page 269)*

## CARAWAY

★ VITAMINS B1, B2, B3; CALCIUM, MAGNESIUM, PHOSPHORUS, POTASSIUM; COPPER, IRON, ZINC; BIOFLAVONOIDS, VOLATILE OIL

✓ ANTIBACTERIAL, ANTIOXIDANT, ANTISPASMODIC, CARMINATIVE, EXPECTORANT, TONIC

Caraway (*Carum carvi*) seeds are used to alleviate upper respiratory-tract problems such as asthma and bronchitis and in a gargle to treat laryngitis. They can also be chewed to alleviate gastro-intestinal disorders, including indigestion, colic, diarrhoea and trapped wind.

**RECIPES** *healing soup (page 244), spicy moroccan soup (page 246), pan bread (page 258), spicy chai (page 270)*

## CAYENNE

★ VITAMINS A, B2, B3; CALCIUM, MAGNESIUM, PHOSPHORUS, POTASSIUM; IRON, ZINC; BIOFLAVONOIDS, VOLATILE OIL

✓ ANTIBACTERIAL, ANTI-CANCER, ANTI-CATARRHAL, ANTIOXIDANT, DIAPHORETIC, STIMULANT, TONIC

! CAYENNE IRRITATES MUCOUS MEMBRANES: HANDLE WITH CARE AND AVOID IN CASES OF GASTRITIS OR STOMACH ULCER

Cayenne (*Capsicum anuum*) is a powerful circulatory stimulant that increases the blood supply to all parts of the body, thus creating a feeling of heat. It is useful for preventing colds, and to deal with general debility in convalescence.

**RECIPES** *spicy moroccan soup (page 246), cold buster (page 268), heart chai (page 269), tea for fever (page 271)*

## CELERY SEED

★ CALCIUM, MAGNESIUM, PHOSPHORUS, POTASSIUM; COPPER, IRON, ZINC; BIOFLAVONOIDS, VOLATILE OIL

✓ ANTIOXIDANT, DETOXIFYING, DIGESTIVE TONIC, URINARY ANTISEPTIC

! SHOULD BE AVOIDED DURING PREGNANCY

Celery (*Apium graveolens*) seeds enhance the elimination of uric acid from the body making them useful in arthritic conditions, particularly gout. They also help in the treatment of urinary-tract infections and stones.

**RECIPES** *tea for joints (page 271)*

## EUCALYPTUS

★ BIOFLAVONOIDS, VOLATILE OIL

✓ ANTIBACTERIAL, ANTIFUNGAL, ANTIOXIDANT, ANTISEPTIC, ANTISPASMODIC, EXPECTORANT, FEBRIFUGE, STIMULANT

Eucalyptus (*Eucalyptus globulus*) is a well-known ingredient in cough remedies, and is useful in treating upper respiratory-tract infections in general. It also acts against urinary-tract infections, and has broad-spectrum antibacterial properties.

**RECIPES** *eucalyptus mix (page 269), lung-cleansing tea mix (page 270)*

## GINGER

★ ZINC; MUCILAGE, PHENOLS, RESIN, VOLATILE OILS

✓ ANTISEPTIC, ANTISPASMODIC, CARMINATIVE, DETOXIFYING, DIAPHORETIC, EXPECTORANT, VASODILATOR

Ginger (*Zingiber officinale*) is a warming and comforting remedy for colds and chills. It stimulates peripheral circulation and helps the body rid itself of toxins.

**RECIPES** *korean kimchi-style salad (page 247), apricot and ginger (page 264)*

## HORSERADISH

★ VITAMIN C; CALCIUM, MAGNESIUM; ZINC; ASPARAGIN, RESIN, VOLATILE MUSTARD OIL

✓ ANTI-ALLERGIC, ANTIBACTERIAL, ANTI-CANCER, ANTIOXIDANT, ANTISEPTIC, DETOXIFYING, DIAPHORETIC, EXPECTORANT, TONIC

! AVOID IN CASES OF UNDERACTIVE THYROID

Horseradish (*Armoracia rusticana*) is a circulatory stimulant, useful for chronic rheumatic conditions, urinary-tract infections, and upper respiratory-tract disorders, such as asthma, bronchial catarrh, hay fever and whooping cough. It also stimulates digestion.

**RECIPES** *beetroot and horseradish salad (page 177)*

## JUNIPER

★ BITTER PRINCIPLES, GLYCOSIDE, TANNIN, VOLATILE OIL

✓ ANTIBACTERIAL, ANTI-CATARRHAL, ANTIFUNGAL, CARMINATIVE, DIURETIC, URINARY ANTISEPTIC

! SHOULD BE AVOIDED DURING PREGNANCY AND BY THOSE WITH KIDNEY DISEASE

A digestive stimulant, juniper (*Juniperus communis*) helps detoxify the body and relieves arthritis and gout. It is also used to treat urinary-tract disorders.

***RECIPES*** *swiss chard and juniper berries (page 259)*

## LIQUORICE ROOT

★ CALCIUM, PHOSPHORUS; BIOFLAVONOIDS, TANNIN, BITTER PRINCIPLES, COUMARINS, GLYCOSIDES, PHYTOESTROGEN, VOLATILE OILS

✓ ANTI-INFLAMMATORY, ANTIOXIDANT, ANTISPASMODIC, ANTI-STRESS, EXPECTORANT, GENTLE LAXATIVE, IMMUNO-STIMULANT

Liquorice (*Glycyrrhiza glabra*) helps the body to cope better in stressful conditions, and has a beneficial effect on the adrenal glands (useful for recovery after steroid therapy). It also relieves bronchial catarrh and coughs, and is a specific treatment for gastro-intestinal ulcers. It has been found to inhibit tumour growth.

***RECIPES*** *cough mixture (page 268), immuni-tea (page 269), liquorice mix (page 270), lung-cleansing tea mix (page 270)*

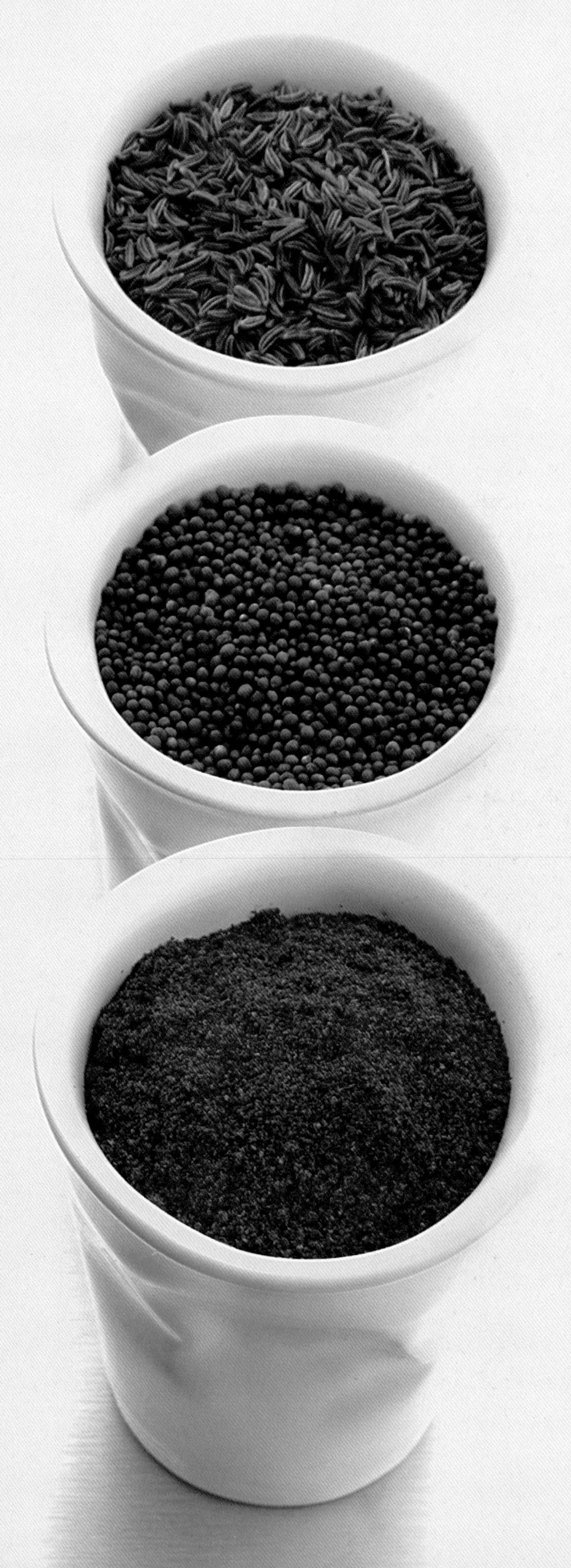

## MUSTARD SEED (BLACK)

★ VITAMINS B1, B2, B3; CALCIUM, MAGNESIUM, PHOSPHORUS, POTASSIUM; IRON, ZINC; MUCILAGE, SINIGRIN, VOLATILE OIL

✓ CARMINATIVE, DIAPHORETIC, DIURETIC, STIMULANT, TONIC

! MUSTARD SEED CAN CAUSE IRRITATION – USE SPARINGLY

Black mustard (*Brassica nigra*) stimulates the circulation and relieves colds, bronchitis, fevers and influenza.

***RECIPES*** *sweet potato curry (page 256), tea for joints (page 271)*

## TURMERIC

★ VITAMIN B3; CALCIUM, PHOSPHORUS, POTASSIUM, MAGNESIUM; COPPER, IRON, ZINC; CURCUMINOIDS, VOLATILE OIL

✓ ANTIBACTERIAL, ANTI-INFLAMMATORY, ANTIOXIDANT

Turmeric (*Curcuma longa*) aids immunity by enhancing the health of the liver. It also mops up free radicals and so helps fight degenerative diseases.

***RECIPES*** *casserole de puy (page 252), paella (page 252)*

# other foods and drinks

## EVENING PRIMROSE OIL

★ VITAMIN E; PHYTOSTEROLS; OMEGA-3 AND -6 FATTY ACIDS

✓ ANTIOXIDANT, HEALING, IMMUNO-STIMULANT

! THIS OIL IS RATHER EXPENSIVE

Evening primrose (*Oenothera biennis*) oil improves the health of body cells, aids normal blood clotting and tissue repair. It is a remedy for eczema and psoriasis, and helpful for multiple sclerosis. It also helps protect against heart disease and some cancers.

**RECIPES** *use in marinades and dressings, or sprinkle on to food*

## GREEN TEA

★ BIOFLAVONOIDS, CATECHINS, THEOPHYLLINE

✓ ANTI-ALLERGIC, ANTI-ASTHMATIC, ANTIOXIDANT, LOWERS BLOOD FATS, LOWERS BLOOD PRESSURE, PREVENTS ABNORMAL CLOTTING

! GREEN TEA CONTAINS CAFFEINE

Green tea is made from the fresh leaves of the tea bush (*Camellia sinensis sp.*). However, unlike the black tea made from the same plant, green tea is unfermented and does not contain the tannins and polyphenolic compounds that inhibit absorption of micronutrients such as iron.

**RECIPES** *green tea with mint (page 269), heart chai (page 269)*

## MISO

★ VITAMINS B2, B3, FOLATE; CALCIUM, MAGNESIUM, PHOSPHORUS; COPPER, IRON, ZINC

✓ ANTIOXIDANT, HEALING, LOWERS BLOOD FATS

Miso is a paste made from fermented soya beans. It can be used as the basis of stews, soups, marinades and sauces. There are several different types, each with a different degree of sweetness and saltiness. It helps keep heart, nerves and muscles healthy, aids liver and red blood cell function, and regulates blood-fat levels.

**RECIPES** *shiitake mushroom soup (page 245)*

## OYSTER MUSHROOM

★ VITAMINS B2, B12; MAGNESIUM, MANGANESE, PHOSPHORUS; IRON, SELENIUM

✓ ANTIOXIDANT

💡 ADD SOY SAUCE TO ENHANCE FLAVOUR

Oyster mushroom (*Pleurotus ostreatus*) enables the body to make full use of the energy stored in the tissues, and helps red blood cells to function properly. It aids liver function, and may help protect against heart disease, cancer and rheumatism.

**RECIPES** *use in recipes in place of shiitake or button mushrooms*

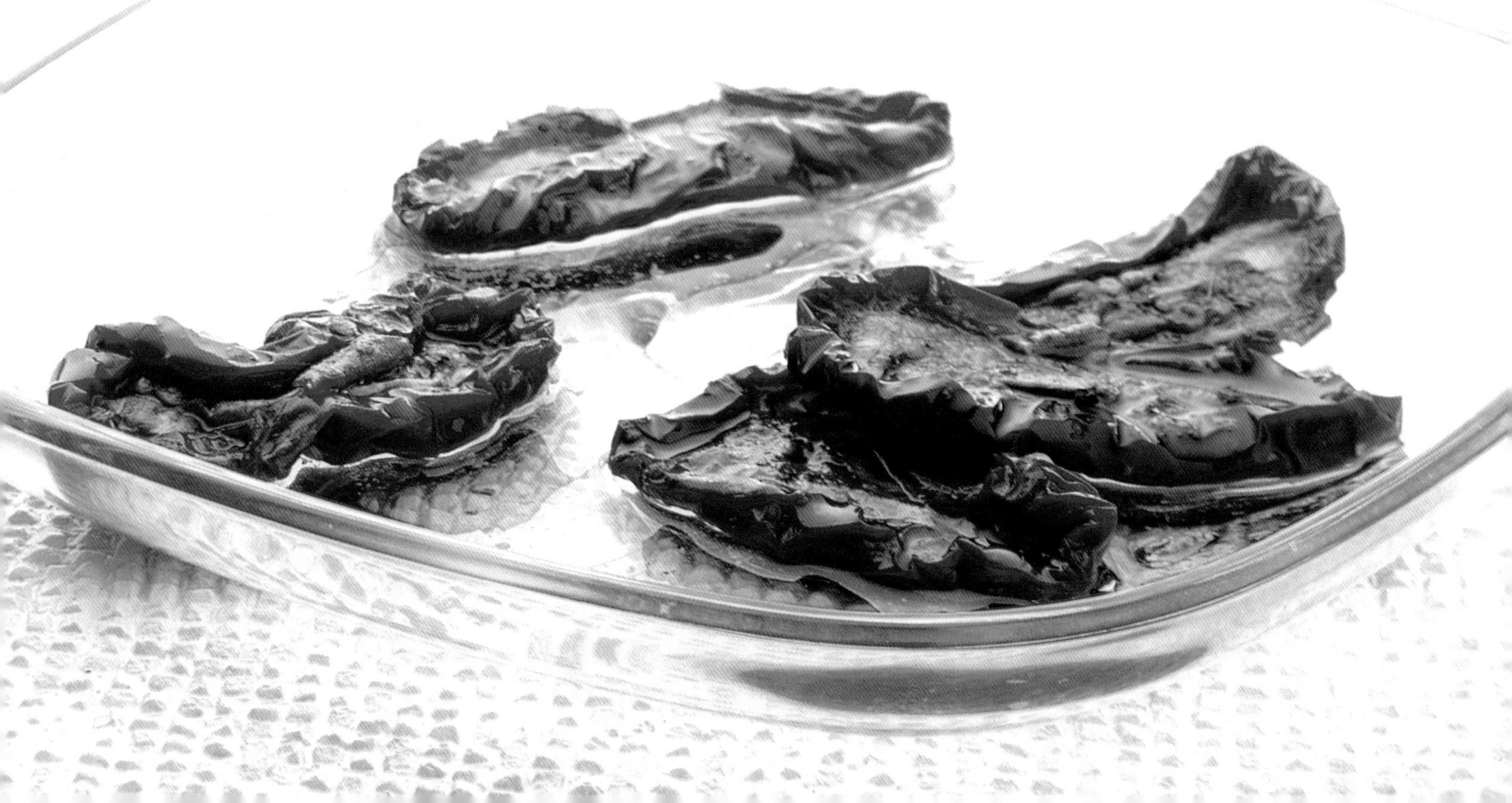

## POLENTA

★ VITAMINS B1, B3; MAGNESIUM, PHOSPHORUS; IRON, ZINC; COMPLEX CARBOHYDRATES, FIBRE, OMEGA-6 FATTY ACIDS, PROTEIN

✓ ANTIOXIDANT, ENERGY-RICH

Polenta is an important energy-rich, savoury, course-ground cornmeal that boosts the body's natural healing capacity. It can taste rather bland on its own, but is an excellent accompaniment to many Mediterranean dishes and a familiar ingredient in Italian country cooking. It is particularly popular as polenta cakes. To make, add boiling water, *herbes de Provence*, sea salt and pepper to pre-cooked polenta to form a stiff dough. Shape the dough into small rissoles and fry in olive oil until golden brown.

**RECIPES** *serve as an accompaniment in place of potatoes or rice*

## SAFFLOWER AND SUNFLOWER OILS

★ VITAMIN E; PHYTOSTEROLS; OMEGA-6 FATTY ACIDS

✓ ANTIOXIDANT, IMMUNO-STIMULANT

Safflower (*Carthamus tinctorius*) and sunflower (*Helianthus annuus*) oils enhance the body's ability to react to injury and repair tissue damage. The omega-6 fatty acids and vitamin E they contain are important for healthy cell membranes, and help ensure normal blood clotting. They also have a beneficial influence on blood pressure and help lower blood-cholesterol levels.

**RECIPES** *safflower oil: baked beetroot salad (page 177), tropical sunshine salad (page 261); sunflower oil: filled avocados (page 193), samosa parcels (page 248), hasselbach potatoes (page 258), carrot 'n' beetroot salad (page 259), raspberry gateau (page 262)*

## SEA VEGETABLE (HIJIKI, IZIKI)

★ VITAMINS A, B12; CALCIUM, MAGNESIUM, PHOSPHORUS; COPPER, IODINE, IRON, ZINC; FIBRE

✓ ANTIOXIDANT, IMMUNO-STIMULANT

💡 IODINE IN THE DIET PROTECTS AGAINST THE ABSORPTION OF RADIOACTIVE IODINE FROM THE ENVIRONMENT

Most of the iodine in the body is found in the thyroid gland. It is an essential component of thyroid hormones, which influence nearly all biochemical reactions in the body and regulate growth, metabolic rate and tissue health. The most reliable sources of iodine in the diet come from the sea, and one of the easiest to use (and most tasty) of the edible seaweeds is sea vegetable (also known as hijiki, or iziki).

**RECIPES** *shiitake with sea vegetable (iziki) (page 215)*

## SUN-DRIED TOMATO

★ VITAMINS A, E; POTASSIUM; COPPER, IODINE, IRON, ZINC; LYCOPENE; ESSENTIAL FATTY ACIDS, PROTEIN, SUGARS

✓ ANTI-CANCER, ANTIOXIDANT

Sun-dried tomatoes (*Lycopersicon esculentum*) promote the health of all body cells (especially the nerves, muscles, skin and mucous membranes). They help prevent the formation of cancer cells and protect against heart disease.

**RECIPES** *brazil nuts and sun-dried tomatoes with beans (page 197), sweetcorn and sun-dried tomato salad (page 260)*

## VEGETABLE MARGARINE

★ VITAMIN E; PHYTOSTEROLS; ESSENTIAL FATTY ACIDS

✓ ANTIOXIDANT, LOWERS BLOOD PRESSURE, LOWERS CHOLESTEROL

! CHOOSE UNSATURATED, NON-HYDROGENATED PLANT MARGARINES

Like the oils it is made from, vegetable margarine helps keep cell membranes healthy, lowers blood cholesterol, and has a beneficial influence on blood pressure.

**RECIPES** *scrambled tofu (page 242), welsh leek and potato soup (page 246), french onion tart (page 255), pear tart (page 263)*

## WHEATGERM OIL

★ VITAMIN E; PHYTOSTEROLS; OMEGA-3 AND -6 FATTY ACIDS

✓ ANTIOXIDANT, HEALING

Wheatgerm (*Triticum sp.*) oil increases the efficiency of the immune response and helps to prevent the immune system from over-reacting to allergens. It increases the health of all cell membranes and may protect against heart disease and cancer. It is also good for skin problems and rheumatoid arthritis.

**RECIPES** *use in salad dressings, and as a replacement for butter or margarine on vegetables*

## YEAST EXTRACT

★ VITAMINS B1, B2, B3, B6, B12, FOLATE; CALCIUM, MAGNESIUM, PHOSPHORUS, POTASSIUM; IODINE, IRON, ZINC

! SOME YEAST EXTRACTS ARE HIGH IN SALT

Yeast extract is a concentrated source of minerals and vitamins, particularly B vitamins. It can help the body to maintain optimum energy levels and improve the health of the blood, bone marrow, nervous system, skin, muscles, mucous membranes and heart. It can be spread on bread or added to soups and stews.

**RECIPES** *italian butterbean soup (page 245)*

# shiitake mushroom

**DELICIOUS AND NUTRITIOUS, SHIITAKE MUSHROOMS HAVE LONG BEEN PRIZED IN THE EAST FOR THEIR ABILITY TO COMBAT INFECTION AND PROTECT AGAINST HEART DISEASE. NOW THE WEST IS DISCOVERING THE AMAZING PROPERTIES OF THIS "FOOD OF EMPERORS".**

## The origin of shiitake

Shiitake mushrooms (*Lentinus edodus*) are native to Japan, China and Korea. Shiitake has a long history of medicinal use in the East, useful in the prevention and treatment of infectious diseases and gastro-intestinal problems, and as a remedy to improve circulation and increase vitality. In China, shiitake mushrooms were once reserved for the emperor and his family. Today, shiitake is one of the most widely produced edible mushrooms in the world.

## Immune-boosting properties

As well as being delicious, shiitake mushrooms are an excellent source of immune-boosting minerals and vitamins, essential amino acids and enzymes. Recent scientific research has concentrated on shiitake's immune-stimulating properties, but Japanese studies have long confirmed its beneficial properties against other common health problems such as atherosclerosis and cancer. Shiitake's ability to stimulate resistance to disease and enhance the immune response is thought to be owing to the fact that the fungus causes the release of interferon and, at the same time, increases the number of macrophages in the blood, enhances phagocytosis, and increases the activity and number of blood lymphocytes. (Lymphocytes and macrophages are two of the most important blood cell types involved in immunity – see page 156.) This combination of actions means that shiitake strengthens the body's first line of defence against infection, by encouraging blood cells to destroy harmful organisms and share information about them with the rest of the immune system, and to clear up cellular debris and waste. In particular, eating shiitake increases resistance to viral infection.

Shiitake's powerful stimulation of immune reaction has kindled interest in the West because of its potential use in the treatment of HIV infections and AIDS. Research suggests that shiitake increases resistance to HIV by blocking initial stages of infection. It is also active against viral encephalitis infection.

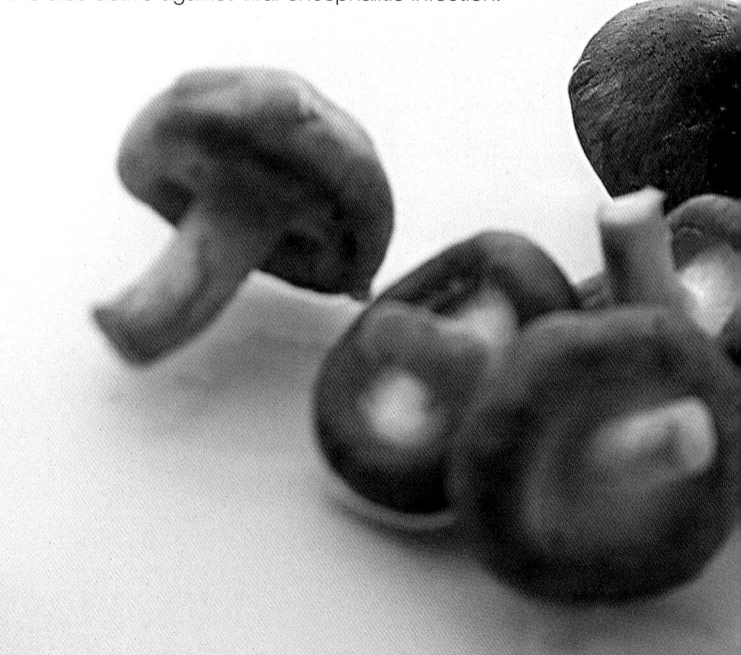

The polysaccharide compound lentinan contained in shiitake has a lowering effect on blood pressure and blood cholesterol, and is beneficial to the whole cardiovascular system, making shiitake a useful remedy in the prevention and treatment of heart disease. It has also attracted considerable attention for its strong tendency to inhibit the growth of tumour cells, and to prevent the spread of metastases (secondaries). However, rather than attacking tumours directly, it works by stimulating the immune system, and boosting the body's own ability to deactivate and eliminate malignant cells.

Shiitake mushrooms are more expensive than the common white field mushrooms, but also very filling – so you need fewer of them in meals. They are widely available, and can be bought fresh, dried or pickled. Fresh or pickled shiitake are prepared and eaten in the same way as white mushrooms. However, dried mushrooms should be rinsed and then soaked for half an hour before use. The stems are hard and should be removed before cooking.

### IMMUNE-BOOSTING PROFILE

★ VITAMINS B1, B2, B3; MAGNESIUM, PHOSPHORUS, POTASSIUM; IRON; BIO-ACTIVE ENZYMES; LENTINAN (POLYSACCHARIDE), PROTEIN

✓ ANTIBACTERIAL, ANTI-CANCER, ANTIVIRAL, LOWERS CHOLESTEROL, IMMUNO-STIMULANT

! SHIITAKE MAY CAUSE DIARRHOEA IF EATEN IN LARGE QUANTITIES

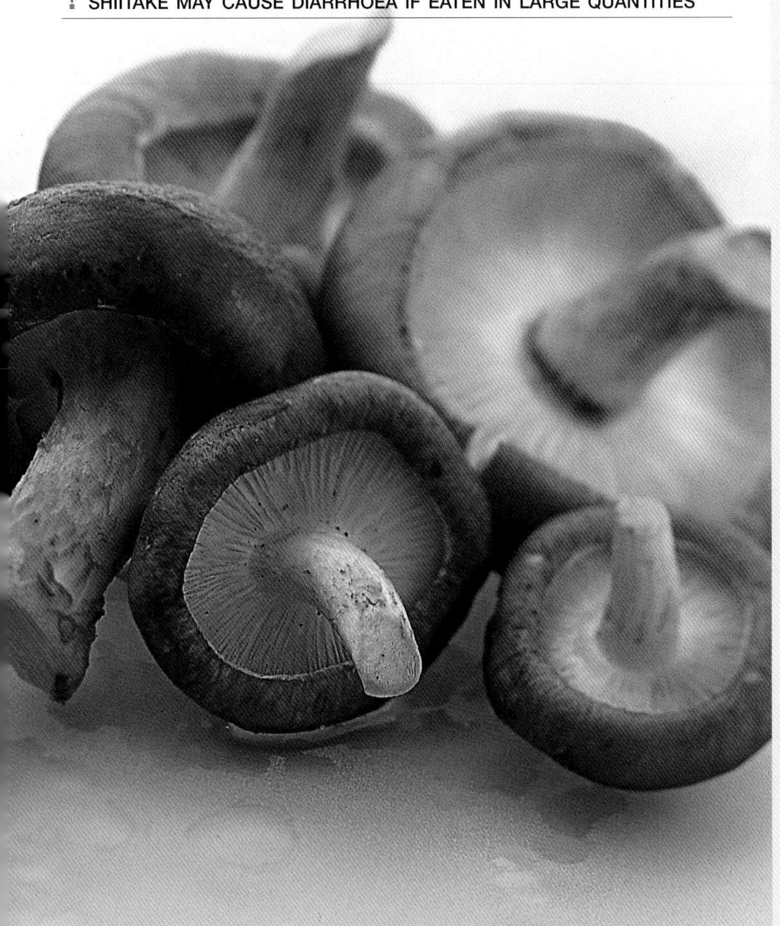

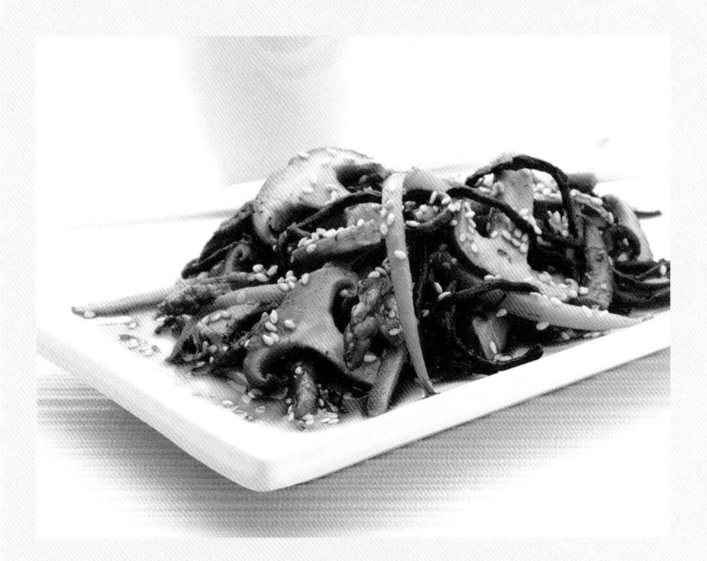

## shiitake with sea vegetable *(above)*

- 150 g dried sea vegetable (iziki)
- 3 tbsp olive oil
- 250 g fresh shiitake mushrooms, cut into strips
- 125 g asparagus
- 4 carrots, cut into julienne strips
- 1 bunch of spring onions
- 200 ml vegetable stock
- 1 tbsp dry sherry
- 2 tbsp soy sauce
- To garnish: 2 tbsp toasted sesame seeds

Rinse the iziki, soak in warm water for 30 minutes, then rinse again. Finely chop the spring onions. Heat the oil in a wok, add the iziki, then the mushrooms, asparagus, carrots and spring onions. Stir-fry for a few minutes, then add the stock, sherry and soy sauce. Simmer gently for 10 minutes. Season to taste. Top with toasted sesame seeds. Serve.

## shiitake salad

- 3 tbsp olive oil
- 250 g smoked tofu, cubed
- 250 g fresh shiitake mushrooms
- 2 tbsp fresh tarragon, finely chopped
- 1 tbsp lime juice
- Salt and pepper to taste
- 1 little gem lettuce
- 1 handful rocket
- 1 handful sorrel leaves

Stir-fry the tofu in oil for a few minutes. Add the shiitake; fry till tender. Add tarragon and lime juice; season. Serve on a bed of green leaves.

## pasta, pesto and shiitake

- 400 g pasta spirals
- 4 carrots, finely chopped
- Kernels of 2 corn cobs
- 4 tbsp green peas
- 300 g fresh shiitake mushrooms
- 1 tsp soy sauce
- 4 tbsp lemon juice

For the pesto:

- 4 tbsp pine nuts, ground
- 2 garlic cloves, crushed
- 1 bunch fresh basil, chopped
- 1 tsp coarse sea salt
- 4 tbsp olive oil

Mix the pesto ingredients and set aside. Cook the pasta in salted water and a splash of oil. After 5 minutes, add the carrots, sweetcorn kernels and peas and cook for 2 more minutes. Drain, place in a bowl and mix in the pesto. Fry the mushrooms (halved) until golden; add a little soy sauce as you turn off the heat. Add the mushrooms to the bowl and mix. Sprinkle with lemon juice and freshly ground black pepper. Serve.

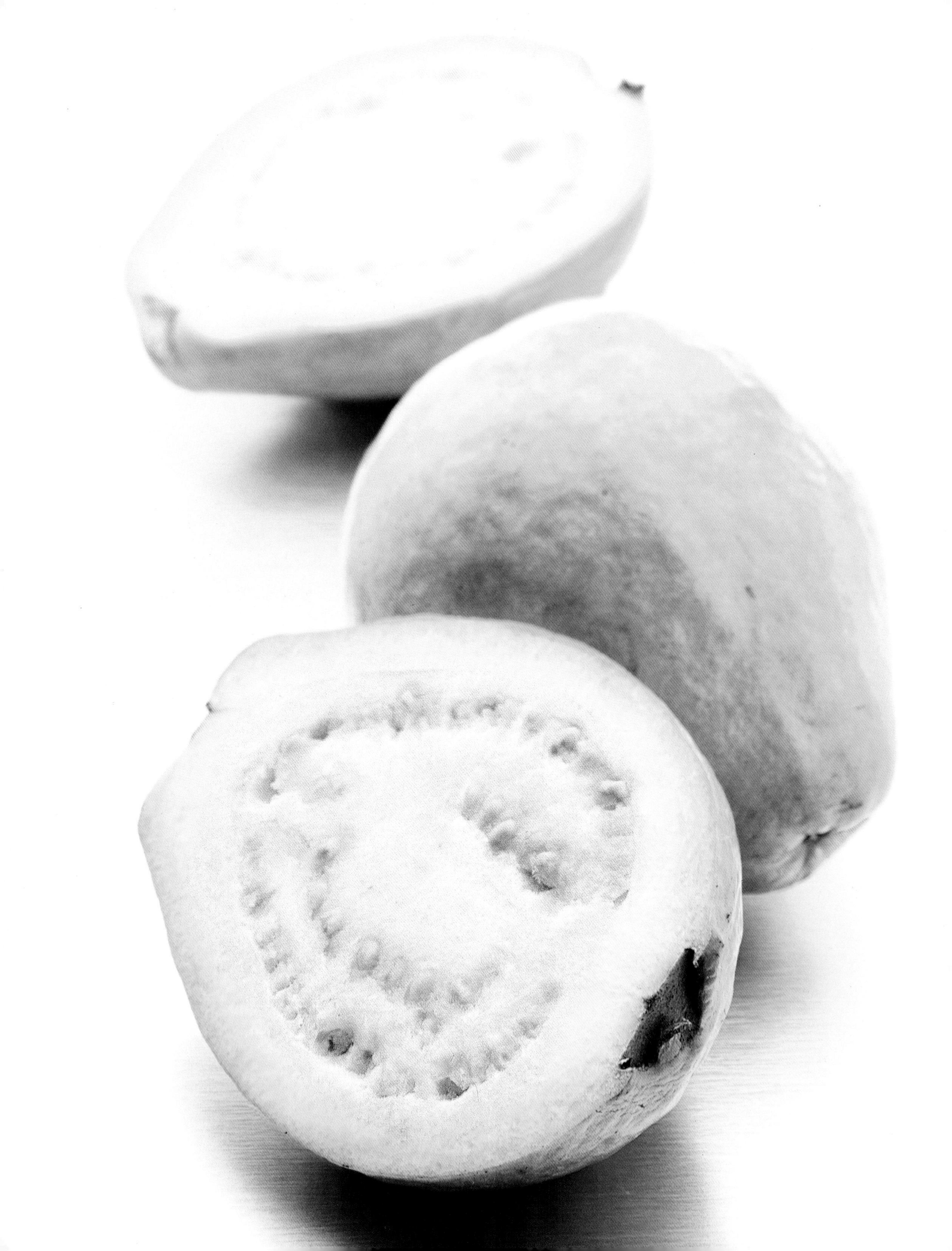

chapter seven

# coping with common ailments

Making the right food choices not only keeps your immune system in tip-top condition but also helps you target specific diseases. The following pages feature some of the common ailments that can develop when the immune system is operating below par, and the steps you can take to avoid or manage such disorders. There is advice on which superfoods to include in your meals, along with page references directing you to mouthwatering recipes that present these foods at their best. There is also advice on problematic products you should avoid, and other simple ways to ensure your immune system is ready for anything that the modern world might have in store.

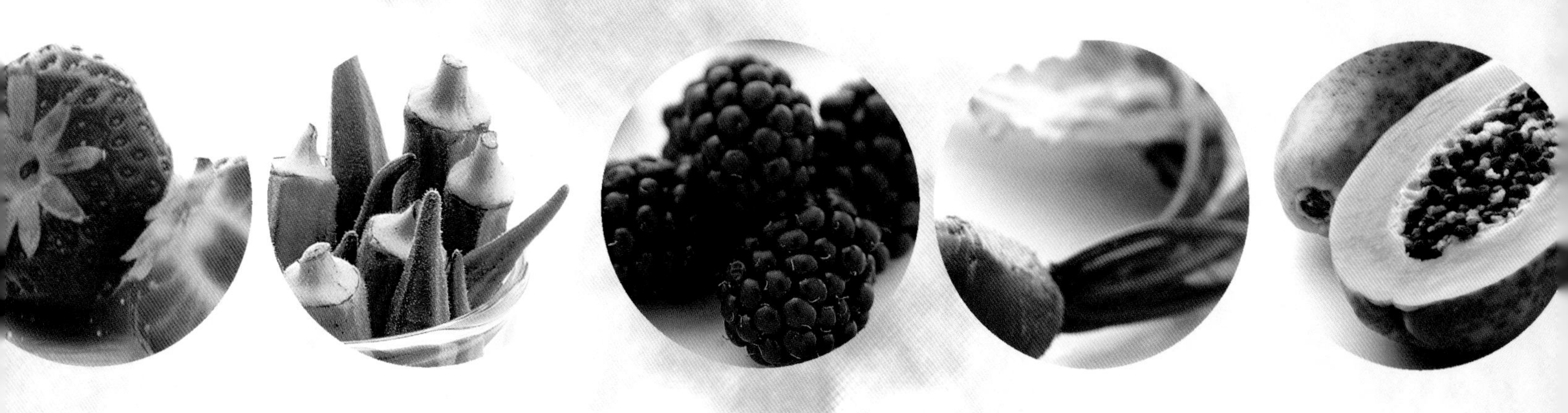

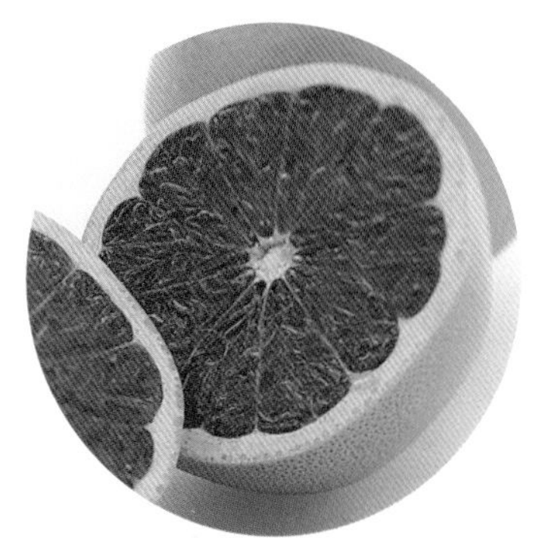

# colds & influenza

**SUPERFOODS FOR COLDS AND INFLUENZA: BLACK MUSTARD, CARROT, CATMINT, CAYENNE, ECHINACEA, ELDERBERRY AND FLOWERS, GARLIC, GINGER, GRAPEFRUIT, GREEN LEAVES, GUAVA, HORSERADISH, LEMON, LINSEED, MELON SEED, NASTURTIUM, NUTS, ONION, ORANGE, PEPPERMINT, ROSEHIP, SUNFLOWER SEED, SWEET POTATO, WILD MARJORAM, YARROW**

Cold and influenza (flu) are viral infections. Both cause runny nose, sore throat, headache, fever and general malaise. Cold symptoms are usually mild at first and develop relatively slowly. In contrast, flu symptoms start abruptly and include aching joints and limbs, high fever, shivering, severe headache and often persistent dry cough. Most flu symptoms last only a few days, but a cough may persist, and depression, lethargy and tiredness often follow and may be long-lasting. Influenza can be accompanied by secondary bacterial infections, such as bronchitis or pneumonia (especially among the elderly), that take advantage of the body's weakened state.

## Prevention

We are constantly surrounded by cold viruses, but if your immune system is strong you are less likely to catch a cold. To strengthen your resistance to colds and flu, ensure good nutrition, manage your stress levels, and try to avoid alcohol, tobacco, recreational drugs, chemicals, excess sugar intake, high levels of dietary cholesterol and other fats, dehydration, or over-exposure to hot or cold. Flu is highly infectious and usually occurs in epidemics that peak in winter. Flu vaccination is only partially effective since the vaccine does not give resistance to all possible strains of the virus. Adverse reactions to the vaccine are common.

## Management

Support the body and let the infection take its course rather than suppressing symptoms that show that the body's defences are at work. The best treatment in the acute phase is sleep and rest, eating very little and drinking lots of liquid in the form of water, weak herbal tea and soup.

Good hydration creates a less favourable environment for the virus while improving the function of the immune system. Because of their natural sugar content, fruit juices and sweetened drinks are not beneficial once the disease gets hold, but thanks to their high antioxidant content, fruit juices are excellent cold and influenza preventives. Dairy products are "mucus forming" and should be avoided altogether.

### SUGGESTED RECIPES FOR COLDS AND INFLUENZA

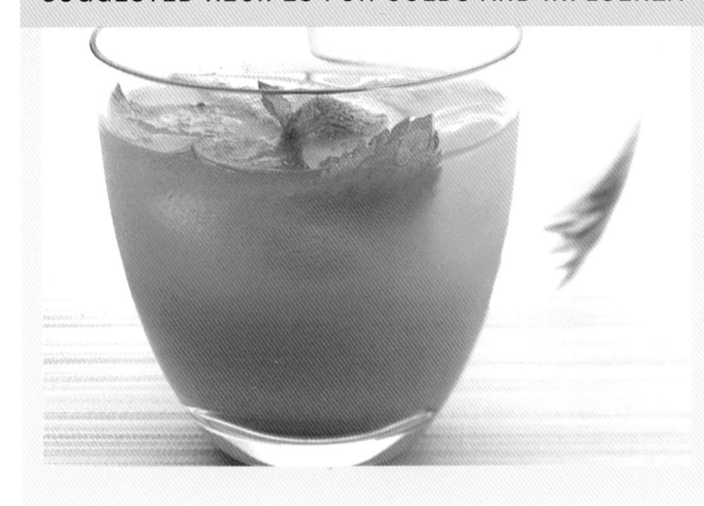

Cool tomato soup (page 244), healing soup (page 244), mint and melon soup (page 245), shiitake mushroom soup (page 245), spicy moroccan soup (page 246), sunrise – *left* (page 267), cold buster (page 268), cough mixture (page 268), eucalyptus mix (page 269), syrup of onion – make in the same way as garlic oxymel (page 269), immuni-tea (page 269), lung-cleansing tea mix (page 270), sage mix for sore throats (page 270), si c (page 270), tea for fever (page 271), tea for headache (page 271).

Cold remedy (tea mixture): Infuse 1 teaspoon each of elderflowers and chamomile flowers in 300 ml boiling water for 10 minutes.

# ear, nose & throat infections

**SUPERFOODS FOR ENT INFECTIONS: ADUKI BEAN, ASPARAGUS, BEETROOT, BILBERRY, BLACKBERRY, CARROT, CHERRY, CHICKPEA, CLEAVERS, CURLY KALE, ECHINACEA, ELDERFLOWER, EUCALYPTUS, GARLIC, GRAPE, GRAPEFRUIT, GREEN LEAVES, GUAVA, HORSERADISH, LEEK, LEMON, MANGO, MARIGOLD, MUESLI, ONION, PEPPERMINT, PUMPKIN, SAGE, SHIITAKE, SPRING GREENS, TAHINI, TEMPEH**

The ear, nose and throat are closely linked by a labyrinth of tubes and passages. This allows infection to spread quickly from one to another. Common ear, nose and throat (ENT) disorders include middle ear and throat infections (including tonsillitis) and sinusitis.

Middle ear infection is especially common in children and often follows colds, flu, tonsillitis, or childhood fevers. It can lead to a build-up of fluid that puts pressure on the eardrum, causing severe earache. The eardrum may perforate, which relieves pressure and pain. Recurrent middle ear infection can lead to otitis media ("glue ear"), a chronic condition causing deafness and learning difficulties.

Sinusitis is inflammation of the cavities in the bones around the nose, causing headache, facial pain and stuffy nose. It is a common complication of colds and flu, and may also be caused by allergy, injury, tooth infection, or poor drainage of the sinuses.

Throat infection can be viral or bacterial, and cause fever, malaise, sore throat and difficulty swallowing associated with inflammation of the lymphoid tissues (tonsils and adenoids) at the back of the throat. Swollen adenoids can cause difficulty breathing, and a tendency to repeated ear or upper respiratory-tract infection.

## Prevention

The best way to prevent ear, nose and throat infections is to strengthen the immune system by eating lots of vegetables and fruit – particularly those high in vitamins A and C, bioflavonoids and zinc. Avoid common allergens, such as dairy foods (including cow's milk in baby formulas), eggs, shellfish, wheat and peanut butter. Avoid repeated upper respiratory-tract infections by following the guidelines on page 218. If you do catch a cold or suffer a bout of flu, take plenty of time to convalesce after the symptoms subside and do not go out and about too early.

## Management

Seek professional help in cases of suspected middle ear infection or if a nose or throat disorder leads to breathing difficulties. Drink lots of fluids (water, herbal tea, diluted vegetable juices and soups). Get plenty of rest, including bed rest if necessary. Avoid suspected allergens and concentrated sources of sugar such as dried fruit, honey, syrups and concentrated fruit juice. Gentle facial massage helps alleviate sinusitis. Herbal gargles can ease throat infections.

### SUGGESTED RECIPES FOR ENT INFECTIONS

Ear infections: green leafy salad (page 181), shiitake mushroom soup (page 245), beetroot and apple (page 264), green party (page 264), cold buster (page 268), tea for ear infections (page 271).

Sinusitis: beetroot and horseradish salad (page 177), curly kale, tomato and broad beans (page 181), spiced nettle soup (page 185), carrot and lemon with garlic (page 264), elderflower spritzer (page 268), eucalyptus mix (page 269).

Throat infection: mint and melon soup (page 245), pumpkin soup (page 245), welsh leek and potato soup (page 246), cool cucumber (page 264), garlic oxymel (page 269), sage mix for sore throats (page 270), si c (page 270), tea for glands (page 271).

Sinusitis remedy (horseradish poultice): Grate fresh horseradish root into a portion of oatmeal (porridge), wrap the mixture in a tea towel and place the compress over the nose, cheeks and forehead (taking care to avoid the eyes).

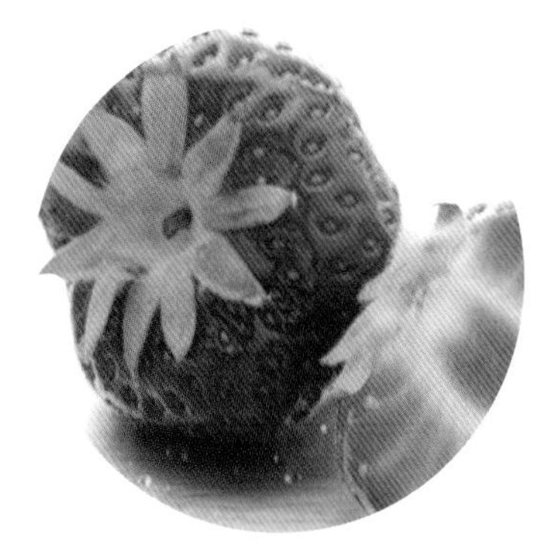

# childhood fevers

**SUPERFOODS FOR CHILDHOOD FEVERS: BLACK MUSTARD, BORAGE, CARROT, CATMINT, CAYENNE, ECHINACEA, ELDERBERRY AND FLOWERS, GARLIC, GINGER, GRAINS, GRAPEFRUIT, GREEN LEAVES, GUAVA, HORSERADISH, LEMON, NUTS, ONION, ORANGE, PEPPERMINT, ROSEHIP, SEEDS, STRAWBERRY, SWEET POTATO, WILD MARJORAM, YARROW**

Childhood fevers are common, especially those arising from colds and other simple upper respiratory-tract infections. They are part of the immune system's natural development and should be managed rather than suppressed. While most childhood fevers resolve quickly, it is vital to exclude serious disorders such as meningitis, so never hesitate to seek medical help in cases of high fever, or if you are worried about a child's condition.

The diseases chickenpox, rubella (German measles), measles, mumps and whooping cough are also common causes of fever in childhood. Chickenpox causes sore throat, headache and rash. Rubella causes runny nose, sore throat, swollen lymph nodes (glands), rash and sometimes joint pain. (Rubella infection in pregnancy may lead to birth-defects.) Measles causes sore eyes, runny nose, dry cough, white spots in the mouth and rash. It may be complicated by middle ear infection, bronchitis, pneumonia, or, less commonly, febrile convulsions (fits). Mumps causes sore throat and painful swelling of the salivary glands. Whooping cough causes distressing bouts of coughing.

## Prevention

A healthy diet aids the proper development and functioning of the immune system and is the mainstay of prevention of childhood fevers. Encourage your children to eat fresh and dried fruit, carrot and cucumber sticks, grapes, tomatoes, grains, nuts and seeds and restrict the availability of sweets, fizzy drinks, burgers and other junk foods. Give children the chance to eat organic foods whenever possible.

## Management

During the acute phase of the fever, bed rest, tender loving care and plenty of fluids (water and weak herbal teas) are the most important steps. When the child's appetite starts to return, offer freshly prepared juices (diluted with water). During convalescence, fruit salads and soups are beneficial and children love pasta dishes, Scandinavian beetroot burgers (page 37) and fruity pancakes (page 103). Avoid sugar, dairy produce, junk foods, and common allergens (wheat, eggs, peanut butter, additives).

## SUGGESTED RECIPES FOR CHILDHOOD FEVERS

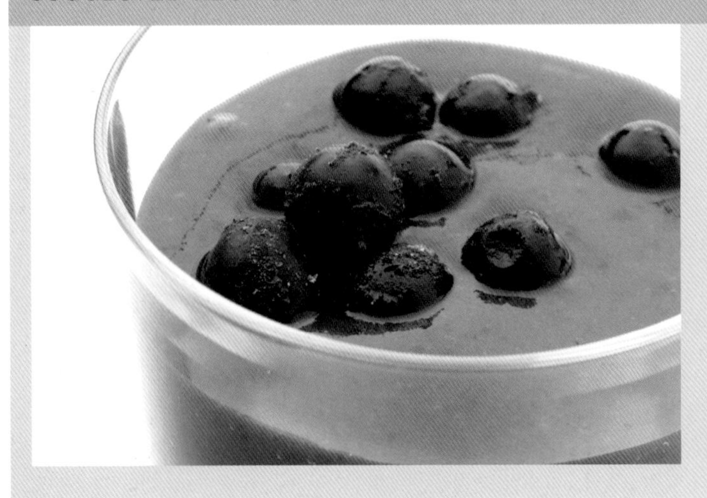

Scandinavian beetroot burgers (page 177), pasta, pesto and shiitake (page 215), fresh fruit salad (page 242), fruity pancakes (page 243), yoghurt with fruit (page 243), mint and melon soup (page 245), black-eye bean and wild marjoram soup (page 245), italian butterbean soup (page 245), tibetan dumpling soup (page 246), raspberry gateau (page 262), tropical fruit salad (page 263), apricot and ginger (page 264), blackberry cream (page 264), caribbean smoothie (page 264), cool cucumber (page 264), creamy mango (page 264), nirvana (page 267), pink pineapple (page 267), soft tutti fruity (page 267), cough mixture (page 268), Si c – *left* (page 270), tea for fever (page 271).

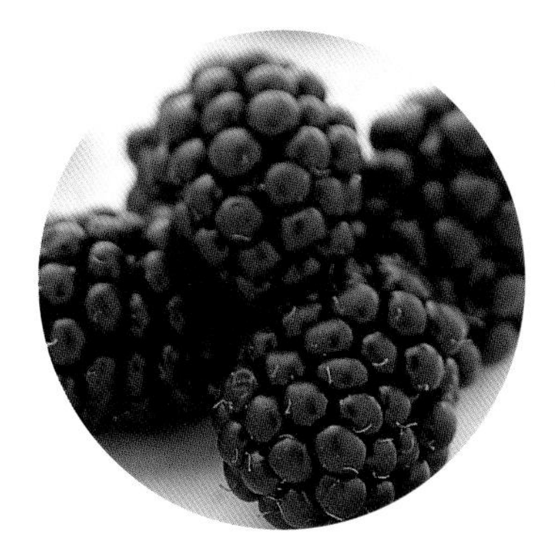

# bronchitis

**SUPERFOODS FOR BRONCHITIS: ADUKI BEAN, AMARANTH LEAVES, ASPARAGUS, BLACKCURRANT, BUTTERNUT SQUASH, CARROT, CHERRY, CHICKPEA, CLEAVERS, CURLY KALE, ELDERFLOWER, GARLIC, GRAPE, GRAPEFRUIT, GREEN LEAVES, GUAVA, HORSERADISH, LEEK, LEMON, LENTIL, MANGO, MUESLI, NASTURTIUM, ONION, SPRING GREENS, SWEET POTATO, TAHINI, THYME, TOFU, SWEET VIOLET, YARROW**

Bronchitis is inflammation of the lining of the bronchial tubes in the lungs. The acute form of bronchitis is usually caused by a viral or bacterial infection and often follows a bout of cold or influenza. The symptoms are cough (initially harsh and dry, later with yellow or green sputum), shortness of breath and fever. Pneumonia is a potentially serious complication of bronchitis, and is particularly dangerous for elderly people. Chronic bronchitis causes persistent or recurrent cough and breathing difficulties and is most common in people with lowered immune function, particularly smokers, drug and alcohol abusers, patients taking immuno-suppressive drugs and those suffering immunodeficiency disorders and cancer. Chronic bronchitis goes hand in hand with structural damage within the lungs called emphysema, which decreases the amount of lung tissue available to absorb oxygen and get rid of carbon dioxide and other waste products. The lungs also develop a rough, thickened lining making breathing very difficult.

### Prevention

The most important step you can take to avoid chronic bronchitis is to quit smoking – or not start in the first place! Keep your weight within optimum limits and eat plenty of foods rich in vitamins A and C, and bioflavonoids and zinc to enhance your immune function. Avoid noxious fumes and immuno-suppressive drugs wherever possible, and breathe fresh air every day. Avoid eating dairy products, which encourage the production of excess mucus.

### Management

Drink large amounts of fluid (water, herbal tea, juice, soup), and drink juices rich in vitamin C – the immune system needs a lot of this nutrient when fighting infection. Garlic, onion and leek have natural antibacterial properties and help avoid the development of complications such as pneumonia. Limit your sugar consumption, particularly added sugar, sweets, fizzy drinks and concentrated fruit juices, and cut out dairy products altogether. Try to avoid suppressing the cough. Herbal expectorants make the cough more "productive" and make it easier to get rid of excess mucus from the airways. A warm poultice (see below) applied to the chest eases breathing. Rest is important but avoid lying flat in bed, which may make breathing more difficult and exacerbate the cough. Use extra pillows or a bolster to prop up your head and upper body.

**SUGGESTED RECIPES FOR BRONCHITIS**

Green leafy salad (page 181), yoghurt with fruit (page 243), spicy moroccan soup (page 246), amaranth and tofu puffs (page 252), provençal mesclun salad (page 259), tropical sunshine salad (page 261), blackberry cream (page 264), carrot and lemon with garlic (page 264), cold buster (page 268), garlic oxymel (page 269), lung-cleansing tea mix (page 270), si c (page 270), tea for fever (page 271).

---

Cough mixture: Pour 1 cup of boiling water over 2 to 3 teaspoons of linseeds (flaxseeds) and leave to infuse for 10 to 15 minutes.

---

Inhalation: Add 1 tablespoon each of chamomile, thyme, eucalyptus and wild marjoram to 600 ml boiling water and infuse for 5 minutes, covered. Wrap a blanket around you and put a big towel over your head. Take the lid off the infusion and gently inhale the steam for about ten minutes. Splash your face with cool water.

---

Mustard poultice: Mix 5 teaspoons of crushed black mustard seeds with a large portion of hot oatmeal (porridge). Wrap the mixture in a tea towel and place this on the chest for 20 minutes; make sure it is not so hot as to cause discomfort, and check from time to time that the mustard is not causing skin irritation.

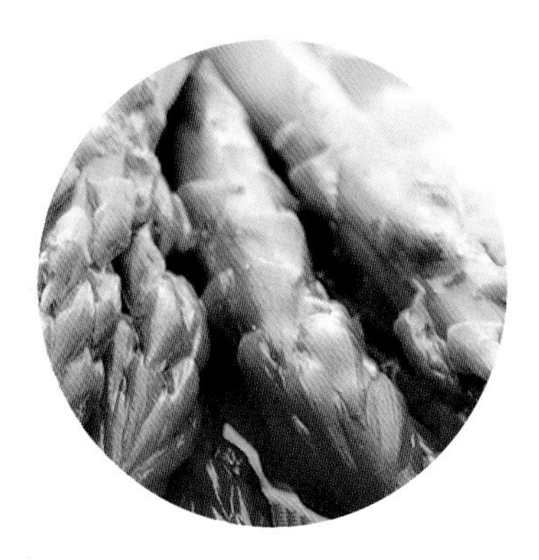

# cystitis

**SUPERFOODS FOR CYSTITIS: ADUKI BEAN, ASPARAGUS, BLACKBERRY, BLACKCURRANT, BRUSSELS SPROUT, BUTTERNUT SQUASH, CARROT, CELERY SEED, CHERRY, CHICKPEA, CLEAVERS, CRANBERRY, CURLY KALE, EUCALYPTUS, GARLIC, GRAPE, GREEN LEAVES, GUAVA, HORSERADISH, LENTIL, MANGO, MUESLI, NETTLE, PASTA, RED PEPPER, RICE, SPRING GREENS, SWEET POTATO, TAHINI, TEMPEH, YARROW**

Cystitis is inflammation of the bladder, most often caused by an infection. The disorder triggers various symptoms including lower abdominal pain, painful and frequent urination, a feeling of urgency to urinate and that the bladder is never completely empty. The urine smells fishy and looks cloudy (maybe with traces of blood).

Cystitis is more common in women than in men (probably because the urethra – the tube that carries urine out of the body – is shorter in women and close to the openings of the vagina and anus, making infection more likely). Cystitis is often associated with pregnancy, sex, sensitivity to cold and mechanical injury (such as catheterization, a medical procedure).

Classical cystitis is caused by bacterial infection, but other organisms, such as chlamydia, are frequently involved. However, many people suffer recurrent symptoms of cystitis without any obvious infective cause, and are given a diagnosis of "urethral syndrome". Some cases of urethral syndrome can be explained by an allergy or sensitivity to materials such as nylon, washing powder, soaps and bubble baths. In bacterial cystitis, serious complications can occur if the infection spreads to the kidneys including acute glomerulonephritis (the symptoms of which are severe malaise, high fever and intense back pain) and chronic reflux nephropathy, which can cause permanent kidney damage.

## Prevention

Eat plenty of fresh foods, mainly of plant origin, and avoid eating too much sugar or drinking too much alcohol or coffee. Keep your meat and dairy intake to a minimum, and avoid junk food and food additives altogether. Include foods that contain plenty of vitamins A and C, and bioflavonoids and zinc. Garlic also has natural antibacterial properties and helps the body to deal with urinary-tract infections. In severe cases, try the detox diet on page 272.

Above all, avoid dehydration and get plenty of rest. Replace coffee and tea with lots of fresh juices, smoothies, herbal teas and water. Avoid acidic foods and drinks (including citrus fruits). Pay attention to personal hygiene, and make sure that you are not allergic to the soaps or soap powders you are using. Avoid douches and intimate deodorants, because they may disrupt the natural bacterial flora and allow harmful micro-organisms to flourish. If you have a tendency to cystitis, it is also important to empty your bladder and wash your genitals before and after sex.

## Management

Cranberry juice can be a highly effective treatment for cystitis. Otherwise, the conventional treatment for cystitis is a course of antibiotics together with high fluid intake, regular bladder emptying and scrupulous hygiene. However, many cases do not respond to this regimen, and repeated or long-term use of antibiotics can bring other problems (such as candidiasis and disturbance of intestinal flora). If you do take antibiotics it is important to allow the body to rebuild its natural defences afterward. Live yoghurt helps the bowel to recolonize with beneficial micro-organisms. Antioxidants including vitamins A, C and E, and zinc, selenium and bioflavonoids help to restore immune function.

### SUGGESTED RECIPES FOR CYSTITIS

Beetroot and horseradish salad (page 177), nettle and sweet potato mash (page 185), avocado smoothie (page 193), pasta, pesto and shiitake (page 215), yoghurt with fruit (page 243), asparagus with ravigote (page 246), korean kimchi-style salad (page 247), tzaziki (page 251), asparagus asian-style (page 253), mushrooms with sage and thyme stuffing (page 256), swiss chard and juniper berries (page 259), catalan salad (page 260), pasta salad (page 260), cranberry spritzer (page 264), vegetable cocktail (page 267), cystitis relief (page 268), immuni-tea (page 269).

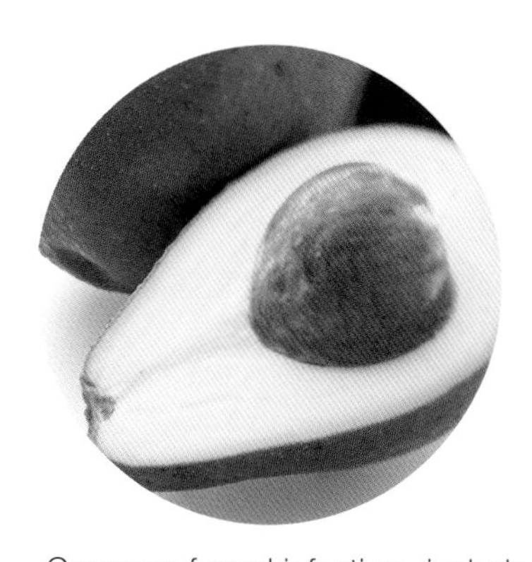

# fungal infections

**SUPERFOODS FOR FUNGAL INFECTIONS:** ADUKI BEAN, AVOCADO, BRAZIL NUT, BROAD BEAN, BUTTERNUT SQUASH, CARROT, CHAMOMILE, CINNAMON, COCONUT, CURLY KALE, ENDIVE, EUCALYPTUS, GARLIC, GINGER, GRAPEFRUIT, LEEK, LEMON BALM, LENTIL, LIVE SOYA YOGHURT, MARIGOLD, PAPAYA, PINTO BEAN, PSYLLIUM SEED, PUMPKIN, RICE, ROSEMARY, SPINACH, SPRING GREENS, SWISS CHARD, THYME, TOFU

Common fungal infections include candidiasis or "thrush" (yeast infection caused by *Candida albicans*); athlete's foot (*Tinea pedis*); and ringworm (*Tinea corporis*). There are two forms of thrush – oral and vaginal. Oral thrush produces thin, white, moist, cottage-cheesy plaques inside the mouth, which rub off to leave red, sore patches. It mainly affects sick babies, the immuno-compromized and the elderly. Vaginal thrush causes abnormal vaginal discharge, irritation and soreness. In managing the disease, it is important to treat sexual partners to avoid a cycle of re-infection. Candida is a common yeast that forms part of our normal gut flora. Drugs (particularly antibiotics and steroids), stress and poor diet can lead to candida overgrowth that affects absorption of nutrients as well as general health, and can lead to serious illness if it spreads to the rest of the body.

Fungal skin infections affect warm, damp places, such as groin creases, and produce clearly demarcated, moist, itchy dark red patches with a few smaller lesions scattered around. Infected finger nails appear thick and brownish. Ringworm appears as a scaly, red patch that enlarges and becomes a raised, scaly circle with a pale centre. It looks as though it has been caused by a burrowing worm, hence the name. It may spread and form more circles and can cause bald patches if it affects the scalp. Athlete's foot often develops between the fourth and fifth toes with the skin becoming itchy, pale, damp, flaky, cracked and mushy.

## Prevention and management

Factors that suppress immunity can increase the risk of fungal infections. These include a diet high in sugar and saturated fat, drugs (antibiotics, steroids, chemotherapy, oral contraceptives, anti-ulcer medication), environmental chemicals, alcohol and stress. Avoiding these is the mainstay of prevention. Papaya contains enzymes that can inhibit yeast proliferation. Cut down on dairy products and, if you have to take antibiotics, eat live yoghurt to help restore a healthy balance of intestinal flora. To manage fungal infection, take plenty of rest and limit your consumption of foods containing yeast (such as bread and yeast extract) and fermented foods (such as cheese, tempeh and vinegar). Avoid known food allergens, alcohol, dairy products and foods high in refined sugar, such as sucrose, fructose, syrup, fruit juice, honey and dried fruits. Take a teaspoon of psyllium seeds in a glass of water after meals.

### SUGGESTED RECIPES FOR FUNGAL INFECTIONS

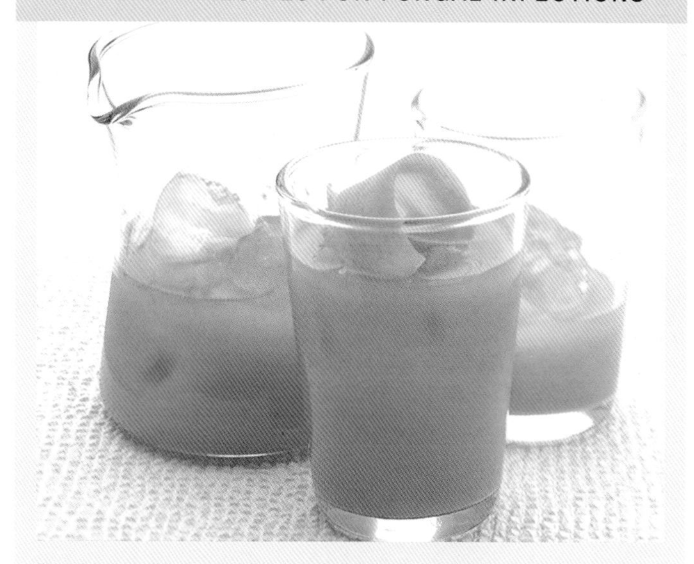

Beetroot and horseradish (page 177), green leafy salad (page 181), stuffed grapefruit (page 189), avocado smoothie (page 193), spicy brazil nut pâté (page 197), scrambled tofu (page 242), korean kimchi-style salad (page 247), guacamole (page 250), tzaziki (page 251), khichuri – rice with lentils (page 257), chinese salad (page 260), apricot and ginger (page 264), carrot and lemon with garlic – *above* (page 264), calming tea (page 268), eucalyptus mix (page 269), spicy chai (page 270), stress relief (page 270), tea for fungal infections (page 271).

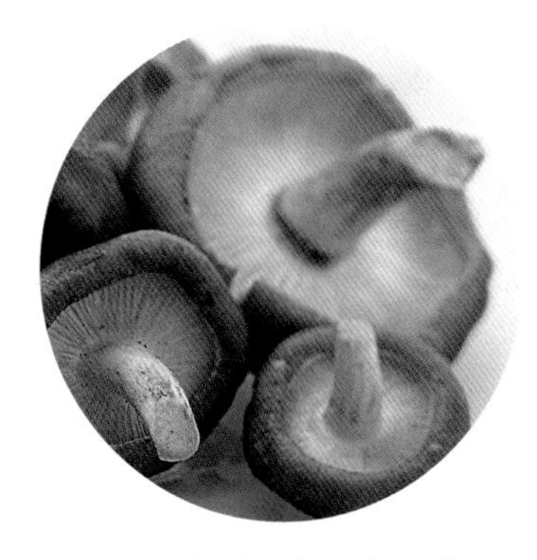

# herpes simplex

SUPERFOODS FOR HERPES SIMPLEX: ADUKI BEAN, AVOCADO, BEETROOT, BRAZIL NUT, CARROT, CHICKPEA, GARLIC, HAZELNUT, LEMON BALM, LENTIL, LIQUORICE ROOT, MACADAMIA NUT, MARIGOLD, MUESLI, PINE NUT, PUMPKIN SEED, SHIITAKE, SPINACH, ST JOHN'S WORT, SUN-DRIED TOMATO, SAFFLOWER AND SUNFLOWER OILS, SWEET POTATO, TEMPEH, TOFU, TOMATO, WALNUT, WHEATGERM, YAM

Herpes simplex is a virus that causes blisters on skin and mucous membranes known as cold sores. The sores commonly appear on the face, fingers, mouth, lips and genitals, and are often accompanied by swollen lymph nodes, itching, stinging pain, fatigue and fever. The virus is transmitted through direct contact with an active cold sore, for example via saliva or sexual fluids.

After the initial infection, the virus lies dormant and may remain unnoticed for long periods of time, until the body's resistance is lowered by colds (hence the name) and other infections, stress, trauma, menstruation or exposure to sun. Cold sores recur near or at the primary site of infection whenever the body is feeling run down. Infection lasts for one or two weeks. Men are generally more prone to cold sores than women.

Herpes simplex infection is a common cause of genital ulcers, but it is important to exclude other, more serious causes such as syphilis and lymphoma. Genital cold sores are also associated with an increased risk of developing cervical dysplasia (abnormal changes in cervical cells that may be a prelude to cancer). However, it is unclear whether the herpes virus is a direct cause of the condition or simply a symptom of a run-down immune response failing to keep cell changes in check.

## Prevention

The best way to avoid infection is to avoid direct contact with active cold sores. The likelihood of infections and the frequency of recurrence are both reduced by maintaining good general health. Resistance to infection depends on having a strong immune system, which in turn depends on good nutrition and having sufficient rest, fresh air and exercise. People suffering from immunodeficiency syndromes, or whose immunity is suppressed by drugs, stress, poor nutrition or chronic disease, are at greater risk of infection. People with eczema are also more susceptible to cold sores and other viral skin conditions.

## Management

Eat foods containing vitamins A and C, and bioflavonoids and carotenoids, which all enhance resistance and inhibit viral attack. Foods rich in zinc reduce the time it takes for sores to heal. Vitamin E-rich foods speed up healing and help reduce pain. Foods with anti-viral properties, such as shiitake, garlic, lemon balm, marigold (calendula), St John's wort, spinach, sweet potato, tempeh, yam and tomato should also be included in the diet. Following a detox diet (see page 272) is a good way to help the body avoid recurring cold sores. Managing stress, avoiding exposure to allergens and limiting refined carbohydrate intake are also important factors.

Carrot, beetroot, liquorice root and lemon balm are all efficient anti-cold-sore remedies. Liquorice root reduces the cell damage caused by herpes simplex infection and inhibits the growth of the sores. A tisane made of liquorice root and lemon balm may decrease the severity and duration of an outbreak if taken regularly (3–4 cups per day) as soon as the first signs of a sore appear. However, liquorice causes an increase in the rate at which potassium is eliminated from the body. So, when taking liquorice, you should also include in your diet plenty of foods that are high in potassium, such as banana, avocado, sweet potato, dried apricot, beans, peas and green leaves.

### SUGGESTED RECIPES FOR HERPES SIMPLEX

Green leafy salad (page 181), oriental salad with tempeh (page 203), shiitake salad (page 215), porridge with dried fruit and quinoa (page 242), muesli (page 243), tofumasalata (page 248), pan amb oli (page 251), sweet potato curry (page 256), winter hot pot (page 256), carrot 'n' beetroot salad (page 259), blackberry crumble (page 263), calming tea (page 268), pick-me-up (page 270), tea for glands (page 271).

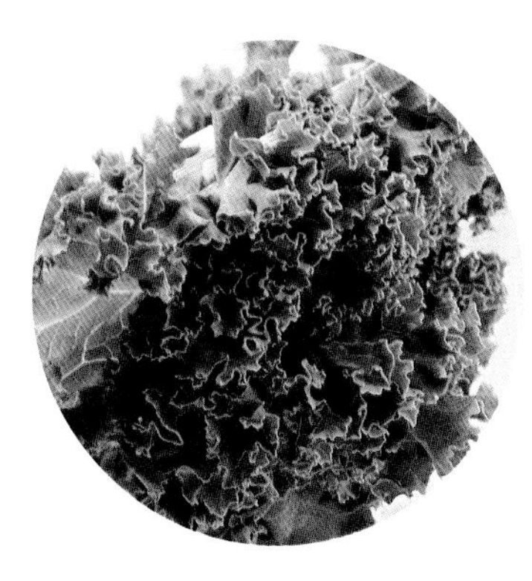

# eczema

**SUPERFOODS FOR ECZEMA: ASPARAGUS, BEANS, BILBERRY, BUTTERNUT SQUASH, CHAMOMILE, CARROT, CLEAVERS, CURLY KALE, ECHINACEA, ELDERBERRY, EVENING PRIMROSE OIL, GRAPE, GRAPEFRUIT, HAWTHORN, LENTIL, LINSEED, MANGO, NETTLE, PEAS, PINE NUT, PUMPKIN SEED, RED PEPPER, SPINACH, SUNFLOWER OIL AND SEED, SWEET POTATO, SWISS CHARD, TEMPEH, TOFU, VIOLET, WALNUT OIL**

Eczema (also called dermatitis) is a very common skin condition characterized by red, itchy, weeping skin patches, which are prone to infection. As time goes by, the skin becomes progressively harder, drier and more brittle because of repeated scratching.

Atopic eczema causes an itchy, sometimes weeping and scaly rash on the face and in body creases. It is common in infants and tends to run in families – two-thirds of eczema sufferers have a family member with the condition and many also develop hay fever and/or asthma. There is also an increased susceptibility to skin infections, including cold sores and warts. Seborrheic eczema causes a crusty rash on hairy skin – especially in the armpits and groin creases and on the face in men. When it occurs on the scalp in babies it is called "cradle cap".

Irritant eczema is caused by direct contact with strong chemicals and usually develops within 24 hours of initial exposure. It causes redness, blisters and cracks in the skin, but does not spread beyond the area exposed to the irritant. Allergic contact dermatitis develops after a second exposure to an allergen such as lanolin, skin cream additives, antibiotic ointments and nickel in jewellery or buttons. The rash is most prominent over the area of initial contact, but can spread all over the body.

## Prevention

Food allergy is a common cause of eczema, and dairy products are the most likely culprits. Stress is also a common factor, and tension can provoke itching. Identifying and eliminating allergens, and dealing with stress are thus the mainstays of prevention.

## Management

It is necessary to eliminate known food allergens. Animal fats and dairy products should be limited in the diet until symptoms subside. Deficiency of essential fatty acids is sometimes a factor in the development of eczema and can be avoided by eating more polyunsaturated oil. Walnut oil is particularly useful because it is both anti-inflammatory and anti-allergic. Evening primrose oil, sunflower oil and seeds, and linseeds (flaxseeds) also help dampen inflammation. Foods containing bioflavonoids are important for controlling inflammation and allergic reactions and enhance the action of vitamin C. Foods containing high levels of zinc and vitamin A are excellent for skin healing and repair.

### SUGGESTED REMEDIES FOR ECZEMA

Tea for the skin (page 271), grapefruit salad (page 189), fresh fruit salad (page 242), spicy moroccan soup (page 246), toasted nuts and seeds (page 248), tomato and cucumber canapés (page 250), tofu balls (page 250), asparagus asian-style (page 253), spinach bouillabaisse (page 255), spring greens and macadamia nuts (page 258), rocket salad (page 259), orange mango salad (page 260), natural beauty (page 266), calming tea (page 268), liquorice mix (page 270).

---

Steroid creams and tablets are common orthodox treatments for eczema, but can carry a risk of side effects after prolonged use. Try a marigold (calendula) ointment or make this compress to reduce inflammation. Pour 600 ml boiling water on to 3 tablespoons of marigold flowers. Cover and allow to cool. Strain and use the liquid to soak a compress before placing it on the affected area. Keep the compress moist and leave in place for one hour.

---

Detoxifying herbs such as nettle, cleavers, violet, chamomile and echinacea aid the digestive system and are an important part of the treatment. Oily ointments can ease discomfort, and barrier creams and gloves can prevent contact with allergens.

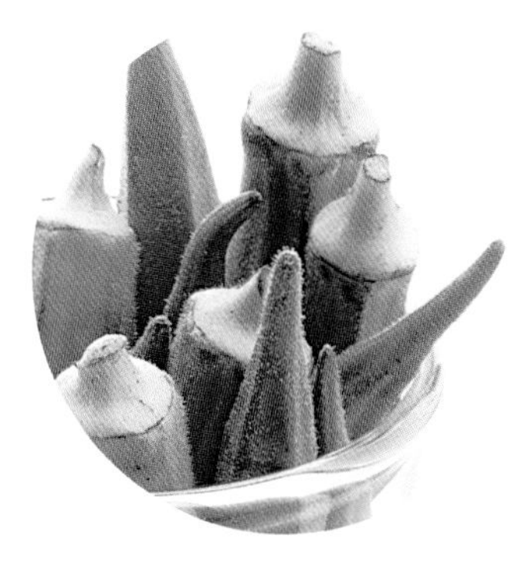

# psoriasis

**SUPERFOODS FOR PSORIASIS:** APPLE, AVOCADO, BANANA, BEANS, BEETROOT, BELGIAN ENDIVE, BERRIES, BRAZIL NUT, BROCCOLI, CARROT, CHAMOMILE, CLEAVERS, CURLY KALE, DRIED FRUIT, GLOBE ARTICHOKE, GRAPE, GREEN LEAVES, LENTIL, LIQUORICE ROOT, MELON, MUSHROOMS, NETTLE, NUTS, OKRA, PAPAYA, PARSNIP, PEAS, PINEAPPLE, PUMPKIN, SPINACH, SQUASH, SWEET POTATO, TOMATO, WHEATGRASS

Psoriasis is a relatively common skin condition that tends to run in families. It is characterized by red, silvery, scaly "plaques" of thickened skin, especially on the scalp, and on the outside of the knees and elbows. These are caused by skin cells dividing at a much faster rate than normal. The scaly plaques can be itchy and may join up to cover large areas of skin. Some sufferers also develop arthritis. Problems with protein digestion, impaired liver function, excess alcohol and animal fats, and psychological factors are all thought to be associated with the development of psoriasis.

## Prevention and management

Both ultraviolet light (from sunlight) and seawater are beneficial – so relaxing on a sunny beach is an excellent preventive and curative measure. Protein digestion can be enhanced by eating foods containing digestive enzymes and vitamin A, such as papaya and pineapple. Detoxing is also important and is encouraged by eating plenty of fruits and vegetables, and foods that encourage liver function such as beetroot, globe artichoke, endive, turmeric and wheatgrass. Foods high in the trace elements chromium and zinc are beneficial. Chromium helps regulate blood-sugar levels and zinc is necessary for skin repair. Foods high in vitamins A, E and folate, and selenium are helpful too. Essential fatty acids found in linseed, walnuts and walnut oil, fatty fish and fish oil inhibit production of inflammatory leukotrienes in the skin. However, avoid animal fats, found in dairy products and meat, which contain substances such as arachidonic acid that increase leukotriene production. Avoid alcohol and high-protein foods, limit sugar intake and try excluding gluten (found in wheat, barley, rye and oats).

Exercise improves circulation and contributes to skin and blood cleansing. Heat therapy in the form of a warm linseed poultice on the affected area may help. Mix a portion of crushed seeds with hot water to make a mushy paste. Spread the paste on to folded muslin or a thin flannel. Wrap the material well around the paste to stop it oozing out. Place the poultice on the affected area and cover with a piece of plastic to keep the moisture in. Leave it in place until it no longer feels pleasantly warm.

### SUGGESTED RECIPES FOR PSORIASIS

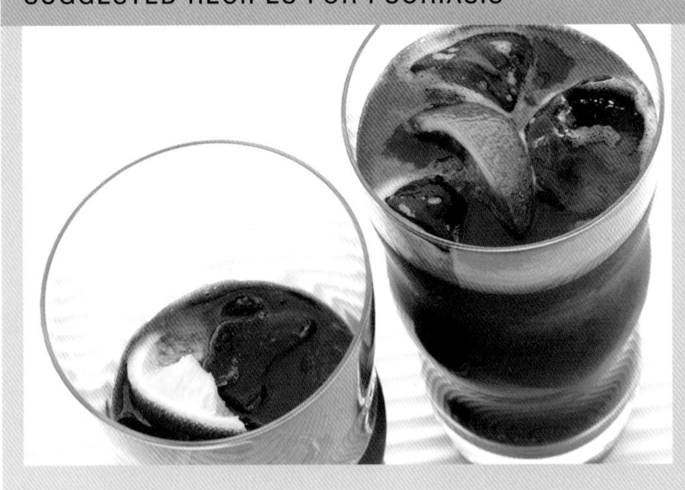

Nettle and sweet potato mash (page 185), grilled endive and brazil nut salad (page 197), spicy brazil nut pâté (page 197), spicy moroccan soup (page 246), tomato and cucumber canapés (page 250), casserole de puy (page 252), butternut squash with red pepper and tomato (page 253), okra in sweet and sour tamarind sauce (page 256), rocket salad (page 259), beetroot and apple – *left* (page 264), papaya power (page 267), pink pineapple (page 267), calming tea (page 268), immuni-tea (page 269), tea for the skin (page 271).

Remedy: Pour a cup of boiling water on to 2 to 3 teaspoons of linseeds; infuse for 10 minutes. Drink a cup morning and evening.

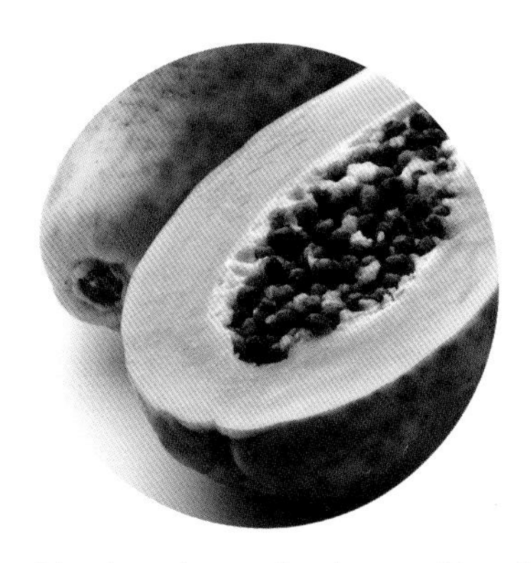

# hay fever

**SUPERFOODS FOR HAY FEVER: ARTICHOKE, AVOCADO, BEANS, BEETROOT, BERRIES, BROCCOLI, BUTTERNUT SQUASH, CARROT, CAULIFLOWER, GREEN TEA, GUAVA, HORSERADISH, LENTILS, MARIGOLD, MUSTARD CRESS, OKRA, PAPAYA, RED PEPPER, SEA VEGETABLE, SHIITAKE, SPINACH, SUN-DRIED TOMATO, SWEETCORN, SWEET POTATO, SWISS CHARD, TEMPEH, VEGETABLE OIL, WHEATGERM OIL, YEAST EXTRACT**

Hay fever is an allergic condition that causes inflammation of the mucous membranes lining the nasal cavity. It is often seasonal. Allergy to tree pollen is worst in spring, allergy to grass and weed pollen is worst in the summer and allergy to moulds occurs mainly in the autumn. Allergy to dust mites and animal dander tends to be worse in the winter when sufferers spend more time indoors with the windows closed. The tendency to develop hay fever often runs in families. When inhaled antigens come into contact with the mucous membranes of the upper respiratory tract, the immune system releases histamine and other chemicals that cause a variety of unpleasant symptoms. These include runny nose, sneezing and itchy eyes. It is also common to feel lethargic.

Allergic reactions are much more frequent and severe if you are over-tired, under stress, recovering from infection, or your immune system is compromised. Common food allergens (such as dairy foods) can lower the threshold for developing hay fever symptoms.

## Prevention

To prevent attacks, aim to strengthen and detoxify the immune system, and minimize exposure to allergens. It is beneficial to avoid additives, such as colourings and preservatives, and common food allergens including eggs, fish, shellfish, nuts (especially peanuts), dairy products, chocolate, wheat and citrus fruits. At the same time, you should include some of the foods and herbs listed above in your daily diet. For the prevention to be effective, start at least a month before the season that your hay fever symptoms occur.

## Management

Eat lots of foods containing vitamins B5, B6, B12 and E, trace elements such as selenium and magnesium, and bioflavonoids and carotenoids. Follow an elimination diet (see page 272) to discover which foods and drinks aggravate your allergy. To strengthen and detoxify your immune system, avoid animal products, coffee, tea, chocolate and refined sugar, and limit your intake of potatoes and citrus fruits. Consider excluding wheat during the hay fever season.

Keep your house as dust-free as possible. For example, consider having wooden or tiled floors with rugs instead of carpets, which trap dust and animal dander. Exclude pets from bedrooms and main living areas. Wash all bedding regularly, using washing powder or perfume-free washing liquid and choose non-feather and low-allergy mattresses, duvets and pillows, and open the windows at least once a day in winter.

### SUGGESTED RECIPES FOR HAY FEVER

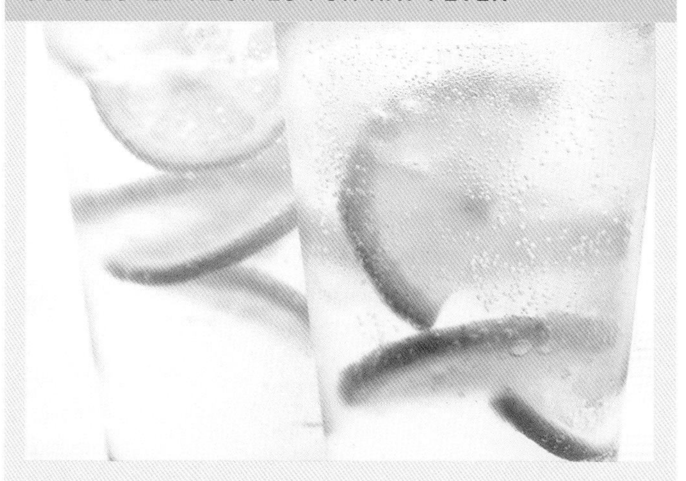

Beetroot and horseradish salad (page 177), artichoke hearts, broad beans and shiitake (page 252), okra in sweet and sour tamarind sauce (page 256), provençal mesclun salad (page 259), green lentil salad (page 260), tropical sunshine salad (page 261), height of passion (page 266), elderberry cordial (page 268), elderflower spritzer – *above* (page 268), syrup of onion (see recipe for garlic oxymel – page 269), green tea with mint (page 269), hay fever relief (page 269), immuni-tea (page 269), pick-me-up (page 270).

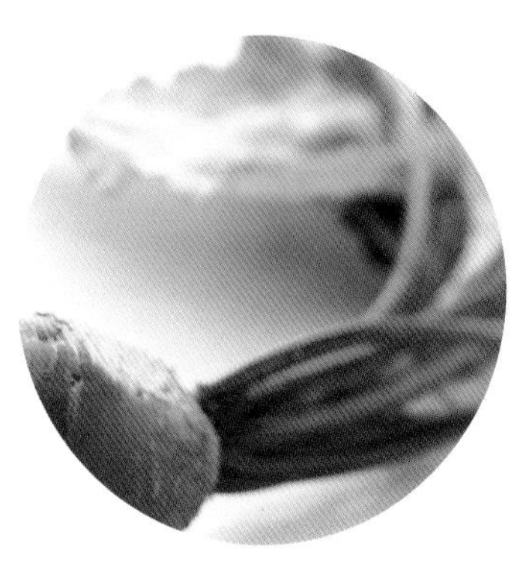

# asthma

**SUPERFOODS FOR ASTHMA: AVOCADO, BEANS, BEETROOT, BERRIES, BLACK CUMIN, BROCCOLI, BUTTERNUT SQUASH, CARAWAY, CARROT, CAULIFLOWER, CAYENNE, CORN, CURLY KALE, DRIED FRUIT, EUCALYPTUS, GARLIC, GREEN TEA, GUAVA, HORSERADISH, LENTIL, LIQUORICE ROOT, NETTLE, OKRA, ONION, PAPAYA, POTATO, RED PEPPER, SEA VEGETABLE, SHIITAKE, SORREL, SWEET POTATO, TEMPEH, THYME, YARROW**

Asthma is a common respiratory disorder causing wheezing, difficulty breathing and dry cough. It is caused by a narrowing of the airways in the lungs as a result of spasm in the bronchial tubes and excess production of thick, sticky mucus. There are two main types: one begins in childhood (especially in families with a history of asthma or allergy) and often clears up with age; the other starts later in life and is often preceded by infection. "Late onset" asthma tends to be chronic and is often harder to treat. Asthma attacks can be triggered by an allergic reaction to dust, pollen, foods, drugs and bacteria, and by exhaustion, excitement, tension, anxiety, exercise, over-exposure to cold air, colds and influenza, or certain drugs (such as beta-blockers). In cases of mild asthma, sufferers usually have no breathing problems between attacks. However, those who have frequent, severe attacks over many years can suffer from constant breathing difficulty.

During an attack it takes tremendous effort to breathe and severe, prolonged attacks can be fatal unless treated with bronchodilators, steroids, oxygen and, if necessary, artificial ventilation. At times like this, most sufferers find they can breathe more easily when sitting up rather than lying down.

### SUGGESTED RECIPES FOR ASTHMA

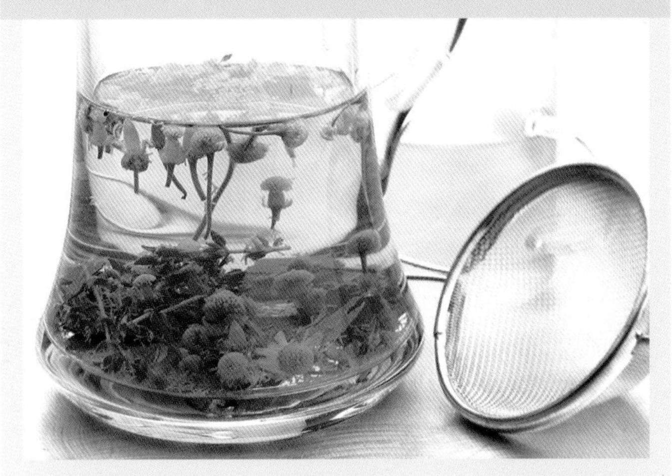

Beetroot and horseradish salad (page 177), curly kale parcels (page 181), curly kale, tomato and broad beans (page 181), nettle and sweet potato mash (page 185), filled avocados (page 193), shiitake with sea vegetable (page 215), italian butterbean soup (page 245), casserole de puy (page 252), butternut squash with red pepper and tomato (page 253), potato salad (page 260), salad with sorrel and tempeh (page 261), eucalyptus mix – *above* (page 269), lung-cleansing tea mix (page 270).

### Prevention

Finding and avoiding the underlying causes and trigger factors is the most important preventive measure. For example, keeping the home as dust-free as possible and washing bedding regularly in perfume-free detergents can help eliminate house-dust mites. Elimination diets are useful for identifying potential food allergens and avoiding them. The most common offenders are: eggs, fish, shellfish, nuts (especially peanuts), milk, chocolate, wheat, citrus fruits, apples and food additives and colouring such as tartrazine, benzoates, sulphur dioxide and sulphites.

### Management

Exclude all meat, fish, eggs and dairy products from the diet, as elimination of animal products has been shown to significantly reduce susceptibility to attacks. Other potential trigger factors that should be avoided include known allergens such as food additives, chlorinated tap water, coffee, tea, refined sugar and added salt, also aspirin and other non-steroidal anti-inflammatory drugs, Limiting the amount of grains in the diet can also be beneficial. Eat plenty of foods containing vitamins B5, B6, B12, C and E, magnesium, trace elements such as selenium, and carotenoids.

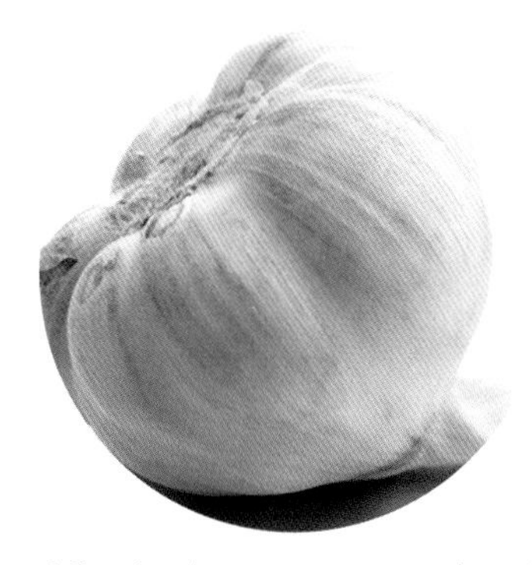

# migraine

**SUPERFOODS FOR MIGRAINE: ADUKI BEAN, BRAZIL NUT, BROAD BEAN, CHAMOMILE, CAYENNE, FEVERFEW, GARLIC, LAVENDER, MARIGOLD FLOWERS, MELON SEED, MUESLI, MUSHROOM, OATS, OKRA, ONION, PASSION FLOWER, PEAS, RICE, ROSEMARY, SWEETCORN, SWISS CHARD, TAHINI, TEMPEH, WALNUT AND WALNUT OIL, WILD MARJORAM**

Migraine is a recurrent and particularly intense form of headache, often accompanied by visual and gastro-intestinal disturbances. The pain always begins on one side of the head, and attacks may start with a visual "aura" (thought to be caused by constriction of cerebral blood vessels). Subsequent dilation of the blood vessels causes a characteristic throbbing headache, often accompanied by nausea, vomiting and sensitivity to light. Migraine often runs in families, and may be associated with a childhood tendency to symptoms such as stomach ache, colic, vomiting, dizziness or travel sickness. Migraine is more common in women than men, and can be triggered by many factors including food allergy. Chronic stress is thought to cause changes to the nervous system that make attacks more likely. Hormonal changes associated with menstruation and the menopause may be a factor in some women. Musculoskeletal disorders such as whiplash injury may be other important triggers.

## Prevention

It may help to keep a diary and make a note of any factors that seem to be linked to an attack, such as particular foods and your emotional state just prior to an attack. Identifying and avoiding allergens can often reduce the number and severity of migraines you suffer. Common offenders include red meat (especially pork), dairy products, wheat, chocolate, eggs, cheese, alcohol (especially red wine, sherry and port), tobacco, coffee, strong tea, tomato, oranges, white sugar, shellfish and food additives (such as nitrates, benzoic acid, tartrazine and monosodium glutamate).

Eating a leaf of fresh feverfew each day over a long period of time may reduce the frequency and/or intensity of the attacks. However, some people are sensitive to the bitter principles in feverfew and can develop small blisters in the mouth after eating the fresh leaves. If you are susceptible to this problem, you can take feverfew in the form of a tisane (place a couple of fresh leaves in a cup, pour boiling water over the top and leave to infuse). Marigold (calendula) flowers offer some protection from the effects of food allergens because they contain quercetin, which dampens down the body's responses to allergens. Foods containing vitamin B3 (niacin) may also be useful in preventing migraine attacks. These include soya products such as tempeh and tofu, muesli, broad beans, brown rice, aduki beans, sweetcorn and mushrooms.

## Management

Many people find the condition is improved by a change of diet such as a reduction in intake of animal produce and increased consumption of fresh fruits and vegetables. Important foods and drinks to eliminate are those containing alcohol, caffeine, cheese, chocolate, shellfish and oranges. Vegetable oils (particularly walnut), cayenne, garlic and onion are all beneficial. Foods high in magnesium (such as Brazil nuts, okra, melon seeds, tahini paste, Swiss chard and brown rice) may also help in the long-term treatment of migraines.

**SUGGESTED RECIPES FOR MIGRAINE**

Green leafy salad (page 181), nettle and sweet potato mash (page 185), spicy brazil nut pâté (page 197), muesli (page 243), khichuri – rice with lentils (page 257), florence fennel salad (page 260), tea for aches and pains (page 271), tea for headache (page 271).

Following a detox and elimination diet (see page 272) can be very useful for identifying and avoiding some of the causes of migraine attacks. After completing the diet, alcohol, cheese, oranges and shellfish should still be avoided until symptom-free for six months. Foods high in animal fats should be kept to a minimum; vegetable oils, garlic and onion should form a regular part of the diet.

# rheumatoid arthritis

**SUPERFOODS FOR ARTHRITIS: ADUKI BEAN, ALFALFA, ASPARAGUS, BEETROOT, BERRIES, CARROT, CELERY, CLEAVERS, CURLY KALE, ENDIVE, FENNEL, FEVERFEW, GARLIC, GRAPES, HARICOT BEANS, HAWTHORN, JUNIPER, LENTILS, LIQUORICE ROOT, MANGO, NETTLE, NUTS, ONION, PAPAYA, PEAS, PINEAPPLE, RICE, SEA VEGETABLE, SUNFLOWER SEED AND OIL, SWISS CHARD, TAHINI, TEMPEH, VIOLET**

Rheumatoid arthritis is a chronic, generalized inflammatory disease that attacks the membranes surrounding joints and tendons, causing pain, swelling, stiffness and loss of movement. It mostly affects adults but can occur in childhood. It commonly begins with weeks of feeling generally unwell, perhaps with weight loss, mild fever, stiffness and pain. The joint symptoms often start in the hands or feet and are worse in the morning. The inflammation may spread to affect all of the joints, leading to increased pain, swelling, stiffness and – in severe cases – deformity. Most sufferers also have some degree of anaemia and vitamin C deficiency.

The condition is an autoimmune disease in which antibodies attack the lining of the joints. What triggers the process is unclear, although it may be associated with genetic factors, nutrition and lifestyle. There is also an association with poor digestion and waste elimination, which can lead to an accumulation of antigenic toxins.

### SUGGESTED RECIPES FOR ARTHRITIS

Curly kale parcels (page 181), nettle and sweet potato mash (page 185), spiced nettle soup (page 185), grilled endive and brazil nut salad (page 197), garlic and savoy cabbage (page 209), yoghurt with fruit (page 243), toasted tempeh with herb salad (page 248), toasted nuts and seeds (page 248), artichoke hearts, broad beans and shiitake (page 252), asparagus asian-style (page 253), spring greens and macadamia nuts (page 258), swiss chard and juniper berries (page 259), florence fennel salad (page 260), tropical sunshine salad (page 261), heart warmer (page 266), green tea with mint (page 269), immuni-tea (page 269), liquorice mix (page 270), tea for joints (page 271).

## Prevention and management

Rheumatoid arthritis is virtually non-existent in cultures where the diet consists mainly of fresh, unadulterated fruits, vegetables, nuts and grains. However, it is relatively common in communities that eat a diet high in sugar, meat, dairy products, saturated fat and refined carbohydrates. Different fats influence inflammation in different ways. Arachidonic acid (from meat and dairy products) increases inflammation but a diet high in polyunsaturated fats and low in saturated fat inhibits inflammation and improves symptoms.

Free radicals are responsible for much of the inflammatory damage caused in arthritis. So eating foods high in antioxidants can be beneficial. Improving digestion with foods such as papaya and pineapple, which contain proteolytic enzymes, alleviates the effect of food allergy and reduces the inflammatory process in the joints. Bioflavonoids block release of histamine and leukotrienes, which are both active inflammatory agents. Foods containing copper reduce arthritic inflammation. Foods high in niacin and tryptophan (components of vitamin B3) dampen arthritic pain.

To aid the elimination of toxins, include natural diuretics in the diet (celery seeds, nettle and cleavers), and support the liver with foods containing bitter principles (globe artichoke, endive and chicory). Taking psyllium seeds helps detoxify the gut and a traditional grape fast (see page 273) can aid general detoxification. Eliminating food allergens can have a beneficial effect on rheumatoid arthritis. Common offenders are dairy products, red meat, pork, wheat, vegetables of the solinacea family (tomato, aubergine, peppers, tobacco – although potatoes are usually fairly well tolerated), shellfish, alcohol (especially red wine and port), oranges and coffee. Other foods to avoid are strawberries, sorrel, currants (red and black), rhubarb, beetroot leaves and spinach.

# inflammatory bowel disease

**SUPERFOODS FOR IBD: APRICOT, ASPARAGUS, AVOCADO, BANANA, BEANS, BEETROOT, BELGIAN ENDIVE, BERRIES, BRUSSELS SPROUT, BUTTERNUT SQUASH, CABBAGE, CAULIFLOWER, CHICKPEA, GRAPE, LEMON, LENTIL, LINSEED, LIVE SOYA YOGHURT, MANGO, NUTS, MUESLI, OKRA, PAPAYA, PARSLEY, PEAS, RICE, SEEDS, SPINACH, SPRING GREENS, SWEETCORN, SWISS CHARD, TAHINI, TEMPEH**

Inflammatory bowel disease (IBD) is a general term for two important digestive disorders – ulcerative colitis and Crohn's disease. Ulcerative colitis involves recurrent inflammation of the large intestine. There is ulceration, leading to bouts of profuse and bloody diarrhoea, fever, abdominal pain, dehydration and often weight loss. There is a risk of life-threatening perforation of the bowel. Crohn's disease involves chronic patchy inflammation of the bowel resulting in diarrhoea (without blood) and fever. It may lead to abscesses, poor absorption of nutrients, bowel obstruction and perforation. IBD may develop at any age, but most often starts between the ages of 15 and 35. Ulcerative colitis is currently the more common of the two, but the incidence of Crohn's disease is rising. The cause is not well understood, but the Western lifestyle and diet, infection, allergy, autoimmune disorders, heredity, and psychosomatic and emotional factors have all been implicated.

### Prevention and management

A balanced diet containing sufficiently good quality calories is one of the most important factors in the prevention and management of IBD. The diet should include foods high in calcium, magnesium, potassium, and trace elements such as zinc and iron. Folate and vitamin B12 are important for the health of the intestinal mucosa and vitamins A, C and E are powerful antioxidants able to inhibit inflammation. Bioflavonoids found in most medicinal herbs have a powerful effect on enzymes involved in the inflammatory response. Inflammation can also be reduced by cutting consumption of animal fats in favour of omega-3 oils found in walnut oil, linseed oil and fish oils. Aim to re-establish the natural gut flora by adding live soya yoghurt and complex carbohydrates to the diet. But avoid wheat bran, sugar and refined carbohydrates, and common food allergens such as wheat, corn and dairy products.

## SUGGESTED RECIPES FOR INFLAMMATORY BOWEL DISEASE

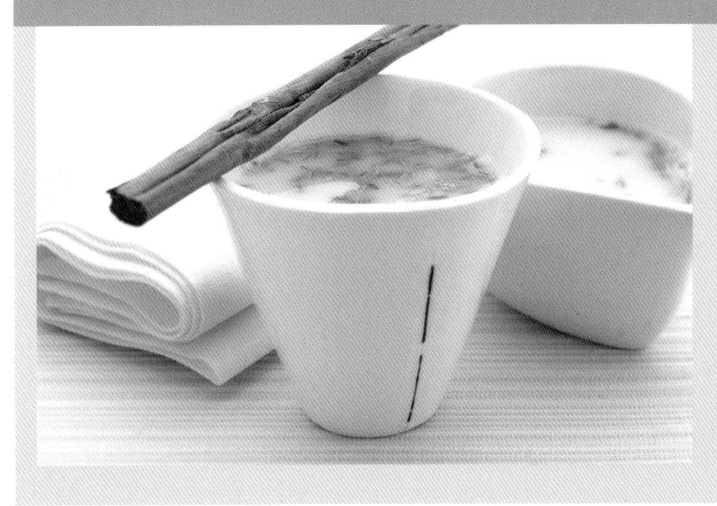

Green leafy salad (page 181), nettle and sweet potato mash (page 185), porridge with dried fruit and quinoa (page 242), muesli (page 243), yoghurt with fruit (page 243), healing soup (page 244), creamy cauliflower soup (page 245), pumpkin soup (page 245), toasted tempeh with herb salad (page 248), tzaziki (page 251), artichoke hearts, broad beans and shiitake (page 252), winter hot pot (page 256), khichuri – rice with lentils (page 257), lemon rice (page 257), carrot 'n' beetroot salad (page 259), florence fennel salad (page 260), green lentil salad (page 260), wild rice salad (page 261), tropical fruit salad (page 263), apricot and ginger (page 264), caribbean smoothie (page 264), calming tea (page 268), spicy chai – *left* (page 270).

# HIV & AIDS

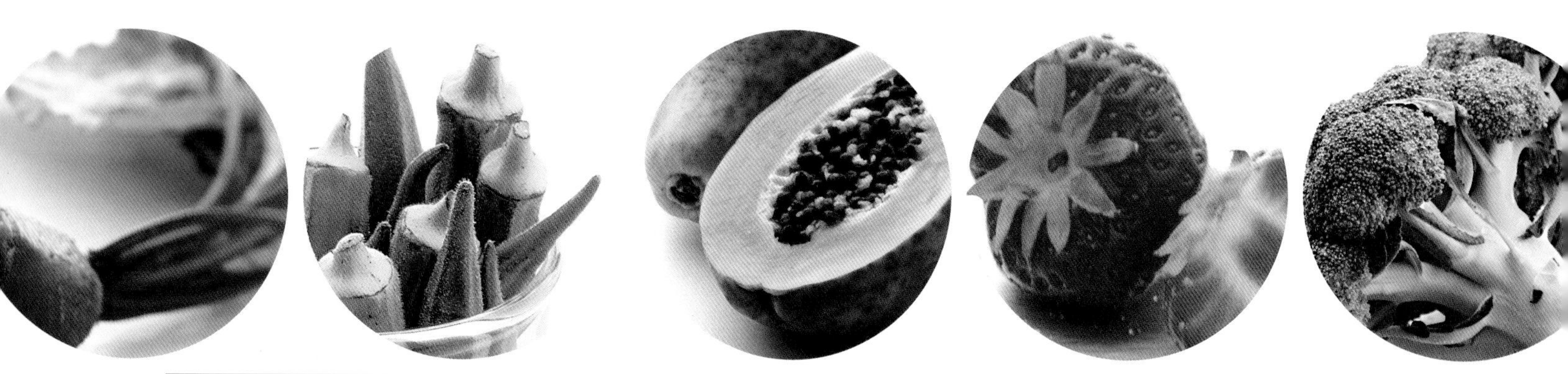

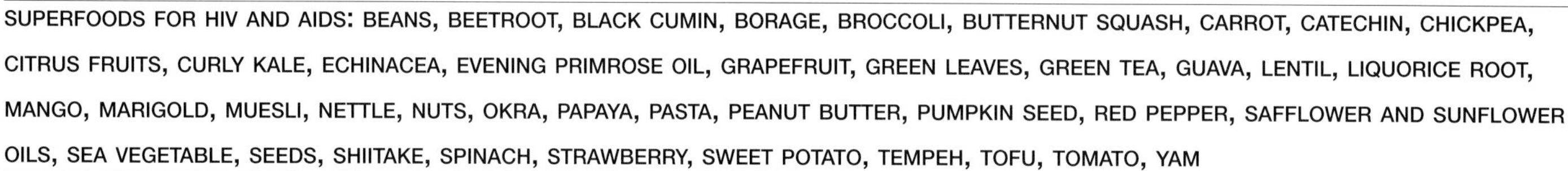

**SUPERFOODS FOR HIV AND AIDS:** BEANS, BEETROOT, BLACK CUMIN, BORAGE, BROCCOLI, BUTTERNUT SQUASH, CARROT, CATECHIN, CHICKPEA, CITRUS FRUITS, CURLY KALE, ECHINACEA, EVENING PRIMROSE OIL, GRAPEFRUIT, GREEN LEAVES, GREEN TEA, GUAVA, LENTIL, LIQUORICE ROOT, MANGO, MARIGOLD, MUESLI, NETTLE, NUTS, OKRA, PAPAYA, PASTA, PEANUT BUTTER, PUMPKIN SEED, RED PEPPER, SAFFLOWER AND SUNFLOWER OILS, SEA VEGETABLE, SEEDS, SHIITAKE, SPINACH, STRAWBERRY, SWEET POTATO, TEMPEH, TOFU, TOMATO, YAM

Acquired immune deficiency syndrome (AIDS) is a group of disorders apparently related to previous infection by the human immunodeficiency virus (HIV). The virus is transmitted via body fluids, during sexual contact, or contaminated blood products. Everyone is potentially at risk of infection, but the most vulnerable groups are people with multiple sexual partners, intravenous drug users who share needles and syringes, and recipients of blood products in countries that do not employ scrupulous screening procedures. The incubation period is 1 to 6 months after infection by the virus. Progression from infection to being "antibody positive" is not well understood. Even though 98 per cent of sufferers have HIV antibodies in their blood, 2 per cent do not! Furthermore, being HIV-positive does not necessarily lead to full-blown AIDS. There are four recognized AIDS-related states:

- antibodies in the blood but no symptoms;
- persistent generalized lymph node enlargement (PGL);
- ARC (AIDS-related complex), which involves the clinical features of chronic disease plus abnormal blood test results;
- full-blown AIDS, involving opportunistic lung infections, skin cancer (Kaposi's sarcoma) and lymphatic cancer.

### Prevention

The most important preventive measure you can take is to use safer sexual practices if your partner's sexual history is unknown to you. This involves taking steps to prevent contact with sexual fluids – for example, by using condoms or avoiding penetrative sex. Intravenous drug users should never share injecting materials. When travelling in developing countries, it is advisable to carry disposable syringes and needles with you, in case of emergency.

Your diet should include plenty of foods that help prevent viral infection, such as garlic, Brazil nut and echinacea, and that strengthen the immune system, such as shiitake and beetroot.

### Management

AIDS is a growing problem all over the world. Although a cure remains elusive, there are simple nutritional and lifestyle changes that are proven to make life easier for sufferers. HIV infection, nutritional status and immune function are intimately connected. The relationship between HIV infection and food is important because strategies that improve nutritional status have a beneficial effect on the course of the disease. The outcome with drug therapy is less hopeful in people with compromised nutrition, whereas good nutrition greatly improves the chances of survival.

In Africa, AIDS was first known as "slim disease" because the condition caused rapid weight loss, leading to early death. The wasting associated with AIDS is caused by inefficient absorption of food, excessive loss of nutrients (mainly through chronic diarrhoea), and less efficient use of nutrients that are absorbed. Once the disorder has been diagnosed, it is possible to maintain the weight of the patient through intensive feeding regimes. When the condition has been stabilized, patients can regain some of the weight they have lost and start to build up the reserves that will make it easier to cope with the condition. Avoiding, reversing or delaying the wasting process requires adopting measures involving all the ways in which food is converted into energy and body mass.

**Food intake** HIV-positive individuals often have a poor appetite, because of inefficient absorption of nutrients, secondary infections, the side effects of certain drugs, fungal infections of the mouth or oesophagus (which makes eating and swallowing difficult), and enlargement of the liver or spleen (which gives a false feeling of fullness). Depression may also be a factor. Therefore, the quality of the food that the patient eats is of vital importance to compensate for the lack of quantity.

**Absorption** The food we eat is broken down in the small intestine, and nutrients are absorbed through the gut wall. This important process can be hampered by HIV infection, and is also disturbed by diarrhoea, which causes food to pass through the digestive system too quickly. Antibiotics used to destroy harmful bacteria may also kill friendly bacteria that live in the gut and support the digestive process by aiding absorption and manufacturing vitamins.

To boost nutrient absorption, it is best to avoid dairy produce and include foods such as apple, grapefruit, chickpea, amaranth leaves, potatoes, fennel, rocket, globe artichoke, Belgian endive and the medicinal herbs peppermint, thyme, catmint and marigold.

**Metabolism** Our metabolic rate determines how quickly we expend the energy we obtain from food. It is often raised in HIV infection and is responsible for much of the fatigue and lethargy felt by people with AIDS. HIV infection alters metabolism, with less protein being manufactured by the liver and more being broken down and used for energy. The result is muscle wasting and a decline in "lean body mass". To maintain energy and stabilize metabolism, the diet should be high in complex carbohydrates, vegetable proteins and fibre and low in fat. All produce should be fresh, organic and unprocessed.

Foods rich in zinc, vitamins A and C, and bioflavonoids are beneficial because they inhibit the activity of viruses and bacteria. Liquorice root and echinacea both support the immune system and enhance many aspects of immune function, as well as inhibiting the spread of viral infection. Grapefruit, pumpkin seed, Brazil nut, nettle, black cumin, borage, sweet potato, yam, tomato and shiitake act specifically against immunodeficiency. Important immuno-stimulants include okra, beetroot, spinach, curly kale, guava, safflower and sunflower oil, evening primrose oil, sea vegetable, peanut butter and marigold.

## The stress factor

The psychological and emotional stress following a diagnosis of HIV may contribute to the progression of the disease because negative emotions have a detrimental effect on the immune response. However, positive emotions enhance appropriate immune responses, so involvement in pleasurable, creative activity and spending more time in the company of close friends and loved ones are both positive ways of improving immune function.

### SUGGESTED RECIPES FOR HIV AND AIDS

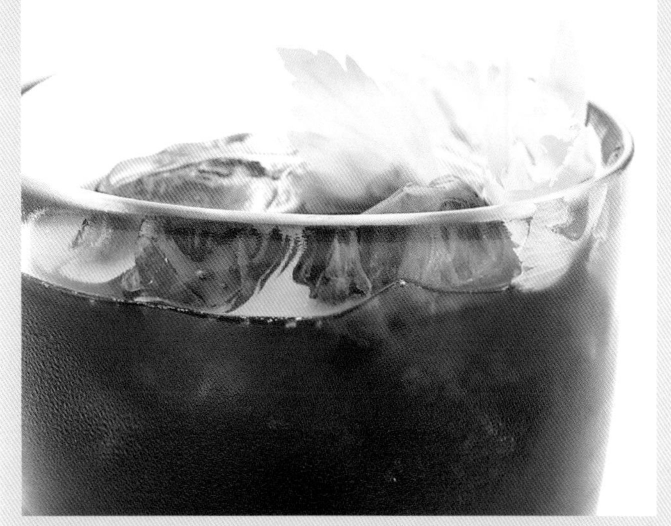

Nettle and sweet potato mash (page 185), nettle and lime tisane (page 185), grapefruit and peppermint fizz (page 189), grapefruit salad (page 189), avocado smoothie (page 193), avocado, watercress and cumin salad (page 193), brazil nuts and sun-dried tomatoes with beans (page 197), grilled endive and brazil nut salad (page 197), shiitake salad (page 215), healing soup (page 244), tofu balls (page 250), artichoke hearts, broad beans and shiitake (page 252), okra in sweet and sour tamarind sauce (page 256), shepherdess' pie (256), carrot 'n' beetroot salad (page 259), tropical sunshine salad (page 261), wild rice salad (page 261), heart warmer (page 266), Vegetable cocktail – *above* (page 267), immuni-tea (page 269), stress relief (page 270).

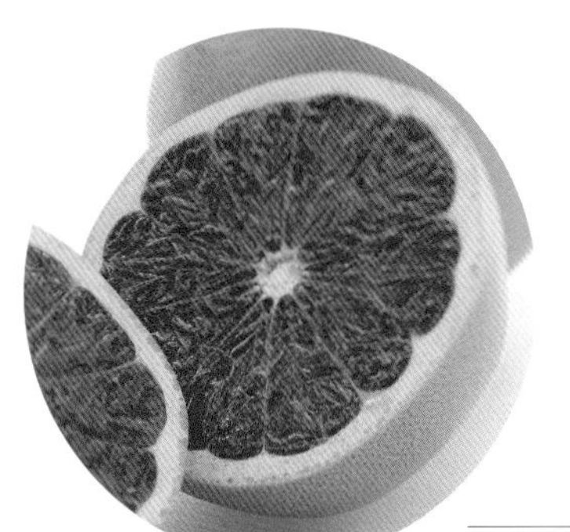

# stress & chronic fatigue syndrome

SUPERFOODS FOR STRESS: BEANS, BORAGE, BROCCOLI, CABBAGE, CARROT, GRAPEFRUIT, GREEN LEAVES, LAVENDER, LEMON BALM, LENTIL, LIQUORICE ROOT, MANGO, MUESLI, NUTS, OATS, ORANGE, PAPAYA, RICE, STRAWBERRY, TEMPEH, TOFU; SUPERFOODS FOR CFS: AVOCADO, BANANA, BEANS, BEETROOT, BLACKCURRANT, BORAGE, CHAMOMILE, CLEAVERS, ECHINACEA, GRAPEFRUIT, GREEN LEAVES, LIQUORICE ROOT, LIVE SOYA YOGHURT, MUESLI, NUTS, OKRA, PAPAYA, PEAS, RED PEPPER, RICE, TEMPEH, TOFU, WHEATGRASS

## STRESS

The relationship between stress and ill health is well documented, but stress levels vary enormously from person to person, as does each individual's ability to cope. To deal effectively with stress, it is necessary to take account of these variations, and to remember that the immune system does not work in isolation. It is affected by thoughts, actions and emotional responses as well as by disease, environment, general lifestyle, age and genetic predisposition.

Stress hormones such as adrenaline and cortisol enable the body to cope with stressful situations, but if they are released in excess or over too long a period, they inhibit (and can damage) the immune response. This means that during periods of chronic stress, exposure to pathogens is more likely to cause disease.

### Prevention and management

Like rest and relaxation, good nutrition can reduce the effects of stress in our lives and enhance immune function. Foods high in vitamins A and C, and zinc and selenium are particularly helpful. Other foods and herbs for stress relief include Belgian endive, cauliflower, artichoke, banana, sesame seed, oats, sweetcorn, wheatgerm, borage, lemon balm, lavender and liquorice root.

## CHRONIC FATIGUE SYNDROME (CFS)

This poorly understood syndrome is also known as myalgic encephalomyelitis (ME) or post-viral syndrome, and may relate to the immune system's difficulty in handling viral infections when already overburdened by "environmental" stress. It does not seem to be related to any specific viral infection, but can persist for months or even years. Common symptoms include severe fatigue after minimal exertion that is not relieved by rest, generalized aches and pains, depressed mood, recurrent sore throats, swollen lymph nodes, headache, mild fever, difficulty adjusting to changes in temperature, and gastro-intestinal disturbance. There may also be a variety of inexplicable neurological symptoms.

### Prevention and management

The best way to prevent or manage the condition is through detoxification, and following a diet rich in foods that enhance resistance to disease and support immune function. To boost the immune system drink plenty of pure water and eat a variety of fresh fruit and vegetables. Choose foods rich in vitamins B6 and C, essential fatty acids, calcium, magnesium and zinc.

### SUGGESTED RECIPES FOR STRESS AND CFS

Stress: spiced nettle soup (page 185), grilled endive and brazil nut salad (page 197), scrambled tofu (page 242), muesli (page 243), creamy cauliflower soup (page 245), samosa parcels (page 248), toasted nuts and seeds (page 248), amaranth and tofu puffs (page 252), artichoke hearts, broad beans and shiitake (page 252), provençale-style kidney beans (page 255), blackberry cream (page 264), creamy mango (page 264), stress relief (page 270).

CFS: grapefruit salad (page 189), shiitake with sea vegetable (page 215), sweet chestnuts and kumquats (page 257), carrot 'n' beetroot salad (page 259), tomato cocktail (page 267), immuni-tea (page 269), sleepy time (page 270).

# depression & anxiety

SUPERFOODS FOR DEPRESSION: AVOCADO, BANANA, BEANS, BORAGE, ENDIVE, GREEN LEAVES, LIQUORICE ROOT, MANGO, MUESLI, PEAS, RED PEPPER, RICE, SOYA PRODUCTS, ST JOHN'S WORT, TAHINI, YEAST EXTRACT; SUPERFOODS FOR ANXIETY: APRICOT, ARTICHOKE, BEANS, BUTTERNUT SQUASH, CAULIFLOWER, CHAMOMILE, GRAPEFRUIT, GREEN LEAVES, LAVENDER, LEMON BALM, OATS, OKRA, PASSION FLOWER, POTATO, RED PEPPER, ROSEMARY, ST JOHN'S WORT, SWEET POTATO, TEMPEH, TOFU, WALNUT, YEAST EXTRACT

## DEPRESSION

There are two forms of depression: psychotic (endogenous) and neurotic (reactive). Psychotic depression is a severe emotional disturbance more common in middle age. The sufferer may become agitated, or profoundly withdrawn and lethargic, and may experience hallucinations and delusions. There are disturbances in bowel habit, appetite and sleep, and a real risk of suicide. Neurotic depression is a reaction to traumatic events such as bereavement and may be accompanied by anxiety, and disturbed appetite and sleep. The underlying causes are not completely understood but contributing factors include physical disorder (such as underactive thyroid), diet, food allergy, smoking, drugs and lifestyle.

### Prevention and management

Measures to prevent or manage depression include taking regular exercise; avoiding cigarettes, alcohol and drinks containing caffeine; using alternatives to oral contraception; eliminating food allergens and additives (particularly aspartame); and eating regular meals with plenty of fresh fruits and vegetables (to stabilize blood-sugar levels). To optimize your nutritional state, eat foods high in B and C vitamins, and magnesium and tryptophan. St John's wort is an effective antidepressant, and herbs that support the adrenal glands, such as borage and liquorice root, are also valuable.

## ANXIETY

Anxiety states are dominated by fast pulse, sweating, butterflies in the stomach, light headedness, and feelings of apprehension and fear. Chronic anxiety takes a toll on the immune system and can lead to physical illness, such as irritable bowel syndrome. The cause can be hormonal, or linked to overactive thyroid and premenstrual syndrome, or a traumatic event. It can also be a symptom of psychiatric illness, such as depression or dementia.

### Prevention and management

Once hormonal imbalance (which needs medical attention) has been ruled out, anxiety states can often be managed with foods that strengthen the nervous system, such as oats, potato, sweet potato, butternut squash, okra, red pepper, Brussels sprouts, cauliflower, artichoke, spring greens, curly kale, apricot, grapefruit, walnut, tempeh, butterbeans, haricot beans, pinto beans and yeast extract. Herbs to calm the nerves include chamomile, lemon balm, rosemary, St John's wort, lavender and passion flower.

**SUGGESTED RECIPES FOR DEPRESSION & ANXIETY**

Depression: pasta, pesto and shiitake (page 215), italian butterbean soup (page 245), hummus with crudités and warm pitta bread (page 246), baba ganoush (page 248), paella (page 252), chinese salad (page 260), baked apples (page 262), calming tea (page 268), liquorice mix (page 270), pick-me-up (page 270), stress relief (page 270).

Anxiety: curly kale parcels (page 181), ruby red melon salad (page 242), porridge with dried fruit and quinoa (page 242), creamy cauliflower soup (page 245), spicy moroccan soup (page 246), rocket salad (page 259), apricot and ginger (page 264), chamomile tonic (page 268), sleepy time (page 270).

# cancer

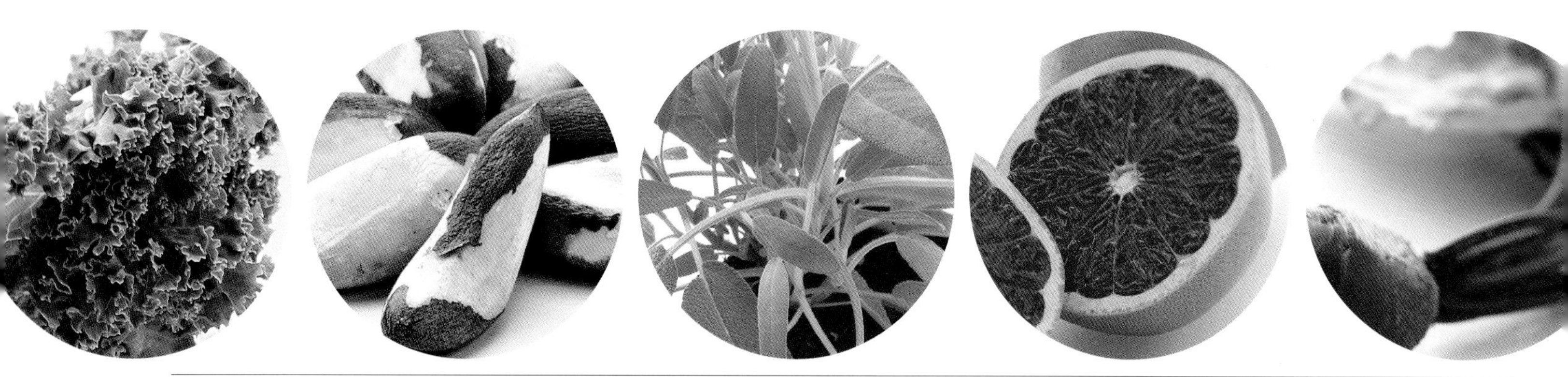

**SUPERFOODS FOR CANCER:** AVOCADO, BEETROOT, BEANS, BERRIES, BRAZIL NUT, BROCCOLI, BUTTERNUT SQUASH, CABBAGE, CARROT, CELERY SALT, CHICKPEA, CLEAVERS, CURLY KALE, ECHINACEA, GARLIC, GRAPE, GRAPEFRUIT, GRAPESEED, GREEN LEAVES, GUAVA, LEMON, LENTIL, MANGO, MARIGOLD, MUNG BEAN SPROUT, NETTLE, NUTS, OLIVE, ORANGE, PAPAYA, PASTA, POTATO, PULSES, RED PEPPER, RICE, SEEDS, SHIITAKE, SPICES, SUN-DRIED TOMATO, SWEET POTATO, TEMPEH, TOFU, VEGETABLE OILS, VIOLET, WHOLEMEAL BREAD, WILD RICE

Research into the nature of cancer has not yet clarified exactly what it is that turns a normal cell into a cancer cell. Although we know that carcinogens such as chemicals, radiation, tobacco, asbestos and viruses can cause tumours, it is not known precisely how or why. But there is growing evidence that nutritional, social, psychological and environmental factors play a role in cancer.

Evidence linking food and nutrition to cancer risk is growing and has been collected over a number of years by comparing different diets with cancer rates. There are big differences in incidence and death from cancer in different parts of the world, but specialists have identified general patterns. Developing countries tend to have high rates of cancers of the upper digestive tract, liver and cervix, whereas developed countries have relatively high rates of hormone-related cancers, and cancers of the colon and rectum.

There is great variation in the length and intensity of exposure to particular environmental carcinogens that will trigger cancerous changes. It is also possible that simultaneous exposure to a combination of carcinogens produces cancer where one alone would have been relatively harmless, and that exposure to stress may alter the body's response to different carcinogens. Genetic factors play a role in some cancers, and some carcinogens – such as free radicals – can originate within the body. Some tumours are benign (non-spreading), but malignant tumours invade surrounding tissues and spread via blood and lymph to form metastases (secondary tumours). There is controversy surrounding the role of viruses in cancer formation. In other mammals (such as rabbits, chickens, mice and cats) several tumours are known to be caused by viruses, but the picture in humans is less clear. However, there is good evidence that viruses may cause some cancers in humans (such as cervical and liver cell cancer, lymphoma and leukaemia).

There are many different types of cancer, each one with its individual features, but all cancers sooner or later disturb normal body function. The danger signals for malignant disease include a change in bowel or bladder habit, sores that won't heal, unusual bleeding or discharge, newly discovered lumps, obvious changes in skin moles or warts, a persistent cough and/or hoarseness, coughing up blood and, very importantly, loss of appetite and unexplained weight loss.

### Prevention

It has been estimated that in the USA 30 per cent of all cancer deaths are related to dietary factors, and that 30 to 40 per cent of cancer cases throughout the world are potentially preventable with simple changes to diet and lifestyle. It is now beyond doubt that the most effective way to reduce cancer risk is to stop smoking, eat plenty of fresh fruit and vegetables, and limit exposure to occupational and environmental carcinogens. Environmental carcinogens are usually man-made and fall into five distinct groups

– additives, dyes and coal tar, pollutant chemicals, fumes and radiation. Not all of these will inevitably trigger cancer in all cases, but it is worth remembering that many carcinogens cause damage by weakening the immune system and so may be indirectly responsible for causing cancerous changes. Therefore, in cancer prevention and management it is very important to keep the immune system as strong as possible by adopting a healthy lifestyle and eating a diet rich in energy and vital nutrients.

For cancer prevention, choose a plant-based diet that includes a rich variety of vegetables, fruits, nuts, pulses, and minimally processed starchy foods. Eat at least five portions of seasonal, organic fresh fruit and vegetables daily, all year round and at least five portions a day of grains, pulses, roots and tubers. Use modest amounts of vegetable oils (mainly olive, walnut, grapeseed, and safflower and sunflower oils), and avoid animal fats altogether. Use herbs, spices, celery salt and soy sauce to season foods, and limit consumption of salted and pickled foods and table salt.

Choose organic foods free of additives, pesticides and other chemicals. Avoid alcohol, meat and dairy products, and if animal protein is eaten, choose fish, organic poultry or meat from non-domesticated animals. Choose minimally processed foods and limit your consumption of refined sugar. Avoid being over- or underweight, stop smoking and take an hour's exercise daily.

Immune system boosters to guard against cancer include garlic, beetroot, grapefruit, curly kale, nettle, avocado, Brazil nut, cleavers, marigold, violet, echinacea and shiitake mushroom, among many others. Also important are foods that contain vitamins A (sweet potato, carrot, red pepper, green leaves, mango, papaya, butternut squash), C (guava, red and green peppers, green leaves, blackcurrant, papaya, mango, lemon, orange, cabbage, broccoli), E (avocado, nuts, sun-dried tomato, sweet potato, sunflower seeds), zinc (aduki beans, tofu, tempeh, lentils, muesli, chickpeas, tahini, pumpkin seeds) and selenium (beans, Brazil nuts, lentils, pasta, sunflower seeds, mushrooms, wholemeal bread), carotenoids (yellow and orange fruits and vegetables), bioflavonoids (especially anthocyanin in dark-coloured berries such as red grape, blueberry, cranberry and hawthorn berry, and quercetin in marigold) and the fatty acids found in walnuts.

### Management

In the early stages of cancer, the most effective dietary approach is to detoxify the system (see detox diet, page 272). Later on in the course of the disease, freshly made juices, smoothies and tisanes are particularly helpful because they contain a high concentration of nutrients (together with antioxidants and other immune system boosters), but are nevertheless easy to digest. Half of the diet should be fresh fruits, especially grapes, which are detoxifying and also contain immune-enhancing anthocyanin. The diet should also be rich in complex carbohydrates – for example, from potatoes, sweet potatoes, rice and wild rice, and essential fatty acids, such as from walnuts. Good sources of protein are pulses, mung bean sprouts, tofu, mushrooms (especially shiitake) and tempeh.

#### SUGGESTED RECIPES FOR CANCER

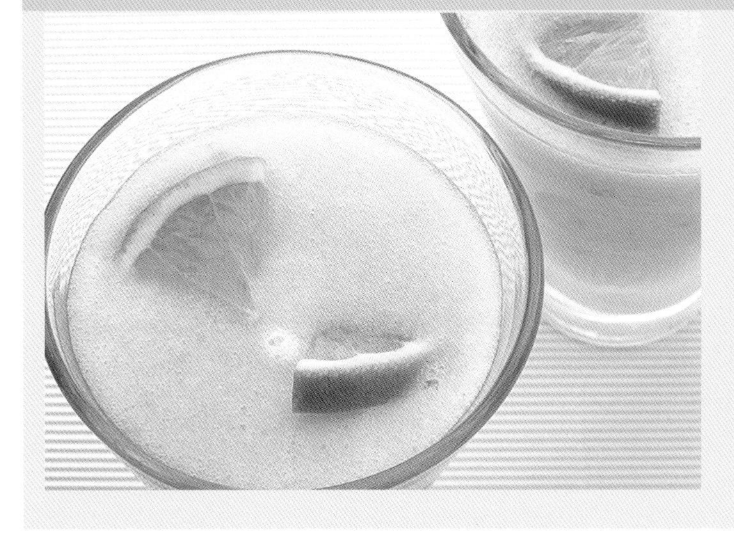

Green leafy salad (page 181), spiced nettle soup (page 185), nettle and lime tisane (page 185), grapefruit salad (page 189), avocado smoothie (page 193), oriental salad with tempeh (page 203), baked tomatoes on toast (page 242), black-eye bean and wild marjoram soup (page 245), shiitake mushroom soup (page 245), tomato and cucumber canapés (page 250), guacamole (page 250), tofu balls (page 250), casserole de puy (page 252), artichoke hearts, broad beans and shiitake (page 252), greek casserole (page 255), carrot 'n' beetroot salad (page 259), rocket salad (page 259), wild rice salad (page 261), tropical fruit salad (page 263), caribbean smoothie (page 264), green party (page 264), guava and apple – *left* (page 266), tea for glands (page 271), tea for the skin (page 271).

# ischaemic (coronary) heart disease

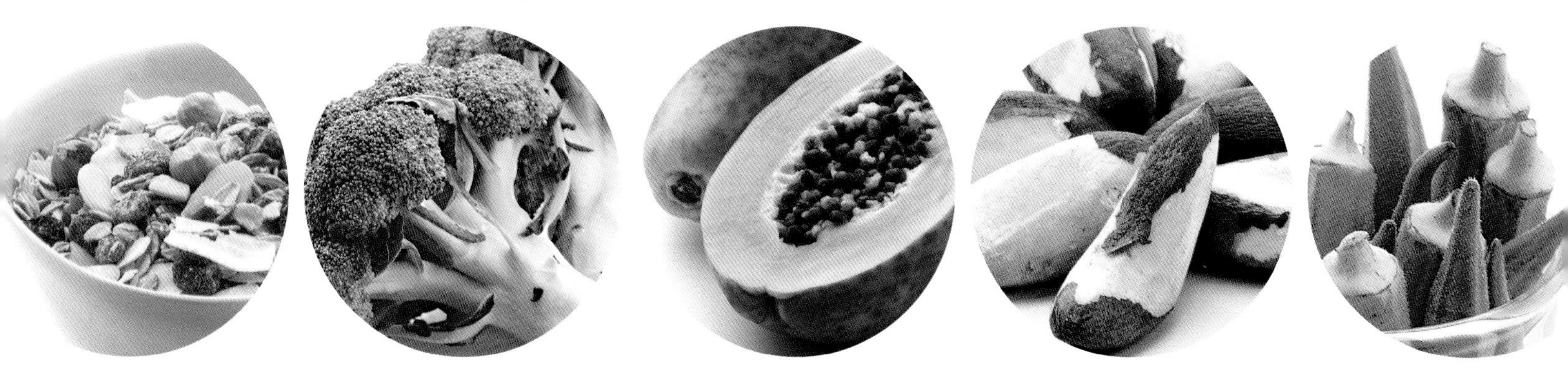

**SUPERFOODS FOR ISCHAEMIC HEART DISEASE:** ALFALFA, ALMOND, APRICOT, BLACK-EYE BEAN, BRAZIL NUT, BROCCOLI, BUTTERBEAN, CANTALOUPE MELON, CHICKPEA, GARLIC, GINGER, GREEN LEAVES, GUAVA, HARICOT BEAN, HAWTHORN BERRY, HAZELNUT, LEMON, LENTIL, LINSEED, MACADAMIA NUT, MANGETOUT PEA, MANGO, MELON, MUESLI, OKRA, ONION, ORANGE, PAPAYA, PINEAPPLE, PINE NUT, PINTO BEAN, PUMPKIN SEED, RED PEPPER, RICE, SESAME SEED, SOYA BEAN, SUNFLOWER SEED, SWISS CHARD, TAHINI, TEMPEH, TOFU, YAM

Ischaemic heart disease is the partial blockage of the coronary arteries by atherosclerosis and thrombosis, leading to poor blood supply to the heart muscle. It is one of the commonest causes of illness and disability and the main cause of death in the Western world. Its major symptom is angina (a crushing pain in the chest spreading up into the neck and down the left arm), and the worst outcome is myocardial infarction (heart attack).

Risk factors include smoking, high blood pressure, high blood cholesterol, a diet high in saturated fats and salt and low in fibre, obesity, diabetes, gout, emotional stress, lack of exercise, social deprivation, oral contraception, genetic predisposition and age.

## Prevention

It is important to avoid smoking, alcohol and coffee completely. Daily gentle exercise, such as walking, is beneficial. Stress is dangerous and should be avoided where possible (or counteracted by allowing plenty of time and space for relaxation). High blood cholesterol, triglyceride (fat) and low- and very low-density lipoproteins (LDLs and VLDLs) are associated with the build-up of fatty deposits in the blood vessels that can lead to coronary artery blockage. Saturated fats (such as animal fats) make things worse, but monounsaturated (mostly oleic acid from olive oil) and polyunsaturated fats (from nuts, seeds and kernels) are associated with more favourable blood-fat levels and thus reduced risk of heart disease. "Trans-fats" (hardened unsaturated fatty acids in meat, dairy and manufactured foods such as margarine) have the same negative effect on blood-fat levels as saturated fats. Obesity, alcohol and refined sugar also contribute to raised blood-fat levels.

Avoiding red meat, eggs, milk and cheese is desirable, and a decrease in overall fat intake by avoiding "table fats" (such as butter) and foods containing invisible fat (such as mayonnaise, cakes and rich sauces and soups) can make a major contribution to long-term cardiac health. The diet should be high in complex carbohydrates and fibre (including oats, linseed and foods high in pectin) and include plenty of fresh fruits and vegetables.

## Management

Angina and heart attack are serious conditions that require professional medical attention. Orthodox management is to encourage gentle exercise and maintain a normal lifestyle while reducing relevant risk factors, and taking drugs such as oral nitrates, beta-blockers, and nifedipine. People at high risk of myocardial infarction may be offered a coronary bypass operation.

There are a number of changes that people can make for themselves to reduce risk and make management easier. The therapeutic goal is to improve blood supply and nutrition to the heart muscle. Healthy eating plays a vital role in the management of heart disease. The aim is to create a diet that provides beneficial nutrients without clogging up the tissues and blood vessels with sugars, fats and additives. Processed and convenience foods are usually high in these but low in nourishment. Making a gradual change and exchanging them for fresh fruits, vegetables, nuts, seeds, pulses and whole grain foods reduces blood-cholesterol levels and improves the blood-fat balance. Alfalfa sprouts and leaves decrease blood-cholesterol levels and reduce fatty plaque formation in blood vessels. Bromelain from pineapple inhibits blood clot formation and also breaks down fatty plaques in the arteries. Onions, garlic and ginger have the same effect, and ginger and garlic also lower levels of blood cholesterol and fat. Magnesium deficiency causes coronary artery spasm and irregular heart beat. Good sources of this mineral include Brazil nuts, okra, melon and sunflower seeds, tahini, Swiss chard, brown rice, muesli, tempeh, tofu and other soya bean products.

**SUGGESTED RECIPES FOR HEART DISEASE**

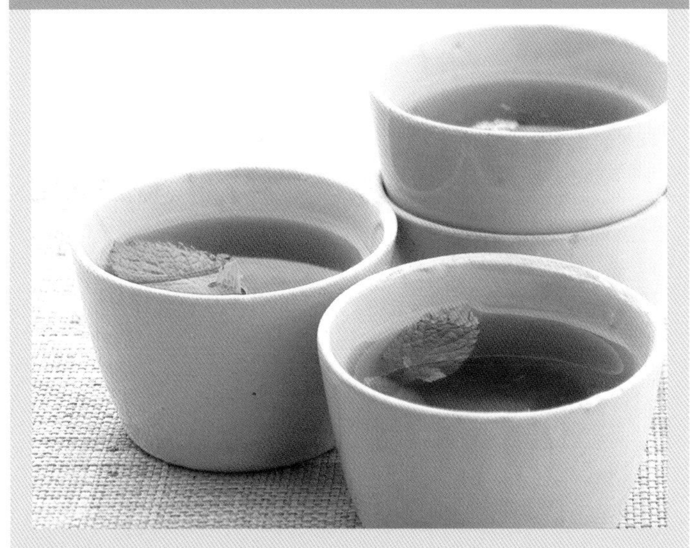

Baked beetroot salad (page 177), brazil nuts and sun-dried tomatoes with beans (page 197), oriental salad with tempeh (page 203), porridge with dried fruit and quinoa (page 242), muesli (page 243), italian butterbean soup (page 245), shiitake mushroom soup (page 245), spicy moroccan soup (page 246), paella (page 252), french onion tart (page 255), okra in sweet and sour tamarind sauce (page 256), provençal mesclun salad (page 259), chinese salad (page 260), orange mango salad (page 260), baked apples (page 262), tropical fruit salad (page 263), mango and lime (page 266), papaya power (page 267), vegetable cocktail (page 267), circulation booster (page 268), green tea with mint – *above* (page 269), heart chai (page 269), si c (page 270).

Carnitine is a vitamin-like compound made in the liver, kidney and brain. It is made from the amino acid lysine (with the help of iron and vitamin C), and is effective in treating heart disease because of its ability to boost the metabolism of saturated fats and cholesterol. The heart normally stores more carnitine than it needs but lack of oxygen in ischaemic heart disease causes depletion of carnitine stores. Foods rich in lysine and iron (such as tempeh, lentils, muesli, peas, tahini, chickpeas, beans, nuts and seeds) help to replenish carnitine. Good sources of vitamin C include guava, red pepper, green leaves, mangetout peas, broccoli, papaya, mango and citrus fruits.

People with heart disease often have a deficiency of coenzymes because their nutritional intake does not keep pace with the increased needs of their tissues. Coenzymes CoA and Q10 are particularly beneficial to the heart because they are involved in the transport of fatty acids to and from cells and in the conversion of fat into energy. Coenzymes have many components in their structure that cannot be synthesized in the body, and which must therefore be supplied in the diet. B-complex vitamins are particularly important in this regard, and good sources of B vitamins include muesli, yeast extract, beans, peas, tahini, soya products such as tempeh and green leaves.

Hawthorn berries and flowering tops are valuable herbal remedies for heart and circulation disorders. They strengthen the heart muscle and lower blood pressure and blood cholesterol levels. They contain anthocyanoid bioflavonoids, which relax the smooth muscle of the artery walls, thus dilating the blood vessels that feed the heart muscle, and increasing the supply of nutrients and oxygen. Garlic is an excellent blood cleanser and thinner, and, if used regularly over a period of time, guards against the formation of fatty deposits in the blood vessels. It can also help to keep blood-cholesterol levels under control.

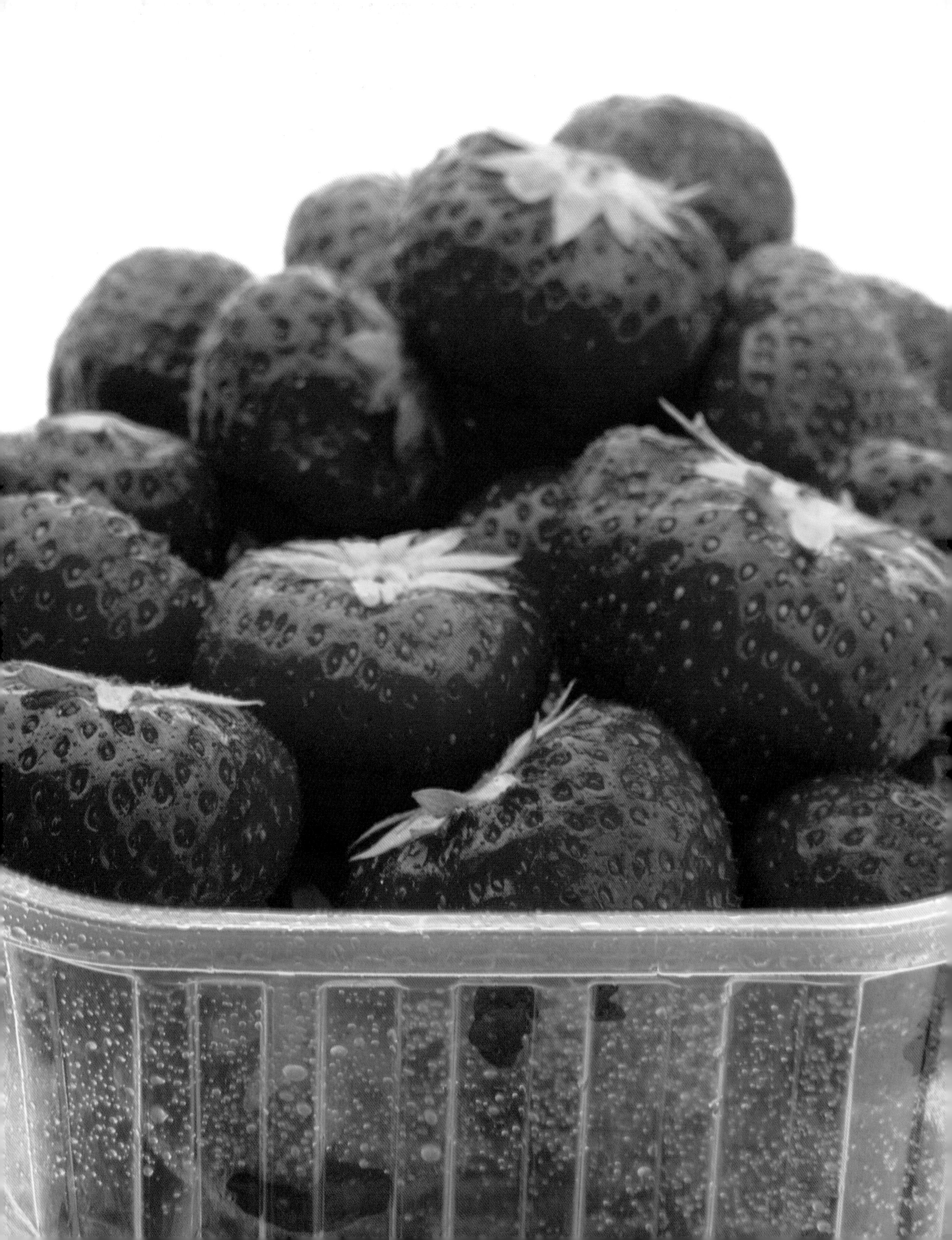

chapter eight

# immune

## foods in practice

Eating is not only the most important route to good health, it is highly enjoyable, too! The most nutritious plant foods are usually also the tastiest. On the following pages we have created a host of delicious recipes that you can enjoy for breakfast, dinner, supper or as tasty snacks. They comprise foods that are packed with vitamins, minerals and other vital nutrients, combined in ways that maximize their health-giving properties.

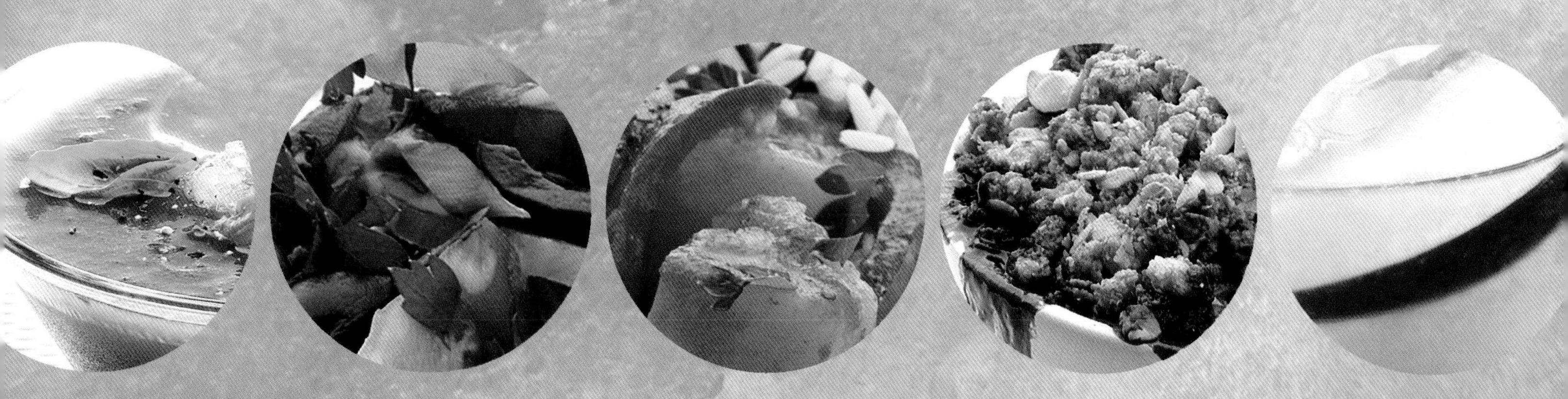

# breakfasts

## baked tomatoes on toast

4 large ripe beef tomatoes
100 g mushrooms, finely chopped
2 garlic cloves, crushed
1 bunch of fresh basil, finely chopped
Breadcrumbs
Sea salt and freshly ground black pepper to taste
Olive oil
4 thick slices of bread, toasted

Preheat the oven to 180°C/gas mark 4. Cut off the bottom of the tomatoes and scoop out the flesh into a bowl. Mix with the mushrooms, garlic and basil. Add enough breadcrumbs to make the mixture hang together. Season with salt and pepper. Fill the tomato shells with the mixture. Sprinkle with a little olive oil. Bake in the oven for about 20 minutes, until the tomatoes are quite soft. Spread a little olive oil on each slice of toast, place a tomato on each and serve immediately.

## scrambled tofu

250 g marinated tofu
4 tbsp soya milk
Sea salt and freshly ground black pepper to taste
30 g vegetable margarine
4 slices of wholemeal bread, to toast
To garnish: fresh rosemary, chopped

Crumble the tofu and mix with the milk. Add salt and pepper to taste. Melt the margarine gently in a saucepan, add the tofu and stir continuously over a low heat until you have a thick, creamy consistency. Meanwhile make the toast. Divide the scrambled tofu on each piece, garnish with rosemary. Serve immediately.

## ruby red melon salad *(far right)*

2 cantaloupe melons, peeled and deseeded
1 pink grapefruit, peeled
To garnish: 12 cherries, halved and stoned
2½-cm piece of fresh ginger root, finely chopped
Maple syrup (optional)

Cut the melon into cubes and divide the grapefruit into segments. Place in individual serving bowls. Garnish with the cherries and the ginger (and add a splash of maple syrup if desired).

## beans and tomatoes on toast

400 g black-eye beans (or haricots), cooked
2 tbsp olive oil
1 red onion, sliced
1 clove garlic, sliced
½ tsp Florence fennel, finely chopped
1 tsp turmeric
1 tsp ground black cumin seed (or ground cumin)
½ tsp cayenne
2 tsp thyme, plus sprigs for garnish
Sea salt and freshly ground black pepper to taste
To garnish: 8 thick tomato slices
4 slices of bread, to toast

Rinse, drain and mash the beans. Stir-fry the onion, garlic and fennel in the oil for 1 minute. Add the turmeric, cumin, cayenne and thyme. Mix in the beans and heat through. Season with salt and pepper. Toast the bread and spread the bean mixture on top. Garnish with 2 tomato slices on each and a little thyme and black pepper. Serve hot.

## fresh fruit salad

2 peaches or nectarines
1 banana
1 kiwi or 2 passion-fruits
1 papaya
1 small bunch of grapes
To garnish: seasonal berries
200 ml unsweetened fruit juice

Peel, deseed and slice the fruit. Place in serving bowl. Add fruit juice and serve.

## porridge with dried fruit and quinoa

150 g rolled oats
4 tbsp quinoa
150 g dried, unsulphured apricots
150 g raisins
150 g each of dried mango, pineapple and apple
To garnish: 8 tbsp soya yoghurt

Soak the oats and the quinoa overnight in a saucepan with 1½ litres water. Place the dried fruit in another small saucepan, cover with water and soak overnight too. In the morning, bring both to the boil (stirring the oats continuously), then cover and simmer each gently for 10–15 minutes. Pour the porridge into separate breakfast bowls. Top with the dried fruit (and liquid) and garnish with two spoonfuls of soya yoghurt. Serve.

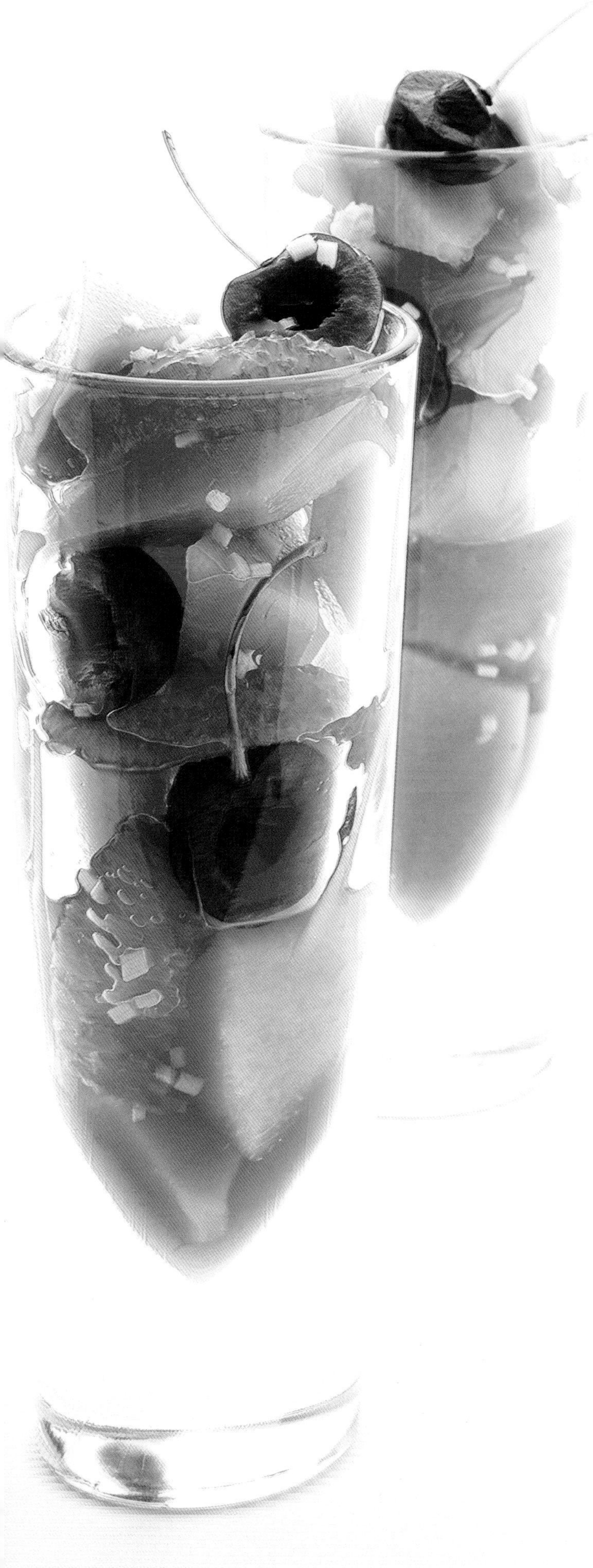

# muesli

125 g rolled oats
2 tbsp each of dried apricots, raisins, dates (chopped)
1 tbsp pecan nuts, chopped
1 tbsp almonds, chopped
1 tbsp sunflower seeds
1 tbsp linseed (flaxseed)
2 tbsp wheatgerm
1 tbsp wheat bran
Soya, rice or almond milk
To garnish: 4 tbsp plain soya yoghurt
4 tbsp fresh seasonal fruit

Combine all the muesli ingredients and serve with your choice of milk. Garnish each serving with a spoonful of yoghurt and a spoonful of seasonal fruit. Serve.

# fruity pancakes

200 g wheat flour
3 tbsp gram flour
2 tsp baking powder
½ tsp salt (optional)
300 ml soya milk
300 ml water
3 tbsp olive oil
Grapeseed oil for frying

For the filling:
150 g dried apricots, chopped
200 ml soya milk
10 strawberries, chopped
100 g raspberries
1 or 2 guavas (or peaches), peeled and sliced
1 banana, chopped
To garnish: ground cinnamon
Maple syrup (optional)

Soak the apricots for the filling in the soya milk overnight. Next day, sift the flours with the baking powder (and salt) and mix well. Add the soya milk and the water a little at a time, stirring continuously with a whisk. Slowly add the olive oil, continuing to stir. Refrigerate for 15 minutes while you combine the filling ingredients. First place the creamed apricots in a bowl and then carefully fold in the other fruit. Cook the pancakes and place a couple of spoonfuls of the fruit filling in the centre of each. Sprinkle with cinnamon (and maple syrup) and serve.

# yoghurt with fruit

500 ml plain soya yoghurt
1 apple, cored and finely chopped
1 mango, deseeded, peeled and finely chopped
4 tbsp blackberries (or other seasonal berries)
1 banana, peeled and finely chopped
To garnish: candied sweet violets (optional)

Divide the yoghurt into individual serving bowls. Then divide the fruit between each bowl, and decorate with candied violets if desired.

# soups, starters, snacks and sauces

## SOUPS

### basic vegetable stock

2 tbsp olive oil
2 onions, chopped
3 garlic cloves, crushed
2 carrots, chopped
1 parsnip or parsley root, chopped
2 carrots, chopped
½ celeriac (celery root), chopped
3 cups of greens, chopped
2 leeks (including green tops), sliced
2 litres water
5 tomatoes, chopped
2 tsp thyme
2 tbsp fresh lovage, chopped
2 bay leaves
2 tbsp fresh parsley, chopped
Sea salt and freshly ground black pepper to taste

Stir-fry the vegetables in the oil. Add water and tomatoes. Bring to the boil and add herbs and salt and pepper. Simmer for 1½ hours. Skim from time to time. Strain, cool, refrigerate, and use diluted to add flavour to soups and stews.

### cool tomato soup *(below)*

1 kg fresh ripe tomatoes, quartered and stalks removed
2 spring onions, finely chopped
4 tbsp fresh (or 4 tsp dried) basil, finely chopped
Sea salt and freshly ground black pepper to taste

Blend the tomatoes. Heat gently in a saucepan. Add the spring onion and basil. Season. Leave to cool and then chill well before serving.

### healing soup

1½ litres water
750 g potatoes, chopped
500 g carrots, chopped
1 tbsp fresh lovage or 1 tsp dried
1 tbsp miso
1 tsp caraway seeds
1 tsp herbes de Provence
Sea salt and freshly ground black pepper to taste

Bring the water to the boil and add the vegetables, lovage, miso and caraway seeds. Simmer gently for 20 minutes. Add the herbes de Provence, blend and heat through. Season and serve with pan bread (see page 258).

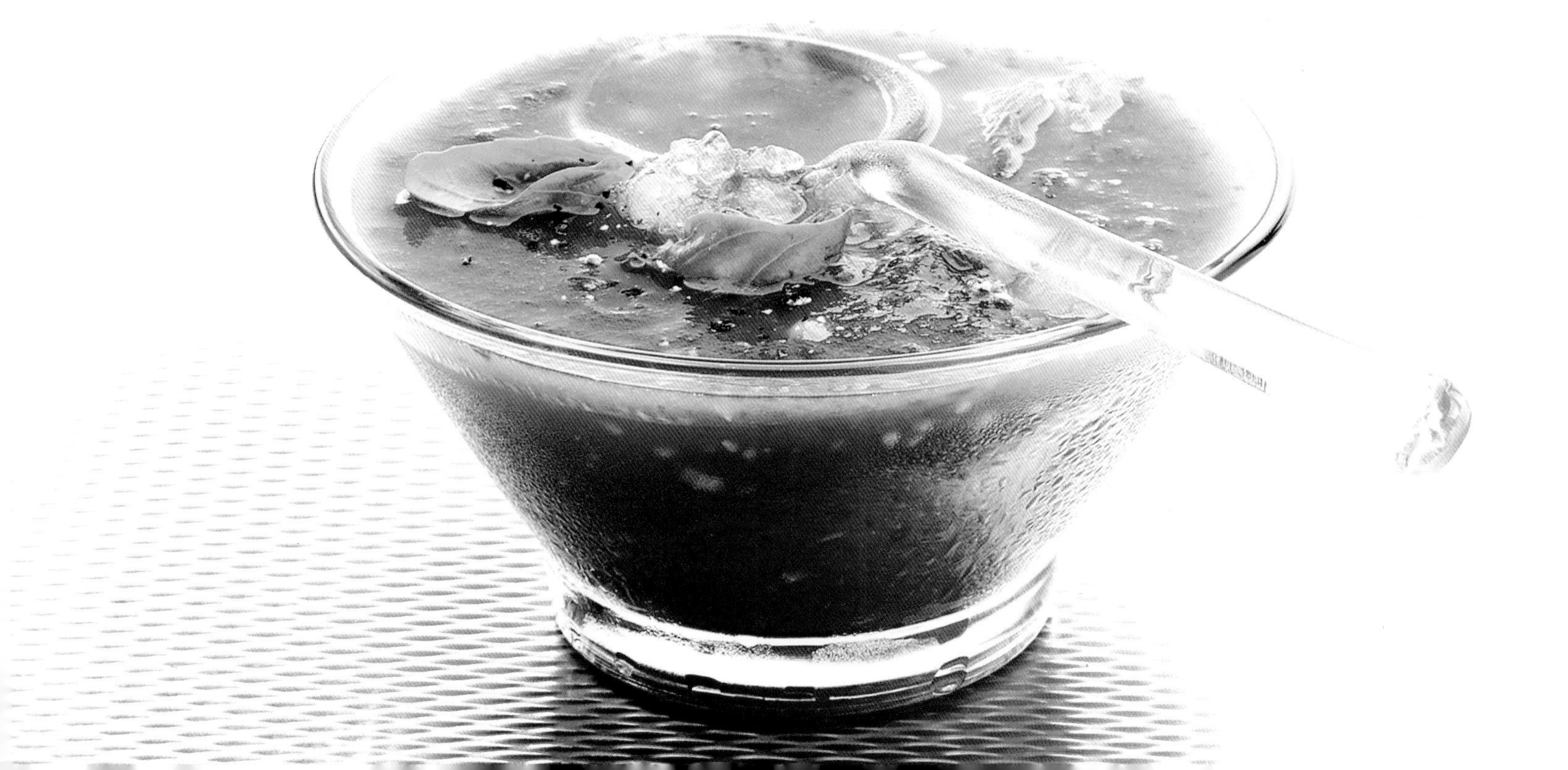

# mint and melon soup

Flesh from 2 cantaloupe melons, chopped
1 cucumber, chopped and peeled
1 tsp maple syrup
1 tbsp lemon rind, grated
200 ml water
3 tbsp fresh mint, finely chopped
Sea salt and freshly ground black pepper to taste
Juice of 1 lemon
To serve: lemon wedges

Heat the melon and the cucumber in a saucepan with the maple syrup, lemon rind and water. Simmer for 10 minutes, stirring from time to time. Add the mint. Blend, season and then add the lemon juice. Allow to cool, then refrigerate for 2 hours before serving. Serve with wedges of lemon.

# black-eye bean and wild marjoram soup

2 tbsp olive oil
2 shallots, chopped
1 garlic clove, crushed
1 tsp fennel seeds
2 tsp ground coriander seeds
1 small fennel, chopped
1 small courgette, chopped
400 g black-eye beans, cooked
500 g tomatoes, skinned and blended
1 litre diluted basic vegetable stock (see opposite page)
2 tbsp tomato paste
3 tbsp fresh (or 3 tsp dried) marjoram, chopped

Gently stir-fry the shallots, garlic, fennel seeds, coriander, fennel and courgette in the oil. Add the beans and the tomatoes, heat through, then add the stock and tomato paste. Bring to boil and add half the marjoram. Cover and simmer for 20 minutes. Add rest of the marjoram. Season with salt and pepper. Serve.

# creamy cauliflower soup

1 cauliflower
2 tbsp olive oil
2 potatoes, chopped
2 shallots, chopped
1 small carrot, chopped
1 litre diluted basic vegetable stock (see opposite page)
200 ml soya milk
Sea salt and freshly ground black pepper to taste
1 bunch of parsley, finely chopped

Cut off the cauliflower florets and steam until tender. Chop up the rest of the cauliflower and stir-fry in the oil together with the other vegetables. Add the stock, bring to the boil and simmer for about 30 minutes. Blend, then add the soya milk together with the florets, seasoning and parsley. Heat through (but don't let it boil) and serve.

# italian butterbean soup

4 tbsp olive oil
1 red onion, finely chopped
2 garlic cloves, finely chopped
4 stalks celery, chopped
400 g butterbeans, cooked
500 g tomatoes, peeled and chopped
1 litre diluted basic vegetable stock (see opposite page)
1 tbsp fresh thyme
1 tsp yeast extract
Sea salt and freshly ground black pepper to taste

Stir-fry the onion, garlic and celery gently in the olive oil. Blend half the cooked beans with the tomatoes and half the stock, then add them together with the whole beans and the remaining stock. Stir well, then add the thyme, yeast extract and salt and pepper. Bring to the boil and simmer for 20 minutes. Adjust the seasoning and serve.

# pumpkin soup

3 tbsp olive oil
1 red onion, chopped
1 garlic clove, chopped
900 g pumpkin, peeled, deseeded and chopped
3 tbsp fresh (or 3 tsp dried) marjoram, plus some to garnish
750 ml diluted basic vegetable stock (see opposite page)
400 ml coconut milk
Sea salt and freshly ground black pepper to taste

Heat the oil gently in a big saucepan. Add the onion, garlic and pumpkin. Stir-fry for 5 minutes, then add the marjoram, stock and coconut milk. Bring to the boil, cover and simmer for 15 minutes or until the vegetables are soft. Add the salt and pepper and blend. Garnish with marjoram and serve.

# shiitake mushroom soup

100 g dried shiitake mushrooms (or 300 g fresh/bottled)
2 tbsp olive oil
2 spring onions, finely chopped
1 garlic clove, finely chopped
1 carrot, finely chopped
2½-cm cube of fresh ginger root, finely chopped
1 tbsp soya sauce
1 tsp maple syrup
1½ litres water with 1 tsp miso
Sea salt and freshly ground black pepper to taste

If using dried mushrooms, soak them in plenty of water for 20 minutes, then discard the stems. Heat the oil gently in a big saucepan and stir-fry the spring onions, garlic, carrot and ginger root for 2 minutes. Add the mushrooms and sauté for another 5 minutes. Add the soy sauce, maple syrup and stock one after the other. Bring to the boil, cover and simmer gently for 30 minutes. Add the salt and pepper and serve.

# spicy moroccan soup

50 g chickpeas
50 g pinto beans (or haricots)
100 g green lentils, rinsed
3 tbsp olive oil
1 garlic clove, finely chopped
1 onion, chopped
1 tsp ground black cumin (or ground cumin)
1 tsp ground coriander
1 tsp caraway seeds
½ teaspoon cayenne
1 tbsp turmeric
2 carrots, chopped
2 potatoes, chopped
3 celery stalks, finely chopped
2½-cm piece of fresh ginger root, finely chopped
500 g tomatoes, blended
1 litre diluted basic vegetable stock (see page 244)
Sea salt and freshly ground black pepper to taste
2 tbsp lemon juice

Rinse and soak the chickpeas and pinto beans overnight. Rinse again and place in a saucepan with the lentils. Add lots of water and cook for 30 minutes. Meanwhile heat the oil gently in a soup pan. Stir-fry the garlic and onion. Add the spices, then carrots, potatoes, celery and ginger. Stir-fry for 5 minutes. Add tomatoes and simmer. Drain the cooking water off the pulses and rinse them. Add the pulses to the pan together with the stock. Bring to boil and simmer for 45 minutes, adding more water if necessary. Season, add lemon juice. Serve.

# tibetan dumpling soup

300 g wholemeal flour
300 g white flour
½ teaspoon salt
2 tbsp olive oil
½ teaspoon fenugreek seeds
1 garlic clove, crushed
1 red onion, sliced
3 tomatoes, chopped
2½-cm piece of ginger root, finely chopped
½ tsp nutmeg, grated
½ tsp turmeric
3 tbsp soy sauce
1 bunch of radishes, sliced
100 g green peas
1½ litres diluted basic vegetable stock (see page 244)
3 spring onions, sliced
Sea salt and freshly ground black pepper to taste

Combine the flours and salt. Add enough water to make a stiff dough. Roll on a floured surface to form a long, finger-thick snake. Cut into 1-cm pieces and sprinkle with flour to prevent them sticking together. Heat the oil in a soup pan and add the fenugreek seeds. Stir-fry until dark brown, then add the garlic and onion. Stir for 3 minutes, then add the tomatoes, spices and soy sauce.
Stir, cover and simmer gently for 5 minutes, then add the radishes and peas. Cook for 2 more minutes. Add the stock, bring to the boil and add the dumplings. Boil for 6–8 minutes until the dumplings are done. Add the spring onions. Season and serve.

# welsh leek and potato soup

50 g vegetable margarine
4 leeks, sliced
4 medium potatoes, chopped into small cubes
1½ litres basic vegetable stock (see page 244)
Sea salt and freshly ground black pepper to taste
To garnish: 1 bunch of chives

Gently sauté the leeks in the margarine, add the potatoes, cook for a few more minutes before adding the stock. Heat through and simmer for 30 minutes. Season, garnish with chives and serve hot. This recipe is also delicious blended.

# STARTERS

## asparagus with ravigote

*(below right)*

2 bunches of asparagus, peeled
1 tbsp lemon juice
Ravigote (see page 251)

Cut off the woody ends of the asparagus. Cook in lightly salted boiling water for about 10 minutes. (One method is to tie the asparagus in a bundle with cotton string and boil with tips sticking out of water.) Serve with ravigote dressing.

## hummus with crudités and warm pitta bread

300 g chickpeas, cooked and drained
2 garlic cloves, crushed
4 tbsp lemon juice
1 tsp sea salt
2 tbsp tahini
To garnish: 1 tbsp fresh parsley, finely chopped
1 tsp paprika
1 tbsp olive oil

For the crudités:
2 carrots and 8 long radishes, sliced into slim sticks
2 celery stalks, sliced into sticks
¼ cucumber, sliced into sticks
8 cherry tomatoes (kept whole)

Blend the chickpeas with the garlic, lemon juice, sea salt and 4 tbsp cold water. Add the tahini and blend again to a smooth paste. Adjust the seasoning and place in a serving bowl. Garnish with parsley and paprika and sprinkle with a little olive oil. Serve with crudités and warmed pitta bread, cut into wedges.

# korean kimchi-style salad

1 small Chinese cabbage, finely chopped
1 tsp unrefined sea salt
2 garlic cloves, finely chopped
2½-cm piece of fresh ginger root, finely chopped
1 fresh chilli pepper, finely chopped
2 tomatoes, finely chopped
1 green pepper, finely chopped
1 carrot, finely chopped
½ cucumber, finely chopped

Place the Chinese cabbage in a bowl. Add the salt and mix well. Add the rest of the ingredients and serve with fresh bread.

# grilled red peppers

3 red peppers, quartered longways and deseeded
Rich garlic dressing (see page 209)

Toast or grill the peppers, with the skin facing the heat, until the skin is charred. Leave to cool in a paper bag. Peel off the skin. Cut into long strips and place in a shallow dish. Sprinkle with rich garlic dressing and serve with French bread.

# vegetable kebabs

*(pictured page 249)*

16 button mushrooms, kept whole
12 cherry tomatoes, kept whole
1 red pepper, cut into chunks
1 green pepper, cut into chunks
2 courgettes, cut into chunks
1 big sweet potato or yam, parboiled and cut into chunks
1 aubergine, cut into chunks
4 shallots, halved
4 bay leaves, halved
4 barbecue skewers

For the marinade (makes ½ litre):
350 g tomato ketchup (see page 251)
150 ml red wine vinegar
Juice of 1 lemon
6 garlic cloves, crushed
2 tbsp raw cane sugar
2 tbsp olive oil
2 tbsp mustard

Mix all the marinade ingredients together in a bowl. Add the prepared kebab ingredients. Mix gently, cover and leave to marinate for 2 hours. Thread the vegetables on to the skewers and brush with marinade. Place the kebabs on a hot barbecue and grill for 10 minutes, turning from time to time. Serve hot.

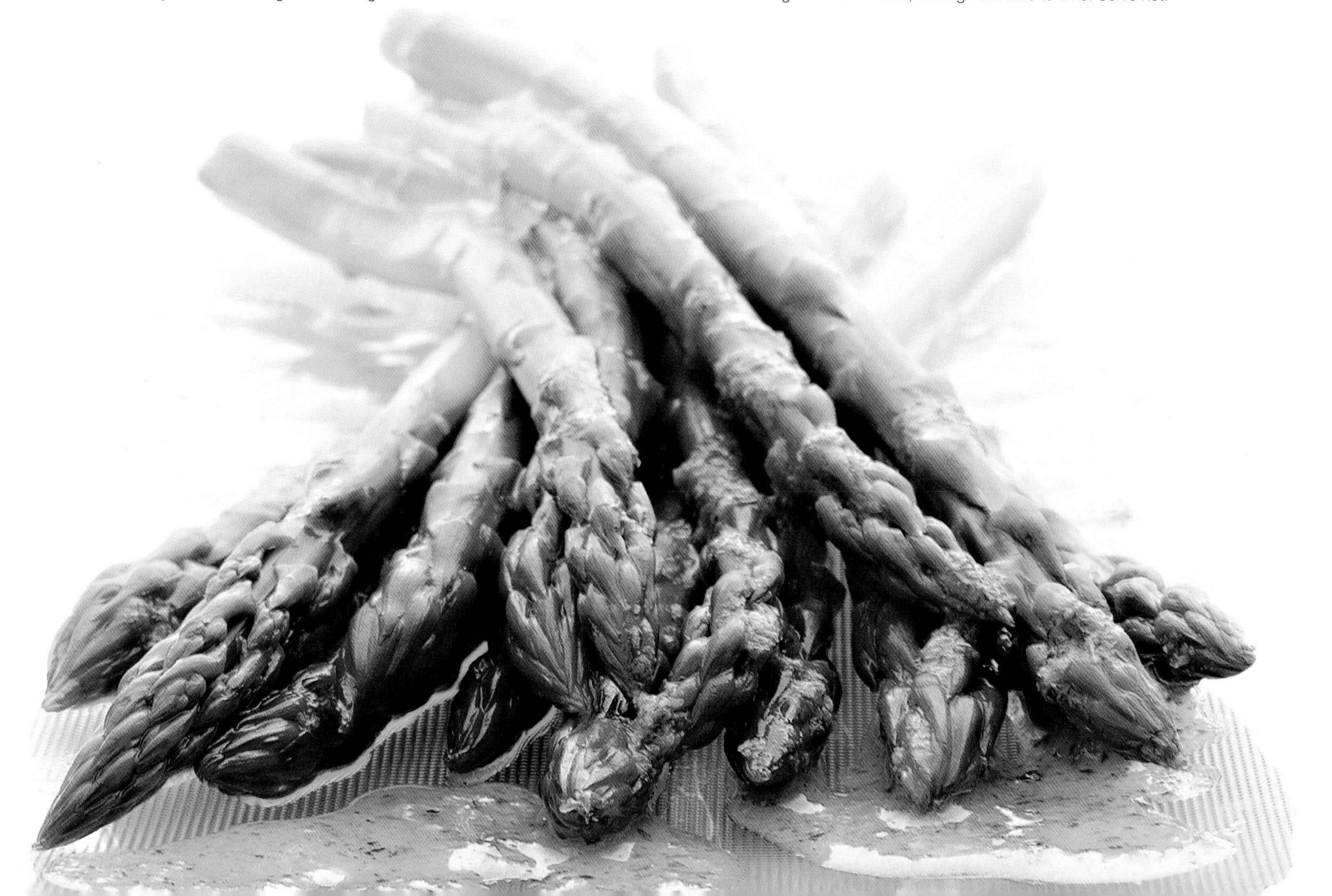

# baba ganoush

1 big aubergine
2 garlic cloves, crushed
4 tbsp tahini
4 tbsp lemon juice
1 tbsp fresh parsley, finely chopped
1 tsp ground black cumin, toasted
Sea salt to taste
To garnish: 1 tsp paprika

Prick the aubergine with a fork. Toast, turning from time to time, until the skin is black and charred. Cool under running water, then cut in half and scoop out the flesh. Chop the flesh finely, place in a bowl and mix in the rest of the ingredients, reserving a little parsley and the paprika to garnish. Adjust the seasoning, garnish, and serve with warm pitta bread, green salad leaves, tomato and cucumber.

# samosa parcels

4 spring onions, finely chopped
1 tbsp fresh ginger root, finely chopped
1 garlic clove, finely chopped
Sunflower oil
250 g marinated tofu, cut into small cubes
2 tbsp soy sauce
250 g filo pastry

Mix the spring onions, ginger root and garlic in a bowl. Gently stir-fry the tofu in a little oil. Turn off heat, add the soy sauce, stir, transfer to the bowl and mix well. Cut the filo pastry into long strips, about 7½-cm wide. Brush each strip with oil. Take the first strip and put 1 teaspoon of filling on one end. Fold the end of the pastry over to form a triangle covering the filling. Keep folding the strip over itself to form a triangular parcel. Repeat with the other strips. Brush the parcels with oil, bake at 220°C/gas mark 7 for 10 minutes or until golden. Serve hot.

# toasted tempeh with herb salad

8 tempeh slices
Sunflower oil
Sea salt
1 small red lettuce
1 bunch of watercress
1 bunch of nasturtium leaves and flowers (optional)
1 carrot, finely sliced
1 bunch chives, finely chopped
To serve: lime dressing (see page 251)

Brush the tempeh slices with oil and toast them on a dry pan till golden. Sprinkle with sea salt and remove from heat. For each serving, arrange some salad and two slices of tempeh on a plate, sprinkle with dressing and serve.

# tofumasalata

200 g smoked tofu
4 tbsp lemon juice
1 tsp grated lemon rind
8 tbsp water
1 shallot, chopped
1 garlic clove, chopped
3 tbsp breadcrumbs
4 tbsp olive oil
1 tsp paprika
Sea salt and freshly ground black pepper to taste

Crumble the tofu and blend with the lemon juice, lemon rind, water, shallot, garlic, breadcrumbs, olive oil and paprika. Add the seasoning and chill before serving with warm pitta, olives and slices of cucumber.

# SNACKS

## marinated olives

300 g olives
4 tbsp olive oil
2 fresh or dried chilli peppers, chopped
½ lemon (unpeeled), quartered and sliced
2 garlic cloves, sliced
1 tsp coriander seeds, crushed
1 tsp dried thyme
1 tsp dried oregano

Gently press the olives with a rolling pin. Place in a bowl with the oil, chilli peppers, lemon, garlic, coriander, thyme and oregano. Mix well, cover and allow to marinate overnight before serving.

## toasted nuts and seeds

1 tbsp cashew nuts
1 tbsp melon seeds
1 tbsp almonds
1 tbsp walnuts
1 tbsp hazelnuts
1 tbsp sunflower seeds
1 tbsp Brazil nuts
Soy sauce
½ tsp sea salt
Few drops of tabasco (optional)

Mix together the cashew nuts, melon seeds, almonds, walnuts, hazelnuts, sunflower seeds and Brazil nuts and dry roast in a heavy frying pan. Turn off the heat. Immediately add the soy sauce, sea salt (and tabasco if desired). Stir well, remove from pan and serve.

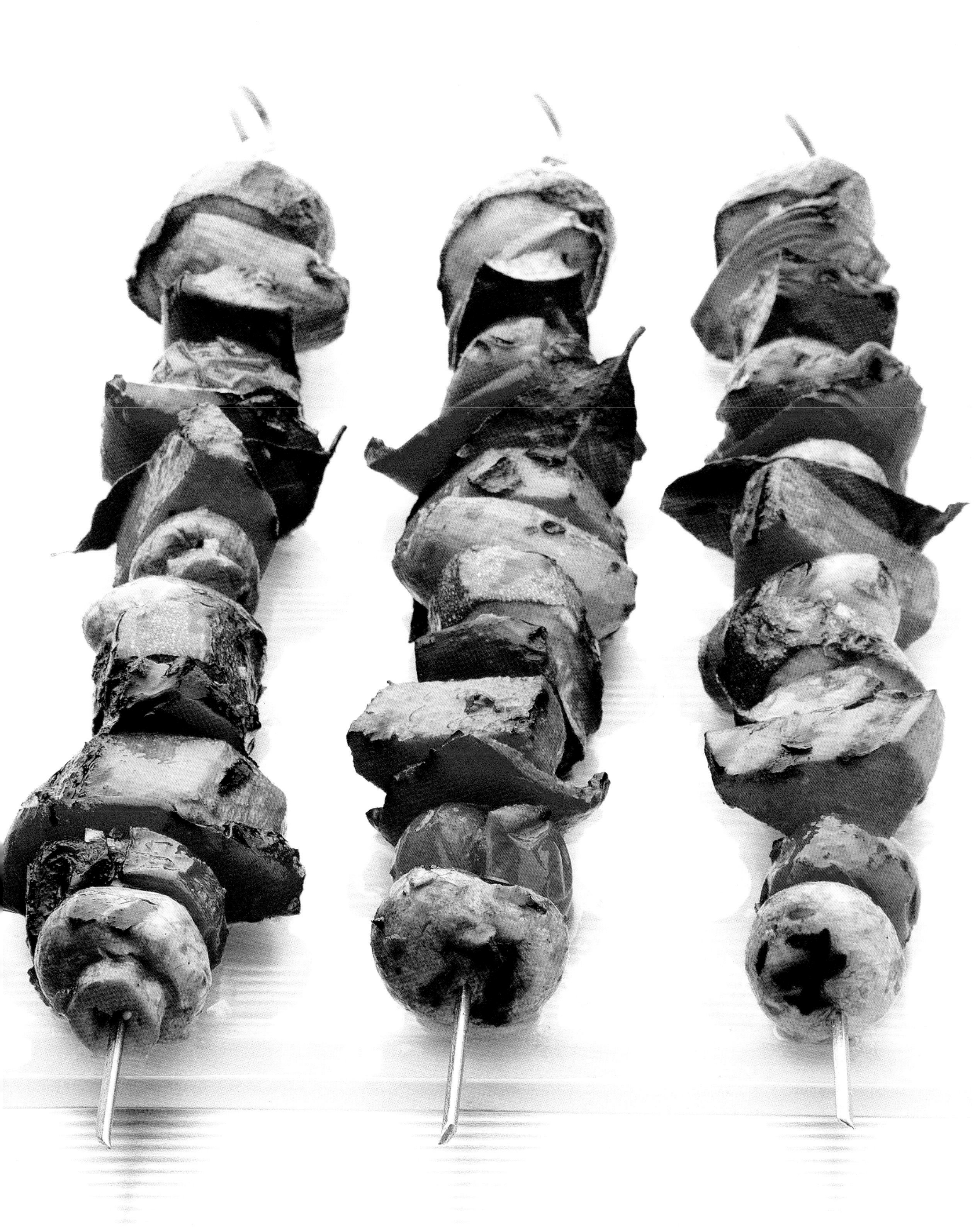

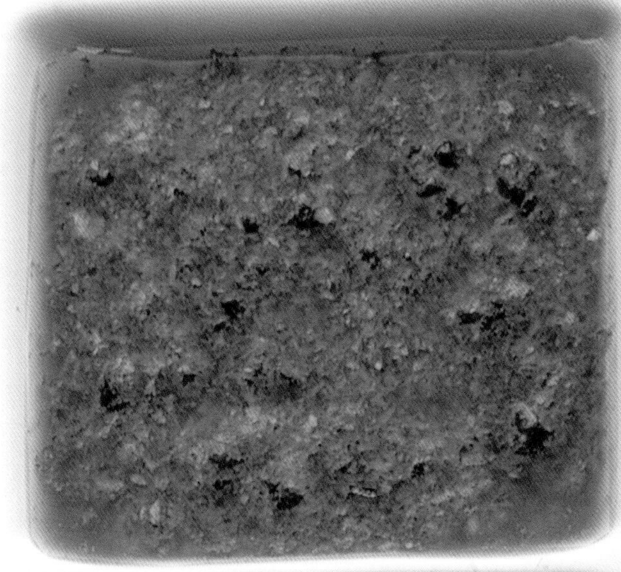

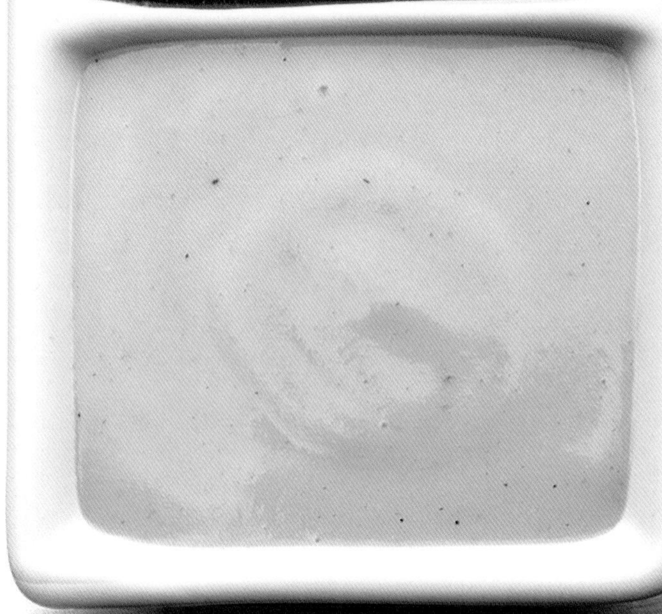

# tomato and cucumber canapés

1 cucumber, thickly sliced
8 cherry tomatoes, halved
200 g walnuts, shelled
1 garlic clove
4 tbsp water
5 tbsp olive oil
Sea salt to taste
To garnish: 1 bunch of fresh parsley, finely chopped

Arrange the cucumber slices and the tomato halves on a large plate. Blend the walnuts, garlic, water and olive oil to a smooth pâté. Season. Place a small spoonful of the pâté on top of each slice of cucumber and tomato. Garnish with parsley and serve.

# guacamole

4 small ripe avocados
2 tsp ground coriander
2 tsp ground cumin
¼ tsp cayenne
4 tbsp lemon juice
2 garlic cloves, finely chopped
1-cm cube of fresh ginger root, finely chopped
2 ripe tomatoes, finely chopped
Sea salt and freshly ground black pepper to taste
To garnish: 1 small bunch of fresh coriander leaves, chopped

Blend the avocados with the coriander, cumin, cayenne, lemon juice, garlic and ginger until almost smooth. Transfer to a bowl, stir in the tomatoes. Season, cover and chill before serving. Garnish with the fresh coriander leaves and serve with tortilla chips and carrot sticks.

# tofu balls

1 onion, grated
1 green chilli, deseeded and finely chopped
500 g tofu, grated or crumbled
2 tsp ground cumin
1 garlic clove, crushed
1 organic lemon, juice and grated rind
1 tbsp olive oil
Sea salt and freshly ground black pepper to taste
Grapeseed oil for shallow frying

Put the onion, chilli, tofu, cumin, garlic, lemon juice and rind, and olive oil in a bowl. Season and mix well. Shape into small balls and shallow fry in the grapeseed oil until golden. Serve with a selection of salad leaves (according to season).

## tzaziki

½ cucumber, finely diced
250 ml plain soya yoghurt
1 tsp olive oil
2 garlic cloves, finely chopped
2 tbsp fresh mint, finely chopped
Sea salt and freshly ground black pepper to taste

Place the cucumber in a bowl along with the yoghurt, olive oil, garlic and mint. Mix well. Cover and chill. Add seasoning. Serve with green salad leaves and warm pitta.

## pan amb oli

4 slices of bread, to toast
2 garlic cloves, halved
2 ripe tomatoes, halved
2 tsp olive oil
Sea salt and freshly ground black pepper to taste

Toast the bread on both sides. Rub one side with the garlic. Squeeze 1 tomato half over the toast and rub in the tomato pulp (discard the skin). Sprinkle with half a teaspoon of oil. Repeat for remaining slices. Season. Serve immediately.

# SAUCES

## lemon tahini dressing

*(far left, bottom)*

2 tbsp lemon juice
1 tbsp tahini
1 tbsp maple syrup
1 tbsp Dijon mustard
7 tbsp olive oil
Sea salt and freshly ground black pepper to taste

Mix together the lemon juice, tahini, maple syrup, Dijon mustard and olive oil, and blend or whisk to a thick, smooth consistency. Add seasoning.

## lime dressing

2 tbsp lime juice
1 tbsp Dijon mustard
1 tsp raw cane sugar
Sea salt and freshly ground black pepper to taste
Olive oil

Combine all the ingredients, except the oil, in a small bowl and whisk together. Add the oil slowly, whisking continuously until you have a smooth dressing. (If you can't get the dressing to emulsify, try adding a little cold water.)

## pesto sauce

*(far left, top)*

2 tbsp pine nuts
1 bunch of fresh basil
2 garlic cloves, crushed
4 tbsp olive oil
1 tsp coarse sea salt

Grind the nuts in a mortar or blender. Add the remaining ingredients and mix to form a coarse paste. Add a little extra oil if necessary.

## ravigote

1 garlic clove
2 tbsp parsley, chopped
2 tbsp chives, chopped
1 tsp tarragon
2 tsp capers
1 tbsp Dijon mustard
1 tbsp red wine vinegar
Pinch of freshly ground sea salt
150 ml olive oil

Blend all the ingredients except the oil. Add the oil very carefully, a little at a time, until the mixture emulsifies, then slowly add the rest of the oil. Serve with cooked vegetables.

## tomato ketchup

*(far left, centre)*

3 tbsp olive oil
250 g onion, finely chopped
500 g red peppers, finely chopped
500 g tomatoes, finely chopped
100 g unrefined cane sugar
3 garlic cloves, finely chopped
1 fresh chilli pepper, deseeded and finely chopped
1 tsp mustard powder
2 tsp paprika
100 ml red wine vinegar
4 whole cloves, crushed
Sea salt and freshly ground black pepper to taste

Stir-fry the onion, red pepper and tomatoes in the oil, then simmer for 45 minutes until they break down. Filter through a sieve. Add the sugar, garlic, chilli pepper, mustard powder, paprika, vinegar and cloves, and simmer very gently for 2 hours until you have a thick paste. Season. (This will keep in the refrigerator for 3–4 days. But if you want to keep it longer, pour the ketchup into clean bottles, put the tops on and place in boiling water for 20 minutes to sterilize the contents.)

# main courses, side dishes and salads

## MAIN COURSES

### amaranth and tofu puffs

30 g vegetable margarine
250 g marinated tofu, cut into small cubes
250 g amaranth leaves (or fresh spinach), chopped
Pinch of nutmeg
Sea salt and freshly ground black pepper to taste
1 packet of puff pastry

Melt the margarine, add the tofu and sauté for a few minutes. Add the amaranth (or spinach) and nutmeg and stir-fry until it goes soft and the water has evaporated. Season and set aside. Preheat oven to 200°C/gas mark 6. Cut the pastry into squares. Dampen the edges. Place a portion of amaranth mixture on each square, fold one side over diagonally to form a triangle, seal well. Place on a greased baking tray and bake for 15 minutes or until golden.

### casserole de puy

100 g lentilles de Puy (brown lentils)
1 bay leaf
3 tbsp olive oil
1 tsp each of coriander, cumin and mustard seeds
1 tsp turmeric
½ tsp cayenne
1 garlic clove, crushed
1 red onion, chopped
1 leek, sliced
250 g button mushrooms
1 potato, chopped
2 carrots, chopped
450 g tomatoes, peeled and chopped
Sea salt and freshly ground black pepper to taste
To garnish: fresh coriander

Put the lentils and the bay leaf on to boil in twice their volume of water. Cover and simmer while you prepare the other ingredients. Heat the oil in a large flameproof casserole dish. Crush the seeds in a mortar and add them with the other spices, then add the garlic, onion and leek. Stir-fry for 2 minutes, then add the mushrooms and stir-fry for a few more minutes. Add the potato, carrots and tomatoes, heat through and add the partially cooked lentils (with the cooking water). Season with salt and pepper, add a little more water to make sure the dish doesn't dry out, then cover and cook in the oven at 180°C/gas mark 4 for 45 minutes. Garnish with fresh coriander. Serve with mashed potato.

### paella

3 tbsp olive oil
250 g long-grain rice
1 tsp turmeric
2 garlic cloves, finely chopped
1 onion, chopped
1 carrot, chopped
250 g artichoke hearts
1 celery stalk, finely sliced
1 red pepper, deseeded and sliced
4 tomatoes, skinned and chopped
500 ml basic vegetable stock (see page 224)
100 g green peas
1 tbsp fresh parsley, finely chopped
1 tbsp fresh marjoram (or 1 tsp dried)
2 tbsp cashew nuts
1 organic lemon, thickly sliced
Sea salt and freshly ground black pepper to taste

Heat the oil in a large deep frying pan and stir-fry the rice until golden. Add the turmeric, garlic, onion and carrot, and stir-fry for a few minutes, then add the artichoke hearts, celery stalk and red pepper, and stir-fry for another 2 minutes. Add the tomatoes and stock. Bring to the boil and simmer for 5 minutes. Add the peas, then simmer until the rice is cooked. Add the herbs, cashews and lemon slices. Season and serve hot.

### artichoke hearts, broad beans and shiitake

2 tbsp olive oil
1 bay leaf
2 tsp ground cumin
1 tsp turmeric
250 g shiitake mushrooms, halved
450 g broad beans (shelled weight)
450 g artichoke hearts, cooked
100 ml water
2 tbsp lemon juice
1 small bunch of parsley, finely chopped
Sea salt and freshly ground black pepper to taste

Heat the oil gently in a large pan. Add the bay leaf and the spices, then the mushrooms. Sauté for a few minutes, then add the broad beans with the artichokes and the water. Heat through, simmer until the beans are tender. Add the lemon juice and the parsley. Season and serve.

# asparagus asian-style

1 bunch of asparagus, ends cut off
2 tbsp olive oil
1 tsp cumin powder
1 stalk lemon grass, finely sliced
2½-cm piece of fresh ginger root, finely chopped
3 medium carrots, cut into julienne strips
1 bunch of spring onions, sliced
1 red pepper, deseeded and finely sliced
2 tbsp tamarind paste, dissolved in 250 ml hot water
1 handful of bean sprouts
2 tbsp soy sauce
1 tbsp maple syrup
1–2 tbsp lemon juice
Sea salt and freshly ground black pepper to taste

Cut the asparagus into 5-cm pieces and set aside. Heat the oil in a wok, add the cumin, lemon grass and ginger, and stir-fry for a few seconds. Add the asparagus, then the carrots, spring onions and red pepper. Stir-fry for another 5 minutes. Add the dissolved tamarind paste. Simmer until the asparagus are cooked. Then add the bean sprouts, soy sauce, maple syrup and lemon juice. Heat through, season and serve with rice or noodles.

# butternut squash with red pepper and tomato

*(below)*

1 butternut squash, deseeded and peeled
2 tbsp olive oil
1 red onion, chopped
1 garlic clove, chopped
1 red pepper, cut into strips
6 ripe tomatoes, skinned and sliced
2 tbsp tomato paste
2 tbsp fresh (or 2 tsp dried) basil, chopped
1 tsp paprika
Sea salt and freshly ground black pepper to taste
To garnish: 2 tbsp parsley, chopped

Chop the butternut squash into chunks. Heat the oil in a large pan, add the onion, garlic and butternut squash, sauté for 2 minutes, and then add the red pepper. Heat through. Add the remaining ingredients (except the parsley), cover and simmer for 20 minutes. Season, garnish with parsley and serve with rice or hasselbach potatoes (see page 258).

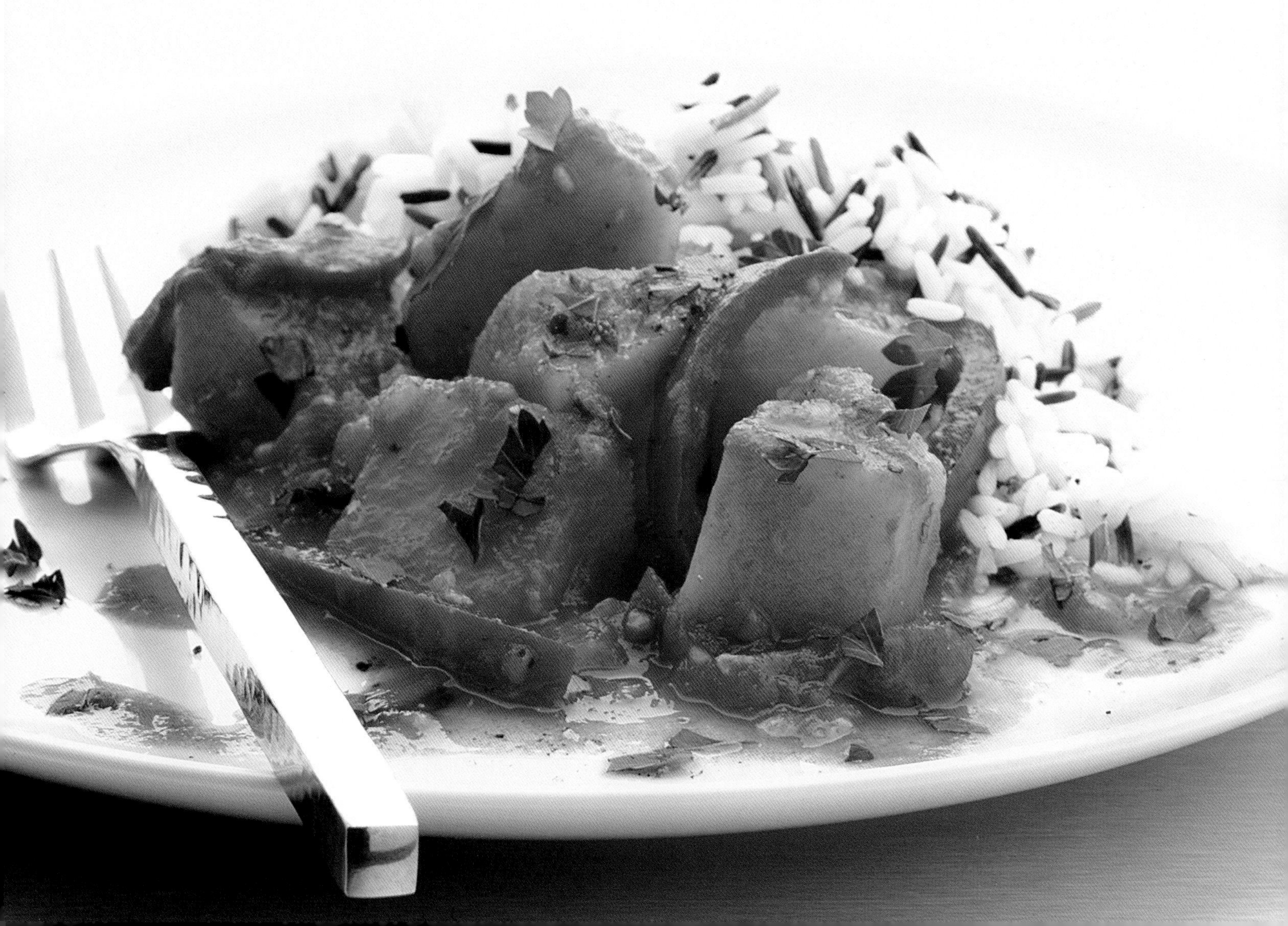

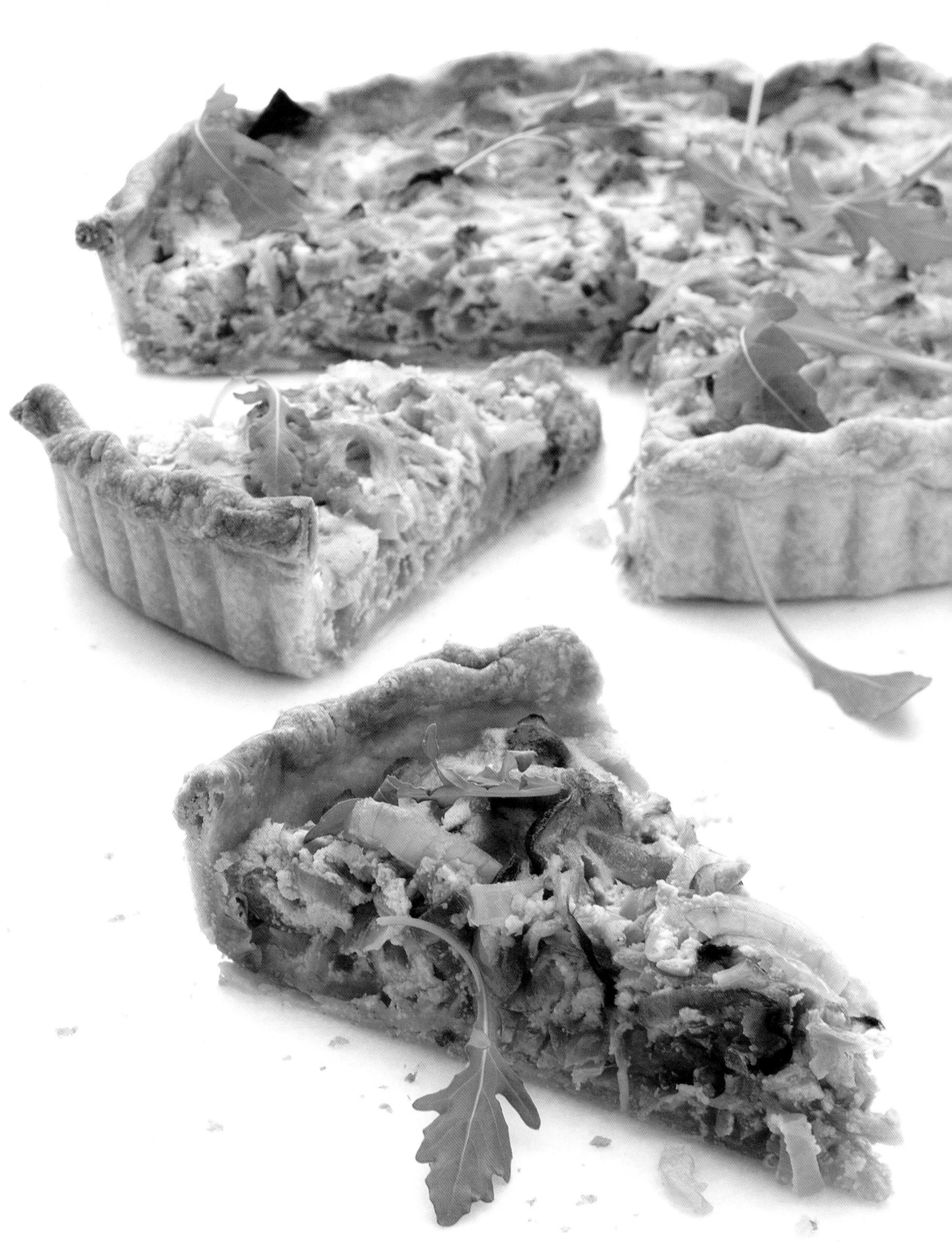

# sweet and sour vegetable parcels

4 thick slices of tempeh, chopped
2 spring onions, sliced into fine strips
2 carrots, cut into julienne strips
2 celery sticks, cut into julienne strips
2½-cm piece of ginger root, cut into fine sticks
10-cm lemon grass stem
1 handful of bean sprouts
8 sheets of filo pastry
Grapeseed oil
1 tbsp soy sauce
2 tbsp lemon juice
1 tbsp vinegar
1 tbsp maple syrup
1 tbsp tomato paste
1 garlic clove, crushed
1 tsp paprika
1 broccoli, cut into florets
100 g baby sweetcorn cobs
1 red pepper, cut into strips

Stir-fry the tempeh. Add the vegetables one at a time in the order above, stir-frying in between. Add the lemon grass and bean sprouts. Stir-fry again and season to taste. Brush the pastry with the oil. Divide the filling between the 8 sheets. Fold the corners of each sheet into the centre and pinch the parcels together. Brush with oil and bake at 200°C/gas mark 6 for 20 minutes or until golden. Meanwhile, mix together the soy sauce, lemon juice, vinegar, syrup, tomato paste, garlic and paprika to make a sauce. Sauté the broccoli, baby sweetcorn cobs and red peppers for 5 minutes. Add the sauce to the vegetables, heat through, and serve with the parcels.

# french onion tart *(left)*

For the short-crust pastry:
250 g wheat flour
½ tsp salt
125 g cold vegetable margarine
75 ml cold water

For the filling:
750 g onions, finely sliced
¾ tsp salt and a pinch of black pepper
250 g tofu, crumbled
200 ml soya milk
1 tbsp flour

Mix the flour and salt. Add the margarine by chopping it into the flour with a knife and spoon until it forms small lumps. Crumble the dough with your hands until it looks like Parmesan (taking care not to let the dough get warm). Add cold water and knead the dough lightly to a smooth lump. Refrigerate until needed. Sauté the onions very gently in some oil. Stir from time to time, taking care not to let them brown. After 10 minutes, add the salt and pepper. Stir, then cover and simmer very gently for 15 minutes. Remove the lid and let the liquid reduce for 5 minutes. Remove from heat. Blend the tofu, soya milk and flour, and mix with the onions. Season to taste. Roll out the dough and place in a greased baking case. Add the filling and bake at 180°C/gas mark 4 for 25–30 minutes.

# provençale-style kidney beans

2 tbsp olive oil
1 red onion, sliced
2 garlic cloves, sliced
1 tin red kidney beans
2 small courgettes, sliced
4 ripe tomatoes, skinned and chopped
100 ml diluted basic vegetable stock (see page 244)
2 tbsp fresh basil, chopped (plus some to garnish)
100 g small niçoise olives
Sea salt and freshly ground black pepper to taste

Heat the oil and sauté the onion and garlic gently for 2 minutes. Add the kidney beans, courgettes and tomatoes, and cook for 2 more minutes, then add the stock and the basil. Bring to the boil and simmer for 10 minutes. Add the olives. Heat through, season, garnish with basil, and serve with wild rice.

# greek casserole

4 tbsp olive oil
250 g tofu, cut into cubes
1 red onion, thickly sliced
1 green pepper, thickly sliced
2 garlic cloves, chopped
1 tbsp wholemeal flour
500 g tomatoes, chopped
1 tbsp tomato paste
2 tsp marjoram
Sea salt and freshly ground black pepper to taste

Stir-fry the tofu cubes in half the oil until they begin to brown. Remove from pan. Add the remaining oil, then the onion. Sauté for a few minutes then add the green pepper and garlic. Sauté for a few more minutes, turn down the heat and mix in the flour. Let it blend in for a minute, then add the tomatoes, turn up the heat and stir well. Add the tomato paste, marjoram and salt and pepper. Stir while you bring the mixture to boil. Add the tofu pieces and mix well. Place in an ovenproof dish and bake, covered, at 180°C/gas mark 4 for about 30 minutes.

# spinach bouillabaisse

3 tbsp olive oil
2 white onions, sliced
2 potatoes, sliced
500 g fresh spinach, chopped
2 garlic cloves, crushed
350 ml diluted basic vegetable stock (see page 244)
Pinch of cayenne
1 tbsp fresh dill, chopped (optional)
1 tbsp fresh parsley, chopped
Sea salt and freshly ground black pepper to taste

Sauté the onion and potato in the oil. Add the spinach and stir until it goes soft, then add the garlic, stock and cayenne. Simmer for 10 minutes, add the dill and the parsley, and season. Heat through and serve with fresh bread.

# okra in sweet and sour tamarind sauce

4 tbsp olive oil
1 tsp black mustard seeds
1 tsp ground cumin
1 tsp ground coriander
Pinch of cayenne pepper
½ tsp turmeric
3 garlic cloves, finely chopped
450 g fresh okra, trimmed
250 ml water
200 g green beans, trimmed
2 tbsp tamarind paste
2 tbsp maple syrup
Sea salt and freshly ground black pepper to taste

Heat the oil gently in a frying pan. Add the mustard seeds, cumin, coriander, cayenne, turmeric and garlic. Stir-fry for ½ minute, then add the okra. Stir-fry for 1 minute then add the water and the beans. Heat through and simmer for 10 minutes, stirring occasionally. Add the tamarind paste and the maple syrup. Simmer again for another 5 minutes. Season and serve with basmati rice.

# shepherdess' pie

120 g lentilles de Puy (brown lentils)
3 tbsp olive oil
1 bay leaf
1 tsp thyme
2 garlic cloves, finely chopped
2 shallots, chopped
2 carrots, finely chopped
300 g mushrooms, quartered
500 g tomatoes, skinned and chopped
150 ml vegetable juice or diluted basic vegetable stock (see page 244)
1 tbsp soy sauce
2 tbsp fresh basil, chopped
Sea salt and freshly ground black pepper to taste

For the topping:
3 large potatoes, chopped
2 sweet potatoes, chopped
60 g vegetable margarine
Soya milk
Paprika

Put the lentils on to boil in three times their volume of water. Boil the potatoes and sweet potatoes in salted water until tender. Meanwhile heat the oil gently and add the bay leaf, thyme, garlic, shallots and carrots. Stir and add the mushrooms. Sauté for a few minutes (until the mushrooms give off their moisture) then add the tomatoes. Drain any remaining cooking water from the lentils and add them together with the stock and soy sauce. Simmer gently for 10 minutes. Add the basil and seasoning. Remove from the heat and place in a large shallow ovenproof dish. Mash the potatoes with the margarine and soya milk. Add seasoning to taste and spread over the filling. Sprinkle with paprika and bake at 240°C/gas mark 8 for 10 minutes or until golden.

# sweet potato curry

3 tbsp olive oil
2 tsp black mustard seeds
1 tsp curry powder
1 red onion, sliced
2 green chillies, sliced
350 g sweet potato, peeled and cubed
250 g sweetcorn kernels
1 spear broccoli, cut into florets
150 g fresh spinach, chopped
400 ml coconut milk
Sea salt and freshly ground black pepper to taste
2 tbsp lime juice
To garnish: 1 bunch fresh coriander leaves, chopped

Heat the oil and add the black mustard seeds and the curry powder and stir-fry until the seeds start to pop. Add the onion and chillies, and stir-fry for another 2 minutes. Add the sweet potato, sweetcorn and broccoli. Stir-fry for 5 minutes then add the spinach and mix well. Add the coconut milk and simmer gently for 10 minutes until the vegetables are soft. Season with the salt, pepper and lime juice. Garnish with fresh coriander and serve with rice.

# mushrooms with sage and thyme stuffing

12–16 large flat open mushrooms
2 tbsp olive oil
3 garlic cloves, crushed
2 tsp thyme
3 tbsp soy sauce
8 tbsp breadcrumbs
4 tbsp fresh parsley, finely chopped

Remove the stalks from the mushroom caps and scrape out the lamellae (gills) with a teaspoon. Place the caps upside down on a greased ovenproof dish or baking tray. Finely chop the mushroom stalks and stir-fry them in the oil with the garlic. Add the thyme and the soy sauce and stir-fry until the mushroom stalks give off their moisture. Add the breadcrumbs and stir until the liquid is soaked up. Remove from heat and add the chopped parsley. Fill the mushroom caps with the mixture and bake at 200°C/gas mark 6 for about 10 minutes.

# winter hot pot

3 tbsp olive oil
1 onion, sliced
2 carrots, sliced
1 parsnip, sliced
1 celery stick, sliced
200 g cooked chickpeas
300 g shiitake mushrooms, kept whole
750 ml basic vegetable stock (see page 244)
Sea salt and freshly ground black pepper to taste
2 big potatoes, thinly sliced

Heat the oil in a deep, ovenproof casserole dish. Add the onion, carrots and parsnip. Sauté for 5 minutes. Add the celery, chickpeas and mushrooms. Stir-fry for another 5 minutes, then add the stock. Heat through, season, and cover with potato slices. Place in a preheated oven and cook at 180°C/gas mark 4 for 45 minutes.

## spicy tofu burgers

1 tbsp olive oil
1 onion, grated
1 carrot, grated
2 tsp ground coriander
1 garlic clove, crushed
2 tsp tomato paste
250 g tofu, crumbled
2 tbsp breadcrumbs
2 tbsp Brazil nuts, finely chopped
Sea salt and freshly ground black pepper to taste
Flour for coating
Grapeseed oil for frying

Heat the oil and gently stir-fry the onion and carrot until soft. Add the coriander, garlic and tomato paste and stir-fry for 2 more minutes. Place in a bowl and mix with the tofu, breadcrumbs and nuts. Season and stir until the mixture sticks together well. Shape into burgers, dip in flour and fry until golden. Drain on paper and serve with steamed vegetables.

## sweet chestnuts and kumquats

500 g fresh sweet chestnuts, shelled (or 350 g dried)
3 tbsp olive oil
1 garlic clove, sliced
1 bay leaf
2 celery sticks, sliced
2 leeks, sliced
3 tbsp wholemeal flour
100 ml red wine
350 ml basic vegetable stock (see page 244)
Juice of 1 tangerine
100 g kumquats
Sea salt and freshly ground black pepper to taste

If using dried chestnuts, soak them for 8 hours before cooking. If using fresh chestnuts, drop them in boiling water and peel them with a sharp knife. Heat the oil in a casserole dish, add the garlic and bay leaf, and stir for a few seconds. Add the chestnuts, celery and leeks. Sprinkle with the flour, mix well, then slowly add the wine, the vegetable stock and the tangerine juice. Heat through, then add the kumquats and season. Cook covered in the oven at 180°C/gas mark 4 for about an hour. Serve with broccoli and wild rice.

# SIDE DISHES

## cucumber, tomato and pepper relish

½ cucumber, chopped
250 g tomatoes, chopped
1 red onion, chopped
2 green chilli peppers, finely sliced
2 tbsp lime juice
2 tbsp fresh coriander leaves, chopped
Pinch of salt
Pinch of unrefined sugar

Mix all the ingredients in a bowl and store in the refrigerator until needed.

## red chilli relish

4 red chillies and 2 red peppers (stalk and seeds removed), chopped
4 ripe tomatoes (stalk removed), chopped
2 garlic cloves, peeled and chopped
3 tbsp lime juice
Sea salt to taste

Blend all the ingredients, store in the refrigerator until needed.

## khichuri – rice with lentils

200 g basmati rice, washed
100 g red lentils, washed
1 bay leaf
5-cm cinnamon stick
1 tsp ground turmeric
1 litre water (approximately)
Sea salt to taste

Place the rice and the lentils in a saucepan with the bay leaf and the spices. Add the water, bring to the boil and simmer until rice is soft (about 30 minutes). Serve.

## lemon rice

300 g basmati rice, rinsed
2 lemon grass stalks, finely sliced
1 litre water (approximately)
Sea salt to taste
3 tbsp lemon juice

Place the rice in a saucepan and add the water and the salt. Bring to the boil. Add the lemon grass and simmer for about 30 minutes until the rice is tender. Sprinkle with lemon juice and serve.

# hasselbach potatoes

1½ kg potatoes, halved
Sunflower oil
Gomassio (sesame salt)
To garnish: 1 bunch of fresh dill, finely chopped

Place the halved potatoes on a chopping board, flat side down, and cut grooves in each (nearly all the way through to the bottom). Then parboil the potatoes in lightly salted water for 5 minutes, drain and cool under running water. Dry gently and place in a lightly greased large roasting tin. Brush well with oil. Bake in a preheated oven at 220°C/gas mark 7 for 25 minutes, or until crisp and golden. Sprinkle with gomassio and garnish with the fresh dill.

# pan bread

250 g wholewheat flour
2 tsp baking powder
½ teaspoon unrefined sea salt
1 tsp caraway seeds (optional)
250 ml water (approximately)

Sift the flour, baking powder and salt together. Add caraway seeds and enough water to form a soft dough. Knead to a smooth consistency. Roll the dough into a sausage and divide it into 12 balls. Roll each ball on a floured surface into 15-cm rounds. Heat a dry heavy frying pan and cook each bread (without oil) for 2 minutes on each side (or until brown spots appear). Serve warm.

# spring greens and macadamia nuts

50 g macadamia nuts
2 tbsp olive oil
1 kg spring greens (or other greens), shredded
100 ml water or diluted basic vegetable stock (see page 244)
1 tbsp lemon juice
Sea salt and freshly ground black pepper to taste

Toast the macadamia nuts in a dry frying pan, then remove from heat. Heat the oil in a large pan or wok, add the spring greens and stir-fry for 5 minutes. Add the water or stock, cover and simmer for another 5 minutes. Add the lemon juice and macadamia nuts, season and serve.

# tomato salsa

500 g ripe tomatoes, finely chopped
2 spring onions, finely chopped
1 red chilli pepper, finely chopped
4 tbsp lime juice
1 bunch of fresh basil, finely chopped
Sea salt and freshly ground black pepper to taste

Mix all the ingredients well in a bowl. Season and serve.

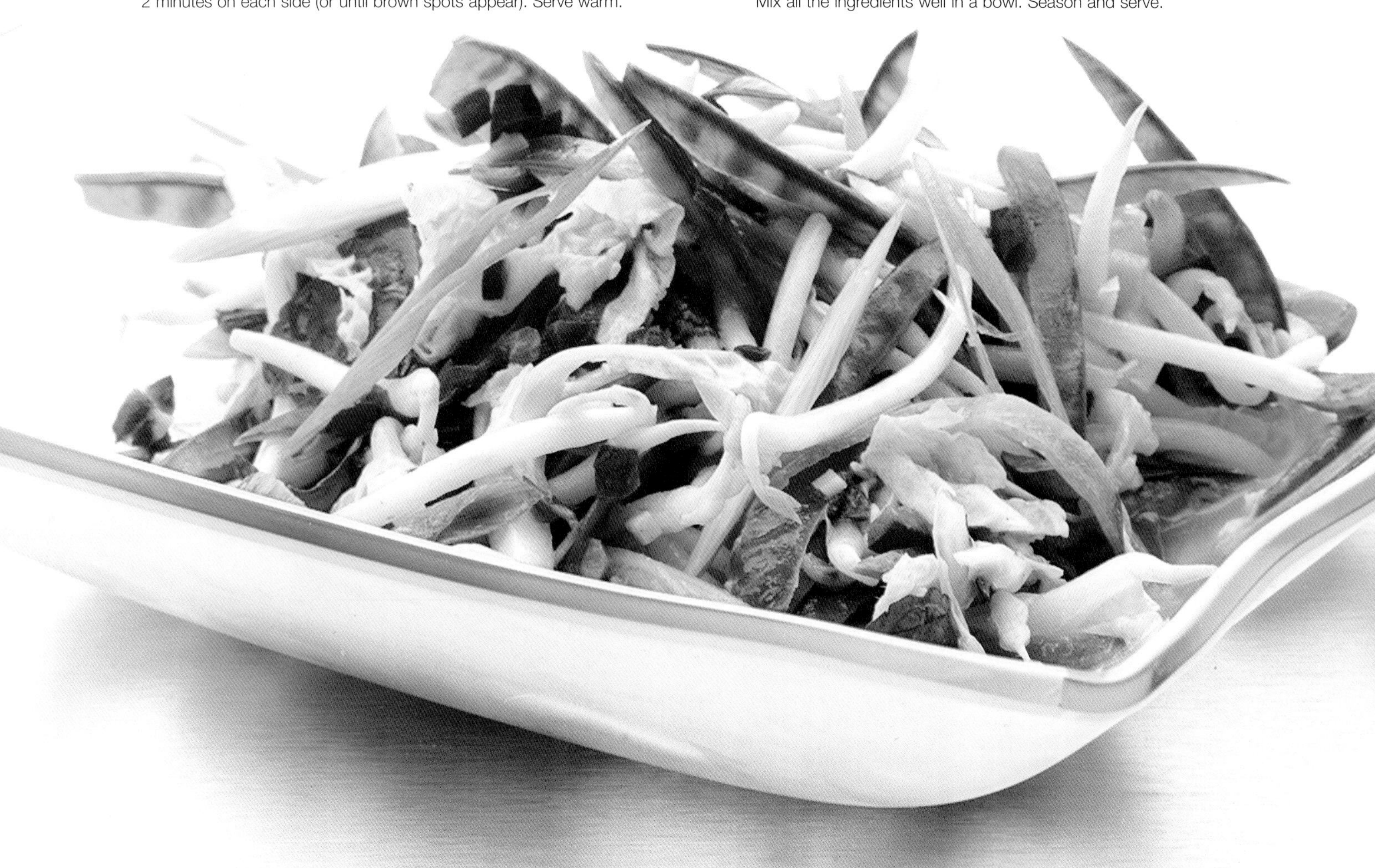

## swiss chard and juniper berries

2 tbsp olive oil
6 juniper berries, crushed
500 g Swiss chard (or other greens), shredded
Sea salt and freshly ground black pepper
100 ml water

Heat the oil gently in a large pan. Add the juniper and stir. Add the greens. Stir-fry for 2 minutes. Add water, cover and simmer for 10 minutes. Season and serve.

# SALADS

## carrot 'n' beetroot salad

300 g carrots, grated
300 g beetroot, grated
1 tbsp fresh ginger root, finely chopped
2 tbsp sunflower oil
4 tbsp lemon juice
100 g bean sprouts
To garnish: 3 tbsp sunflower seeds, roasted
3 tbsp pumpkin seeds, roasted

Mix the grated carrots and beetroot with the ginger. Add the oil and the lemon juice, and mix well. Add the bean sprouts and mix gently. Garnish with the seeds.

## salad niçoise

100 ml olive oil
2 tbsp white wine vinegar
1 tbsp lemon juice
1 tbsp Dijon mustard
1 tbsp maple syrup
Sea salt and freshly ground black pepper to taste
200 g new potatoes in their skins, boiled in lightly salted water
125 g marinated tofu, cut into small cubes
Soy sauce
250 g green beans, topped, tailed and steamed
250 g tomatoes, cut into boats
½ cucumber, chopped into sticks
½ iceberg lettuce
4 tbsp small niçoise olives
2 tbsp fresh basil, finely chopped
2 tbsp fresh parsley, finely chopped

Combine the oil, vinegar, lemon juice, mustard and maple syrup in a bowl, whisk or hand-blend, then season to taste. Cut the cooled potatoes in half and add them to the dressing. Mix well and set aside. Sauté the tofu in a little oil, turn off the heat and add a few drops of soy sauce. Add to the potatoes. Leave to cool a little, then add the rest of the ingredients and serve with French bread.

## bulgur wheat salad

250 g bulgur wheat, cooked and cooled
1 bunch of spring onions, sliced
2 tomatoes, chopped
1 green pepper, deseeded and cut into strips
½ cucumber, chopped
1 garlic clove
2 tbsp fresh coriander leaves, chopped
2 tbsp fresh mint, chopped
2 tbsp fresh parsley, chopped
4 tbsp olive oil
3 tbsp lemon juice
Sea salt and freshly ground black pepper to taste

Place the bulgur in a salad bowl and mix with other ingredients. Serve cold.

## artichoke salad

8 artichoke hearts
4 big ripe tomatoes, cut into boats
1 red onion, sliced
100 g green olives
450 g flageolet beans (cooked weight)

If using fresh artichokes, prepare them by breaking off the outer "petals". When you get to the softer inner ones, cut them off with a sharp knife as close to the heart as possible. Scrape out the "choke" with a teaspoon. (Leave the hearts in cold water while you prepare the others, to avoid discolouration.) Plunge the hearts into boiling water and cook for about 20 minutes (or until tender). Cool and place with the other ingredients in a salad bowl. Serve with French bread and lemon tahini dressing (see page 251).

## provençal mesclun salad

1 butterhead lettuce, shredded
A small handful of the following green leaves and herbs:
Rocket, sorrel, radicchio, mustard cress, nasturtium leaves and flowers, parsley, mint and/or basil
Rich garlic dressing (see page 209)

Place the shredded lettuce in a large salad bowl, add the green leaves and herbs, mix lightly and add the dressing just before serving.

## rocket salad

4 handfuls of rocket, shredded
1 small red onion, finely chopped
4 small ripe tomatoes, cut into boats
Lime dressing (see page 251)
To garnish: 4 tbsp walnuts, roughly chopped

Place the rocket in a salad bowl, add the onion and tomato, and the dressing. Garnish with the walnuts and serve with fresh crusty bread.

# catalan salad

1 kg potatoes, boiled in their skins and allowed to cool
1 broccoli, cut into florets, steamed and allowed to cool
1 avocado, sliced
1 red pepper, deseeded and sliced
1 yellow pepper, deseeded and sliced
1 spring onion, chopped
4 tbsp olives
3 tbsp capers
3 tbsp fresh parsley, finely chopped
1 tbsp fresh thyme
Lime dressing (see page 251)

Cut the potatoes into thick slices. Place in a salad bowl and combine with the other ingredients. Add the dressing and serve.

# chinese salad *(pictured page 258)*

¼ Chinese cabbage, finely sliced
1 tsp fresh ginger root, finely chopped
1 tsp garlic, finely chopped
1 small red chilli pepper, deseeded and finely chopped
1 small bunch of watercress, chopped
250 g bean sprouts
100 g mangetout peas, trimmed
2 spring onions, finely sliced
Lime dressing (see page 251)

Place the Chinese cabbage in a salad bowl and add all the other ingredients. Mix well, add the dressing and serve.

# florence fennel salad

1 bulb Florence fennel, thinly sliced (keep tops to garnish)
1 avocado, thinly sliced
100 g pecan nuts
100 g green olives
1 cucumber, thinly sliced
Rich garlic dressing (see page 209)

Mix all the ingredients with the dressing. Garnish with fennel tops and serve.

# green lentil salad

50 g green lentils (dry weight), cooked and cooled
200 g yellow beans, steamed and cooled
1 small cauliflower, cut into florets
2 carrots, cut into peelings
200 g green peas, shelled
1 young courgette, thinly sliced
1 bunch of watercress, chopped
Lemon tahini dressing (see page 251)

Mix all the ingredients with the dressing and serve.

# orange mango salad

1 orange, peeled and chopped
2 mangos, peeled and chopped
2 carrots, cut into peelings
1 handful of radicchio, finely shredded
1 red chilli, deseeded and finely sliced
1 tsp ginger root, finely chopped
3 tbsp lemon juice

Mix all the ingredients in a salad bowl and serve.

# pasta salad

350 g three-coloured pasta twists, cooked
1 courgette, grated
2 tomatoes, cut into boats
1 bunch of asparagus, trimmed, cooked and cut into pieces
1 bunch of fresh basil, finely chopped
Lime dressing (see page 251)

Cool the pasta and place in a salad bowl. Add the other ingredients, then add the dressing and serve.

# potato salad

1 kg new potatoes, boiled in their skins
300 ml plain soya yoghurt
1 shallot, finely chopped
1 small red pepper, finely chopped
2 tbsp capers
1–2 tbsp lemon juice
Sea salt and freshly ground black pepper to taste
To garnish: 1 small bunch of chives, finely chopped,

Allow the potatoes to cool and cut them into thick slices. Combine the rest of the ingredients to make the dressing. Place the potatoes in a salad bowl and add the dressing, mix gently, season, garnish with the chives and serve.

# sweetcorn (maize) and sun-dried tomato salad

4 sweetcorns, cut into chunks and boiled for 3 minutes
50 g sun-dried tomatoes, cut into strips
1 handful of rocket
1 small lettuce, shredded
2 tbsp fresh basil, chopped
4 tbsp walnut oil
2 tbsp balsamic vinegar
Sea salt and freshly ground black pepper to taste

Put the sweetcorn in a bowl on a bed of tomatoes, rocket, lettuce and basil. Whisk together the oil and vinegar and toss with the salad. Season and serve.

# salad with sorrel and tempeh

2 tbsp olive oil
8 tempeh rashers
1 handful of young sorrel leaves, shredded
1 little gem lettuce, shredded
Rich garlic dressing (see page 209)

Fry the tempeh in the olive oil until crisp and golden. Sprinkle with salt then cut into bite-size pieces. Place the sorrel and lettuce leaves in a bowl and add the tempeh. Pour the dressing over and mix gently. Serve.

# tropical sunshine salad

3 carrots, cut into peelings
1 avocado, sliced
1 mango, peeled and sliced
1 pomegranate, peeled and cut into segments
1 handful of nasturtium leaves and flowers
4 spring onions, sliced
1 garlic clove, finely chopped
2½-cm piece of ginger root, finely chopped
3 tbsp safflower oil
3 tbsp lime juice
Sea salt and freshly ground black pepper to taste

Combine all the ingredients in a salad bowl and mix well. Season and serve.

# wild rice salad *(below)*

50 g wild rice (dry weight), cooked and cooled
1 bulb Florence fennel, steamed, cooled and sliced
1 red pepper, grilled and skinned (see grilled red peppers – page 247)
2 tomatoes, cut into boats
2 spring onions, sliced
1 celery stalk, sliced
100 g black olives, stoned
2 garlic cloves, crushed
Lemon tahini dressing (see page 251)
To garnish: 2 tbsp fresh basil, finely chopped
2 tbsp fresh parsley, finely chopped

Place the rice and fennel in a salad bowl, then add the rest of the ingredients. Add the dressing, garnish with the fresh herbs and serve.

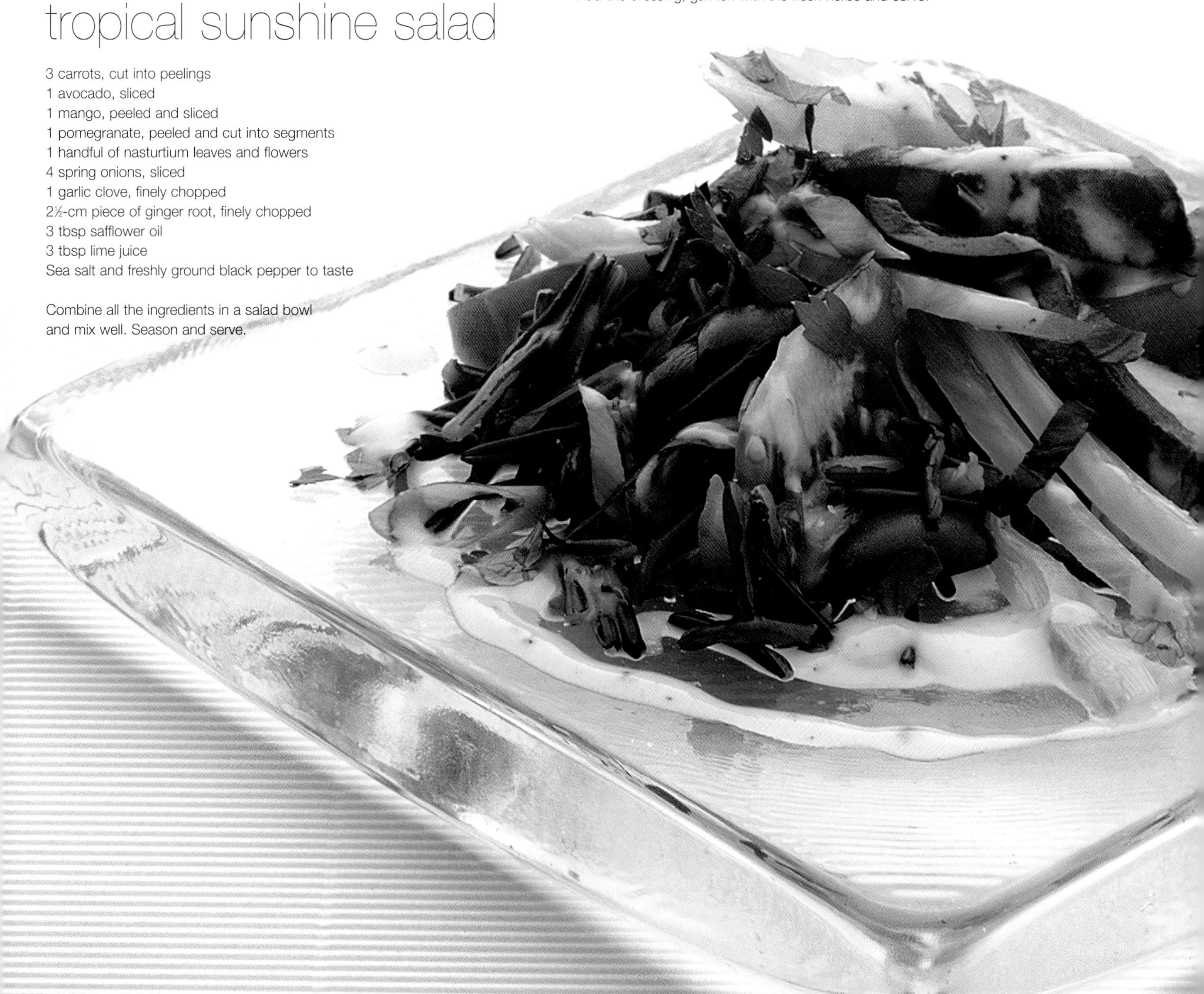

# desserts

## raspberry gateau

250 g wholewheat flour
1 tbsp baking powder
50 g ground almonds
125 g raw cane sugar
100 ml sunflower oil
2 tbsp malt extract
½ tsp vanilla (or almond) essence
250 ml warm water

For the topping:
200 ml plain soya yoghurt
50 g blanched almonds, finely chopped and lightly toasted
350 g fresh raspberries
3 tbsp maple syrup (optional)

Sift the flour and baking powder together. Add the ground almonds and sugar. Preheat the oven to 180°C/gas mark 4. Grease a round cake tin with oil and sprinkle with flour. Combine the oil, malt, vanilla (or almond) essence and warm water and quickly add the mixture to the flour. Mix as quickly as possible. Pour the mixture into the cake tin, smooth the top and bake for 20–30 minutes (until it doesn't stick to a skewer). Leave to cool a little, then remove from tin and place on a round serving plate and spread the yoghurt evenly over it. Arrange the almonds and the raspberries over the yoghurt (and sprinkle with maple syrup).

## baked apples

4 cooking apples, cored
4 bananas, mashed
10 dates, stoned and chopped
4 tbsp macadamia nuts, chopped
3 tbsp tahini
3 tbsp lemon juice
100 ml maple syrup

Preheat oven to 180°C/gas mark 4. Cut a line horizontally around the middle in the skin of each apple. Mix half the mashed banana with the chopped dates and stuff the mixture into the apple. Sprinkle the nuts on top. Bake for 20 minutes. Mix the tahini with the rest of the banana, lemon juice and maple syrup. Add a little water and stir to a rich sauce. Pour over the baked apples.

## passion-fruit sorbet *(far right, back)*

300 ml passion-fruit pulp, blended
125 g raw cane sugar
100 ml water

Heat the water and the sugar gently in a small heavy-based pan until the sugar dissolves. Stir gently from time to time to loosen the sugar from the base of the pan. Bring to the boil and simmer for 1 minute. Cool, then mix with the passion-fruit. Stir well then freeze the mixture in a shallow non-metal container until solid (4–6 hours). Just before serving, break up the frozen mixture into chunks and blend until smooth. Serve immediately.

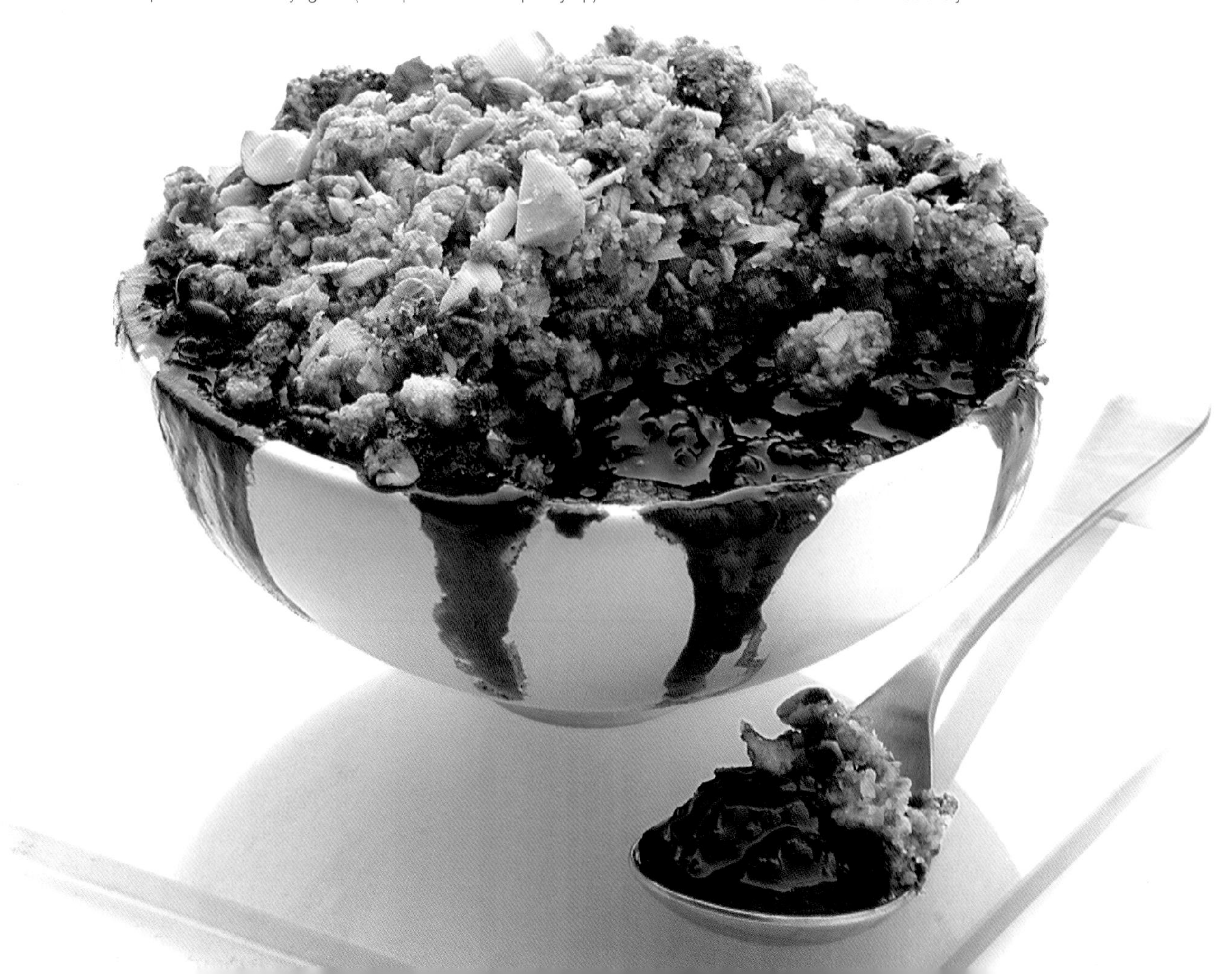

# blackberry crumble *(below left)*

1 kg blackberries (or bilberries, mulberries, raspberries or blueberries)
3 tbsp raw cane sugar
2 tbsp white flour

For the topping:
100 g wholemeal flour
100 g rolled oats
4 tbsp chopped nuts
150 g vegetable margarine
4 tbsp honey

Preheat oven to 200°C/gas mark 6. Mix the blackberries with the sugar and flour in a pie dish. For the topping, mix the flour, oats and nuts in a bowl, then rub in the margarine and honey. Cover the berries with crumble mixture and lightly smooth the surface. Bake for 30 minutes or until golden. Serve warm or cold.

# nectarine surprise

4 nectarines, thinly sliced
4 tbsp maple syrup
1 tsp fresh ginger root, grated
To garnish: 1 tbsp fresh mint, finely chopped

Place the sliced nectarines in a bowl. Heat 100 ml water and add the maple syrup and ginger. Cool and pour over the nectarines. Leave to marinate in the refrigerator for a couple of hours before serving, garnished with the mint.

# raspberry sorbet *(right, front)*

300 ml raspberries, juiced
100 ml water
175 g raw cane sugar

Heat the water and the sugar gently in a small heavy-based pan until the sugar dissolves. Stir gently from time to time to loosen the sugar from the base. Bring to boil and boil for 1 minute. Cool before mixing with the raspberry juice. Stir well, then freeze in a shallow non-metal container until solid (4–6 hours). Just before serving, break into chunks and blend until smooth. Serve immediately.

# tropical fruit salad

2½-cm cube of ginger root, finely chopped
4 tbsp maple syrup (optional)
1 lemon, juice and grated rind
100 ml pineapple juice
8 lychees, peeled and stoned
1 pineapple, peeled, cored and sliced
1 mango, peeled and cut into cubes
4 kiwis, peeled and sliced
1 papaya, peeled, deseeded and sliced

Put the ginger, syrup and juices in a pan. Heat gently and simmer for 1 minute. Pour into a bowl. Cool. Add the fruit and serve.

# pear tart

4 big ripe pears, peeled, halved longways, cored and deseeded
Marzipan (optional)

For the short-crust pastry:
250 g wholewheat flour
½ tsp salt
60 g raw cane sugar
125 g cold vegetable margarine

Mix the flour, salt and sugar, and chop in the margarine with a knife and a spoon until it forms small lumps. Crumble the mixture with your hands until it looks like Parmesan (taking care not to let the dough get warm). Add 5 tbsp cold water and knead the dough lightly into a smooth lump. Refrigerate until needed. Preheat the oven to 200°C/gas mark 6. Divide the pastry in two, roll out one half and place in a greased flan case. Press a lump of marzipan, if using, into the core of each pear half, then place the pears, face down, in the flan shell. Cover with the other half of the pastry. Press lightly down between the pears and firmly around the edge. Bake for 20–30 minutes or until golden. Serve warm or cold.

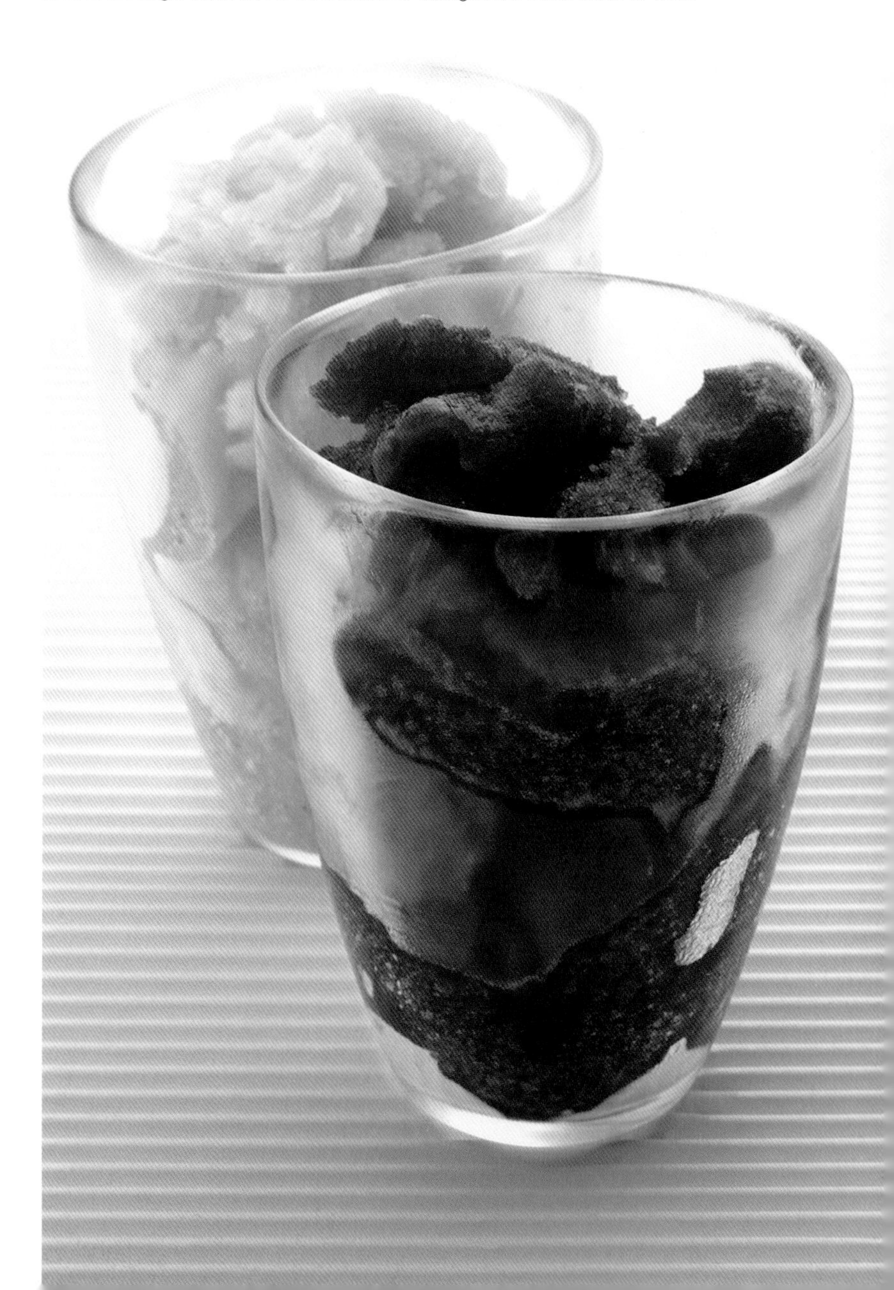

# juices

## apricot and ginger

5 apricots, stones removed
1 tsp fresh ginger root, chopped
100 ml apple juice
100 ml soya milk

Blend all the ingredients and serve with ice.

## autumn fruit

2 apples, cored and quartered
2 pears, cored and quartered
½ grapefruit, peeled

Process all the ingredients in a juicer and serve with ice.

## beetroot and apple

250 g fresh beetroot, quartered
3 apples, cored and quartered
To garnish: 1 slice of lime

Juice the beetroot and the apple and mix well. Pour into a tall glass and garnish with a slice of lime.

## blackberry cream *(far right, front)*

100 g blackberries
1 ripe banana
1 pear, cored and quartered
100 ml plain soya yoghurt
1 tbsp sunflower seeds

Blend all the ingredients in a blender and serve chilled.

## caribbean smoothie

¼ pineapple, peeled, cored and chopped
½ mango, peeled and chopped
1 banana, peeled

Blend all the ingredients and serve chilled.

## carrot and lemon with garlic

250 g carrots
1 garlic clove, peeled
Juice of ½ lemon

Press the garlic through the juicer together with the carrot. Mix with the lemon juice and serve.

## cool cucumber

1 cucumber
1 tomato
1 green pepper, quartered and deseeded
1 garlic clove, peeled
2 sprigs of fresh dill

Juice the ingredients, reserving a little dill to garnish. Serve chilled.

## cranberry spritzer

300 g cranberries (or 100 ml cranberry juice)
100 ml fizzy water
To garnish: 1 slice of lemon

Juice the cranberries and mix with the fizzy water. Garnish with lemon and serve.

## creamy mango *(right, back)*

1 mango, stoned, peeled and cubed
1 banana, peeled
1 wedge of fresh coconut
Juice of 1 orange

Blend the mango, banana and coconut. Add the orange juice, mix well and serve.

## green party

2 celery stalks with leaves
¼ bulb Florence fennel
1 handful of rocket leaves (or other green leaves)
½ cucumber
1 tomato
Few sprigs of fresh basil
To garnish: 1 slice of lime

Juice the celery, fennel, green leaves, cucumber, tomato and basil. Garnish with lime and serve cool.

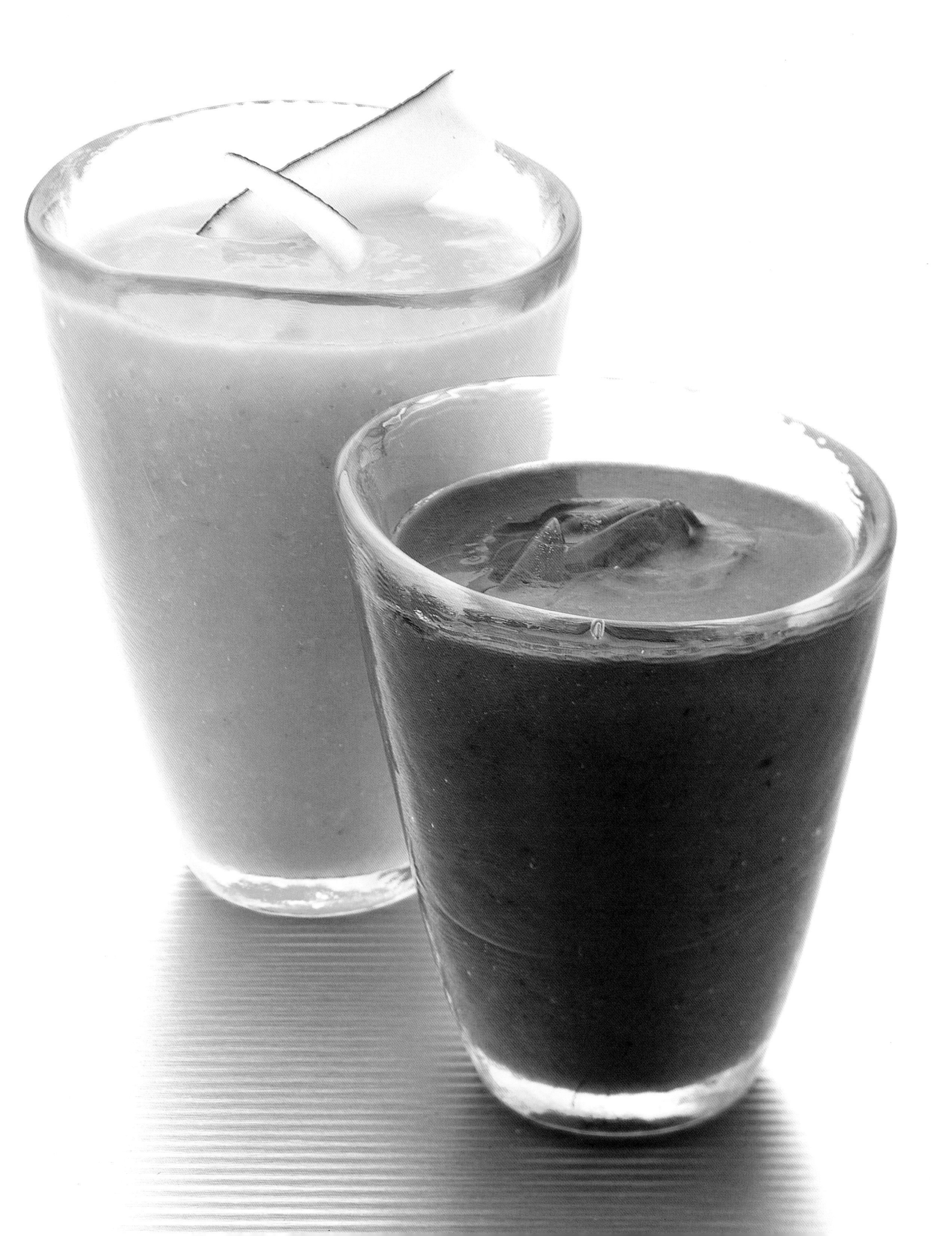

# guava and apple

1 guava, peeled
150 ml apple juice
To garnish: 1 slice of orange

Blend the guava with the apple juice. Serve in a tall glass garnished with a slice of orange.

# heart warmer

100 g carrots
100 g beetroot
2 celery sticks with leaves
2 garlic cloves, peeled
2½-cm piece of ginger, peeled
Juice of ½ lemon

Juice the carrot, beetroot, celery, garlic and ginger. Add the lemon juice, mix well, and serve.

# height of passion

3 passion-fruits, peeled
½ mango, peeled
¼ pineapple, peeled

Juice the fruits and serve with ice.

# mango and lime

1 mango, peeled and stoned
100 ml almond milk
Juice of 1 lime
To garnish: pinch of cinnamon

Blend all of the ingredients, garnish with cinnamon, and serve chilled.

# melon and orange

200 g cantaloupe melon, deseeded and peeled
Juice of 1 orange

Blend the melon with the orange and serve with ice.

# natural beauty *(far right)*

2 apples
½ cantaloupe melon

Process the fruits in a juicer and serve.

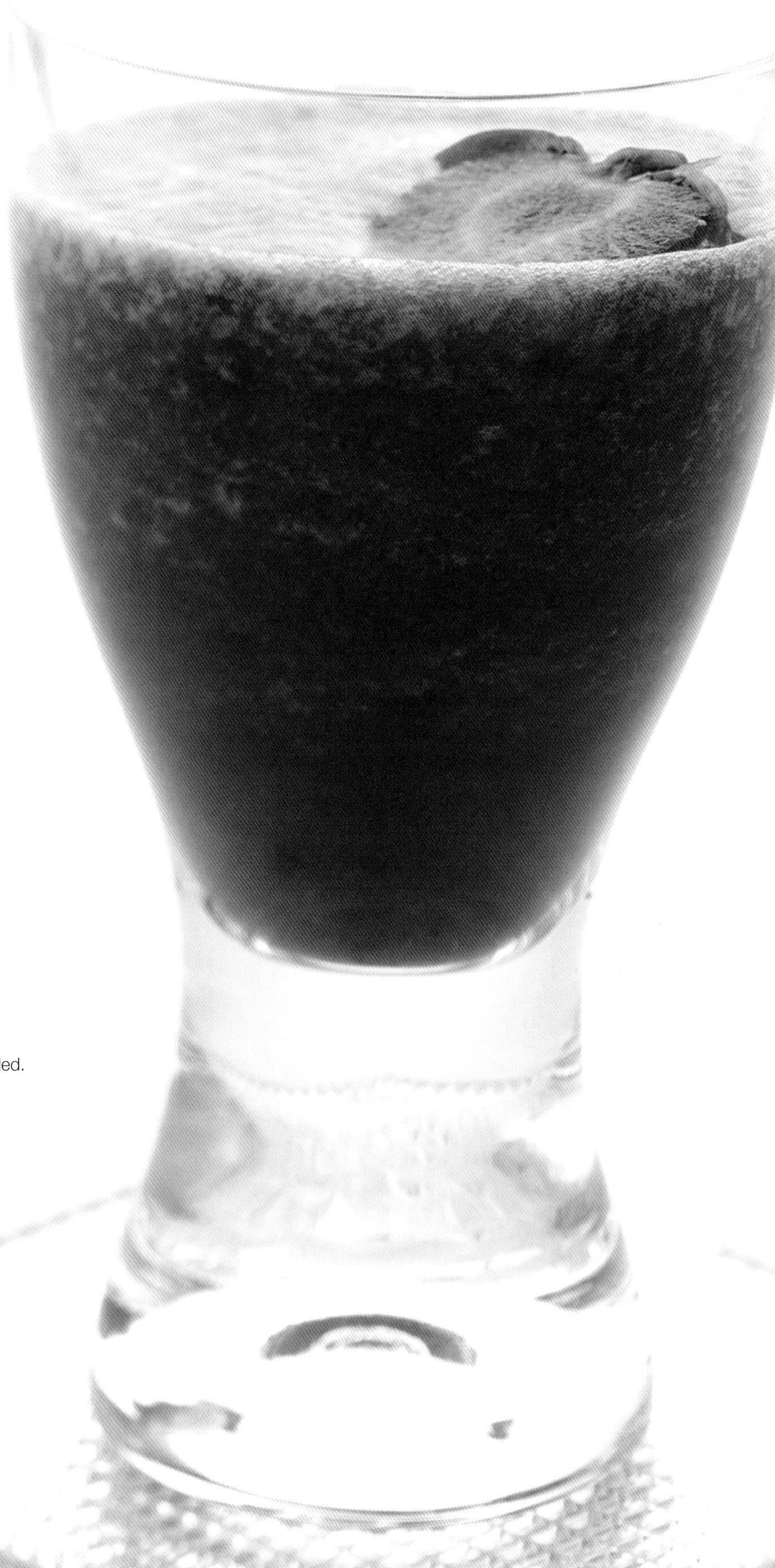

# nirvana

1 ripe pear
6 strawberries
4 apricots
1 peach
To garnish: 1 slice of tangerine

Juice the fruits and serve garnished with a slice of tangerine.

# papaya power

1 papaya, peeled and stoned
Juice of 1 lemon

Blend the papaya with the lemon juice and serve with ice.

# piña colada

½ pineapple, peeled, cored and chopped
4 tbsp coconut milk
1 tsp lime juice
2 tsp maple syrup

Process all the ingredients in a blender and serve with ice.

# passion and lime

2 passion-fruits
1 tbsp maple syrup
Juice of 1 orange
Juice of ½ lime
2 tbsp plain soya yoghurt
Pinch of vanilla powder
Fizzy water to taste

Blend the first 6 ingredients. Pour into a glass and add fizzy water. Serve with ice.

# tomato cocktail

200 g tomatoes, quartered
1 carrot
1 small beetroot, quartered
3 lettuce leaves
3 spinach leaves
6 sprigs of watercress
4 sprigs of parsley
1 celery stalk with leaves
Pinch of celery salt
Few drops of tabasco (optional)

Juice the first 8 ingredients. Pour into a glass and mix well, add a pinch of celery salt, and a few drops of tabasco if desired. Stir, and serve garnished with lemon.

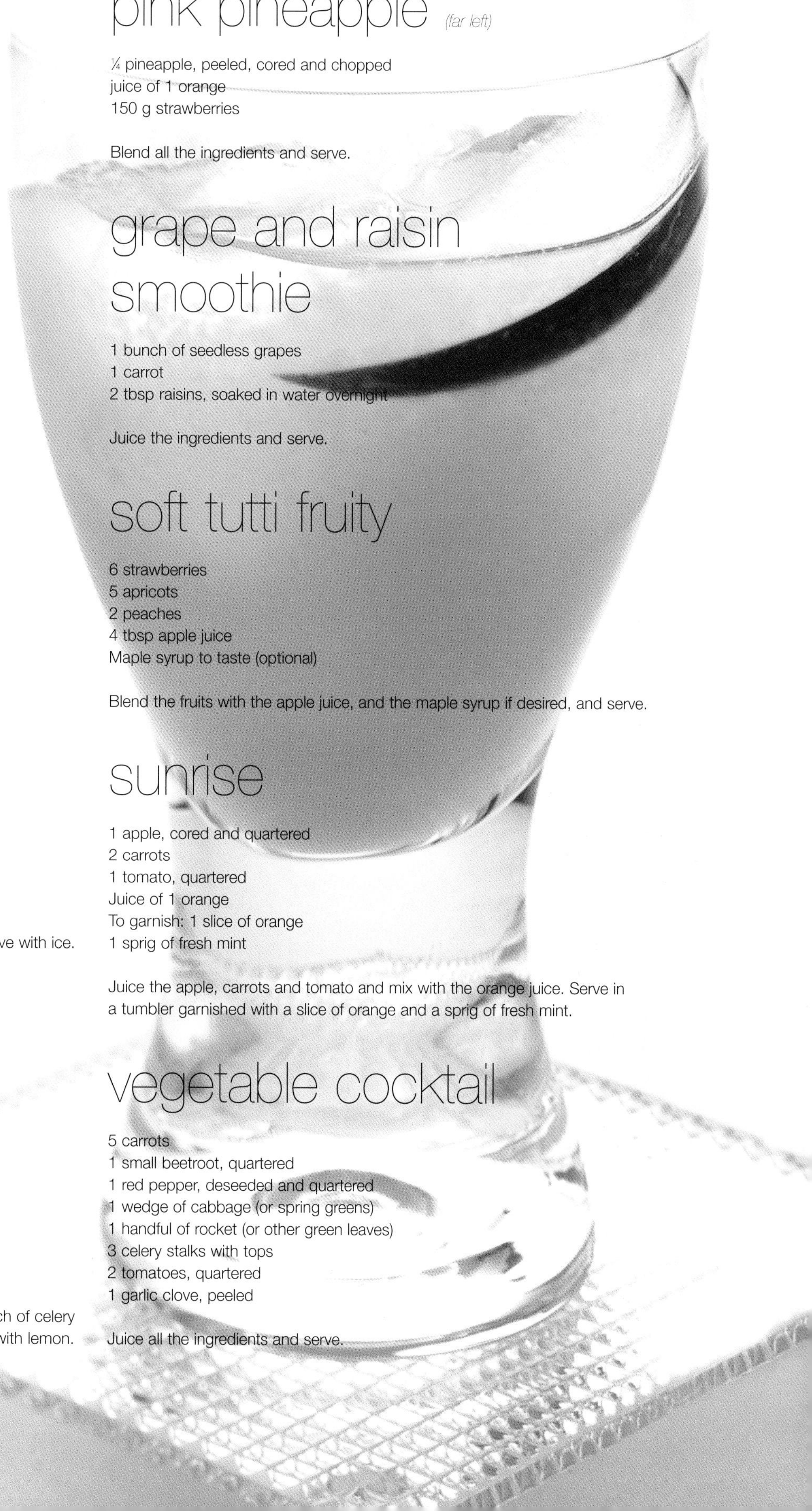

# pink pineapple *(far left)*

¼ pineapple, peeled, cored and chopped
juice of 1 orange
150 g strawberries

Blend all the ingredients and serve.

# grape and raisin smoothie

1 bunch of seedless grapes
1 carrot
2 tbsp raisins, soaked in water overnight

Juice the ingredients and serve.

# soft tutti fruity

6 strawberries
5 apricots
2 peaches
4 tbsp apple juice
Maple syrup to taste (optional)

Blend the fruits with the apple juice, and the maple syrup if desired, and serve.

# sunrise

1 apple, cored and quartered
2 carrots
1 tomato, quartered
Juice of 1 orange
To garnish: 1 slice of orange
1 sprig of fresh mint

Juice the apple, carrots and tomato and mix with the orange juice. Serve in a tumbler garnished with a slice of orange and a sprig of fresh mint.

# vegetable cocktail

5 carrots
1 small beetroot, quartered
1 red pepper, deseeded and quartered
1 wedge of cabbage (or spring greens)
1 handful of rocket (or other green leaves)
3 celery stalks with tops
2 tomatoes, quartered
1 garlic clove, peeled

Juice all the ingredients and serve.

# herbal drinks and syrups

## calming tea

1 part chamomile
1 part lavender flowers
1 part lemon balm
1 part St John's wort

Mix the herbs well. Use 1 teaspoon of herb mixture per cup of boiling water. Place the herbs in a warmed teapot and pour boiling water over them. Cover and leave to infuse for 10 minutes.

## chamomile tonic

60 g chamomile flowers
750 ml organic white wine
3 tbsp honey
2 tbsp lemon juice

Mix all the ingredients in a bowl. Cover and leave in a cool, dark place for 10 days. Strain through a cheesecloth and store in sterile bottles.

## cold buster

½ tsp elderflowers
½ tsp wild marjoram
½ tsp yarrow
Small pinch of cayenne
1 cup boiling water
2 tbsp lemon juice
Honey to taste

Place the herbs in a mug in a tea filter or strainer. Add boiling water. Cover and leave to infuse for 10 minutes. Remove the herbs, add the lemon juice and honey. Drink hot.

## cough mixture

1 tsp sweet violet
½ tsp borage
½ tsp liquorice root
½ tsp thyme
½ tsp wild marjoram
200 ml boiling water
1 tsp honey
Squeeze of lemon juice

Place the herbs in a warmed teapot. Add the boiling water, cover and leave to infuse for 10 minutes. Pour into a mug, add honey and lemon juice, and serve.

## circulation booster

3 parts hawthorn flowers or berries
2 parts yarrow
1 part black mustard seeds

Mix the herbs. Use 1 teaspoon of herb mixture per cup of boiling water. Place the herbs in a warmed teapot and pour boiling water over them. Cover and leave to infuse for 10 minutes.

## cystitis relief

1 part celery seeds
1 part cleavers
1 part echinacea
1 part sweet violets
1 part yarrow

Mix the herbs well. Use 1 teaspoon of herb mixture per cup of boiling water. Place the herbs in a warmed teapot and pour boiling water over them. Cover and leave to infuse for 10 minutes.

## elderberry cordial

1 kg ripe elderberries (with stalks removed), rinsed
500 ml spring water
2 tbsp lemon juice
1 tsp citric acid (optional)
350 g unrefined cane sugar

Place the berries in a saucepan with the water, lemon juice, and citric acid if using. Bring to boil and simmer gently until the berries burst. Strain through a cheesecloth, add the sugar and bring back to the boil. Simmer again for 5 minutes. Skim and pour into sterilized, warm glass bottles. Seal and store in a cool, dark place. Drink diluted with hot water.

## elderflower spritzer

1 head of fresh elderflowers
1 slice of lemon
100 ml boiling water
1 tsp honey
100 ml fizzy water

Place the elderflowers and the lemon slice in a small bowl. Add the boiling water and the honey. Cover and leave to cool. Strain and pour into a tall glass filled with ice, add the fizzy water, and serve immediately.

# eucalyptus mix

3 parts eucalyptus leaves
2 parts chamomile
2 parts thyme

Mix the herbs well. Use 1 teaspoon of herb mixture per cup of boiling water. Place the herbs in a warmed teapot and pour boiling water over them. Cover and leave to infuse for 10 minutes.

# garlic oxymel *(below)*

200 ml red wine vinegar
3 tbsp fresh garlic, chopped
2 tsp black cumin seeds
250 g honey

Place the vinegar, garlic and cumin in a small saucepan. Bring to the boil, cover, and simmer for 5 minutes. Strain and add the honey. Bring to the boil and simmer again, very gently, for another 5 minutes. Remove from heat and store in a clean jar. Take 1 tablespoon at a time.

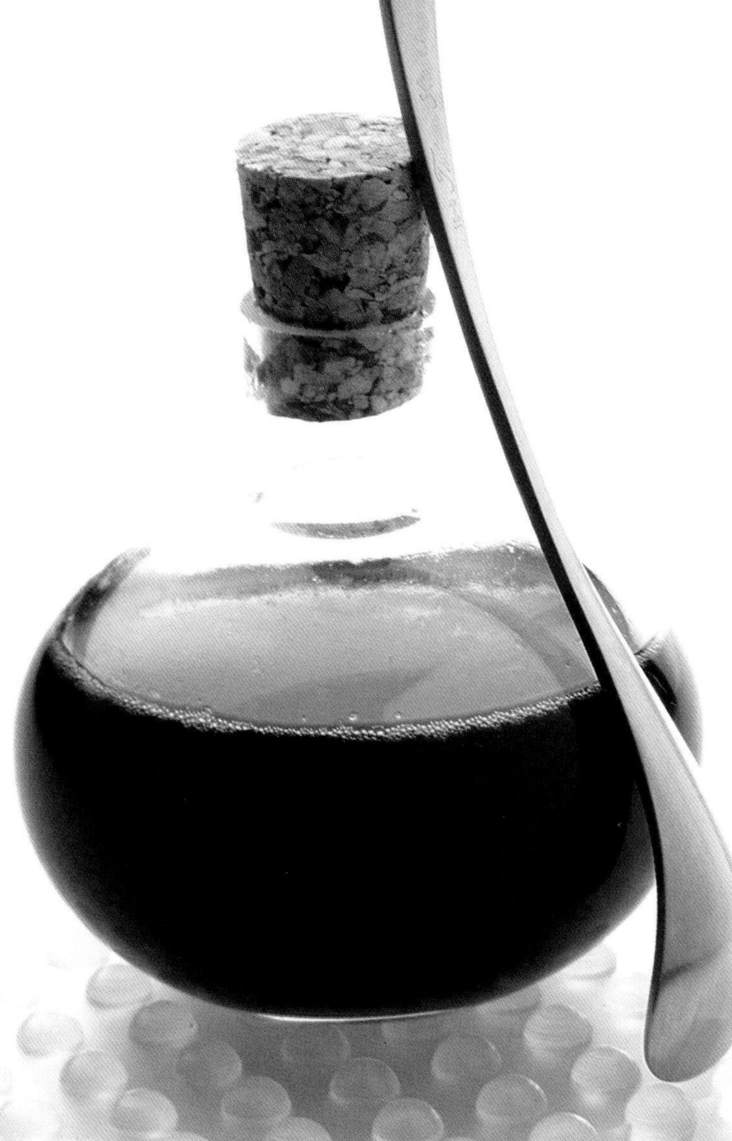

# green tea with mint

1 tsp green tea
1 tbsp fresh mint, chopped
200 ml boiling water

Place the green tea and the mint in a warmed teapot. Add the boiling water, cover and leave to infuse for 5 minutes. Serve hot or chilled.

# hay fever relief

1 tsp fresh horseradish, grated
1 tsp honey
1 glass of water

For the tisane:
2 parts elderflowers
1 part chamomile
1 part echinacea
1 part eyebright
1 part liquorice
1 part peppermint

Mix the grated horseradish with the honey and take with a glass of water. Make the tisane by mixing the herbs and adding 1 teaspoon of the herb mixture per cup of boiling water to a warmed teapot. Cover, and leave to infuse for 10 minutes.

# heart chai

1 tsp green tea
1 tsp black cumin seeds
1-cm piece of cinnamon stick
1 tsp lemon balm
Small pinch of cayenne
300 ml soya (or rice) milk
1 tsp honey (optional)

Place all the ingredients, except the honey, in a small saucepan, bring to the boil and simmer gently for 2 minutes. Strain into a large cup, add the honey if desired, and serve.

# immuni-tea

2 parts nettles
1 part borage
1 part cleavers
1 part echinacea
1 part liquorice
1 part thyme

Mix the herbs well. Use 1 teaspoon of herb mixture per cup of boiling water. Place the herbs in a warmed teapot, add the boiling water, cover, and leave to infuse for 10 minutes.

# liquorice mix

1-cm piece of liquorice root, chopped
1-cm piece of cinnamon stick
½ tsp fennel seeds
½ tsp fresh ginger root, chopped
200 m water

Place all the ingredients in a small saucepan and bring to boil. Simmer gently for 5 minutes. Strain and serve.

# lung-cleansing tea mix

1 part elderflowers
1 part eucalyptus leaves
1 part liquorice root
1 part thyme
1 part peppermint
1 part sweet violets

Mix all the herbs well. Use 1 teaspoon of herb mixture per cup of boiling water. Place the herbs in a warmed teapot. Add the boiling water. Cover and leave to infuse for 10 minutes.

# pick-me-up

2 parts rosehips
1 part jasmine tea
1 part lemon balm
1 part lavender
1 part oats, whole grains, crushed
1 part rosemary

Mix all the ingredients together. Use 1 teaspoon of mixture per cup of boiling water. Place the ingredients in a warmed teapot. Add the boiling water. Cover and leave to infuse for 10 minutes.

# rosehip syrup

125 g rosehips
500 ml water
125 g raw cane sugar

Place the rosehips and water in a saucepan. Bring to the boil, remove from heat and leave to cool. Strain through several layers of cheesecloth to make sure seeds and fine hairs are discarded with the fruit. Bring the liquid back to the boil, add the sugar and simmer gently until the volume is reduced by a third. Stir gently from time to time. Pour into sterile bottles and store in a cool, dry place.

# sage mix for sore throats

1 tsp sage
½ tsp cleavers
½ tsp fresh ginger root, finely chopped
300 ml boiling water

Place the sage, cleavers and ginger in a warmed teapot, add the water, and leave to infuse for 5 minutes.

# si c

1 guava, peeled
½ papaya, peeled and deseeded
1 banana, peeled
100 g blackcurrants
100 g strawberries

Blend the ingredients and serve with ice.

# sleepy time

2 parts passion flower leaves
1 part catmint
1 part chamomile
1 part lavender

Mix all the herbs well. Add 1 teaspoon of herb mixture per cup of boiling water to a warmed teapot. Cover, and leave to infuse for 10 minutes.

# spicy chai

1-cm piece of cinnamon stick
½ tsp black mustard seeds
½ tsp fennel seeds
½ tsp liquorice root
¼ tsp caraway seeds
300 ml rice milk
1 tsp honey (optional)

Place all the ingredients in a small saucepan and bring to the boil. Simmer for a few minutes. Pour into a mug, add the honey if desired, and serve.

# stress relief

1 part basil
1 part borage
1 part lavender
1 part lemon balm
1 part peppermint

Mix all the herbs well. Add 1 teaspoon of herb mixture per cup of boiling water to a warmed teapot. Cover, and leave to infuse for 10 minutes.

# tea for aches and pains

2 parts meadowsweet
2 parts St John's wort
1 part rosemary

Mix all the herbs well. Add 1 teaspoon of herb mixture per cup of boiling water to a warmed teapot. Cover, and leave to infuse for 10 minutes.

# tea for ear infections

1 part cleavers
1 part echinacea
1 part elderflowers
1 part liquorice root
1 part peppermint
1 part rosehips
1 part St John's wort

Mix all the herbs well. Add 1 teaspoon of herb mixture per cup of boiling water to a warmed teapot. Cover, and leave to infuse for 10 minutes.

# tea for fever

½ tsp borage
½ tsp catmint
½ tsp chamomile
Small pinch of cayenne
1 cup boiling water

Place the herbs in a warmed teapot. Add the boiling water. Cover and leave to infuse for 5 minutes.

# tea for fungal infections

2 parts echinacea
1 part cleavers
1 part lemon balm
1 part marigold (calendula)

Mix the herbs well. Use 1 teaspoon of herb mixture per cup of boiling water. Place the herbs in a warmed teapot and pour the boiling water over them. Cover and leave to infuse for 10 minutes.

# thyme syrup

3 tbsp dried thyme
500 ml water
350 g unrefined cane sugar

Bring the water to the boil in a small saucepan. Add the thyme and remove from heat. Cover and leave to infuse for 20 minutes. Strain and add the sugar. Heat gently until sugar dissolves. Pour into sterile bottles and store in the refrigerator.

# tea for glands

1 part borage
1 part cleavers
1 part echinacea
1 part marigold (calendula)

Mix all the herbs well. Add 1 teaspoon of herb mixture per cup of boiling water to a warmed teapot. Cover, and leave to infuse for 10 minutes.

# tea for headache

1 part feverfew
1 part marjoram
1 part peppermint
1 part rosemary

Mix all the herbs well. Use 1 teaspoon of herb mixture per cup of boiling water. Place the herbs in a warmed teapot. Add the boiling water. Cover and leave to infuse for 10 minutes.

# tea for joints

1 part black mustard seeds
1 part celery seeds
1 part elderflowers
1 part nettles
1 part St John's wort

Mix all the herbs well. Use 1 teaspoon of herb mixture per cup of boiling water. Place the herbs in a warmed teapot. Add the boiling water. Cover and leave to infuse for 10 minutes.

# tea for the skin

1 part cleavers
1 part echinacea
1 part nettles
1 part sweet violets
½ part marigold (calendula)

Mix all the herbs well. Use 1 teaspoon of herb mixture per cup of boiling water. Place the herbs in a warmed teapot. Add the boiling water. Cover and leave to infuse for 10 minutes.

# winter tonic

200 g ripe mulberries (or blackberries)
1 banana
2 tbsp maple syrup
100 ml almond milk

Blend the ingredients and serve.

# diet plans

## detox and elimination diet

If you suffer from any serious medical disorders, including cancer, diabetes mellitus, depression, eating disorders, severe asthma, or epilepsy, it is not advisable to undertake an elimination diet without medical supervision. The idea of this diet is to eat only things to which you are unlikely to be allergic – which may take a lot of willpower and support! Follow it for two weeks to give your system time to eliminate any offending food allergens.

If you suspect you have a food allergy, but you are unsure to what you are allergic, one way to find out for sure is to keep a diet diary. Take seven pieces of A4 paper and mark each one with a different day of the week. Carry the relevant piece of paper around with you everywhere each day for the following week, and record EVERYTHING you eat and drink and the time you had it. (It is easy to forget what you've eaten if you don't write it down immediately.)

At the end of each day, write down how (and where) you've been that day, whether you've had any allergy symptoms (such as migraine or stomach ache) and, if you are suffering from arthritis, whether your arthritis was better or worse (on a scale of 1 to 10) that day. Food allergy symptoms can start up to 24 hours after the allergen was consumed, so keeping a diet diary enables you to look back and identify possible offenders more easily.

If after a week it is clear that you have "good" days and "bad" days according to what you eat (and provided you feel well when you wake up the next morning after a good day), you can start to plan your own elimination diet by keeping your diet diary up to date and eliminating the foods you have found are not good for you.

If your symptoms are not that clear cut, try the following elimination diet plan to discover which things to leave out of your diet (you can always reintroduce them after a while, to see if you still react to them). Choose a time when you haven't got too many commitments – choosing different foods from those you are used to is inevitably time consuming.

When following this diet plan, you may experience symptoms of withdrawal and detoxification (such as nausea, headache, the feeling that your teeth and tongue have a furry coat, and even diarrhoea) but these symptoms should diminish after a couple of days, leaving you feeling fresher and more alert. Eat and drink (water or mild herbal tea) every 2–3 hours and have plenty of the foods on the "allowed" list. Keep a record of everything you consume and note any reaction you experience. Avoid using toothpaste during the diet – use salt or baking powder instead.

### DAY ONE

Cut out all stimulants (tea, coffee, chocolate, cigarettes, alcohol), processed "convenience" foods, and foods containing additives.

### DAY TWO

Cut out all dairy products, wheat, buckwheat and sugar (including honey and syrups), and any foods containing these.

### DAY THREE

Cut out all meat, fish, and shellfish.

### DAY FOUR

Cut out all corn, nuts and pulses, and foods containing these.

### DAY FIVE

Cut out all foods belonging to the nightshade family (*solinaceae*): potato, aubergine, peppers, chillies, cayenne, paprika and tomatoes. Eat only steamed or raw vegetables, rice and fruit.

### DAY SIX

Cut out all citrus fruits (lemon, orange, grapefruit, lime, tangerine, kumquat, mandarin, clementine). Eat only vegetables and those fruits not belonging to the citrus and nightshade families.

### DAY SEVEN

Drink only water, fruit and/or vegetable juices. Make your own mixtures according to taste.

### DAY EIGHT

Eat vegetables and fruits, except citrus fruits and members of the nightshade family.

### DAY NINE

Eat vegetables, fruits and rice. Drink water and juices. Reintroduce foods from the nightshade family. Observe any reaction.

### DAY TEN

Eat vegetables, fruits and rice. Drink water and juices as on day seven. Reintroduce citrus fruits. Observe any reaction.

### DAY ELEVEN

Eat vegetables, fruits and rice. Drink water and juices as on day seven. Reintroduce corn, nuts and pulses. Observe any reaction.

### DAY TWELVE

Eat vegetables, fruits and rice. Drink water and juices as on day seven. Reintroduce wheat, sugar, and fish. Observe any reaction.

### DAY THIRTEEN

Eat vegetables, fruits and rice. Drink water and juices as on day seven. Reintroduce dairy products. Observe any reaction.

### DAY FOURTEEN

Eat vegetables, fruits and rice. Drink water and juices as on day seven. Reintroduce shellfish. Observe any reaction.

### DAY FIFTEEN

Start eating "normally" again, but note your reactions carefully when you reintroduce meat, stimulants and food additives. Review your diet diary and take note of the food groups to which you reacted negatively. Base your future diet on what you have discovered.

## traditional grape fast

A grape fast is cleansing and detoxifying. The best time to do it is at the end of the summer when grapes are fresh, cheap and plentiful. Choose organic grapes and eat as many as you like on the "grape" days. You should also drink plenty of clean water and have unsweetened organic grape juice, little and often, throughout. Take plenty of time to rest, too. Avoid smoking during the fast.

### DAYS ONE, TWO AND THREE

Eat only grapes and drink only water and grape juice.

### DAY FOUR

Eat nothing but drink plenty of water and grape juice.

### DAYS FIVE, SIX AND SEVEN

Eat only grapes and drink only water and grape juice.

## gentle healing diet

If you are suffering from a chronic illness, or have been through a period of physical, mental, emotional or spiritual stress, a gentle healing diet is a necessity to provide resources for healing. It is made up of foods that are highly nutritious, easily digested, and easily absorbed and used by the body. The diet contains the right amount of protein for growth and repair, and plenty of complex carbohydrates for sustained energy. It is low in fat but contains all the necessary essential fatty acids, and it is high in vitamins, minerals and other healing phytochemicals. Eat as many of the following foods as you like, and in any combination that suits you.

### COMPLEX CARBOHYDRATES

Grains, roots and tubers – rice, pasta, couscous, bulgur, parsnips, celeriac (celery root), carrots, potatoes, sweet potatoes, beetroot.

### VEGETABLE PROTEIN

Beans, peas, grains and green leaves. (Meat is not suitable for this gentle healing diet because it is a very concentrated food containing no fibre, and it may contain residues of hormones, antibiotics, nitrates and other additives or harmful substances.)

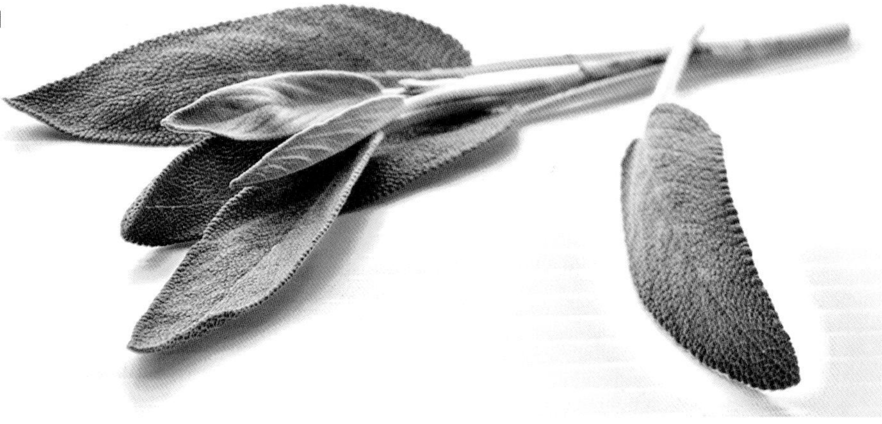

### VITAMINS, MINERALS AND PHYTOCHEMICALS

Organically grown vegetables, either raw or cooked, boiled, baked, or steamed depending on your taste, your state of health and your digestion. Start with cooked vegetables if you find raw foods hard to digest and add some raw ones little by little. Organic vegetables contain more nutrients and less water than those produced by intensive farming methods, and they are not contaminated by sprays and fertilizers, which the body needs energy to deal with.

Fruit is also a very healthy food, and you should eat one or two pieces each day. But in this diet the emphasis is on building up resources by eating food that provides steady energy without too many short bursts upsetting blood-sugar levels. Most fruits contain simple sugars (disaccharides) that are digested and absorbed into the blood stream more quickly than the complex carbohydrates (polysaccharides) found in grains and many vegetables. Eat fruits that are in season, and particularly fruits that improve digestion, such as papaya, pineapple, banana and grapefruit. Lemons contain a lot of vitamin C and not too much sugar.

### UNSATURATED FAT

Nuts, seeds and olive oil all contain unsaturated fatty acids that are beneficial to health.

### DRINKS

The aim is to build up resources by eating nutritious foods and keeping the digestive load to a minimum. Drinks should follow the same guidelines and be limited to water, vegetable juices (without sugar), and herbal teas (avoid the artificially flavoured ones).

### SUGGESTED MENU (CHOOSE ONE FROM EACH CATEGORY)

### BREAKFAST

baked tomatoes on toast (page 242)
scrambled tofu (page 242)
beans and tomatoes on toast (page 242)
porridge with dried fruit and quinoa (page 242)
muesli (page 243)

### SALAD AND SOUP LUNCH

grilled endive and brazil nut salad (page 197)
oriental salad with tempeh (page 203)
carrot 'n' beetroot salad (page 259)
salad niçoise (page 259)
bulgur wheat salad (page 259)
artichoke salad (page 259)
rocket salad (page 259)
catalan salad (page 260)
florence fennel salad (page 260)
green lentil salad (page 260)
potato salad (page 260)
sweetcorn (maize) and sun-dried tomato salad (page 260)
wild rice salad (page 261)
healing soup (page 244)
black-eye bean and wild marjoram soup (page 245)
creamy cauliflower soup (page 245)
italian butterbean soup (page 245)
spicy moroccan soup (page 246)
tibetan dumpling soup (page 246)
welsh leek and potato soup (page 246)

### DINNER

#### Starters

asparagus with ravigote (page 246)
hummus with crudités and warm pitta bread (page 246)
korean kimchi-style salad (page 247)
grilled red peppers (page 247)
vegetable kebabs (page 247)
baba ganoush (page 248)
tofumasalata (page 248)

#### Main course

scandinavian beetroot burgers (page 177)
amaranth and tofu puffs (page 252)
casserole de puy (page 252)
paella (page 252)
provençale-style kidney beans (page 255)
greek casserole (page 255)
spinach bouillabaisse (page 255)
shepherdess' pie (page 256)
sweet potato curry (page 256)
mushrooms with sage and thyme stuffing (page 256)
winter hot pot (page 256)
sweet chestnuts and kumquats (page 257)

### SNACKS

spicy brazil nut pâté (page 197)
toasted nuts and seeds (page 248)
marinated olives (page 248)
tomato and cucumber canapés (page 250)
guacamole (page 250)
tzaziki (page 251)
pan amb oli (page 251)

### DRINKS

Pure water, herbal tea, freshly made vegetable juices, dandelion or chicory coffee substitutes.

### FOODS TO AVOID

- All sugars and foods containing added sugar
- All refined or processed foods and junk foods
- Fruit juices
- Stimulants (such as tea, coffee, alcohol, chocolate, fizzy drinks)
- Non-prescription drugs and supplements
- All foods containing saturated fats
- Additives
- Dairy products
- Meats
- Fish

If you suffer from an arthritic condition, this healing diet may bring you relief from symptoms and pain. If it does not, you should consider modifying your diet to exclude the following: wheat, potatoes, tomatoes, peppers, aubergines, acidic fruits and vinegar.

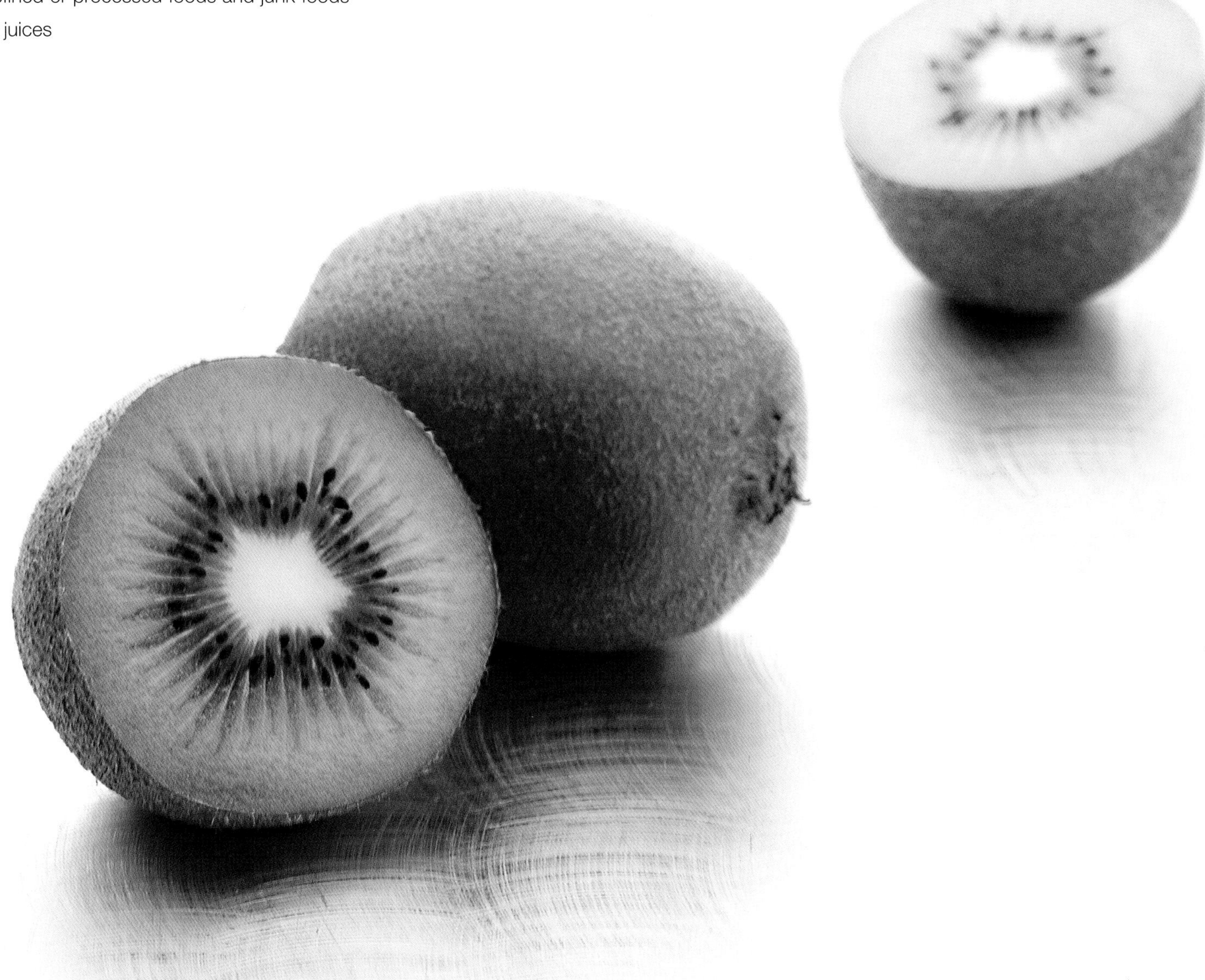

# glossary

Words in **bold** type also appear in this glossary.

**ACETYLCHOLINE** a chemical messenger needed for normal functioning of the central and autonomic nervous systems.

**ANTHOCYANINS** dark-blue **antioxidants** that may reduce the "stickiness" of blood platelets and help prevent blood clots.

**ANTIBIOTIC** a treatment for infectious disease that works by killing, or inhibiting the growth of, infecting organisms.

**ANTI-CATARRHAL** a substance capable of reducing secretions from mucous membranes.

**ANTICOAGULANT** reduces the tendency of the blood to clot.

**ANTIOXIDANT** a substance that inhibits and controls the harmful action of **free radicals**. Vitamins C and E and the trace elements selenium and zinc are important antioxidants.

**ANTISCORBUTIC** prevents scurvy – a beneficial property of any food containing vitamin C (ascorbic acid).

**ASTRINGENT** causes binding and drying, for example to treat bleeding and diarrhoea.

**BENZOIC ACID** an antiseptic primarily used to treat urinary-tract infections and as a preservative in cordials and pickles.

**BETA-SITOSTEROL** a plant sterol that lowers blood cholesterol levels and is also believed to reduce tumour growth, particularly in the colon.

**BIO-ACTIVE COMPOUNDS** chemical substances, such as **antioxidants**, that are found in foods and are known, or believed to have, beneficial effects on human health.

**BIOFLAVONOIDS** also known as flavonoids, a group of **bio-active compounds**, including **quercetin**, **kaempferol**, **rutin** and hesperidin, with **antioxidant**, **diuretic** and other wide-ranging properties. They reduce blood-cholesterol levels, and may protect against heart disease and some cancers.

**BITTER PRINCIPLES** a group of plant chemicals with a distinctive bitter taste. They stimulate secretion of digestive juices, activate the liver and may act as natural **antibiotics**, antifungals and anti-cancer agents.

**BROMELAIN** a protein-digesting enzyme found in pineapple. It mimics the action of pancreatic enzymes and may reduce inflammation and swellings.

**CAMPHOR** a component of some volatile oils with warming, numbing, pain-relieving and insecticidal properties.

**CARMINATIVE** relieves intestinal wind (flatulence).

**CAROTENE** a **carotenoid** in orange-coloured plant foods.

**CAROTENOIDS** pigments with strong **antioxidant** properties found in brightly-coloured plant foods. They are converted into vitamin A in the body.

**CHLOROPHYLL** a green pigment responsible for photosynthesis in plants that stops the growth of bacteria and soothes inflammation.

**CITRIC ACID** a plant acid that gives the distinctive sharp taste to lemons, limes, unripe oranges, currants and raspberries. It has a cooling, thirst-quenching effect.

**COUMARINS** phytochemicals with natural anti-blood-clotting properties. May protect against stomach and breast cancer.

**CRUCIFEROUS** a member of the Cruciferae family of plants that includes cabbage, kale, mustard greens, turnip and swede. Cruciferous plants are rich in **glucosinolates**.

**CURCUMINOIDS** yellow pigments found in turmeric with anti-inflammatory properties. They enhance the action of adrenal hormones and are beneficial to the liver.

**CYANOGLYCOSIDES** **bio-active compounds** found in some plants and may have medicinal properties.

**DECOCTION** a medicinal preparation made by boiling plant material (such as roots, wood, bark, nuts or seeds) in water, usually for 10 to 15 minutes.

**DEPURATIVE** encourages the body to eliminate impurities.

**DIAPHORETIC** encourages sweating.

**DIURETIC** increases the flow of urine.

**ESSENTIAL OILS** also known as volatile oils, these are strong-smelling oils that give plants their characteristic odour and have many pharmacological actions.

**EXPECTORANT** provokes the expulsion of mucus and impurities from the lungs.

**FEBRIFUGE** a remedy that cools fever.

**FLAVONOID** see **bioflavonoid**.

**FOLATE**, or folic acid, a type of B-vitamin so called because it is found in foliage.

**FOLIC ACID** see **folate**.
**FORMIC ACID** an irritant acid found in nettles.
**FREE RADICALS** by-products of metabolism that can cause damage to cell membranes by oxidation of fatty acids. Free radicals are neutralized by **antioxidants**.
**GLUCOKININ** a chemical found in various plants including blueberry and garlic that lowers blood-sugar levels.
**GLUCOQUINONE** a chemical found in nettle that may help lower blood-sugar levels.
**GLUCOSINOLATES** a group of more than 20 chemicals (including indoles and isothyocyanates) found in edible plants such as cabbage, cauliflower and broccoli. They increase the activity of enzymes that help the body eliminate potential carcinogens and thus help to protect against cancer. However, glucosinolates may inhibit iodine uptake by the thyroid gland if eaten in large quantities.
**GLUTATHIONE** a **free-radical** "scavenger" dependent on selenium for its **antioxidant** activity.
**GLUTEN** a protein contained in cereals such as wheat, barley, rye and oats. Components of gluten called gliandins can provoke the immune reaction that causes coeliac disease.
**GLYCOSIDES** compounds made up of a combination of sugars and non-sugars, found widely in nature, many of which have powerful medicinal actions (such as digitalis in foxglove).
**HISTAMINE** is derived from the amino acid histidine and found in the tissues of animals and plants. It has various powerful effects on the body (including dilating small blood vessels, constricting the bronchial tubes and stimulating the production of gastric juice), and is responsible for urticaria ("nettle rash").
**HYDROGENATED FATS** found in many processed foods, these are made by adding hydrogen to **polyunsaturated fats** in a process known as hydrogenation. Hydrogenated and partially hydrogenated fats are more solid at room temperature than polyunsaturated fats (or oils), but the chemical and physical techniques used to produce them cause unwelcome changes, such as the production of unhealthy "trans" fats.
**IMMUNO-STIMULANT** boosts the body's natural defences.
**INFUSION** a remedy made by steeping plant material (usually flowers and leaves) in hot water.
**ISOFLAVONES** a group of **bio-active compounds** found in cereals and pulses (including soya) that are structurally similar to human oestrogen. Isoflavones may protect against breast cancer, but there is continuing debate about the effect of phytoestrogens on infants fed on soya-based formula foods.
**KAEMPFEROL** a **bioflavonoid** found in many plant foods.
**LACTOBACILLI** a bacterial species that forms part of the body's healthy microbial ecology. Also found in live yoghurt.
**LECITHIN** a complex phospholipid fat found in many body tissues, particularly the brain and nerves. It is also found in various foods. Plant lecithin may help the body to deal with excess cholesterol and help prevent abnormal blood clotting.
**LENTINAN** a polysaccharide found in shiitake mushrooms that enhances the immune response by stimulating T-helper cell activity. It is now being investigated as a possible treatment for AIDS (in conjunction with other drugs) and cancer.
**LEUKOTRIENE** one of the eicosanoid family of chemicals, derived from arachidonic acid. It causes contraction of smooth muscle and is involved in the inflammatory response to injury.
**LINOLEIC ACID** one of the "essential" fatty acids (so called because they cannot be made in the body and thus have to be consumed in the diet). It is found in vegetables, nuts, grains, fruits, plant oils, eggs and fowl, and is one of the **omega-6** family of **polyunsaturated fats**. It can be converted in the body to gamma-linolenic acid and arachidonic acid, both of which have powerful effects on immune function, the inflammatory response and cell metabolism.
**LINOLENIC ACID** an essential fatty acid necessary for normal health. One of the **omega-3** family of **polyunsaturated fats**, linolenic acid is found in abundance in linseed, mustard and pumpkin seeds, soya and walnut oils, green leafy vegetables, meat and meat products. It is converted in the body to eicosapentaenoic acid (EPA – also found in fish oil) and docosahexaenoic acid (DHA – also found in fish oil and some algae), both of which have beneficial effects on blood-fat levels and inhibit blood clotting.
**LUTEIN** an **antioxidant carotenoid** in many plant foods.
**LYCOPENE** an **antioxidant carotenoid** found in tomatoes. It is released from tomatoes when they are cooked, and its absorption into the body is improved by the presence of small amounts of oil or fat in the meal.
**MONOUNSATURATED FAT** a type of fatty acid that contains one chemical double-bond in its carbon chain. Olive oil is particularly rich in monounsaturated fat, which is found also in many animal, fish and vegetable fats.

**MUCILAGE** a complex carbohydrate found in many plants. It has a slimy texture when dissolved in water. Herbal remedies containing mucilage soothe inflamed mucous membranes.
**OLEIC ACID** one of the omega-9 family of unsaturated fats.
**OMEGA-3** a group of unsaturated fatty acids containing **linolenic acid**, EPA and DHA.
**OMEGA-6** a group of unsaturated fatty acids containing **linoleic acid** and arachidonic acid.
**OXALATE** also known as oxalic acid, a chemical found in various foodstuffs, including tea, rhubarb and spinach, which, when present in the body in large amounts, encourages the formation of urinary stones. People suffering from urinary stones (or any form of gastro-intestinal malabsorption) should avoid foods containing oxalates.
**PAPAIN** a substance obtained from the juice of the papaya that mimics the action of digestive juices, thus aiding digestion.
**PECTIN** a soluble non-starch polysaccharide (NSP) found in fruits and plants and used as a gelling agent in jams and preserves. Soluble NSP in the diet helps protect against diseases associated with high blood cholesterol, such as coronary heart disease and gallstones.
**PHENOLIC ACIDS** substances found in wines, teas and freshly picked vegetables and fruits, which encourage detoxification and inhibit the formation of cancer cells.
**PHYTOCHEMICALS** **bio-active compounds** found in foods of plant origin with health-enhancing effects. They include allium compounds, **carotenoids**, **coumarins** and **bioflavonoids**.
**PHYTOHORMONES** plant-derived chemicals, such as phytoestrogens, that mimic the action of human hormones.
**POLYSACCHARIDES** large carbohydrate molecules made up of chains of simple sugar molecules linked together. Starch is a type of polysaccharide.
**POLYUNSATURATED FAT** a type of fatty acid containing two or more double bonds in its carbon chain. It is found mainly in plant oils and is an essential part of a healthy diet.
**PORPHYRINS** pigments found in the blood and tissues of animals and also in plants and micro-organisms.
**POULTICE** a hot pack applied to the skin, prepared by mixing herbs (such as oats, linseed or comfrey) with hot water and wrapping the mixture in a piece of linen or muslin.
**PROTEASE INHIBITORS** proteins found in plants, such as cereals and pulses, that may help protect against cancer.
**QUERCETIN** a **bioflavonoid** found in foods such as onions, tomatoes, apples, berries and tea. An **antioxidant**, it is thought to act as an antihistamine, to treat allergies and prevent heart disease and cancer, but there is, at present, little evidence to support these claims.
**QUINIC ACID** a sugar compound found in fruits, such as apples, peaches, pears, plums and some vegetables, that has antiviral and neuroprotective properties.
**RUTIN** a **bioflavonoid** with a reputation for toning and healing peripheral blood vessels.
**SACCHARIDE** another name for carbohydrate. Complex carbohydrates, fruit sugar and glucose are also known as polysaccharides, disaccharides and monosaccharides, respectively.
**SALICYLATE** also known as salicylic acid, a chemical of plant origin that forms the basis for the drug aspirin. Plants containing salicylate have antiseptic, painkilling and anti-inflammatory effects.
**SAPONINS** **bio-active compounds**, traditionally used for their **expectorant**, **diuretic** and anti-inflammatory effects. They are found in many foods and herbs, including soya beans, oats, liquorice, violet, yarrow, asparagus and other vegetables.
**SATURATED FAT** a type of fatty acid containing the maximum number of hydrogen atoms. Saturated fats are usually solid at room temperature. Animal fats (including butter, lard and suet) contain a high proportion of saturated fat, as do solid vegetable fats like coconut oil. Saturated fats can be made in the body and so are not needed in the diet.
**SULPHUR** a mineral found in some food plants and medicinal plants that has a cleansing, anti-rheumatic effect.
**TANNIN** a plant constituent that causes tissue to contract by precipitating proteins. Traditionally used to make leather by tanning animal hides, and used therapeutically to reduce secretions and discharges. It has an **astringent** action.
**TARTARIC ACID** a fruit acid found in grapes.
**THYMOL** a volatile oil with strong antiseptic properties.
**TRYPTOPHAN** an amino acid that can be converted into vitamin B3 in the body.
**VALERIANIC ACID** a volatile oil with sedative properties.
**VASODILATOR** a substance that causes the blood vessels to widen (dilate), thereby enhancing blood flow.
**VOLATILE OIL** see **essential oils**.

# top ten foods

The following lists give the top ten sources of vitamins, minerals and trace elements. In each case foods are listed according to amount per portion, beginning with the highest.

## WATER-SOLUBLE VITAMINS

**VITAMIN B1** (thiamin): peas, brown rice, yeast extract, potato, muesli, sunflower seed, pinto bean, cabbage, tahini paste, leek

**VITAMIN B2** (riboflavin): yeast extract, tempeh, muesli, avocado, seaweed, oyster mushroom, sweetcorn, mushrooms, peas, mustard leaf

**VITAMIN B3** (niacin – including proportion converted from tryptophan): yeast extract, tempeh, muesli, broad bean, peas, peanut butter, brown rice, soya bean, potato, wheat bran

**VITAMIN B5** (pantothenic acid): broad bean, avocado, mushrooms, tempeh, Brussels sprout, purple broccoli, endive, sweetcorn, sweet potato, potato

**VITAMIN B6** (pyridoxine): tempeh, muesli, potato, avocado, red pepper, banana, Brussels sprout, leek, lentil, curly kale

**VITAMIN B12** (cobalamin); (f) = fortified: yeast extract (f), vegetable stock (f), vegetable margarine (f), soya milk (f), breakfast cereals (f), tempeh, seaweed, sourdough bread, shiitake mushroom, soy sauce

**FOLATE**: black-eye bean, Swiss chard, Savoy cabbage, spinach, broad bean, pinto bean, endive, Brussels sprout, curly kale, okra

**BIOTIN**: tempeh, soya bean, hazelnut, peanut, almond, muesli, black-eye bean, mushrooms, avocado, mangetout

**VITAMIN C**: guava, red pepper, spring greens, blackcurrant, green pepper, Brussels sprout, curly kale, papaya, strawberry, purple broccoli

## FAT-SOLUBLE VITAMINS

**VITAMIN A**: sweet potato, carrot, red pepper, butternut squash, Swiss chard, spinach, curly kale, spring greens, mango, cantaloupe melon

**VITAMIN D**: Although a number of foods are fortified with vitamin D, only a few foods contain vitamin D naturally. The best way to ensure adequate vitamin D is to spend some time each day in the open air, as we all produce vitamin D internally by the action of sunlight on our skin

**VITAMIN E**: wheatgerm oil, sun-dried tomato, sweet potato, sunflower oil, safflower oil, sunflower seed, avocado, hazelnut, almond, butternut squash

**VITAMIN K**: broccoli, spinach, parsley, cabbage, curly kale, spring greens, cauliflower, peas, soya-based margarine, vegetable oil

## MINERALS

**CALCIUM**: tofu, okra, spring greens, spinach, curly kale, tempeh, sesame seed, purple broccoli, spring onions, dried fig

**MAGNESIUM**: Brazil nuts, okra, melon seed, Swiss chard, brown rice, tempeh, sunflower seed, sesame seed, beans, spinach

**PHOSPHORUS**: brown rice, tempeh, tahini, muesli, peas, beans and lentils, nuts and seeds, sweetcorn, tofu, sweet potato

**POTASSIUM**: avocado, potato, sweet potato, dried apricots, squash, beans, banana, spinach, courgette, Brussels sprout

## TRACE ELEMENTS

**IRON**: tempeh, lentil, potato, muesli, spring greens, endive, peas, tahini paste, cumin seed, dried peach

**ZINC**: aduki bean, tofu, tempeh, lentil, muesli, pasta, wheat bran, chickpea, tahini paste, brown rice

**MANGANESE**: oyster mushroom, brown rice, muesli, tempeh, pine nut, tofu, blackberry, macadamia nut, hazelnut, aduki bean

**COPPER**: tempeh, brown rice, aduki bean, pigeon pea, mushrooms, melon seed, sunflower seed, cashew nut, tahini, soya bean

**IODINE** (the most reliable sources come from the sea): fish, seaweed, sea salt and iodized salt. The amount in plants varies depending on iodine levels in the soil

**SELENIUM**: Brazil nut, lentil, wholemeal bread, pasta, sunflower seed, pinto bean, red kidney bean, cashew nut, mushrooms, soya bean

# index

**Bold** numbers indicate main entries in this book.